KU-784-839

Contraceptive Research and Development

Looking to the Future

Polly F. Harrison and Allan Rosenfield, *Editors*

Committee on Contraceptive Research and Development

Division of Health Sciences Policy

INSTITUTE OF MEDICINE

NATIONAL ACADEMY PRESS
Washington, D.C.   1996

National Academy Press • **2101 Constitution Avenue, N.W.** • **Washington, D.C. 20418**

NOTICE: The project that is the subject of this report was approved by the Governing Board of the National Research Council, whose members are drawn from the councils of the National Academy of Sciences, the National Academy of Engineering, and the Institute of Medicine. The members of the committee responsible for the report were chosen for their special competences and with regard for appropriate balance.

This report has been reviewed by a group other than the authors according to procedures approved by a Report Review Committee consisting of members of the National Academy of Sciences, the National Academy of Engineering, and the Institute of Medicine.

The Institute of Medicine was chartered in 1970 by the National Academy of Sciences to enlist distinguished members of the appropriate professions in the examination of policy matters pertaining to the health of the public. In this, the Institute acts under both the Academy's 1863 congressional charter responsibility to be an adviser to the federal government and its own initiative in identifying issues of medical care, research, and education. Dr. Kenneth I. Shine is president of the Institute of Medicine.

This project was funded by the Contraceptive Research and Development (CONRAD) Program, the Andrew W. Mellon Foundation, the National Institute of Child Health and Human Development of the National Institutes of Health, the Rockefeller Foundation, and the United States Agency for International Development. USAID does not take responsibility for statements or views expressed in this report.

Library of Congress Cataloging-in-Publication Data

Contraceptive research and development : looking to the future / Polly
    F. Harrison and Allan Rosenfield, editors ; Committee on
    Contraceptive Research and Development, Division of Health Sciences
    Policy, Institute of Medicine
        p.   cm.
    Based on two workshops held in 1994-1995.
    Includes bibliographical references and index.
    ISBN 0-309-05442-7
    1. Contraception—Research—Congresses. 2. Contraception—
Forecasting—Congresses. I. Harrison, Polly F. II. Rosenfield,
A. (Allan) III. Institute of Medicine. Committee on Contraceptive
Research and Development.
    [DNLM: 1. Contraception—methods—congresses. 2. Contraceptive
Devices—congresses. WP 630 C753 1996]
    RG133.C66   1996
    613.9′4—dc20
    DNLM/DLC
    for Library of Congress   96-26149
                                                                              CIP

The serpent has been a symbol of long life, healing, and knowledge among almost all cultures and religions since the beginning of recorded history. The serpent adopted as a logotype by the Institute of Medicine is a relief carving from ancient Greece, now held by the Staatlichemuseen in Berlin.

Acknowledgments

There are many to thank. A study of this sort is a process and, as it goes forward and initial assumptions crumble and seemingly straightforward objectives ramify, the complexity of the process requires an ever-larger network of helpers.

This study was organized around two major activities.* The first was a workshop on the prospects of the science underlying the development of new contraceptives, held at the National Academy of Sciences in December 1994. We were honored to have as invited presenters at that workshop: Nancy Alexander, Deborah Anderson, Mina Bissell, William Bremner, Egon Diczfalusy, Mahmoud Fathalla, Susan Fisher, Judah Folkman, Frank French, Henry Gabelnick, David Garbers, Walter Gilbert, David Hamilton, Jeffrey Harris, John Herr, Bertil Hille, Aaron Hsueh, William Lennarz, Bruce Lessey, Jiri Mestecky, Walter Moos, Andrés Negro-Vilar, Bert O'Malley, David Page, Paul Primakoff, JoAnne Richards, Patricia Saling, Neena Schwartz, Roy Smith, Allan Spradling, Robert Stein, Jerome Strauss, Paul Van Look, Geoffrey Waites, Debra Wolgemuth, and Lourens Zaneveld.

The second major activity was a workshop on the opportunities, challenges, and strategies for private-sector participation in contraceptive research and development, held at the Academy in May 1995. This activity consisted of panel discussions and presentations by representatives from the legal, policy, regulatory communities, and large and small pharmaceutical industry, and our thanks

---

*Please see Appendix E for list of participants and their affiliations.

v

are especially due to Philip Corfman, Robert Essner, Ellen Flannery, Jacqueline Forrest, David Garbers, Michael Kafrissen, William Sheldon, and Hans Vemer. We thank as well the many other representatives of the pharmaceutical industry who joined us to participate in what was intended to be the beginning of a dialogue across sectors. We most particularly thank two individuals who were instrumental in this component of the study: Alan Goldhammer of the Biotechnology Industry Organization (BIO) who executed a survey of BIO members to help identify potential interest in that community in contraceptive research and development; and Laura Tangley, the science writer who so effectively summarized the proceedings of our first workshop as grist for the second and who did much of the later work on Chapters 3 and 4.

We are also eager to thank others who contributed written material for this report. Deborah Anderson, David Hamilton, John Herr, Alison Quayle, Patricia Saling, Kevin Whaley, and Lourens Zaneveld who, together with the scientists on the study committee—Horacio Croxatto, Michael Harper, Donald McDonnell, and Wylie Vale—authored the scientific papers that constitute the appendixes summarized in Chapter 4. We also want to thank Andrés Negro-Vilar, who provided much material for Chapter 3, and Ellen Flannery, our legal bulwark for Chapter 7.

There were others who gave us all manner of guidance and information along the way: Sarah Brown and Leon Eisenberg, whose work on the 1995 Institute of Medicine study, *The Best Intentions: Unintended Pregnancy and the Well-Being of Children and Families*, was so illuminating for this study; James Cavanaugh, who helped us begin a journey through unfamiliar waters; Steven Canafy and his tour of the current legislative environment; Lisa Kaeser's excellent analysis of contraception in the context of managed care; Olivia Judson, our link to current thinking in the United Kingdom about contraceptive technology; Luigi Mastroianni, Jr., chair of the 1990 National Research Council and Institute of Medicine study, *Developing New Contraceptives: Obstacles and Opportunities*, the wisest of historians; Bert Peterson, who helped us understand some of the implications of sterilization; James Trussell, a fount of information and clarification; as well as a number of staff members from the Alan Guttmacher Institute; the Population Council; the Program for Appropriate Technology in Health; and WHO's Special Programme for Research, Development, and Research Training in Human Reproduction. We thank Decision Resources, The Wilkerson Group, and Frost and Sullivan for permission to use information on the contraceptives market that would not otherwise have been available to us. All were extremely generous and prompt with whatever information we needed at whatever moment.

We also express gratitude for the help of the Board on Health Sciences Policy in identifying study committee members, and to Institute of Medicine staff, Timothy Kanaley, research assistant; Sharon Scott-Brown, project assistant; and Linda DePugh, administrative assistant. We thank May Tang, who spent her Washington semester internship from Pomona College with us and developed the Glossary, constructed tables, and assisted greatly with preparation of the manuscript for review and publication; without her, completion of this project would have been far more difficult. We thank Valerie Setlow, director of the Division of Health Sciences Policy, for her support and administrative creativity; Nancy Diener, for her patience with the financial realities of executing a large and complex study; Claudia Carl, for her combination of compassion and rigor in shepherding the report through the review process; and Mike Edington, for getting this report to the press in rapid and good condition and for finding Andrea Posner as our copy editor.

Finally—but far from last in importance—there are the sponsors: the Rockefeller Foundation, the Andrew W. Mellon Foundation, the Contraceptive Research and Development Program, the National Institute of Child Health and Human Development, and the United States Agency for International Development. The consensus around funding this study was formed in a climate of fiscal austerity, a climate in which tradeoffs among possible investments are typically difficult, especially around a topic that remains sensitive, controversial, and even somewhat unfashionable. The Institute of Medicine is, therefore, particularly earnest in its expression of appreciation for the confidence of the study sponsors, their patience, and their unfailing encouragement.

Polly F. Harrison, *Senior Study Director*
Allan Rosenfield, *Chair*

Contents

Contraceptive
Research
and
Development

Summary

This study began with three questions.

The first was: Is there really a need for new contraceptives and, if so, why?

The second was: If, as has been said, the field of contraceptive research and development has somehow lost the energy that characterized it at the time of what is called the "first contraceptive revolution," are there new prospects in the science that could reenergize it?

The third was: Given such prospects, would they be sufficient to accomplish that revitalization? The committee sensed early in its deliberations that, as exciting as scientific opportunity might prove to be, the climate for development would constrain it. Thus, the committee opted not only to explore the prospects in the new science, but to examine the context for collaboration between the public and private sectors that would be essential to meeting the need and demand for new contraceptive options.

THE EXISTENCE OF NEED AND SOME FUNDAMENTAL CONCEPTS

Other questions surfaced early in the committee's work: Was there really a need for new contraceptives, why, and what kind of contraceptives? The committee pressed itself to answer those questions and concluded that there is not only a need for new contraceptives but evidence of a real market for them. While the existing array of contraceptive options represents a major contribution of science and industry to human well-being, it fails to meet needs in significant populations and the costs of that failure are high, for societies, for families, and for individuals.

Throughout its work, the committee sought to frame the issues around contraceptive research and development in a way that might offer a fresh outlook on the subject. Four concepts seemed to merit integration into such a framework: the idea of a "woman-centered agenda," the challenges of unintended pregnancy, consideration of contraceptives from both the perspective of need and market demand, and new possibilities for collaboration between the sectors.

The Idea of a "Woman-centered Agenda"

For many years, women's health groups and advocates, as well as some researchers, have called for more safe and effective contraceptives that would better meet the needs of both women and men. In 1989, Carl Djerassi, a major figure in the development of the first contraceptive pill, suggested a list of priorities for new contraceptives. In order of descending priority, they were: (1) a new spermicide with antiviral properties, (2) a "once-a-month" pill effective as a menses-inducer, (3) a reliable ovulation predictor, (4) easily reversible and reliable sterilization for males, (5) a contraceptive pill for males, and (6) an antifertility vaccine for males or females or both.

Over the half-decade since then, a construct referred to as a "woman-centered agenda" has evolved, its source an expanding dialogue within a number of national and international women's groups, and between some of those groups and scientists working in reproductive and contraceptive research. The agenda reflects a more expansive view of contraception that attempts to integrate concerns for contraceptive efficacy into concerns for the overall reproductive health and general well-being of the primary users of contraceptives, that is, women. The notion of a woman-centered agenda for contraceptive research and development does not imply that there is some "universal woman" or some necessary, unitary view of women's preferences; it is simply that the field should refocus itself toward approaches in areas where the needs of women are still unmet by existing methods.

At the top of that agenda are three types of methods that were included in that 1989 agenda. Slightly restated, these are contraceptives that are also protective against sexually transmitted diseases (STDs), including human immunodeficiency virus (HIV); menses-inducers and monthly methods targeted at different points in the menstrual cycle; and contraceptive methods for males that would both expand their range of contraceptive choice and their sharing of the responsibility for contraception.

There is also a subtext for the agenda that has two themes: One is women's concern for control over their own bodies, including control over the occurrence and timing of pregnancy; the other concern is for equity in terms of physical safety and well-being. The basic message from research around these topics is that, as a general matter, women want contraceptives that are safe and efficacious, with minimal side effects. However, some women also assign value to methods that are discreet, easy to use, and nonsystemic. For still others, it is important that they themselves control method use, in other words, methods that are not controlled by a partner or unduly dependent on a provider. And, as reflected in the agenda, many women want full protection against sexually transmitted infection.

No single contraceptive can ever satisfy all these criteria simultaneously. Nor is that required since individual needs will always vary personally and situationally. At the same time, the present array of contraceptive technologies does not respond adequately to these criteria for many women and couples, many of whom would be willing and able to pay were there a fuller range of contraceptive options. In more and more societies, rich with technological diversity and replete with seemingly endless permutations of consumer goods, it is odd indeed that these particular options, central to the lives of so many individuals, families, and societies, are so limited.

The Challenge of Unintended Pregnancy

A recently published report by the Institute of Medicine made the following its lead recommendation: "To begin the long process of building national consensus around this norm, the committee recommends a multifaceted, long-term campaign to (1) educate the public about the major social and public health burdens of unintended pregnancy; and (2) stimulate a comprehensive set of activities at the national, state, and local levels to reduce such pregnancies." Similar objectives have motivated public statements by the United Nations Population Fund and the Alan Guttmacher Institute that underscore concerns about unintended pregnancy as a global problem.

This committee finds the central ideal of this proposed campaign—"every child a wanted child"—compelling, for women, for children, and for families. Attainment of this ideal is far too critical to be left to chance or the passage of time. It requires a thoughtful and deliberate response, a pivotal part of which must be the increased, careful, and consistent use of some form of contraception or, for the highly motivated, the exercise of periodic abstinence. Thus, greater knowledge about reproductive health and, in that context, contraception, is essential for providers, consumers, and the public at large, if fully informed, free, and appropriate choices are to be made about fertility regulation and sexuality. In turn, the proper use of contraceptive technologies for fertility regulation is linked both to the availability of quality contraceptive services providing a full range of safe, approved methods of contraception and an earnest and continuing search for more and better methods for more people.

In this connection, the committee finds understanding both in the United States and the developing world about the extent, causes, and consequences of unintended pregnancy and sexually transmitted disease to be seriously incomplete. The committee views this distressing situation as due largely to three relentlessly interacting factors: a welter of conflicting messages about sexuality and responsibility, inadequate education, and constrained access to a range of contraceptive alternatives that are suitable for those who most need them.

The committee agrees that the large numbers of unplanned and unwanted pregnancies in the world are not due solely to inadequate contraceptive methods. It is surely true that substandard health services; lack of public education; inadequate provider training; misunderstandings about risks and poor understanding of how people calculate risk; and social, cultural, and religious influences on family planning behavior, all can play a role in whether contraception is used and whether it is used appropriately and properly. Still, the committee finds ample indication that new technologies would improve the overall effectiveness of contraception in ways that currently available contraceptives do not and in ways that enhanced access and education, in themselves, alone, cannot.

Need and Market Demand

There are two categories of need for new contraceptive technologies. These overlap somewhat, but each has distinctive implications. The first category comprises public health needs that, left unanswered, generate further problems that are often quite costly, to individuals and to societies. Yet, as irrefutable and sizable as these needs may be, for a number of reasons they may not evoke a disposition, either by societies or individuals, to pay for their satisfaction.

The second category consists of needs that are recognizable in public health terms and, in addition, can elicit a disposition, either by society or individuals, to invest in resolving them. In other words, again for a number of reasons, these needs are of enough concern to produce market demand.

Indicators of Public Health Needs

Unintended Pregnancy   Unintended pregnancy is both a fundamental notion underlying the rationale for contraception and a measure of a fundamental public health need in today's world. Nearly 60 percent of all pregnancies in the United States and anywhere from 24 to 64 percent of all pregnancies worldwide are unintended, either because they were mistimed or because they were not wanted at all. Despite reigning stereotypes, unintended pregnancies are not confined to adolescents, minorities, or developing countries. While a majority of pregnancies among teens under age 19 are unintended, women of all ages and marital status—everywhere—face difficulties planning and preventing pregnancy. In the United States, of the 6.3 million pregnancies in 1987, 3.5 million were unintended; of these, 2 million occurred among women over age 20. Half of those unintended pregnancies occurred among women who had unprotected sex despite having no intention to become pregnant; slightly under half occurred among women who were, in fact, using contraception that either failed or was used improperly.

The committee contemplated the prospect of attempting to discern what portion of the unintended pregnancies in the world might be averted by new contraceptive technology. While not a totally impossible task, it is certainly a large and difficult one, well beyond the committee's mandate and capabilities. The task of determining what percentage of women who used no contraceptive at all would have done so had there been new technologies available is particularly daunting; one would have to know that the reason no contraceptive had been used was rejection of the available methods. It may be more informative to consider those women who were contracepting but became pregnant because the method failed or because it was used improperly. Either case may reflect lack of knowledge or some limitation in the efficacy and ease of use of a method; in some instances, both kinds of deficiency are at work.

Abortion Approximately one-third of the 190 million pregnancies in the world in 1995 ended in abortion; that same proportion applies in the United States. Clearly, those millions of women who choose to terminate a pregnancy, many submitting to unsafe and illegal procedures that can be life-threatening, attest to the need for improved access to and utilization of existing contraceptive methods and the need for new and improved contraceptive options. Furthermore, the evidence is overwhelming that, in most countries, children from unwanted conceptions, and their mothers, tend to be at greater medical risk and may become socioeconomic burdens—on society, on their families, and on their own life chances. In developing countries, unsafe abortion is a leading cause (perhaps as high as 20 percent) of the more than 500,000 maternal deaths that occur annually. Contraception is the first line of defense against unintended pregnancies, and any contraceptive option that will diminish the proportions of mistimed and—especially—unwanted pregnancies should be considered essential to societal and individual well-being.

Population Growth A focus on women's reproductive health and a woman's agenda for contraceptive research and development does not mean that other consequences of contraception suddenly do not matter. Family planning is an option for individuals that may benefit the larger community as well. Slower population growth is believed by many to contribute significantly to the healthy sustainability of the planet. Were only unwanted births prevented, the global number of live births would fall from 139 million a year to 122 million and the global rate of population growth would drop by 19 percent. There is also growing and powerful evidence that users can drive the demographics: It has been suggested that family planning programs that truly enable individuals to achieve their reproductive objectives actually have more impact on reducing fertility than do programs driven solely by demographic goals.

Unmet Need and Unserved and Underserved Populations   While contraceptive prevalence has risen impressively worldwide, new analytical approaches to the definition and measurement of the "unmet need" for family planning have produced estimates of from 120 million to 228 million women who can be defined as lacking effective contraceptive protection. These are the women most critically in need, that is, who do not want to be pregnant but who are not using any kind of contraception or who are using methods that are, for one reason or another, problematic.

The available contraceptive array is limited in the extent to which it can respond to variability in individual and family situations, to cultural differences, to specific health problems and shifting personal preferences, and to life cycle stages and changing reproductive intentions across those stages. Nor does the present array respond to the lengthening of the time during which women are at risk of unwanted conception, a lengthening that has resulted from earlier initiation of sexual relations, multiplicity of partners, and smaller family size ideals. The contraceptive needs of adolescents, sexually-active single or postpartum women, women who are lactating or in their later reproductive years, and—very importantly—men of any age, remain substantially unmet. Adolescents are of special concern, not only by virtue of their youth and vulnerability but because the contraceptives that are most appropriate to their age and health status are few in number and require meticulous use to be fully effective. The fact of these unserved and underserved populations is an indicator of both public health needs and market demand.

Indicators of Market Demand

Contraceptive Side Effects, Failure, and Discontinuation   Like any medical intervention, all contraceptive methods have side effects, some of which are burdensome, some unacceptable. The most popular forms of reversible contraception are hormonally based, namely, oral, injectable, and implant contraceptives. Although these are safe and have many benefits and few risks, they also have side effects that result in frequent discontinuation of their use. These side effects are generally not life-threatening complications, but rather symptoms such as spotting and irregular bleeding, weight gain, nausea, and mood changes, annoying to some women, very distressing to others. Together with myths and rumors about methods, side effects account for much of method discontinuation or misuse and will persist as obstacles to more widespread and effective use of reversible hormonal contraceptive methods.

Somewhat different, but equally difficult problems lead to much less use than might be expected of the very effective intrauterine devices (IUDs) currently available. These include the very negative impact that endures as a consequence of the publicity generated by the infections and deaths attributable to the Dalkon Shield IUD, misconceptions about IUDs and their association with infection, and side effects of bleeding and cramping experienced by some women. Furthermore, except for sterilization, IUDs, implants, and injectables, the factors of inherently low efficacy and/or imperfect use limit the contraceptive effectiveness of most of the currently available methods, although in widely varying measure. It is unrealistic to expect that there will soon be a contraceptive technology that is fully efficacious, with no side effects, for all users, under all conditions. Still, each additional method expands the spectrum of possibilities to an ever-larger number of users, as does the series of improvements that are inevitably made to all medical technologies after their first market introduction.

Sterilization Sterilization is the most used contraceptive in virtually all the world's regions, including the United States. While the method is most satisfactory for individuals who consider their families complete, many women are resorting to sterilization at unexpectedly early ages simply because they have found no reversible method to be satisfactory. Sterilization is clearly an excellent choice for women and men who are certain that they wish no more children; it is unsuited to the great majority of younger individuals. Studies have clearly demonstrated that the younger a man or woman is when a sterilization procedure is performed, the greater the chances that there will be later regret and a request for a reversal of the sterilization, a procedure that is complex, costly, and subject to failure. More effective and acceptable reversible contraceptive methods would allow for sterilization procedures to be used primarily by those who have truly completed childbearing. While sterilization can stand as an indicator of willingness to spend a considerable sum to terminate childbearing, that reading is somewhat compromised by the fact that, in many cases and particularly in the United States, some third-party payer is willing to assume the costs for the intervention, yet not willing to assume the costs for provision of reversible contraceptives.

Sexually Transmitted Disease, Including Human Immunodeficiency Virus (HIV) An important focus in this study was on the science and policy implications of the interface between sexually transmitted disease (STD) and contraception, since sexual contact, usually sexual intercourse, is necessary for both. In the past, attention to these two sets of concerns has generally proceeded on parallel tracks, guided by the correct perception that sexual activity and reproduction do not inevitably coincide and the incorrect perception that the populations requiring protection from STDs and from conception are utterly distinct. The STDs were viewed as a matter of no concern for the normative majority, that is, married couples creating families, for whom the risk of sexually transmitted infections was considered trivial. The facts of today's world must persuade us that this norm is much eroded and that the dynamics producing the erosion have altered the composition and greatly increased the size of the global population at risk, of which a sizable proportion is—simultaneously—vulnerable to possibly unwanted conception and surely unwanted infection. Though it is true that there are important biologic and behavioral differences between STDs and unintended pregnancy, it is hard to justify continued separation of the two, either programmatically or scientifically. Because of the spread of heterosexual transmission beyond groups typically considered high risk, because of greater female physiological vulnerability to infection and to more severe sequelae, and because of the potential of vertical transmission from mother to fetus, both society and individuals confront very high costs as the prevalence of sexually transmitted disease (STD) rises.

Only the condom provides protection against both conception and STD transmission. Because the female condom is not yet widely used and research has not yet been completed on the protection it provides against STDs, the single method now available for protection against both STDs and conception is the male condom—a method not controlled by women. Nor is there yet any single *non-*contraceptive technology that eliminates the risk of infection by the full gamut of pathogens that are transmitted sexually. Growing double-method use and increases in condom sales volumes indicate that the risk and urgency of this large problem are more appreciated and that individuals are willing to pay for protection. The market signals would seem to be quite clear.

Costs   Almost all the world's health systems are being driven to contain costs and look far more attentively at preventive approaches and economies of scale. The short- and long-term costs of unintended pregnancy and sexually transmitted disease are high; the cost-effectiveness of all contraceptive methods is excellent. Furthermore, availability of a good method mix has an independently positive effect: The addition of even a single major method to a family planning program can account for significant increase in contraceptive use-prevalence and reduction in crude birth rates. As health systems worldwide restructure and, hopefully, recognize the savings to be derived from prevention, contraception as an integral part of reproductive and family health should attract greater support. Beyond this, there are benefits to health that are less easily quantifiable but no less real, including substantial benefits from contraceptive methods themselves, such as protection against ovarian and endometrial cancer, benefits which can have a positive bearing on consumer decision-making. In less precise but commonsensical terms, experience indicates that a larger number of options will enhance overall acceptability and greater utilization across a wider range of individuals from different cultural backgrounds.

In sum, this committee finds an authentic need for development of new contraceptives and related reproductive health technologies. It believes that the nature of some of the need for such technologies is such that it represents a large and potentially profitable market. The committee also finds an agenda for contraceptive research and development that is "woman centered" to be reasonable, just, and also market worthy. The challenge is to find creative ways to elicit the best response from the scientific and industrial communities in a conducive climate that protects the integrity of inquiry and the safety of consumers.

The issue of climate is central. The aspects of context that press on every effort to provide safe and effective contraceptive technologies are complex and reflective of deeply rooted differences and deeply held beliefs. In addition, there is the current atmosphere of fiscal austerity in so much of the world, an atmosphere that cannot be ignored. At the same time, what is to be done about real, urgent, and unmet needs that affect public health and well-being everywhere? The committee has opted for a set of recommendations that are neither glamorous nor sweeping. They are, instead, unified by their practicality, located in the middle ground of policy, and intended to respond to what seem to be the needs of a significant majority.

THE PROSPECTS OF THE SCIENCE

The next question was whether there are possibilities that have been generated through the insights and mechanisms unfolding in contemporary science that would offer fresh, exciting, and plausible leads for a whole new generation of contraceptives. The committee dedicated vigorous effort to this question, reviewing a large body of evidence and expert testimony about possible leads to new contraceptive technologies, with special emphasis on those that respond to priority needs and might also evoke market demand.

It is the nature of science to pursue lines of inquiry that may turn out to be unrewarding for all sorts of reasons, no matter how plausible or broadly enticing they may have seemed; the ability to predict such eventualities is always limited. Nevertheless, basic research has been the wellspring of all quantum leaps in contraceptive technology so far and it will continue to be the wellspring for any significant innovations in the future. It is of interest in this regard that emphasis in AIDS and cancer research has very recently been retargeted toward fundamental issues in cell and immunobiology. New technologies, such as computer modelling, combinatorial chemistry and rational drug design, *in vitro* screening systems, and molecular biology, now provide tools for pursuing new leads in a meaningful and perhaps more rapid fashion. This gives hope that the progress of contraceptive development can be accelerated, that previously intractable problems will be much more susceptible to solution, and that discriminations can be made further upstream.

The committee concluded that there are, indeed, good prospects in the science that fit—or can be made to fit—the environment of both need and demand. Some of this promise could be realized in the nearer term; some, as is always the case early in the discovery process, must be seen as more distant possibilities. There is, however, no dearth of ideas, no lack of potential targets.

Criteria for Decision-making

A Woman-centered Agenda

Women—and men, if they are to share more of the responsibility for contraception and protection of themselves and their partners against infection—have many different requirements. These will vary according to many factors, including age, the nature of intimate relationships, ability to pay for methods, and access to health services, but the overall need is great and urgent. The committee has concluded that a vigorous and honest attempt to be responsive to a woman-centered agenda fulfills objectives that have potential benefits to all parties. At the same time that there is no "universal woman" to whom the information in this report and its recommendations are meant to apply in some inevitable, culture-blind fashion, there are two principles that are arguably universal: (1) the goal of enhancing women's control over their own bodies, including control over the occurrence and timing of pregnancy; and (2) equity for women's physical safety and well-being.

> **Recommendation 1. The committee recommends that priorities for new research be assessed against the preference criteria presented in a new "woman-centered agenda" and that existing public-sector contraceptive research and development portfolios be reassessed similarly. Such an approach highlights the need for improvements and new advances in contraceptives for women, and in areas where there are few or inadequate options, namely:**
>
> **• Methods that act as chemical or physical barriers to conception and to transmission of sexually transmitted diseases, including the human immunodeficiency virus (HIV);**
> **• Menses-inducers and once-a-month methods targeted at different points in the menstrual cycle;**
> **• Methods for males that would expand their contraceptive choices and responsibility.**

It is also the case that some existing contraceptive methods, such as the current oral contraceptives, condoms, and spermicides, have major health benefits above and beyond those produced by contraception. In strategies for future contraceptive development, the possibility of other health benefits should be assessed and, where such can be identified, those methods should be accorded priority. It is clear, however, that it may be difficult to establish *a priori* that there will be any such benefits. However, new contraceptive methods for which such benefits cannot be predicted should not be discarded from consideration when they meet the criteria of need, efficacy, safety, and acceptability.

Specificity of Targets

The committee is sensitive to the global atmosphere of austerity and pressures for cost containment, as well as the ambivalence toward basic science in the United States. It sought, therefore, to establish some foundation for making some *a priori* judgment about priorities for new directions. One area of consensus was around the matter of specificity of targets. Another had to do with points of intervention in the menstrual cycle and how the most controversial of those might be addressed.

The committee and the panel of scientists at the workshop it convened on New Frontiers in Contraceptive Technology had reservations about pursuit of targets that make for interesting biology but are less likely as candidates for attack because they are not specific enough. At the same time, there are likely to be many genes whose products are truly specific; that is, the interruption of these products will not affect anything but that cell. In this connection, the committee noted the particular concerns of some women's groups about immunocontraception and its long-term, systemic effects on other aspects of reproductive function. For these and related reasons, it would seem desirable that priority be given to new directions that focus on peripheral rather than central processes, since products that act centrally, such as oral contraceptives, are already available and specificity is more likely to be achieved by concentration on peripheral targets.

Recommendation 2. Modern scientific methods now exist that can identify genes whose products are involved solely in reproduction and are therefore prime targets for inhibition of conception. Fundamental research on the cells, tissues, and organs that contribute to conception can now be carried out with a new and incisive precision using tools of modern biology. The committee recommends, therefore, that priority be accorded to work with genes whose products are truly specific and urges attention to the fact that investment in basic research in contraception will be essential if work with these elements is to proceed with reasonable dispatch. Absent such investment, it is hard to see where innovative new approaches to contraception will come from.

The science is also potentially responsive not only to the requirements of contraception but to the additional imperative of addressing the mounting burden of the sexually transmitted diseases, including HIV. Because sexual relations can "transmit" both conception and infection, the design of new reproductive technologies must consider how to protect women against both, sometimes independently and sometimes together. The technologic and practical challenges of simultaneous protection against conception and infection are daunting. Clinical trials will present special technical and ethical challenges for developers, regulators, and trial participants, and industry will have to make some hard market

choices. Nonetheless, there are indications in the science that such double protection is not an implausible objective and the attempt is a matter of great urgency.

Few of the approaches presented immediately below will lead to new products in the short term and, indeed, many are long term. Nevertheless, if there are
to be radically new and more specific contraceptives and anti-infective agents in
the next century, the work must begin now.

Approaches to New Contraceptive Methods for Females and for Males

**Recommendation 3. Toward development of new contraceptive meth-
ods for females and for males, the areas of specific research that have
come to light during this study and that this committee believes deserve
the greatest attention in the shorter and longer terms are presented in
Boxes S-1 and S-2.**

The Contributions of Immunology to Contraception and
Prevention of Infection

There has been much discussion of the desirability of curtailing investment
in immunocontraception, primarily in response to concerns expressed by some
women's groups and by individual analysts, that immunocontraception will not
prove to be a biomedically appropriate contraceptive option for women in general
and that research and development investment in that area would be better placed
elsewhere. Nonetheless, curtailment at this point seems premature: It is not yet
clear that immunocontraceptive research cannot produce a safe, efficacious, reversible, medium- to long-term contraceptive that will expand the current range
of options in a way that a significant proportion of women and men will find
useful and desirable.

The field also has the power to provide insights into fundamental immunologic and physiologic structures and mechanisms that could enrich development
of other applications. The committee discerns three distinct possibilities: (1)
more complete knowledge of the structure and function of sperm immunogens
that could lead to development of chemical barrier methods efficacious in preventing both conception and infection; (2) better understanding of the surface
proteins instrumental in cell signaling prior to fertilization and implantation, for
applications in fertility and infertility research, and (3) the possibility that the
search to understand immunogenicity and assure reversibility of immunocontraceptives could uncover novel application and delivery approaches and new paradigms in pathogenesis. Still, given the plethora of potential antigens and paucity
of available funds, regular review permitting crucial decisions about selection
among candidates would be advisable.

Box S-1
Approaches to New Contraceptive Methods for Females

Vaginal Methods (Barriers)

Short-to-medium term:

• identifying agents that are spermiostatic rather than spermicidal
• developing antifertility agents that inhibit virus and/or other pathogenic organisms in the vagina
• modifying mucous secretions from cervical epithelial cells to prevent sperm passage

Monthly Methods and Menses-inducers

Short term:

• evaluating combinations of antiprogestins, antiestrogens, and inhibitors of enzymes involved in steroid synthesis to induce menses

Long term:

• understanding factors involved in blastocyst implantation
• developing specific luteolytic agents

Inhibition of Ovulation

Long term:

• inhibiting ovulation using nonpeptide GnRH antagonist/hormone combinations
• understanding the mechanism controlling follicular rupture as a way to prevent ovulation while permitting development of the corpus luteum

Inhibition of Fertilization

• inhibiting sperm-egg fusion, acrosome reaction induction, and sperm transport
• understanding the molecular basis of follicular atresia and luteinization, to provide leads for specific induction of atresia in the dominant follicle

---

Recommendation 4. The committee believes that the field of immuno-contraception holds promise: for contraception, for innovative approaches to barriers to infection, and for areas of science with broader applications. The committee recommends the emphases presented in Box S-3.

Box S-2
Approaches to New Contraceptive Methods for Males

Short term:

• inhibiting LH and FSH secretion by combinations of progestin/androgen as long-acting injectables or implants

Long term:

• targeting spermatogenesis using inhibition of FSH secretion, or FSH action using receptor blockers
• inhibiting meiosis
• affecting epididymal function to disrupt sperm maturation
• inducing premature acrosomal activation
• identifying genetic loci that affect gamete development or behavior, and developing inhibitors of these functions

---

Box S-3
Approaches to Immunologic Contraception for Females and Males

• pursuit of multideterminant sperm immunogens and early conceptus antigens
• increased research on antibodies to reproductive hormones and their receptors
• increased research on the local immune response of the female reproductive tract
• emphasis on immunologic methods protective against HIV (human immunodeficiency virus), HSV (herpes simplex virus), and HPV (human papilloma virus)

Monthly Methods and Menses-inducers

The area of menses-inducers or, more generally, postimplantation technologies, is one of the most complex of those discussed in this report. Due at least in part to the pressures brought to bear by groups opposed to abortion, the French pharmaceutical company, Roussel-Uclaf, decided against bringing its antiprogestin product RU 486 (mifepristone) to market in the United States, transferred rights to the Population Council, and is said to have curtailed its research in the general area of endocrinology. Similarly, two other major European companies that have developed effective drugs with antiprogestin properties, have left them on the shelf with no present intentions of bringing either to the market. This suggests at a minimum that it is unlikely that there will be major private sector pharmaceutical investment in this area.

At the same time, postimplantation technologies, including menses-inducers, can play an important role in the reduction of maternal mortality and morbidity and in the promotion and protection of reproductive and infant health. In addition, since a woman is not aware of any physiologic changes associated with pregnancy until after implantation and since, naturally, many pregnancies fail during this same period, agents that would prevent implantation are an attractive target for a monthly method. Furthermore, for many who accept the medical and legal definitions of the establishment of pregnancy as occurring only after implantation, this sort of contraceptive would not be construed as an abortifacient.

The committee recognizes that, among some groups, there are political and social sensitivities concerning menses-inducers, particularly postimplantation technologies, that place pressures on both the public and the private sectors to abjure research in this area. Yet there are also sensitivities among groups who feel that postimplantation alternatives are appropriate and necessary. Because of persistent controversy, the development of postimplantation technologies is unlikely to attract the capital and research efforts of most large pharmaceutical firms, either in the United States or in Europe, nor is it likely that U.S. public sector entities can play a significant role in developing these methods independently. There is evidence, nonetheless, that some small biotechnology firms, at least partly because they lack the "deep pockets" of the large integrated companies, are able and willing to work in this area. Public/private sector partnerships in other industrial or developing economies may offer promise for the development of these important and urgently needed products. Nonprofit organizations have had significant interest in this area in the past and continue to be relevant partners in research and development toward postimplantation technologies.

Recommendation 5. The committee urges that the research and development of anti-implantation and postimplantation methods be pursued as a response to a major public health need and to evidence of demand. Nonetheless, because the area of postimplantation is so controversial and thus unlikely to attract investment by large pharmaceutical companies, partnerships between smaller firms and nonprofit organizations may represent the most appropriate avenues for research, in the United States and elsewhere. The committee recommends this area of research and development as a priority for funders for whom this controversy is not constraining. Research on monthly methods up to and including implantation should also have high priority.

TRANSLATING UNMET NEED INTO MARKET DEMAND

The committee then asked itself: Given good prospects in the science, would they be sufficient to accomplish that revitalization; if not, why not; and what sort of climate and resources would be required for that to happen? The purpose of this set of questions was to scan the environment in which contraceptive research and development transpire and to identify what factors would act either to further or impede efforts to launch a "second contraceptive revolution."

It is tempting to seek one prime explanation for why things are the way they are in this field. This committee sought to find—if it could—the lead factor responsible for the difficulties that seem to have become chronic in contraceptive research and development and has concluded that such a factor does not exist. Rather, the elements that intervene in the field form a complex set of interacting factors, with the dominance of any one over the others being a function of context, the nature of a product, timing, and coincidence. Liability, economic factors, the size and character of an industrial firm, regulations, politics and ideology, and the attitudes and behaviors of individuals, independently and together, act in unpredictable ways. It is this unpredictability that is, for investors and developers, a feature of the landscape that may be accepted as inevitable but must still be kept as small as possible.

Even though the committee believes that there is considerable unmet need for new contraceptive technologies in the industrial and developing economies of the world; even though a compelling public health case can be made for the development of a broader portfolio of contraceptive options for women and men; even though contraceptives are highly cost-effective; and even though there are likely to be large savings to be realized from the prevention of sexually transmitted diseases; that may not be enough. The response of industry is conditioned by how all this can be translated into a strong, profitable, politically safe, and reasonably predictable market for prospective products. The high costs and risks of committing to development of a specific product are such that no firm will undertake commercialization of a new medical technology without at least a strong belief in the existence of a substantial market of consumers able and willing to pay for it, in other words, the existence of market demand. Even given a very large market, all pharmaceutical investments must compete for scarce investment dollars with other products that may have larger or more profitable markets or both. The fundamental issue is economic, an issue to which other conditions and events may contribute. For example, the impact of regulatory requirements on being first to market; the unpredictable, potentially high, and sometimes arbitrary costs of liability; and the effects of political intimidation and consumer boycott on the reputation of a given firm and the safety of its employees; are all important.

Support for the Provision of Contraceptives

The benefits and savings from preventing unintended pregnancies are reaped by whoever is already footing the bill for *not* preventing them. This can be the individual, but it is increasingly likely that the primary burden of cost will fall either on the public sector in countries where that sector contributes substantially to the cost of health care (for instance, Medicaid and various social welfare programs in the United States) or on third-party payers (e.g., health management organizations and private insurance carriers). It makes economic and medical sense to invest in programs for curbing smoking, drunk driving, drug addiction, and infectious disease, because such programs benefit all parties directly involved. Thus, the same would seem to be true of any program that would reduce the gap between the unmet need and the market demand for contraceptives and anti-STD agents. However, for a profit-oriented health service this is not necessarily the case, since returns to investment in prevention may end up benefiting the next plan or plans in which a given individual enrolls. Nonetheless, because an unintended pregnancy occurs in a much shorter time frame than, for instance, development of lung cancer in a smoker, the payoff to a health plan's investment in prevention of an unintended pregnancy is quicker by far.

Despite the powerful cost-reducing benefits of contraception, there is very limited coverage of contraceptives by many health insurance plans and many health maintenance organizations in the United States. For another large portion of the prospective market for new contraceptive products in the United States, Western Europe, and the developing world, publicly financed health programs are similarly incomplete in what they cover; in the United States, that coverage has been declining steadily over the past decade. This limited support, combined with low-cost existing substitutes for prospective new products, acts as a constraint on demand. In the committee's judgment, the development of new contraceptive technologies will depend, among other things, on assurance of a substantial market for both existing and new technologies. Thus, broader provision of third-party coverage for contraceptive services could be important to the maintenance of a strong market demand. In other words, contraception could be an important cost-containment mechanism for both the public and private sectors.

Recommendation 6. The committee recommends that, to make a full range of contraceptive products accessible to consumers and to increase demand for contraceptive products to something closer to the level of unmet need, there should be continued and sufficient government support of contraceptive services—for males as well as females—particularly for low-income individuals and particularly in developing countries. The committee also recommends that third-party payers, who bear the costs and may reap the benefits of the health status of their covered populations, include contraception as a covered service. Ideally, family planning services and the management of sexual health would be integrated components of comprehensive reproductive health services.

The significant difference between the industrialized and developing countries in this regard is that, as in the case of new vaccines, translation of scientific potential into new products that can meet the needs of these markets is difficult at the prices consumers (or governments) are typically able to pay. The characteristic solution has been that international bilateral and multilateral external assistance programs procure large quantities of contraceptive commodities from developers or manufacturers at a public sector contract price sufficient (given large volumes and low distribution and marketing costs) to cover developers' costs, with a modest profit. Prices charged to developing country governments, however, can be substantially lower, thus ensuring substantial demand and overcoming economic impediments to widespread adoption of these products in those countries. Creation of some sort of multilateral "purchasing pool" for new contraceptives could rely on industrialized-country agencies or firms to fund a two-tiered pricing and distribution system that would be profitable for pharmaceutical firms and feasible for developing economies. Manufacturers could compete to develop and produce pilot lots of contraceptives that met specifications developed by these agencies as especially relevant to the needs of developing countries. The winning firms would be eligible for large-scale purchases of their products by the sponsoring agencies for distribution at a lower price in developing economies. The prospect of a large procurement commitment should attract the interest and, possibly, entry by firms not now pursuing the development of contraceptives for industrial or developing country markets.

> **Recommendation 7. The committee recommends that consideration be given to a multilateral approach that would enlist the participation of public agencies and private philanthropic organizations toward support for an extension of the Global Contraceptive Commodity Programme that would create incentives for the development of new contraceptives. Since contraceptive procurement is already tiered and since both purchasers and vendors appear to accept that as a fact of life, an additional tier might be constructed for volume commitments for procurement of new contraceptives at prices that would constitute an incremental attraction to industry and still be feasible for countries able and willing to expand the range of contraceptives available to their populations.**

Direct Funding for Contraceptive Research and Development

The committee recognizes the difficulties international agencies face in obtaining additional funding for contraceptive research and development at a time of fiscal austerity. Still, the committee's scrutiny of funding for contraceptive research and development over the past 15 years indicates that it has, at best, remained flat in constant dollars and may actually have diminished. This means that cuts of any size have major implications, since targeted financial support from the public sector, notably on the part of the U.S. Agency for International Development and the National Institute for Child Health and Human Development, has been critical in drawing U.S. university and not-for-profit institutional researchers into the field of reproductive biology and in catalyzing and sustaining the creative research partnerships that produced the advances in contraceptive research and development over the past two decades. The public sector also has particular strength and expertise in supporting the later stages of contraceptive research and development, for example, the clinical trials necessary to obtain the data required by the drug regulatory process.

An increasingly frequent pattern of work in the contemporary pharmaceutical industry is a sequence of "virtual partnerships" and contract research arrangements at different junctures in the research and development processes. This is not an unfamiliar pattern for contraceptive research and development; in fact, the willingness of small companies to risk engagement, and the willingness of the public and non-profit sectors to venture along with them, have been pivotal in advances in the field. It is possible that the power and speed of combinatorial chemistry and high-speed computer modelling of compounds may make it more plausible for these sorts of collaborations to occur earlier in the research sequence. The partial nature of such early commitments might be attractive to biotechnology companies and might also mean that large pharmaceutical companies, wary of involvement in full product launch, would be willing to engage in different kinds of collaboration "closer to the bench." Any function that can expeditiously catalyze these sorts of ad hoc mechanisms across and within sectors could provide considerable value added. The reverse is also true; that is, any function impeding the healthy growth of such mechanisms is value lost.

Recommendation 8. The committee strongly endorses continued public sector support of, first, basic research in innovative areas of reproductive biology as a source of new leads for contraceptive research and development and, second, in the applied research that will bring the most promising leads to fruition. The committee believes that the greatest value added will accrue to strategies focused on attracting investment in those smaller domestic and foreign firms able and willing to do early-stage research in contraceptives or in a fundamental reproductive mechanism of particular promise. In this connection, the committee calls attention to the new Consortium for Industrial Collaboration in Contraceptive Research, whose purpose is to catalyze funding for feasibility studies and matching industry investment in early-stage contraceptive research and development in priority areas of the woman-centered agenda. The committee believes this initiative to be a creative and potentially high-payoff mechanism for sponsor investment.

TOWARD A MORE TEMPERATE CLIMATE

The Need for New Guidelines

Inevitably, regulatory factors are taken into account when a pharmaceutical or biotechnology firm decides whether or not to proceed along a given research and development trajectory. Responses to the requirements of the U.S. Food and Drug Administration (FDA) take time, and time is money, either in the form of additional "burn time," perhaps involving the costs of more trials, or in the form of delay in being early to market. The FDA has been working on the problems of delays in its approval processes and a number of internal reforms and procedural modifications have been implemented. In its contacts with industry, the committee encountered no generalized sentiment for diluting the rigor of FDA approval processes; in fact, any possibility that pending tort reform legislation might include a federal product liability statute giving contraceptive manufacturers credit for FDA approval of contraceptive drugs and devices argued against such dilution.

The committee found that, in general, industry wants clear *a priori* guidelines on drug regulatory requirements for new contraceptives, to reduce uncertainty and wasteful error. Because contraceptives constitute a global market, it is crucial that these regulations be internationally harmonized. Although it lacks regulatory authority, the World Health Organization has, in the past, convened cross-sectoral symposia on guidelines for contraceptives; these efforts seem to have constituted a strong contribution to guidelines development and to have been appreciated by the FDA and industry. Comparable efforts are urgently needed in the area of vaginal microbicides and spermicides, since industry will need clear guidance if it is to enter this high-priority field. The committee recognizes the difficulty of anticipating all possible contingencies in any set of guidelines, particularly in the case of truly pioneer products, but finds such guidelines to have been generally conducive to industry investment; they are not, of course, a guarantee of such investment.

Recommendation 9. The committee recommends that approval guidelines be developed as quickly as possible for the high-priority area of vaginal microbicides and spermicides, as a first step toward clarifying requirements for clinical trials and monitoring of novel contraceptives in general. A consensus conference on this topic is recommended, perhaps convened by the World Health Organization. Of special concern in this specific context are guidelines for what would constitute clinically significant levels of anti-infective efficacy, as well as risk of possible fetal exposure.

Product Liability

Contraceptives, like vaccines, therapies for drug addiction, and diagnostics and therapies for a number of infectious diseases, particularly the diseases unique to the developing world, are "social products." That is, their benefits, intended or unintended, go beyond the prevention and cure of disease in individuals, such that they also have considerable benefits for the health of the public. However, for various reasons, the large majority of these products do not generate enough margin of profit for industry to justify investment in their development. This is particularly so when that margin is affected by other contextual issues that not only reduce its size but produce other negative consequences such as damage to a firm's reputation, stockholder unhappiness, and threats to the prosperity of its other product lines.

With respect to contraceptives, factors of this genre have generated what might be called "The Contraceptive Paradox": that is, the disconnect between the consensus around the need for the widest possible offering of contraceptive methods, and the disappearance of some contraceptive options that have made it to market. Several contraceptive advances—the Today sponge, Norplant implants, Depo-Provera, and RU 486 (mifepristone) and other antiprogestins—are either unavailable or in some way besieged. Despite major improvements that have made intrauterine devices appropriate for a large number of women, the method has not yet overcome its difficult history and regained its former acceptability, at least in the United States. The newly introduced Depo-Provera, approved by the FDA only after much controversy and opposition by several women's groups, has also come under further attack. The Today sponge is no longer on the market, and the Norplant implant, which became the method of choice for many women quite quickly after its introduction, has experienced a dramatic decline in use because of removal problems in a small percentage of women and the large amount of negative publicity deriving from widely publicized class action lawsuits related to problems with breast implants. There have also been concerns that any contraceptive made with silicone and analogous biomaterials might become scarce or disappear from the market altogether or, perhaps for a time at least, become prohibitively expensive. This could affect the new two-rod Norplant II implant system, new female barrier methods now in clinical trials, hormone-releasing IUDs made with silicone, new male and female barrier methods made with silicone and analogous polymers, and tubal ligation clips, not to mention the loss of options in connection with other conditions such as cardiovascular disease.

The committee encountered mixed views on the relative impact of liability on pharmaceutical innovation, in general, and contraceptive research and development, in particular. For some firms it is more of an issue than for others, but in no case is the current tort situation in the United States considered trivial. Where it is not costly in dollar terms, it can be costly in terms of company reputation; the time, energies, and concerns of staff; and an overall disposition to enter, reenter, or remain in the field of contraceptive research and development. What is also costly—and not always taken into account—are the costs to the large majority of consumers when a product is removed from the market entirely or for long periods of time.

In its 1990 report, the National Research Council and Institute of Medicine Committee on Contraceptive Development recommended that the U.S. Congress enact a federal product liability statute that would give contraceptive manufacturers credit for approval of contraceptive drugs and devices (and their labeling) by the FDA. The gist of such a defense—termed the government standards, FDA, or regulatory defense—is as follows: If it is established that an injury-causing aspect of a contraceptive drug or device was in compliance with all applicable requirements of U.S. federal food and drug law at the time that drug or device was made or sold, then a manufacturer or seller of a contraceptive drug or device would not be liable under any of the relevant legal theories (misrepresentation, warranty, negligence, or strict liability) for any injury related to design, nor liable for failure to provide adequate warning or instruction regarding any danger associated with its use, nor liable if the FDA had *not* asserted that the contraceptive drug or device was *not* in compliance. The defense would *not* be available if a claimant were able to establish that the manufacturer should have made design modifications or given different or additional warnings or instructions; if the manufacturer or seller knew or should have known of studies showing increased risk of harm from the contraceptive drug or device that indicated increased likelihood of serious injury; or if the claimant established that the FDA was not informed of dangers regarding the contraceptive drug or device that were known to the manufacturer or seller, and that the injury to the claimant or persons sharing the claimant's medical characteristics was attributable to such dangers.

The arguments for the FDA defense are that punitive elements of damage awards are meant to punish egregious behavior, not to punish companies that comply with the strict rules of the regulatory system and could not have predicted the side effects alleged to have caused the injury. The arguments against it are that the proposed legislation would protect irresponsible corporations at the expense of people victimized by faulty products. In general, manufacturers of all types of products have sought to limit their liability exposure and consumer groups have generally opposed these efforts. The pivotal issue appears to be that proposals for some kind of government standards defense have generally overlooked the widely held public belief that people are entitled to compensation for harm, particularly harm caused by negligence. Nonetheless, it is critical to note that the argument for some kind of government standards defense does not do away with liability. FDA compliance is, indeed, a shield, but noncompliance— importantly including concealment of data by the manufacturer—makes that shield worthless.

The committee is comfortable in, first, arguing that liability is still a significant disincentive to contraceptive research and development and, second, in reaffirming the recommendation of the 1990 NAS committee that a government standards defense is a necessary, though not sufficient, condition for unfettering the field. The committee has noted the facilitating effect on the vaccines field of the National Vaccine Injury Compensation Act and, while that is not a fully analogous example, it does suggest that, for controversial products that contribute importantly to the public health yet produce only modest profit margins, some parameters on liability can act as an incentive to research and development.

Recommendation 10. The committee reiterates the 1990 NRC/IOM committee recommendation that the U.S. Congress enact a federal product liability statute that gives contraceptive manufacturers credit for FDA approval of contraceptive drugs and devices. When the FDA has considered the relevant health and safety data on a contraceptive product, has approved the product, and has required warning and instructions to accompany it, it is sound national policy to make this approval available to manufacturers as a limited defense and not to penalize them for something they could not have known at an earlier point. Because the statute would interact with postmarketing surveillance efforts, this recommendation would be more compelling were formal postmarketing surveillance studies to be generally required. This said, the committee adds emphatically that it endorses a government standards defense only in the context of existing levels of rigor and scrutiny in approval processes and presentation of all relevant data by manufacturers.

Informed Choice

Since this committee was convened, the array of available contraceptives has been affected by the liability cloud around Norplant implants, the related crisis around biomaterials deriving from silicone breast implants, and the 20 years of controversy before Depo-Provera was approved for contraceptive use in the United States. At present, all three products have successfully met approval standards required by the U.S. Food and Drug Administration and regulatory agencies in many other countries. The committee also recalls the fate of IUDs in the United States after the widely publicized Dalkon Shield affair. No matter how suitable the newer IUDs have proved to be for many women, no matter how innocent of associated wrongdoing, and no matter how devoted their following, they have never regained their status in the mind of the consumer public. It seems that once there is adverse publicity about an approved contraceptive product, it is hard for that product to maintain or regain significant market share.

It may also be that, in some cases, a product is used by individuals for whom it is inappropriate and/or who have expectations that there will be no risk involved in the use of that particular contraceptive method. No pharmaceutical product is right for all patients and all pharmaceutical products have side effects, slight for some individuals, significant for others; contraceptives are no exception, although they bear a special cargo of cultural freight and skepticism toward those who develop and produce them. It is also true that, as with vaccines, contraceptives are used by presumably healthy people whose tolerance for side effects is lower than it is for the products they use when they are ill. These experiences are unfortunate: for the immediate user; for developers and potential manufacturers, because of the loss of the time and resources invested; and for other putative users, for whom the method in question might be quite appropriate yet whose options are now diminished. Each such case naturally affects women's feelings about contraception and the willingness of science and industry to pursue new investments in the field.

The term "informed choice" has been accumulating currency in the family planning community and among women's advocacy groups. As in legal understandings of informed consent, the principles of patient autonomy and adequacy of information are pivotal in informed choice. However, the emphasis is on information for the protection of the patient or client, a desirable objective even if there were no threat of liability. That protection is achieved by avoiding injury; injury, in turn, is avoided largely by fully informing potential users about all aspects of a product they are considering and encouraging them *not* to use a product if they find any of those aspects unacceptable. A key element is the informing process itself. The assumption is that provision of correct information is not enough; presentation, intelligibility, and confirmation that the information was understood are necessary to insure that individuals assess and select among options in an informed way.

Concurrent with the worldwide search for cost-effectiveness in health services, including preventive interventions that are cost-effective in the shorter term, is the promotion of ideas about the "educated patient," patient autonomy, health promotion, client-centered care, and the significance of client-provider information exchange. In the context of contraceptive use and family planning, these have become standard themes. The point is often made that at least some of the failure rates associated with contraceptive methods (e.g., barrier methods) are a function of inadequate information and support or, as in the case of emergency contraception, an almost total lack of communication from provider to client. There is also ample evidence that women everywhere, to a varying extent, are inadequately prepared by providers for the possibility of contraceptive side effects, their implications, and appropriate response.

The core implication of all this is that accuracy of information and its completeness, intelligibility, and overall effectiveness are more critical than ever to health care in general and to reproductive health in particular. The media through which this information must flow obviously include radio, television, and the printed page. They also include consumer education initiatives at different informational levels and at different stages of development: the international dialogue among women's groups and scientists, the U.S. campaign to reduce unintended pregnancy, and the design of informed consent and informed choice protocols for specific contraceptive methods. The committee applauds these efforts, urges support for them, and suggests one more area for development, that is, the untapped potential and often counterproductive medium of product labeling and packaging.

The Role of Packaging Information

The packaging and labeling of contraceptives—the "software"—could play a much more useful role in educating clinicians and consumers about contraceptive technology—the "hardware"—than they now do. At present, the labels and inserts in contraceptive packaging are daunting visually and technically, a fact often attributed to FDA demands and to concerns about liability. At the same time, the FDA only has jurisdiction to approve package inserts as accurate statements of the safety and efficacy of their contents; they are not in the business of approving new, perhaps more effective ways of informing consumers and clinicians.

Labeling can be dismissed as a small matter, or at least smaller than other forces that impinge on the availability and use of contraceptives, such as the media, advocacy groups, and the ideas, information and, sometimes, misinformation that flow through them. Still, a single categorical location where intelligible, accurate information about the technical aspects of individual contraceptive technologies—their risks, side effects, contraindications, benefits, and proper use—is consistently available, could anchor the information base. It is also the case that the media pay attention to package labels; an apparent misreading of the label on the Reality female condom, published in a major trade journal, sent the manufacturer's stock plummeting.

The technical complexity, regulatory considerations, legal implications, and what might be called the pedagogy and artistry of labeling are extensive. Even assuming that the method in question is physiologically and socially appropriate for use by a given population, there will always be some part of that population for whom newly accessible information will make no direct difference, either because it does not fit into the ways they calculate risk, or because they receive the information inadequately transmitted through an intermediary. Nor is there any easy way to calculate the costs and benefits of better labeling. Revising labeling in some generic way would inevitably impose costs, but these would seem unlikely to be crippling for large companies. In a clinic setting, helping individuals make informed choices takes time and effort, both at a premium for busy health care providers who may also have patient load quotas. A well-informed consumer may decide not to use a product after all, and a possible sale does not occur, yet another cost. Still, these costs must be arrayed against others: the possible harm to a user or a user's progeny, the costs of compensating that harm, the costs to the reputation of the firm, and the costs to other appropriate consumers of losing an option when a contraceptive method is withdrawn from the market.

> **Recommendation 11. The committee believes that users of contraceptives have a right to information about them that is balanced, accurate, and intelligible. Significant sources of such information are the labels and inserts that are integral to pharmaceutical packaging. The legal, regulatory, educational, sociocultural, scientific, and even artistic aspects of these packaging elements are large and complex, so that modifying them significantly will require cross-disciplinary and cross-sectoral effort. The committee urges that this topic be addressed soon, for two reasons. First, balanced, accurate, and intelligible contraceptive packaging is of potential benefit to contraceptive users, health providers, manufacturers, and entities concerned with public health and welfare, since it could contribute to the more appropriate and wiser use of contraceptive technologies. Second, the activity in itself offers the opportunity for much-needed dialogue within and across sectors, genders, classes, and systems of belief.**

CLOSING COMMENT

Despite the undeniable richness of the science that could be marshaled to give the women and men of the world a broader, safer, more effective array of options for implementing decisions about contraception, childbearing, and prevention of sexually transmitted disease, dilemmas remain. These dilemmas have to do with laws and regulations, politics and ideology, economics and individual behavior, all interacting in a very complex synergy that could lead to the conclusion that nothing can be done to resolve the dilemmas because everything needs to be done.

This committee examined the development of vaccines for the world's children as an experience with many analogies to contraceptive research and development. That experience informs us that the dilemmas around controversial medical products, whatever the sources of controversy, tend to be incremental and systemic in their resolution. Modification of the terrain for vaccine research and development took time—two decades of working groups charged with solving "the vaccine problem," a decade of legislative attempts to construct a passable bill, and close to a decade for industry to perceive that the legislative remedy was effective. Change came from several sources—from a surge of discovery in the science, from legislative action that modified public policy, from leadership at national and international policy levels, and from the decision of a major international donor to seek outside guidance in assessing its processes and their impact.

This does not mean that the same amount of time will be needed for improvement in the contraceptive landscape, nor will the solutions be the same. The central implication is that there is not likely to be a "silver bullet" solution to the dilemmas faced by the field of contraceptive research and development. Each piece of the dilemma will have to be tackled in cumulative fashion as part of a coherent strategy, each resolution improving matters somewhat and eventually amassing enough weight to tip the balance in a more positive direction. What this study committee has tried to do is identify a relatively small set of emphases and changes that, altogether, could turn the field around, but that, even partially implemented, could open up the field to freer, more equitable access to those who require its fruits.

1

Introduction

This report is about the need for new contraceptive technologies, the potential of contemporary science to respond to that need, the context in which that need will or will not be met, and the prospective roles of the private and public sectors in meeting it. The study that culminated in this report responded to a request that the Institute of Medicine explore these questions as an element of the Rockefeller Foundation's "Contraception 21" initiative: a search for ways to set the research agenda for the contraceptives of the twenty-first century and to mobilize the resources of all sectors toward a "second contraceptive revolution."[1]

THE FIRST CONTRACEPTIVE REVOLUTION

A pivotal dimension of family and child well-being and of female reproductive health is the ability to regulate fertility. A critical component of that ability is the availability of safe and effective contraceptive methods, both reversible and irreversible. Before 1960, that availability, for men and for women, was limited to the irreversible options of male and female sterilization and the reversible methods of the condom and withdrawal for men, a few barrier methods for women, and periodic abstinence, all of which had relatively high failure rates when not used consistently and carefully. The "contraceptive revolution" which began in the 1950s changed that picture with the invention of oral contraceptives and the reintroduction[2] of intrauterine devices, innovations which, for the first time, separated reversible contraception from the act of coitus (Rockefeller Foundation 1993).

The 1970s and 1980s brought infusions of funding for contraceptive research by the U.S. government and other governments, motivated by demographic concerns. Support was made available for improvements in the delivery of hormonal contraception, as well as for the development of new delivery modalities such as implants and injectables, so that the quality and range of contraceptive options were considerably enhanced. Contraceptive use in the developing world rose from less than 10 percent of couples (31 million) in the early 1970s to current levels of 50–60 percent (446 million) by the late 1980s (United Nations, forthcoming). Use of the technologies emerging from the first contraceptive revolution accounted for the great preponderance of that increase: Despite significant regional differences, as of 1995 most of the world's women who use any contraception are selecting modern contraceptive methods (Guttmacher Institute 1995a).

THE CHANGING STRUCTURE OF CONTRACEPTIVE NEEDS

While currently available contraceptives are obviously adequate for many individuals, there is ample evidence that they can only inadequately respond to the changing structure of contraceptive needs. The character of those needs, as we will discuss in detail in the next chapter, is variable, complex, and different in several important ways from the needs that characterized the period of the first contraceptive revolution. The fact that those needs are presented sequentially in the following paragraphs should not be interpreted as evidence of priority; all are of great importance and each is in some way related to the others.

First, there is the sheer volume of need. Minimum estimates of what is defined as "unmet need" range from 120 million to 238 million women worldwide who are at risk of unintended pregnancy because of nonuse of contraception, misuse, or contraceptive failure (Guttmacher Institute 1995a; Institute of Medicine [IOM] 1995a; Robey et al. 1992). Nearly half of the pregnancies defined as "unintended" in the United States as of 1987 had occurred among the 90 percent of women who were, in fact, using some contraceptive method (Forrest 1994).

Second, there are the 52 million pregnancies that women decide to resolve in abortion, approximately 28 percent of all pregnancies worldwide (Guttmacher Institute 1994; WHO 1994). Somewhere around 21 million of those abortions are performed under unsafe and septic conditions, and the burdens of mortality and morbidity they generate are high (WHO 1994). In the United States, of the 6.3 million pregnancies estimated to have occurred in 1987, over half were unintended at the time of conception and, of those, approximately half ended in abortion (Harlap et al. 1991). In the current array of contraceptive methods, there is no method that is explicitly intended to prevent pregnancy in women who have been exposed to unprotected sex, thereby obviating the possible need to confront the dilemmas of abortion.

Third, there is the high proportion of women who opt for sterilization, now the most used method in most of the world's regions, including the United States where over one-third of women using contraception have made that choice (Forrest and Fordyce 1993; Ingrassia et al. 1995; Marquette et al. 1995; Mosher and Pratt 1990). Women may elect this essentially irreversible method, even at unexpectedly young ages and earlier than they themselves might wish, because no alternative reversible method is seen as satisfactory.

Fourth, there remain large subpopulations whose contraceptive requirements remain insufficiently addressed, significantly those of males in general, to whom the first contraceptive revolution brought no new reversible contraceptive options, as well as the requirements of special times and circumstances across the female life span, notably adolescence, lactation, and the perimenopausal period.[3]

Fifth, there is the virtually undisputed reality that no existing contraceptive method can meet the requirements, intentions, and preferences of all individuals in all circumstances over entire reproductive lifetimes. Nor can any method be totally without side effects, risks, or trade-offs in terms of safety, efficacy, convenience, usability, and appropriateness (Fathalla 1994). In fact, it is difficult to envision any prospective method that could respond to all these variable requirements. Furthermore, for many women it is also important, even vital, that their contraceptive method be "user-controlled," that is, that it permit them to be the primary decision-makers about utilization. All this argues for the broadest possible range of available options.

Sixth, of particular concern in the United States, is the fact that the range of contraceptive options, rather than becoming more generous in an era when so many other medical technologies are proliferating, is actually narrowing and, in fact, is more constrained than in other industrialized countries. The reasons for this are diverse and complicated, their net effect most worrisome.

Seventh, and of mounting urgency, there is the need to address the growing burden of the sexually transmitted diseases and the ways in which they intersect—or do not intersect—with contraception. At present, only abstinence from sexual intercourse provides absolute protection against both infection and conception. For those choosing to be sexually active, while some forms of contraception reduce the possibility of either pregnancy or infection, they do not eliminate it. The male condom can provide good protection against both, but its efficacy depends on perfect use and on decisions which do not inevitably rest with women.

NEW CONCEPTS: REPRODUCTIVE HEALTH AND THE "WOMAN-CENTERED AGENDA"

Over the past 15 years, as a consequence of thought and advocacy on the part of internationally oriented activist groups, funding agencies, research organizations, and policy makers concerned with women's health, the concept of "population control" has moved toward a perspective which contemplates contraception within the more ample framework of "reproductive health." That framework is a comprehensive, more inclusive model of female health and well-being that encompasses fertility and infertility, contraception, abortion, childbearing, maternal morbidity and mortality, sexuality, sexually transmitted diseases, menstruation, and menopause and, for some theorists, child survival and male reproductive health as well (Behrer 1993; Dixon-Mueller 1993; Ford Foundation 1991; Germain and Ordway 1989; Lane 1994; Ruzek 1993). At its most expansive, the model also takes into account the social, political, and economic context of reproductive health and women's general empowerment (Lane 1994) and the ways in which each of these complements and reinforces the others (Bongaarts 1994; Germain and Kyte 1995; Guttmacher Institute 1995b; UNFPA 1994).[4]

The central themes informing this framework, that is, the concepts of women's control over their own bodies and equity for women's physical safety and well-being, have now taken root in the United States. The general subject of the health of U.S. women is now a focus of priority concern and has provoked attention to the necessity of including women in clinical trials for new preventive and curative therapies, long focused mainly on men. In response, the U.S. National Institutes of Health established in 1990 an Office of Research on Women's Health and recently launched a ten-year Women's Health Initiative. All this has fueled the interest of pharmaceutical companies, several of which have established female health care research departments (Bhargava 1992).

A significant component of this new rationale and, within that, contraception, is the accumulated body of evidence that just meeting the individual family planning desires of women (their "unmet need") would go a good distance toward meeting the demographic goals of those countries that have set such goals (Sinding 1994). The principal reason for this dynamic is that family planning approaches that are "woman centered," dedicated to quality of care, provision of a full range of contraceptive options and the informational basis for making informed choices among them, and generally satisfying clients are simply more effective in terms of adoption and continuation (Bongaarts and Bruce 1995; Bonnie et al. 1991; Bruce and Jain 1995; Germain 1987; Potts and Rosenfield 1990). It is individual women, with full access to better information and better tools, who determine the outcomes of population programs, rather than population programs determining women's behavior (Miller and Rosenfield 1996). This represents a shift away from the rationale that drove much of public funding for contraceptive research during the 1970s and 1980s, rooted as it was in the demographic concerns of governments (Brown 1995). It also lies at the heart of the Programme of Action that was articulated at the 1994 United Nations International Conference on Population and Development in Cairo. In this context, individuals decide to limit or space births for a variety of personal and family reasons, even though many individuals may well include among those reasons a recognition of the societal implications of having very many children.

Finally, the shift has laid the foundation for a new "woman-centered" approach, not only in services but in deciding on priorities for contraceptive research and development (R&D)(Fathalla 1994; Khanna et al. 1994). At the most general level, the approach calls for an agenda centering on methods more directly under women's control so as to enhance their autonomy, enable them to shield themselves from sexually transmitted disease, diminish their dependence on the medical system and on the agreement of a partner for use of a contraceptive or anti-infective, and provide them with entirely new access to a range of methods that can be used postcoitally. While it might seem counterintuitive, another component of that agenda is development of contraceptive choices for men that will permit them to share more of the responsibility for contraception.

There does appear to be consensus on these broad areas as appropriate and necessary orientations for new contraceptive research and development. There also seems to be agreement that the current array of available contraceptives must be expanded, though the point is often made that it is necessary to improve the availability of those contraceptive methods that presently exist, as well as the ways in which they are made available. Important among those ways is assuring much better informed contraceptive users.

At a more specific level, however, there is no "universal woman," nor is there some unitary view of women's contraceptive preferences. There are differences among women's health advocates—as well as between those advocates and scientists—about the meaning of each of these focal areas, their relative importance, and the proper criteria for setting research and development priorities (Barroso 1994; Correa 1993; Dixon-Mueller and Germain 1993; Germain 1987; Marcelo and Germain 1994; WHO/HRP 1991; Women's Global Network for Reproductive Rights 1993). Most of the energy in the debate centers on perceptions of the risk and benefits of contraceptive technologies and on the definitions and relative weights of their safety, efficacy, affordability, and acceptability (Snow 1994). The details of this debate are reflected in Chapter 2 and Chapter 5 of this report since, as significant features in the current climate surrounding contraceptive research and development, they affect the determination of needs in the field and, by extension, the market.

CONTRACEPTION AND SEXUALLY TRANSMITTED DISEASE

A question raised before this committee was the appropriateness of including the sexually transmitted diseases (STDs)[5] in a study of the current scientific prospects for contraceptive technology. The question is natural enough: The fields of family planning and the prevention and cure of STDs, including HIV/AIDS, have traditionally operated independently, surely in the case of research and development, only slightly less so in the delivery of clinical services (Cates 1994). The operating assumption has long been that the STDs have to do with sexual activity, and contraception with reproduction. The implication was that the STDs were not a concern for the normative majority, that is, married couples creating families, for whom the risk of sexually transmitted infections was considered trivial.

The epidemiologic and sociologic facts of today's world must persuade us that this norm is much eroded and that the dynamics producing the erosion have altered the composition and greatly increased the size of the global population at risk, of which a considerable proportion is—simultaneously—vulnerable to possibly unwanted conception and surely unwanted infection (Brunham and Embree 1992; WHO 1995). This is so despite the fact that sexual activity is not necessarily concurrent with reproduction or contraception: sexual activity continues much longer than reproductive activity, may occur during pregnancy and lactation, and may involve a variety of partners and types of sexual activity that do not have reproduction as their primary objective. The dimensions of these phenomena are discussed in Chapter 2 from the perspective of needs for new technology, and in Chapter 3 from the perspective of the market.

Another point of relevance is the existing technologic intersection between contraception and disease prevention. The condom has long been used as a contraceptive and as a barrier to STDs. While other contraceptives have also been found to provide some protection against infections, none protect against all STDs; any protection is highly dependent on perfect use and is variable by gender; double protection is ideally required; and some contraceptives, individually and used concurrently with other methods, may even enhance susceptibility to the risk of certain infections. Unfortunately, those contraceptives that best prevent pregnancy provide minimal protection against STDs. In all instances, there are many unanswered questions which jointly affect the fields of sexually transmitted disease and family planning and involve questions of safety, contraceptive use, and the nature of the need for new contraceptive methods (Antrobus et al. 1994; Cates and Stone 1992). The fact that some existing contraceptives— barrier and non-barrier—bestow any protection at all suggests that scientific exploration of this intersection is not only necessary but plausible (Claypool 1994; Elias and Heise 1993; Stratton and Alexander 1993).

THE NEED FOR A SECOND CONTRACEPTIVE REVOLUTION

By the late 1980s, many of the factors that had been driving the research agenda of the 1970s and 1980s had changed drastically. The mission's clarity had become blurred by the debate about whether it was population growth, or inequitable access to economic and social opportunity, that was the world's major problem. There was also the widespread misconception that, with oral contraceptives, the "problem" had been solved. From the standpoint of the science, the promise of reproductive endocrinology was diminishing, funding opportunities were decreased, and new scientists were not being attracted by the field. And, largely for legal, political, sociocultural, and ultimately economic reasons, there was relentless retrenchment from the field of contraceptive research by most major pharmaceutical companies. In the 1960s, a dozen large pharmaceutical companies had been active in contraceptive research and development; nine of those were in the United States. By the mid-1980s, just four such firms continued to have significant contraceptive research and development programs; three were in Europe, just one in the United States.[6] Had it not been for public-sector commitment during these years, the field might well have fallen into utter scientific oblivion (NRC/IOM 1990; Rockefeller Foundation 1993).

The net effect of this stalling of the first revolution was that there has been no real scientific breakthrough in contraceptive technology, for either men or women, in over three decades. The sole exception has been the antiprogestins, arguably the greatest breakthrough in fertility regulation technology since the discovery of oral contraceptives (Brown 1995; IOM 1993b). Modification of hormonal contraceptive delivery through injectable and implant technologies and dramatic improvement in intrauterine devices (IUDs) were significant developments, but they were not significant breakthroughs from the perspective of fundamental science. Because development of new contraceptive technologies typically takes 10 to 20 years, contraceptive products that are now emerging from the pipeline tend to fit the earlier demographically driven paradigm and respond only in a limited way to newer thinking (Brown 1995). Although recent surveys of contraceptive research and development indicate that there are close to 100 product leads being pursued around the world, most are incremental improvements—modifications in dosage, form, or delivery—and all but one are hormonally based (PATH 1993). Such improvements have been important and necessary but the argument might be made that, absent any shared, coherent set of priorities, large gaps will persist in contraceptive research and development. At best, contraceptive needs will be filled erratically and slowly, impairing wise and effective allocation of resources under conditions of increasingly probable scarcity (IOM 1993a).

In sum, the advances in cell and molecular biology and biotechnology that have been opening new frontiers in other areas of the medical and biological sciences have been exploited in only limited ways in contraceptive research. There are at least two possible explanations. One is that the new science, as much as it has contributed to innovation in other domains, is not, in fact, as applicable to development of novel contraceptives and the new leads that have been identified are not scientifically enticing enough to industry. The other is that there are other historical and current factors, outside the science, that are holding back contraceptive research. This study explores both possibilities.

THE ENVIRONMENT FOR CONTRACEPTIVE RESEARCH AND DEVELOPMENT AND THE OBJECTIVES OF THIS STUDY

In January 1990, the Committee on Contraceptive Development of the National Research Council (NRC) and the Institute of Medicine released a report on two years of analysis of barriers facing the development of new contraceptive methods.[7] The committee concluded that contraceptive development was indeed stalled; that the most problematic obstacles were the political and ideologic climate in the United States, the organization of resources available for research, some of the federal regulatory requirements, and the specter of product liability. Absent public policy changes that would lower at least some of these obstacles, the committee predicted that contraceptive choices in the next century would not be appreciably different than what they were at the time of that study (NRC/IOM 1990).

The present study, undertaken over five years later, began with the premise that contraceptive development continues to be largely stalled, but that the factors previously considered formidable barriers were no longer viewed by the pharmaceutical industry as the primary deterrents to its involvement in the field. In an analysis of industry perceptions commissioned by The Rockefeller Foundation as part of its Contraception 21 initiative, the Program for Appropriate Technology in Health (PATH) determined that the major obstacles for industry are, instead, economic (PATH 1995). In general, the analysis concluded, the pharmaceutical industry does not seem to perceive either sufficiently enticing new product ideas or an adequately large, interested, and financially rewarding market that would justify the sizable investments required for development of fundamentally new contraceptive methods.

It seemed logical, therefore, to put our study emphasis, first, on fresh leads that might emerge from the rapid advances in the biomedical sciences and, second, on changes in the character of the market, in the hope that, together, the science and a differently perceived market might motivate at least some industrial players to return to the field. Nonetheless, we must note that, although there have been some helpful regulatory modifications since the 1990 report, the political and ideologic climate in the United States continues to be critical in the domains of law and resource investment and remains, therefore, of high economic relevance for industry. Although the charge to the committee did not ask that we analyze that climate, it continues to so influence the field that we could not justify ignoring it. The matter of the sociopolitical climate is addressed in Chapter 7 as part of the cluster of reasons that "explains" why industry perceives engagement in contraceptive research and development as problematic, a cluster that importantly includes matters of product liability.

Of comparable relevance is the fact that the technical adequacy of contraceptives does not, in itself, guarantee wide social acceptance. The decisions to use contraception, plan a family, or practice safer sex are rarely just pragmatic, intellectual matters or issues of biologic function. Rather, they are profoundly rooted in personal identity and sense of control, roles and expectations, feelings about sexuality, concepts of risk, and peer and partner influences (Hatcher et al. 1994; IOM 1995a). In turn, each of these individual factors is rooted in religious beliefs, family and group traditions, and values; knowledge and education; and the contemporary play of larger socioeconomic and cultural forces. Important among the latter are the ethnic, cultural, regional, and religious diversity within a growing number of national populations, shifting as those populations urbanize and are increasingly linked to global communications media; the effects of economic variables on fertility, perceptions of personal opportunity, family structure, and access to reproductive health care; and divergent views on sexuality and appropriate sexual behavior, gender roles and relative power, and contraception and abortion. Within each of these independently weighty variables, there is contradiction, ambivalence, and volatility which, despite a fair amount of analysis and despite a sizable literature, is neither systematically or deeply understood (IOM 1995a). We consider aspects of these variables in Chapter 5 in the context of the women's agenda and attitudes toward contraception and contraceptive methods.

International and Domestic Perspectives

This report is admittedly uneven in incorporating both the international and domestic dimensions of contraceptive research and development. We have done so in Chapter 2 in the contexts of unintended pregnancy, abortion, maternal mortality, the public health dimensions of sexually transmitted diseases, and male involvement in contraception. In Chapter 5, we do so in relation to contraceptive use, side effects, failure and discontinuation; sexually transmitted disease as a focus for research and development; and contraceptive commodity supply and cost-effectiveness. Chapter 6 focuses primarily on the role of the U.S. biopharmaceutical industry and public and nonprofit sectors, but does not exclude international actors and notes the relevance of the globalization of industry. Chapter 7 is oriented clearly toward U.S. regulatory and legal matters, alluding nonetheless to the far less litigious climate elsewhere; the chapter also comments on commonalities, for instance, the effects of more conservative positions and ideologies on contraception. Finally, while some of the conclusions and recommendations in Chapter 8 have to do with U.S. policy, which the IOM is chartered to inform and advise, other conclusions and recommendations do have implications well outside U.S. national borders.

STUDY METHODOLOGY

The primary objectives for the study were, first, to attempt to identify new scientific leads for the next generation of contraceptives and, second, to consider ways to attract significant involvement by the private sector, including the pharmaceutical and biotechnology components of industry, in contraceptive research and development.

The audience for the study report was defined as leaders of the public- and private-sector policy and scientific research communities, both in the United States and abroad; legislators and regulators concerned with the frameworks that foster or impede the movement of scientific discovery to the world community of clients; and those active in the fields of family planning and reproductive health generally.

In meeting the charge, the committee and staff used several methods to gather needed information. They reviewed published data and analyses and canvassed the field of science; talked informally, during committee meetings and at other times, with experts on the various topics under study; held five meetings of the full committee over a 13-month period (August 1994 through July 1995); surveyed 170 biotechnology companies to ascertain their involvement and interest in contraceptive research and development; conducted smaller, informal surveys of scientists to refine priorities for potential research leads; canvassed a small sample of pharmaceutical companies concerning their experience with litigation concerning contraceptive methods; and developed a mini-case study as the basis for a follow-on workshop at the end of the study.

Study Workshops

Finally, two workshops were held. The first, in December 1994, convened two groups of scientists: (1) scientists engaged in what are considered frontier areas of contraceptive research, with emphasis on male contraception, methods protecting against sexually transmitted diseases (including HIV/AIDS), menses-inducers, and a rather loose category entitled "other, female-controlled methods"; and (2) scientists *not* engaged in contraceptive research but conducting cutting-edge basic biological research that might have potential for producing new leads in the next decades. The former group updated the latter about progress in contraceptive research; the latter talked about how developments in their respective fields might lead to significant breakthroughs for the general field of contraceptive research (IOM 1995b).

The second workshop convened representatives from the pharmaceutical industry and from the biotechnology sector to examine the proceedings from the first workshop, reviewing areas of possible contraceptive research and development; to discuss incentives and disincentives to moving contraceptive research and development forward; and to consider how the "next dollars" might be spent most effectively and how younger scientists might be attracted toward relevant areas of research (see Appendix E for workshop agendas and rosters).

The Bellagio Conference

Another component of the Rockefeller Foundation's Contraception 21 Initiative, in which some committee members and IOM staff participated, was a conference on "Public/Private-Sector Collaboration in Contraceptive Research and Development" held under Rockefeller Foundation auspices in April 1995 in Bellagio, Italy. The four-day meeting, which brought together a mix of representatives from the private and public sectors,[8] had three objectives: to establish and promote dialogue between public-sector programs and private industry; to review experiences in public- and private-sector collaboration and identify constraints; and to make recommendations for promoting a partnership between the public and private sectors, all in the field of contraceptive research and development. The subject of this conference was particularly relevant to the charter of this committee, and some of the rich discussion the conference engendered is woven into this report and so identified.

The primary conclusion of the conference was that private/public-sector collaboration was utterly essential to accelerating action on behalf of the woman-centered agenda for contraceptive research and development, most importantly with respect to the development of woman-controlled vaginal spermicides and microbicides, male methods of fertility regulation, and menses-inducers. The consensus of the meeting was that such collaboration was necessary for mobilizing more resources from industry toward investment in these areas and for getting new, safe, and effective products into the market with maximum speed.

Consensus was also reached on a set of recommended activities, all intended to enhance cross-sectoral involvement. The first was that there be a review of the research and development portfolios of public-sector programs from an industry perspective, in the conviction that the current duplication of effort, continuation of work on lines that were essentially unpromising, and development of products of no potential interest to an industrial partner would do little to advance the field. The second dealt with training clinical investigators from selected developing country centers so as to expand participation of those centers in industry-sponsored clinical trials of new contraceptives to standards approved by the U.S. Food and Drug Administration. The third had to do with initiation of special studies of drug regulatory requirements for vaginal microbicides/spermicides, public-sector pricing structure, and comparative analysis of product liability experiences and solutions.

The final recommendation was a proposal for initiating a program of collaborative effort between the public sector and private industry in the early stages of development, when product viability is still in doubt and investment is still seen as high risk, with the rationale that risk-sharing in those stages might tip the balance in industry investment. The program will match, not necessarily on a 50/50 basis, the investment of industry—large and small industry, as well as industry in emerging-economy and developing countries—in research at not-for-profit research institutions in areas of priority for the woman-centered contraceptive agenda. Special consideration is to be given to developing-country centers and an affiliated consortium of donors might also provide early-stage support to those same not-for-profit entities. The hope is that this focused, directed plan might serve both to make investment by industry in the contraceptive research and development field more attractive and to prime a stream of funding from different sectors. The Rockefeller Foundation has already taken first steps toward its implementation (Rockefeller Foundation 1995).

Antecedents and Relationships

In addition to the Bellagio Conference, this report follows and builds on other international and U.S. domestic activities in a less direct but significant fashion. While the scale and purposes of these activities differ, all are germane to the report's process, content, and implications. These include the 1984 International Conference on Population (Mexico City); the 1993 International Symposium on Contraceptive Research and Development for the Year 2000 and Beyond; the 1993 Science Summit on World Population (New Delhi); and, most centrally, the previously mentioned International Conference on Population and Development held in Cairo in September 1994.

There is also a "family relationship" with two other IOM studies. One, already mentioned, was the 1990 study, *Developing New Contraceptives: Obstacles and Opportunities*, a report of a study committee under the chairmanship of Luigi Mastroianni. The other, *The Best Intentions: Unintended Pregnancy in the United States*, was completed in May 1995 by an IOM committee under the chairmanship of Leon Eisenberg. As the reader will discover, we have profited considerably from both studies.

The Cairo Conference

While the entire Programme of Action that emerged from the Cairo conference is relevant to this report, the portion of the Programme that addresses "Technology, Research, and Development" (Chapter XII) is of primary relevance and we reproduce it partially here:

> Research, in particular biomedical research, has been instrumental in giving more and more people access to a greater range of safe and effective modern methods for regulation of fertility. However, not all persons can find a family-planning method that suits them and the range of choices available to men is more limited than that available to women. The growing incidence of sexually transmitted diseases, including HIV/AIDS, demands substantially higher investments in new methods of prevention, diagnosis and treatment. . . . In spite of greatly reduced funding for reproductive health research, prospects for developing and introducing new contraceptives and regulation of fertility methods and products have been promising. Improved collaboration and coordination of activities internationally will increase cost-effectiveness, but a significant increase in support from governments and industry is needed to bring a number of potential new, safe and affordable methods to fruition, especially barrier methods. This research needs to be guided at all stages by gender perspectives, particularly women's, and the needs of users, and be carried out in strict conformity with internationally accepted legal, ethical, medical and scientific standards for biomedical research. . . .

> Governments, assisted by the international community and donor agencies, the

private sector, nongovernmental organizations and the academic community, should increase support for basic and applied biomedical, technological, clinical, epidemiological and social science research to strengthen reproductive health services, including the improvement of existing [methods] and the development of new methods for regulation of fertility that meet users' needs and are acceptable, easy to use, safe, free of long- and short-term side effects and second-generation effects, effective, affordable and suitable for different age and cultural groups and for different phases of the reproductive cycle. Testing and introduction of all new technologies should be continually monitored to avoid potential abuse. Specifically, areas that need increased attention should include barrier methods, both male and female, for fertility control and the prevention of sexually transmitted diseases, including HIV/AIDS, as well as microbicides and virucides, which may or may not prevent pregnancy. . . .

To expedite the availability of improved and new methods for regulation of fertility, efforts must be made to increase the involvement of industry, including industry in developing countries and countries with economies in transition. A new type of partnership between the public and private sectors, including women and consumer groups, is needed that would mobilize the experience and resources of industry while protecting the public interest. National drug and device regulatory agencies should be actively involved in all stages of the development process to ensure that all legal and ethical standards are met. Developed countries should assist research programs in developing countries and countries with economies in transition with their knowledge, experience and technical expertise and promote the transfer of appropriate technologies to them. . . . (UNFPA 1994)

REPORT ORGANIZATION

This report has three principal parts. The first comprises Chapter 2, with its focus on the dimensions of need for contraception and for new contraceptives, on unintended pregnancy and its consequences, and on the linkages between sexually transmitted infection and contraception.

The second part of the report consists of Chapters 3 and 4. Chapter 3 discusses contraceptive technologies that, all things being equal, could conceivably become available in the relatively near future. Chapter 4 summarizes the potential that lies at the more distant scientific frontier, potential that is discussed in detail in supporting Appendices A (Female Methods), B (Male Methods), C (Immunologic Contraception), and D (Barrier Methods) and their extensive references. A glossary is also provided which defines the technical terms used in Chapters 3 and 4—though not the technical terms used in the appendixes, since we assume that the readers of those sections will be primarily scientists for whom the terminology will be quite familiar—as well as technical terms used in other chapters.

The third part of the report takes up different facets of the environment around contraceptive research and development. Chapter 5 examines the current contraceptive market; the limitations of currently available contraceptives; specific contraceptive needs as market opportunities; consumer perspectives; and possible financial incentives for investment, including the role of subsidy and the cost-effectiveness of contraception. Chapter 6 analyzes the roles of the private and public sectors in contraceptive research and development, emphasizing the adaptations of the biopharmaceutical industry to health sector restructuring and the meaning of those adaptations for developments in reproductive health in general and contraception in particular. The chapter also examines patterns of funding for contraceptive research over time, beginning in 1970. Chapter 7 scrutinizes the regulatory and legal context for the field, as well as some of the sociopolitical and cultural forces which affect that context. Chapter 8 presents the report recommendations.

REFERENCES

Alan Guttmacher Institute. Hopes and Realities: Closing the Gap Between Women's Aspirations and Their Reproductive Experiences. New York: The Alan Guttmacher Institute. 1995a.

Alan Guttmacher Institute. The Cairo consensus: Challenges for U.S. policy at home and abroad. Issues in Brief, March, 1995b.

Alan Guttmacher Institute. Clandestine Abortion: A Latin American Reality. New York: The Alan Guttmacher Institute. 1994.

Antrobus P, A Germain, S Nowrojee, eds. Challenging the Culture of Silence: Building Alliances to End Reproductive Tract Infections. New York: International Women's Health Coalition and Women and Development Unit, University of the West Indies. 1994.

Barroso C. The alliance between feminists and researchers. IN Contraceptive Research and Development 1984 to 1994: The Road from Mexico City to Cairo and Beyond, PFA Van Look, G Pérez-Palacios, eds. Delhi: Oxford University Press. 1994.

Behrer M. Population and family planning policies: Women-centered perspectives. Reproductive Health Matters 1:4–12, May 1993.

Bhargava SW. Finally, a healthy interest in women. Business Week, pp. 88–89, 20 July 1992.

Bongaarts J. Population policy options in the developing world. Science 263:771–776, 1994.

Bongaarts J, J Bruce. The causes of unmet need for contraception and the social content of services. Studies in Family Planning 26(2):57–75, 1995.

Bonnie K, A Germain, M Bangser. The Bangladesh women's health coalition. Quality 3(1), 1991.

Brown GF. Long-acting contraceptives: Rationale, current development, and ethical implications. Special Supplement, Hastings Center Report 25(1):S12–S15, 1995.

Bruce J, A Jain. A new family planning ethos. The Progress of Nations. New York: United Nations Children's Fund. 1995.

Brunham RC, JE Embree. Sexually transmitted diseases: Current and future dimensions of the problem in the Third World. IN Reproductive Tract Infections: Global Impact and Priorities for Women's Reproductive Health. A Germain, KK Holmes, P Piot, JN Wasserheit, eds. New York: Plenum. 1992.

Cates W Jr. Family Planning and STDs: Some Differences Between the Disciplines. Presentation at the 31st Annual Meeting of the Association of Reproductive Health Professionals, Atlanta, GA, 6–8 October 1994.

Cates W Jr, KM Stone. Family planning: The responsibility to prevent both pregnancy and reproductive tract infections. IN Reproductive Tract Infections: Global Impact and Priorities for Women's Reproductive Health. A Germain, KK Holmes, P Piot, JN Wasserheit, eds. New York: Plenum. 1992.

Claypool LE. The challenges ahead: Implications of STDs/AIDs for contraceptive research. IN Contraceptive Research and Development 1984 to 1994: The Road from Mexico City to Cairo and Beyond. PFA Van Look, G Pérez-Palacios, eds. Delhi: Oxford University Press. 1994.

Correa S. Population and Reproductive Rights Component: Platform Document, Preliminary Ideas. Paper prepared for the International Conference on Population and Development [Cairo 1994]. Development Alternative with Women for a New Era. February 1993.

Dixon-Mueller R. Population Policy and Women's Rights: Transforming Reproductive Choice. Westport, CT: Praeger. 1993.

Dixon-Mueller R, A Germain. Four Essays on Birth Control Needs and Risks. New York: International Women's Health Coalition. 1993.

Djerassi C. The bitter pill. Science 245:354–361, 1989.

Elias CJ, L Heise. The Development of Microbicides: A New Method of HIV Prevention for Women (Working Papers No. 6). New York: The Population Council. 1993.

Fathalla M. Fertility control technology: A woman-centered approach to research. IN Population Policies Reconsidered: Health, Empowerment, and Rights. L Chen, A Germain, G Sen, eds. Cambridge, MA: Harvard University Press. 1994.

Ford Foundation. Reproductive Health: A Strategy for the 1990s. New York: Ford Foundation. 1991.

Forrest JD. Preventing unintended pregnancy: The role of hormonal contraceptives. American Journal of Obstetrics and Gynecology 170(5; Part 2):1485–1489, 1994.

Forrest JD, RR Fordyce. Women's contraceptive attitudes and use in 1992. Family Planning Perspectives 23:175–179, 1993.

Gelijns AC, CO Pannenborg. The development of contraceptive technology: Case studies of incentives and disincentives to innovation. International Journal of Technology Assessment in Health Care 9(2):210–232, 1993.

Germain A. Reproductive Health and Dignity: Choices by Third World Women. Technical background paper prepared for the International Conference on Better Health for Women and Children Through Family Planning, Nairobi, Kenya, October 1987.

Germain A, R Kyte. The Cairo Consensus: The Right Agenda for the Right Time. New York: International Women's Health Coalition. 1995.

Germain A, J Ordway. Population Control and Women's Health: Balancing the Scales. New York: International Women's Health Coalition and the Overseas Development Council. 1989.

Guttmacher Institute. See Alan Guttmacher Institute.

Harlap S, K Kost, JD Forrest. Preventing Pregnancy, Protecting Health: A New Look at Birth Control in the United States. New York: The Alan Guttmacher Foundation. 1991.

Hatcher RA, J Trussell, F Stewart, et al. Contraceptive Technology: 16th Revised Edition. New York: Irvington Publishers. 1994.

Ingrassia M, K Springen, D Rosenberg. Still fumbling in the dark—Contraception: With all the condoms, pills and foams, why are so many women getting sterilized? Newsweek, 13 March 1995.

Institute of Medicine (IOM). The Best Intentions: Unintended Pregnancy and the Well-Being of Children and Families. S Brown, L Eisenberg, eds. Washington, DC: National Academy Press. 1995a.

IOM. Summary of Proceedings: Workshop on Contraceptive Research and Development and the Frontiers of Contemporary Science, 9–10 December 1994. Washington, DC: Division of Health Sciences Policy. Unpublished document. 1995b.

IOM. Applications of Biotechnology to Contraceptive Research and Development: New Opportunities for Public-/Private-Sector Collaboration. Washington, DC: Division of Health Sciences Policy. Unpublished concept paper. 1993a.

IOM. Clinical Applications of Mifepristone (RU 486) and Other Antiprogestins: Assessing the Science and Recommending a Research Agenda. MS Donaldson, L Dorflinger, SS Brown, and LZ Benet, eds. Washington, DC: National Academy Press. 1993b.

Khanna J, PFA Van Look, PD Griffin, eds. Challenges in Reproductive Health Research: Biennial Report 1992–1993. Geneva: World Health Organization, Special Programme of Research, Development and Research Training in Human Reproduction. 1994.

Lane SD. From population control to reproductive health: An emerging policy agenda. Social Science and Medicine 39(9):1303–1314, 1994.

Marcelo AB, A Germain. Women's perspectives on fertility regulation methods and services. IN Contraceptive Research and Development 1984 to 1994: The Road from Mexico City to Cairo and Beyond. PFA Van Look, G Pérez-Palacios, eds. Delhi: Oxford University Press. 1994.

Marquette CM, LM Koonin, et al. Vasectomy in the United States, 1991. American Journal of Public Health 85(5):644–649, 1995.

Miller K, A Rosenfield. Population and women's reproductive health: An international perspective. Annual Review of Public Health 17:359–382, 1996.

Mosher WD, WF Pratt. Contraceptive use in the United States, 1973–88. Advance Data from Vital and Health Statistics of the National Center for Health Statistics 182: 20 March 1990.

National Research Council and Institute of Medicine (NRC/IOM). Developing New Contraceptives: Obstacles and Opportunities. L Mastroianni, PJ Donaldson, TT Kane, eds. Washington, DC: National Academy Press. 1990.

Potts M, A Rosenfield. The fifth freedom revisited: I, Background to existing programs. Lancet 336:1227, 1990.

Program for Appropriate Technology in Health (PATH). Contraceptive research and development update. Outlook (Special Issue) 13(20), June 1995.

PATH. Outlook 11(2), 1993.

Robey B, et al. The reproductive revolution: New survey findings. Population Reports, Series M, No. 11. Baltimore: Johns Hopkins University, Population Information Program. 1992.

Rockefeller Foundation. Public-/Private-Sector Collaboration in Contraceptive Research and Development: A Call for a New Partnership. Report from the Bellagio Conference, 10–14 April 1995. New York: Rockefeller Foundation. 1995.

Rockefeller Foundation. Mobilization of Resources to Launch a Second Contraceptive Technology Revolution: A Concept Paper. Unpublished document. New York: The Rockefeller Foundation. 1993.

Ruzek SB. Editorial: Toward a more inclusive model of women's health. American Journal of Public Health 83(1):6–7, 1993.

Sinding SW. Women's demands and demographic goals. Planned Parenthood Challenges. 1994/1.

Snow R. Each to her own: Investigating women's response to contraception. IN Power and Decision: The Social Control of Reproduction. G Sen, R Snow, eds. Cambridge, MA: Harvard School of Public Health. 1994.

Stratton P, NJ Alexander. Prevention of sexually transmitted infections. Infectious Disease Clinics of North America 7(4):841–859, 1993.

United Nations. Levels and Trends of Contraceptive Use as Assessed in 1994. New York. In press.

United Nations Population Fund (UNFPA). Report of the International Conference on Population and Development (A/CONF.171/13). New York: United Nations. 1994.

World Health Organization (WHO). An Overview of Selected Curable Sexually Transmitted Diseases. (WHO/GPA/STD/95.1). Geneva: WHO/Global Programme on AIDS. August 1995.

WHO. Abortion: A Tabulation of Available Data on the Frequency and Mortality of Unsafe Abortion, 2nd edition. (WHO/FHE/MSM/93.13). Geneva: Maternal Health and Safe Motherhood Programme, Division of Family Health. 1994.

WHO, Special Programme of Research, Development and Research Training in Human Reproduction, and the International Women's Health Coalition. Women's Perspectives on the Selection and Introduction of Fertility Regulation Technologies: Report of a Meeting between Women's Health Advocates and Scientists, Geneva, 20–22 February 1991.

Women's Global Network for Reproductive Rights. Population and development policies: Report on the International Conference on Reinforcing Reproductive Rights, Madras, India, May 1993. Newsletter 43, April–June 1993.

NOTES

1. The term "Second Contraceptive Revolution" was coined by Mahmoud Fathalla and has been adopted by the Rockefeller Foundation as a central concept in the population and environment component of its portfolio. The term has acquired a certain currency in the field and describes the hoped-for revitalization of research and investment in the development of a new generation of contraceptive technologies.

2. The first modern IUDs were developed independently in Germany and Japan in the 1920s and 1930s, but fell into disrepute in the Western industrialized countries because of substantial numbers of cases of pelvic inflammatory disease (PID) and peritonitis. In the late 1950s, the time seemed ripe for its rehabilitation and the Population Council invested in the further development of the method (Gelijns and Pannenborg 1993).

3. Traditionally, the perimenopausal period has been defined as the few (three to five) years around menopause. Current thinking is that it should be viewed as beginning as early as the mid-thirties, coincident with onset of decline in ovarian function.

4. Bongaarts (1994) makes the point that even were family planning programs in the developing world perfectly able to *supply* all the unmet need for contraception, they would still not be able to reduce population growth to zero in countries where, on average, desired fertility still exceeds two children and thereby have significant effect on the momentum of population expansion. From this perspective, family planning programs are part of a set of complementary and mutually reinforcing approaches such as education, empowerment of women, implementing public health measures to reduce infant and child mortality, and delaying childbearing, that tend to raise the *demand* for family planning. He notes that "investment in family planning programs produce larger reductions in unwanted fertility when social conditions such as education and gender equality are favorable" (Bongaarts 1994).

5. The reproductive tract infections (RTIs) have been broadly defined to include sexually transmitted infections and infections that are nonsexually transmitted, and comprise three types of infection: (1) sexually transmitted diseases (STDs), such as chlamydia, gonorrhea, trichomoniasis (which may or may not be sexually transmissible), syphilis, chancroid, genital herpes, genital warts, and human immunodeficiency virus (HIV) infection; (2) endogenous infections, caused by overgrowth of organisms that can be present in the genital tract of a healthy woman, such as bacterial vaginosis and vulvovaginal candidiasis; and (3) iatrogenic infections, associated with medical procedures, such as female genital mutilation, poor delivery practices, cesarean section, unsafe abortion, and improperly performed pelvic examinations and IUD insertions (Brunham and Embree 1992). Of the three types of reproductive tract infections—sexually transmitted, endogenous, and iatrogenic—the majority are sexually transmitted in direct fashion (Brunham and Embree 1992). However, the iatrogenic infections are also important because they are linked to contraception, or the lack of contraception, through sepsis during the medical procedures cited above. Of the eight major STD pathogens producing RTIs, four are bacterial (chancroid, chlamydia, gonorrhea, syphilis) and four are viral (HIV, human papilloma virus/HPV, herpes simplex type 2/HSV-2, and hepatitis B/HBV).

6. The sole remaining U.S. firm was Ortho Pharmaceutical Corporation (a subsidiary of Johnson and Johnson); the three European firms were Organon International, Schering AG, and Roussel-Uclaf (a subsidiary of Hoechst Pharmaceuticals). The U.S. firms that for all practical purposes had abandoned significant efforts on new contraceptive research as of the mid-1980s included: Syntex Laboratories; G.D. Searle and Company; Parke-Davis and Company; Merck Sharp and Dohme Company; the Upjohn Company; Mead Johnson; Wyeth-Ayerst Laboratories; and Eli Lilly and Company (Djerassi 1989; NRC/IOM 1990).

7. The committee that generated the report (National Research Council and the Institute of Medicine. Developing New Contraceptives: Obstacles and Opportunities. Washington, DC: National Academy Press. 1990) included physicians; public health, policy, and legal experts; pharmaceutical company executives; reproductive biologists; economists; and demographers.

8. Public sector participants came from WHO's Special Programme in Human Reproduction and Training, the Population Council's Center for Biomedical Research, the U.S. Agency for International Development, the Contraceptive Research and Development Program (CONRAD), the Center for Population Research of the U.S. National Institute of Child Health and Development of the National Institutes of Health, the U.S. Food and Drug Administration, and the Program for Appropriate Technology in Health (PATH). The private sector was represented by eight firms: Finishing Enterprises, Ortho Pharmaceutical Corporation (Johnson and Johnson), and Wyeth-Ayerst Laboratories, from the United States; Gedeon Richter, Organon, Pharmacia-Leiras, and Schering AG, from Europe; and Silesia, from Brazil.

2

The Need and Demand for
New Contraceptive Methods

ISSUES OF TERMINOLOGY

In the context of family planning and contraception, the terms "need" and "unmet need" are applied, qualitatively and quantitatively, in several overlapping and intersecting ways, depending on the purposes of their application. They may incorporate the notions of "demand," "unmet demand," or "potential demand" or even be used interchangeably with those terms; and all terms are almost inevitably entangled with various conceptualizations of "preferences" and "intentions." The definition and computation of who "needs," "demands," "prefers," and "intends" what, and under which circumstances, have been debated for well over a decade. The debate is, however, far from an arid academic exercise: Its results have always been significant for the design, implementation, and evaluation of family planning programs. Because the terminology debate is vitally connected to the commodities, that is, the fertility regulation technologies that are essential to family planning, it has large and necessary implications for the pace and direction of contraceptive research and development, as well as for the involvement of industry in R&D processes.

Accordingly, this chapter begins with issues of terminology and its quantitative implications, as a basis for thinking about the personal and public health components of current needs for contraceptive technologies in the United States and worldwide. Some of these needs are *general*, in the sense that they are needs for *contraception*; others, addressed more fully in Chapter 5, are *specific* needs for *new contraceptive technologies* which have, in the eyes of this committee, clear implications for the market. "General needs" include the consequences of

General Needs for Contraception	Specific Needs for New Contraceptives	Shared Needs/ Shared Market
To avoid consequences of unintended pregnancy, including:	Contraceptive failure and/or side effects	Postcoital and postovulatory methods
• high rates of induced abortion • high rates of maternal morbidity and mortality (particularly in developing countries)	High rates of sterilization among young women Increased prevalence of sexually transmitted diseases (STDs), including HIV/AIDS	Methods protective against sexually transmitted diseases (STDs) and/or conception, especially woman-controlled methods
To adapt to longer reproductive life spans worldwide and to the needs of special populations, importantly the youngest sexually-active age groups	Limited involvement of males, in contraception and in protection against STDs	More contraceptive options for males

FIGURE 2-1 General needs for contraception, specific needs for new contraceptive methods, and the market created by these shared needs.

unintended pregnancy, notably abortion and maternal mortality, and the changing requirements of the reproductive life span. "Specific needs" include sexually transmitted reproductive tract infections; lack of involvement of males in contraception; and contraceptive failure and side effects. Figure 2-1 presents this breakdown in graphic form.

MARKET DEMAND

In economics, "demand" has both volitional and authoritative dimensions, since it comprises the notions of desire to purchase and possess, as well as the power to do so. In classical microeconomic theory, demand has an iterative relationship with supply, a relationship that is mediated by the market, which transmits information about prices, quantities, and elasticities in each.

However, application of traditional supply-and-demand concepts to understanding the role of demand in processes of technological innovation has not been very illuminating (Lotz 1993; Mowery and Rosenberg 1982). A more rewarding perspective is offered by marketing research, which distinguishes between "needs," "wants," and "demands" in ways that are useful for thinking about development of new medical technologies in general and contraception in particular. In one analysis, a human *need* is defined as "a state of felt deprivation of some basic satisfaction," *wants* as "desires for specific satisfiers of these deeper needs," and *demands* as "wants for specific products that are backed up by an ability and willingness to buy them." The more explicitly needs are articulated as demands, the higher the likelihood that the "demander" will be willing to pay for satisfaction of those needs (Kotler 1988).

The concept of market demand introduces the important notion of "signals," or expressions that come from a potential user—or third-party population—with both the willingness and ability to pay for satisfying needs and wants that are assumed to be in some way "unmet" (Lotz 1993; Nelson and Winger 1977). These may be (a) very specific signals about product specifications; (b) signals about a roughly described product; (c) signals about product class; (d) signals about demand for some kind of functions; or (e) no signals whatsoever, even if demands exist. The degree to which these can be determined will have a lot to do with the probabilities that investment will be attracted and that innovation will occur (Teubal et al. 1976). The sending and receiving of signals and the overall influence of demand factors on investment—in this case, investment in medical innovation—is not at all straightforward or linear; on the contrary, it is highly iterative (Gelijns and Pannenborg 1973; Lotz 1993; Mowery and Rosenberg 1982). It is also highly dependent on knowledge about the "owners" of the needs, that is, the "users," their preferences, and the expression of those preferences in patterns of adoption.

In this framework, the populations that are germane to conceptualizing the market for the outputs from contraceptive research and development are

1. the population that
   (a) has been defined as having an unmet need for family planning, and
   (b) has evidenced a desire to actively use contraception in response to that need; and
2. the subset of that population (or some third party) which can—and will—pay for the satisfaction of those needs and desires.

Thus, the "market demand" population is always the smallest subpopulation in the set. If it cannot be identified somehow as substantial, there is no incentive for a potential product developer or seller to invest in this particular market. Therefore, from a commercial perspective it is crucial to determine what fraction of the "unmet need" population represents a true market opportunity.

CALCULATING THE UNMET NEED FOR CONTRACEPTIVES

Like "demand," "unmet need" is an elusive concept, changing according to how survey questions are posed, what assumptions are made, and the criteria used for exclusion and inclusion (Dixon-Mueller and Germain 1992). All these elements affect quantification of the ultimate size of the population defined as needing contraceptive protection, as well as estimates of what is needed in the way of services and commodities. The definition of unmet need is surely crucial for computing the market for contraceptive technologies.

Over the past 15 years, there have been numerous alternative calculations of the need and demand for contraceptives. The most generally accepted have been those authored by Westoff (e.g., Westoff and Ochoa 1991), which have been enormously useful in defining national family planning policies and prioritizing the need for international assistance. However, these approaches have been revisited recently from a women's health perspective and revised in a way that defines the base population more broadly (Dixon-Mueller and Germain 1992 and 1994; Guttmacher Institute 1995a; Wulf 1995) (see Table 2-1). The rationale for "casting a wider net" is that conventional definitions, which essentially restrict the unmet-need concept to married women[1] and nonusers of contraception, respond neither to the contemporary realities of women's (or men's) lives, nor to the statistical realities concerning contraceptive utilization, effectiveness, and appropriateness.

The expanded definition adds to the basic conventional definition the following population groups:

- sexually active, unmarried women;
- women with postpartum amenorrhea;
- women who are using a less effective contraceptive method but who definitely want to avoid or postpone childbearing;
- women who are using a more effective method but who are using it incorrectly, are dissatisfied, or should not be using it for health reasons;
- women with unwanted pregnancies; and
- women with related reproductive health problems (Dixon-Mueller and Germain 1994).

Both the conventional and expanded definitions can be used to calculate need in national population subgroups by residence, age, and even subculture, and to compare countries in terms of magnitudes and characteristics of need and the ability of women in those countries to realize their reproductive wishes. Nonetheless, the effects of their different premises on calculation of unmet need can be strikingly large in the aggregate, ranging from an estimated 120 million (Ketting 1994; Robey et al. 1992) to 228 million women at risk of unplanned pregnancy even though they do not want to have a child (Guttmacher Institute 1995a).

REPRODUCTIVE PREFERENCES

Reproductive preferences have been a routine part of fertility and family planning surveys from their inception, as these surveys have sought to quantify and measure fertility norms (desired or ideal number of children), reproductive intentions (intentions to postpone or terminate childbearing), spacing intentions (preferred length of the next birth interval), and wanted and unwanted births (intendedness).

Reproductive preferences are also integral to defining unmet need. While preference data were for a long time viewed as the "soft" part of demographic surveys, recent methodological research has raised confidence in their predictive validity, although that is variable. For example, using the "ideal" or "desired" number of children has been thought to lack any particularly predictive utility, because it reflects societal norms more than it truly reflects individual intentionality. However, though there may be some erosion in individual preferences in response to personal, family, or societal pressures (Freedman 1990), the percentage of women who state that they want no more children is a good short-term predictor of fertility rates (Westoff 1991). As such, it is a reasonable indicator for purposes of user-based market analysis, despite the inevitable divergence between the number of children women say they wanted or would want in the future and the number they actually have (the "KAP [knowledge, attitudes, and practices] gap").[2]

Since there have been some dramatic changes in fertility levels worldwide during the past two decades, it is reasonable to assume that there has been some kind of fit between women's preferences and their actual behavior. The fact that the fit is imperfect does not invalidate the measure. At the same time, even the most meticulously shaped definition of either unmet need or unmet demand omits a number of qualitative variables that are crucial to conceptualizing the market for new contraceptive technologies. Discounting the force of various dimensions of local culture—for example, politics, gender roles, and the values assigned to fertility—and assuming that women everywhere will behave in the same ways given equivalent knowledge, resources, and options, is as risky for calculating a market as it is for implementing family planning programs.

THIRD-PARTY AND PUBLIC HEALTH PERSPECTIVES

Having defined a population with an unmet demand for contraception, it is then possible to address the question of what fraction of that population represents true *market* demand. As suggested at the beginning of this chapter, there are two very different subpopulations to be accounted for: Subpopulation 1, consisting of those able and willing to spend their own resources; and Subpopulation 2, consisting of those for whom some third party is prepared to pay. This latter, "third-party" category contains considerable variety: private insurance companies, managed care organizations, hybrid network arrangements, and government programs for the poor in the United States and other developed nations, as well as national family planning and public health sector programs in develop-

TABLE 2-1 Comparison of Two Approaches to Calculating Unmet Need for Family Planning

Population Characteristics	Westoff and Ochoa (1991) Include as Having an Unmet Need for Contraception:	AGI (1995) Includes as Having an Unmet Need for Contraception:	Assumptions Underlying AGI Calculations
Union status	All women currently in union	All women of reproductive age	Many single women also have a need to avoid pregnancy
Age	Aged 15–49	Aged 15–44	Women aged 45–49 are probably infecund in any event
Pregnancy	All women who did not want most recent pregnancy and were not contracepting at time of that conception	All women who do not want current pregnancy, whether or not contracepting at time of that conception	Some women are unable to use any method effectively or are using a method with high failure rates
Amenorrhea postpartum	All women who did not want most recent pregnancy and were not contracepting at the time of that conception	All women who do not want another child, soon or ever, and are not using an effective method of contraception	All have a need even if, technically, they cannot conceive at the moment
Use of postpartum abstinence	Women using postpartum abstinence		Although the abstinence may not be intended to prevent pregnancy, it nonetheless has assured contraceptive effect, so that women maintaining postpartum abstinence are not in need
Method use		Women using traditional methods of contraception (rhythm, withdrawal, etc.)	Traditional methods can have high failure rates and thus do not offer effective protection from unintended pregnancy

	Excludes:	Excludes:	
Fecundity	All women married for at least 5 years, not contracepting, and who have not had a child during that time	Only women who themselves say they cannot have a child; women who do not so indicate are defined as "in need"	Unless women indicate that they have been infecund during this period, they might actually have conceived during a period assumed to be infecund and then had an abortion

NOTE: "Includes" means that women with these characteristics are included in the pool of women considered to have an unmet need for contraception. "Excludes" means that women with these characteristics are *not* included in that pool, since either their need is viewed as satisfied or they are not considered at risk of conception.

SOURCES: Alan Guttmacher Institute (AGI). Hopes and Realities: The Gap Between Women's Aspirations and Their Reproductive Experiences. New York: The Alan Guttmacher Institute. 1995. Westoff CF, LH Ochoa. Unmet Need and the Demand for Family Planning. DHS Comparative Studies, No. 5. Columbia, MD: Institute for Resource Development. 1991. Wulf D. The Unmet Demand for Family Planning. Unpublished paper. New York: Rockefeller Foundation, 1995.

ing and industrializing countries, often at least partly subsidized by overseas development assistance.

These subpopulations also have slightly different perspectives regarding the "value" or cost-effectiveness of contraception. Individuals, who do not as directly bear some of the broader social costs of increased population size that result from less-than-optimal levels of contraception, give primary emphasis to efficacy, side effects, out-of-pocket costs, and personal concerns such as convenience and autonomy. In contrast, third-party payers are more likely to be sensitive to the costs of unintended pregnancies, in terms of the cost and risks of abortion and the costs and risks of carrying unintended pregnancies to term.

In the developing world, there is more heterogeneity in perspectives on family planning and contraception, depending on the history of a given country, its culture and religions, and where it is demographically, economically, and epidemiologically. Some countries, particularly those whose fertility rates remain high, must continue to worry about population growth rates, sizes, and densities. A growing number of other countries, further along in the demographic and epidemiologic transitions, must address both an "unfinished agenda" of high mortality, infectious disease, and malnutrition and a swelling agenda of noncommunicable and chronic diseases in adults and the elderly (Mosley et al. 1993). All countries, sooner or later, will find themselves obliged to somehow add to their priorities the new agenda, articulated at Cairo and ratified at Beijing, relating to the empowerment of women and their reproductive health and rights. The fact that these economies must take into account all these valid and pressing agendas and must do so with persistently constrained health sector resources means that they, like the established market economies and the formerly socialist economies of Europe, are also having to focus hard on issues of cost containment, cost-effectiveness, and cross-sectoral externalities and trade-offs in development investment (World Bank 1993). But here, too—and this is important—individuals have the same concerns and needs as do individuals in developed countries: they do not voluntarily choose to use contraception primarily because of national demographic or macroeconomic concerns.

There is a third area where individual and societal health needs coincide because their nature is such that, left unsatisfied, they incur costs of some kind which can be quantified, albeit in different ways. The costs of contraception can then be compared to the costs of nonsatisfaction of these shared individual and public health needs so that, in some cases, it is possible to develop cost-benefit or cost-effectiveness ratios. At a minimum, it is possible (though not necessarily simple) to calculate the various costs of a given case of "nonsatisfaction" to whoever the payer is: the society at large, some third-party payer, or an individual. These shared unmet needs include unintended pregnancy, abortion, maternal mortality and morbidity, and sexually transmitted disease, needs which can be especially acute and especially costly in populations of particular vulnerability owing to such covariates as age, parity, ethnicity, or socioeconomic status.

The societal costs of all of these are high and, in some instances, can only increase, either because the magnitude of the need itself increases, or because it will simply become more expensive to deal with, or both. Contraception offers very cost-effective and risk-reducing alternatives to unwanted pregnancies, whether those pregnancies are terminated by abortion or allowed to go to term, as well as to morbidity (Lee and Stewart 1995; Trussell et al. 1995). At present in the United States, a majority of third-party payers would seem to be missing a major investment by not offering a broad range of contraceptives as a cost-containment strategy that has potential economic payoff well in excess of many other forms of health care. We will argue in Chapter 5 that contraception that includes or is accompanied by protection against sexually transmitted diseases is even more cost-effective and surely risk-reducing. As more and more third-party payers assume long-term responsibility for covering large, stable populations over a long period of time for a broad range of health care services, it is reasonable to assume that they will look to those savings that can be derived from prevention and, therefore, see the economic value and consequent logic of substantially increasing their investment in contraceptive and reproductive health services as a major cost-containment tool. This will not be an overnight process. Ongoing restructuring of the managed care industry and the current mobility of subscribers shopping for the best care at the best price will, for a while, affect the potential for a given HMO to realize a payback from investment in prevention. At the same time, the payback from pregnancy prevention, with its rapid "turn-around" and transparent causal attribution, can be realized much faster than, for instance, the payback from nutrition education and prevention of high-cost chronic diseases.

A LIFE SPAN PERSPECTIVE

There is a growing constituency in the public health community for a more inclusive and integrative model of individual and family health and well-being, and use of the phrases "life cycle" and "life span" to define a perspective have acquired a certain currency, particularly in connection with women's health and well-being. The basic premise of this perspective is that human health and illness are not a haphazard affair, but express the accumulation of conditions that begin early in life, in some respects before birth. A second premise is that the factors that favor good health and precipitate ill health are not purely genetic or biological but can be social, economic, cultural, and psychological, and can work together or against one another across the span of an individual's life in ways that we are only beginning to understand. The third premise is that no reasonable public health strategy can ignore these dynamics and what constitutes a continuity of risk over an entire lifetime (Institute of Medicine [IOM] 1996; Tinker et al. 1994; UNFPA 1994; World Bank 1994). The importance of the life span concept to this report is straightforward enough: At different points across their life spans, women have different reproductive intentions, different pressures on their lives, different needs for contraception, and different overall reproductive health requirements. Contraceptive research and development has to take all of these life span dimensions into account since, to a large extent, they shape the structure of demand.

In developed countries, the portion of the female life span that can be described as the "potential reproductive years," that is, the years between menarche and menopause, constitutes about half of a woman's total life span; in developing countries, where life expectancies are generally shorter, that portion can be well over half. This means that a typical woman in the United States is at biological risk of pregnancy for approximately 36 years (Hatcher et al. 1994). Fourteen percent of those potential reproductive years (or years at biological risk of pregnancy) is spent in Stage 1, the years between menarche and first intercourse, and 19 percent in Stage 2, the years between first intercourse and marriage; during these two stages, the large majority of women will be trying to avert or postpone pregnancy. Stage 3 comprises the years between marriage and first birth, or 5 percent of the years at risk, during some part of which some women will be averting or postponing pregnancy. Stage 4, the years between first birth and attainment of desired family size, represents 11 percent of the potential reproductive years, during which the emphasis for most women is on spacing births. The years that follow, that is, the years between attainment of desired family size to menopause (Stage 5) occupy 51 percent of the whole span of potential reproductive life. This span of years consists of two periods, the boundary between which is typically blurred except for women who are surgically sterile. The first is the period between the age of intending no more children and presumed[3] sterility, during which many women will want to avert pregnancy; the second comprises the years from presumed sterility to menopause, when there is no concern for contraception. Nevertheless, during Stage 5 and into the postmenopausal period (Stage 6), many women will still require protection from sexually transmitted infection, as is increasingly the case for many women throughout their reproductive years (Forrest 1993).

For women who want a certain number of children, these proportions change somewhat to account for the years spent in pregnancy, postamenorrheic abstinence or infecundity, or sexual inactivity. The hypothetical woman who is sexually active between ages 20 and 45 and wants two children will need protection from pregnancy for approximately 20 years, that is, 82 percent of her 25-year reproductive life. The woman who wants four children will need protection for about 16 years, or 64 percent of her reproductive life. Even the woman who wants six children will need nearly 12 years of protection, or 46 percent of her reproductive life (see Table 2-2). For women who begin childbearing in their teenage years, these estimates are, of course, conservative. The general rule is that, for all women, everywhere, the younger they are when they begin their reproductive lives, the older they are at menopause; the fewer children they want,

TABLE 2-2 Proportions of Female Reproductive Life During Which Protection from Pregnancy Is Needed

Number of Children Wanted by Hypothetical Woman	Number of Months Wanting Pregnancy	Number of Months Being Pregnant	Number of Months Postpartum Protection	Number of Months Not Wanting Pregnancy	Number of Years Not Wanting Pregnancy	% of Total Reproductive Life
2	24	18	12	246	20.5	82.0
4	48	36	24	192	16	64.0
6	72	54	36	138	11.5	46.0

NOTE: Reproductive life span is hypothesized to be 300 months, or 25 years, from age 20 to age 45.

SOURCE: Alan Guttmacher Institute. Hopes and Realities: Closing the Gap Between Women's Aspirations and Their Reproductive Experiences. New York: The Alan Guttmacher Institute. 1995.

the longer they must spend in need of some kind of contraception (Guttmacher Institute 1995a).

The stages in the potential reproductive years can be further characterized according to the ways they differ from one another biologically, socially, and psychologically, as well as in the balance required among prevention of pregnancy, protection from disease, and preservation of fertility (Fathalla 1992; Forrest 1993; Fortney 1989; King and Smith 1994). Obviously, transition from stage to stage is not uniform among women or among societies. Women do not transit at the same age or in the same order, and some women in some situations may even skip a stage or advance into a next stage in ways that can be biologically or socially worrisome. Unduly early or unduly late pregnancies are prime examples: The fact that many women in the world have their first baby while they are still adolescents can have high costs: Even when prepregnancy disadvantages are taken into account, early childbearing appears to have a causal and adverse effect on the health and social and economic well-being of children and, in varying measure, on their mothers (IOM 1995; Kubicka et al. 1995).[4]

Table 2-3 examines each stage of female reproductive life in terms of a few key biological, social, and psychological variables; fertility goals, sexual behavior, and contraceptive use; and the qualities of contraception that are particularly necessary at certain times. The table includes the postmenopausal years even though this period lies beyond what are biomedically defined as the reproductive years, since many women continue to be sexually active; because of menopause-associated physiological changes (e.g., structural changes in vaginal tissues), those women remain vulnerable to sexually transmitted infections. This means that continued protection against those infections may be required later in the course of women's lives than is usually thought to be the case, a dimension that is appropriate to thinking about prospects for new reproductive technologies.

The principal message that emerges from this scrutiny of the texture of the female reproductive life span is that, at various points in their lives, women everywhere have different reproductive intentions and, consequently, different needs for family planning and the maintenance of their reproductive health. This means that, first of all, contraceptive services need to offer a full range of methods that are responsive to these changing requirements. Second, viewing contraceptive technology from the perspective of the overall reproductive life span makes it clear that there are periods of that span that are not now served well or appropriately by the current array of methods; most strikingly, there are considerable limitations in what is available for very young women and for women later in life who wish to preserve their fertility but who cannot use the long-term, high-effectiveness methods that are currently on the market.

PREFERENCES AND INTENTIONS

Over the past four decades in the United States, as part of the National

Survey of Family Growth (NSFG) and its predecessors,[5] a series of questions has been regularly asked of women about the timing and intentionality of their pregnancies. Efforts to capture responses of this type are difficult at best, and many vulnerabilities and complexities intrude. The fragility of human recall, changes in circumstance, ambivalence, differences of meaning, shifts in intensity of feeling, all come into play. However, the NSFG has developed very specific terminology and definitions to measure "unintended pregnancy," using the following definitions of "intended" and "unintended":

- *intended* at conception: wanted at the time, or sooner, irrespective of whether or not contraception was being used; or
- *unintended* at conception: if a pregnancy had not been wanted at the time conception occurred, irrespective of whether or not contraception was being used.

Among *unintended* pregnancies, a further distinction is made between *mistimed* and *unwanted*:

- *mistimed* conceptions are those that were wanted by the woman at some time, but which occurred sooner than they were wanted; and
- *unwanted* conceptions are those that occurred when the woman did not want to have any more pregnancies at all (IOM 1995).

These definitions have been applied in a large number of national and international surveys in ways that are similar enough to be considered comparable. As suggested in the preceding section, by these definitions almost all women—and this is true worldwide—are at risk[6] for unintended pregnancy throughout most of their reproductive years (Forrest 1994). The next sub-sections present the ways in which these various elements of unintended pregnancies are expressed, internationally and in the United States.

Unintended Pregnancy Worldwide

Everywhere in the world, there is often a gap between the number of children women say they want and the number they actually have. Substantial percentages of women report everywhere that they have had all the children they want or that they do not want another pregnancy for at least two years. Many also report that their most recent birth was unwanted or mistimed.[7] And, for many of the world's women, the alternative to carrying an unintended birth to term, whether that birth was mistimed or unwanted, was abortion (see Figure 2-2).

The ranges of each of those categories of intention, preference, and action differ from region to region and from country to country, as one would expect (Table 2-4 and Table 2-5). The highest regional percentage of wanted births, 76

TABLE 2-3 Life Span Factors in Women's Reproductive Lives

	Stage 1 Menarche–Intercourse	Stage 2 Intercourse–Marriage
Biologic variables	Menarche	First intercourse High reproductive capacity High risk of exposure to STDs
		High risk of unintended pregnancy High maternal/child mortality and morbidity from too-early pregnancy
Social variables	Politically most contentious stage Restricted provision of family planning services Constrained access to information about sexuality and contraception	Politically contentious Laws governing age at marriage Restricted provision of family planning services
Psychological variables	Limited future orientation/ ability to judge risks/conse- quences/defer gratification Heightened sense of unique invulnerability Need to establish adult identity/peer intimacy Constrained ability to negotiate use of coitus- related methods Ambivalence	Constrained ability to negotiate use of coitus- related methods Ambivalence
Fertility goals: Childbearing	Postpone	Postpone
Future fertility	Preserve	Preserve (high need)

Stage 3 Marriage–1st Birth	Stage 4 1st Birth–Attainment of Desired Family Size	Stage 5 Menopause	Stage 6 Postmenopause

Marriage
High reproductive
  capacity
Possible fetal
  wastage/ectopic
  pregnancy/infertility
	Intend no more children
	High reproductive
	  capacity
		Sterility/infertility	

			Increased incidence
			  and severity of
			  many gynecologic
			  problems

	Parity requirements for sterilization	Irrelevant	

Greater intellectual/
  emotional maturity/
  ability to judge
  consequences
		Heightened maturity	

Postpone	Space	Stop	
Preserve (high need)	Preserve (diminishing need)	Irrelevant	

continued on next page

TABLE 2-3 Continued

	Stage 1 Menarche–Intercourse	Stage 2 Intercourse–Marriage
Sexual behavior:		
No. of partners	Variable	Variable to higher
Frequency of intercourse	Variable	Variable to higher
Coital predictability	Low	Moderate to high
Contraceptive use	None	Erratic use/high discontinuation
Most common methods	Pill	Pill
Next most common	Condom	Condom
Importance of method characteristics:		
Conception prevention	High	Moderate
Reversibility	High	High
Not coitus-linked	High	Low
STD prevention	High	Moderate (if monogamous)
Safety during breastfeeding	High	High

NOTE: STDs = sexually transmitted diseases.

SOURCES: Modified from Forrest JD, Timing of reproductive stages, American Journal of Obstetrics and Gynecology 82:110, 1993, and Hatcher RA, J Trussell, F Stewart, et al. Contraceptive

Stage 3 Marriage–1st Birth	Stage 4 1st Birth–Attainment of Desired Family Size	Stage 5 Menopause	Stage 6 Postmenopause
Variable	Variable Challenge to discern infidelity/self-protect against STDs	Variable	Variable
Variable	Variable	Variable	Variable
High	High	High	High
Sterilization	Sterilization	Irrelevant	
Pill, condom			
High	Irrelevant	Irrelevant	
Low	Low to irrelevant	Irrelevant	
Moderate	Irrelevant	Irrelevant	
Low (if monogamous)	Low (if monogamous)	Low (if monogamous)	Low (if monogamous)
Moderate	Irrelevant	Irrelevant	

Technology, 16th revised ed., New York, Irvington Publishers, 1994. We have added Stage 6, the postmenopausal period, since many women remain sexually active despite termination of fertility, and may require protection from sexually transmitted infections.

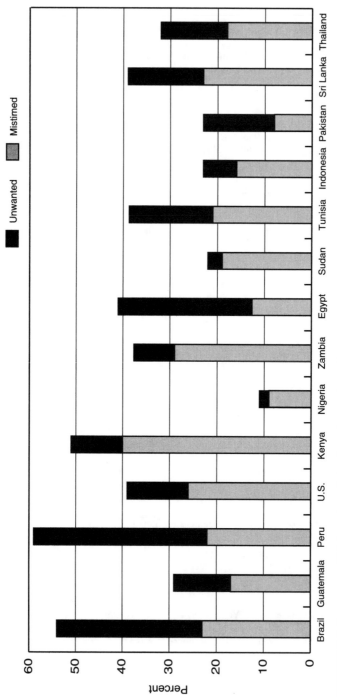

FIGURE 2-2 Percentage of births unintended, selected countries, 1985–1992. Source: Alan Guttmacher Institute. Women, Families, and the Future: Women and Reproductive Health (Regional Fact Sheet). New York: The Alan Guttmacher Institute. 1994.

TABLE 2-4 Distribution of Pregnancies by Outcome, Selected Developing Regions and Developed Countries (various dates, in percentages and millions of pregnancies)

Region	Number of Pregnancies[a]	Wanted		Mistimed		Unwanted		Abortion	
		%	No.[a]	%	No.[a]	%	No.[a]	%	No.[a]
Sub-Saharan Africa (1994)	28.9	76	22.0	10	2.9	3	0.9	11	3.2
North Africa and Middle East (1994)	11.6	58	6.7	12	1.4	18	2.1	12	1.4
South and Southeast Asia (1994)	65.4	63	41.2	10	6.5	9	5.9	18	11.8
Latin America (1994)	16.4	38	6.2	15	2.5	19	3.1	28	4.6
China (1990)	40.4	47	19	13	5.3	10	4.0	30	12.1
Japan (1992)	1.9	36	0.68	36	0.68	3	0.06	25	0.47
France (1991)	1.1	66	0.73	12	0.14	3	0.03	19	0.21
United States (1988)	6.5	43	2.8	19	1.2	9	0.59	29	1.9

[a]All numbers are in millions.

SOURCES: This table was derived from a graphic presentation in: Alan Guttmacher Institute, Hopes and Realities: Closing the Gap Between Women's Aspirations and Their Reproductive Experiences, p. 25, New York, Alan Guttmacher Institute, 1995. That graphic was, in turn, constructed from the following sources:

For the developing regions of the world, the number of abortions and live births: Alan Guttmacher Institute, Women, Families and the Future, New York, 1995.

For China, the number of abortions: Henshaw SK, Induced abortion: A world review, Family Planning Perspectives 22:76–89, 1990; the number of live births: United Nations, World Population Prospects: The 1994 Revision, New York, 1995.

For France, the number of abortions and live births: Council of Europe, Recent Demographic Developments in Europe, 1993.

For Japan, the number of abortions: Ministry of Health and Welfare, The Report on the Statistics Relating to Eugenics Protection, Tokyo, 1993; the number of live births: Vital Statistics of Japan 1992, Tokyo, 1994.

For the United States, the number of abortions: Henshaw SK, J Van Vort, Abortion services in the United States, 1987 and 1988, Family Planning Perspectives 22:102–109, 1990; the number of live births: National Center for Health Statistics, Monthly Vital Statistics Report, Vol. 38, No. 6, 1989.

TABLE 2-5 Planning Status, Last Birth, and Preferences for Next Birth (selected countries, various survey years)

Country and Survey Year	Average Number of Children			% Whose Last Birth Was Unplanned			% Who Want to Stop or Postpone		
	Wanted	Have[a]	"GAP"	Mistimed[b]	Unwanted[c]	TOTAL	Stop[d]	Postpone[e]	TOTAL
Cameroon, 1991	6.7	5.5	–	17	5	22	45	14	59
Nigeria, 1990	5.9	6.2	+	9	3	12	53	9	62
Pakistan, 1990–1991	5.3	5.9	+	8	16	24	21	40	61
Jordan, 1990	4.9	5.4	+	12	26	38	28	53	81
Guatemala, 1987	4.2	5.1	+	16	13	29	40	47	87
Kenya, 1993	3.8	6.0	++	36	20	56	33	52	85
Egypt, 1992	3.5	3.7	+	9	33	42	19	67	86
Indonesia, 1991	3.4	2.8	–	16	8	24	32	54	86
Mexico, 1987	3.2	3.0	–	24	27	51	18	62	80
Philippines, 1992	3.2	3.8	+	26	21	47	25	63	88

China, 1987-88	2.8	2.0	–	u	u	u	17	64	81
Thailand, 1987	2.8	2.1	–	18	15	33	23	66	89
Colombia, 1990	2.6	2.6	=	17	21	38	20	64	84
Japan, 1992	2.6	1.5	–	48	4	52	7	82	89
United States, 1988	2.6	2.1	–	26	13	39	23	64	87
France, 1994	2.3	1.7	–	15	4	19	u	u	u

NOTES: u = Data unavailable; + = have more children than wanted; – = have fewer children than wanted; = = have number of children wanted.

aUnited Nations estimate of total fertility rate.
bPercentage of women 15–49 who had a child in the previous five years and whose last birth was not planned at that time.
cPercentage of women 15–49 who had a child in the previous five years and whose last birth was not planned at any time.
dPercentage of women 15–49 who want no more children.
ePercentage of women 15–49 who want to delay the next birth.

SOURCE: Derived from Appendix Table 5 (Columns 1 and 5, 18 and 19, and 20 and 21), Alan Guttmacher Institute, Hopes and Realities: Closing the Gap Between Women's Aspirations and Their Reproductive Experience, New York, The Alan Guttmacher Institute, 1995.

percent, was reported by Sub-Saharan Africa, the next highest by South and Southeast Asia with 63 percent, followed by North Africa and the Middle East with 58 percent, and a low 28 percent of wanted births in Latin America. Although these are huge aggregations, it is worth noting that in Sub-Saharan Africa, where fertility norms are high, about one-fourth of most recent births were nonetheless unwanted. In the North Africa–Middle East region, close to half of recent births were unwanted, with most of that percentage deriving from unwanted rather than mistimed births. The highest regional abortion rates were in South and Southeast Asia, where 18 percent of all recent births were so terminated.

There is inevitably variation among countries in almost all respects. First, there is gap between the family size women say they want and the family size they actually have: the "KAP gap." In some countries, for example, Colombia, Egypt, and Nigeria, women are close to having the total number of children they want; in fact, in Colombia, women say they are having exactly the number they want. (At the same time, 38 percent of Colombian women reported that their latest birth had been unintended, with intentionality divided almost equally between unwanted and mistimed births.) In contrast, in Guatemala, Jordan, Kenya, Pakistan, and the Philippines, the gap between the total number of children women want and the number they actually have was large. Not surprisingly, in countries where national policies discourage more than two children per family, notably China and Indonesia, some women would like more children than they actually have. However, the same was true in countries where there are no constraining policies—France, Japan, Mexico, Thailand, and the United States (Guttmacher Institute 1995a).

The structure of unintendedness of the most recent birth varies internally according to the percentage of mistimed as opposed to unwanted pregnancies. The highest rates of overall unintendedness were reported by Japan, Kenya, Mexico, the Philippines, and Egypt, where close to half of latest births were unintended; Colombia, Jordan, Thailand, and the United States were close behind, with at least one-third of all births unintended. Within this structure, however, ranges differed. Rates of *unwanted* pregnancies ranged from 48 percent in Japan to 8 and 9 percent in Egypt, Nigeria, and Pakistan. The range for *mistimed* pregnancies was narrower, from 33 percent in Egypt to 3 and 4 percent in Nigeria, France, and the United States. Of the countries and regions for whom percentages of births ending in *abortion* were calculated, the highest rates were reported in China (30 percent), the United States (29 percent), Latin America (28 percent), Japan (25 percent), and France (19 percent); the lowest rates were in Sub-Saharan Africa (11 percent) (Guttmacher Institute 1995a).

In sum, the large majority of women in virtually every country surveyed have indicated that they somehow wish to control future childbearing, either by not having another pregnancy (stopping) or postponing the next pregnancy for at least two years (spacing). The proportion of women actively wanting to become pregnant was very low—less than one in five—in developing and most developed countries. In the same sample analyzed in Table 2-4, the lowest percentages of women who want to either stop childbearing altogether or postpone it were in Sub-Saharan Africa yet, even there, these percentages were two-thirds of all women surveyed. Everywhere else, the percentages of women who wanted to control the occurrence or timing of their next pregnancy ran around 80 to 90 percent. Nevertheless, even in a number of countries where unintendedness rates were high (France, Japan, Thailand, and the United States, for example), the average woman nonetheless indicated that she would—overall—like slightly more children than she actually had. This suggests that attitudes toward family size are often ambivalent and highly sensitive to circumstance (Guttmacher Institute 1995a), so that timing of births and the ability to determine their spacing are crucial. Another message from these figures is related to the global nature of unintendedness. The Guttmacher Institute analysis notes: "If these proportions are an indication of the success with which women plan their pregnancies, many women in the developed world appear to be doing no better than women in developing regions" (Guttmacher Institute 1995a).

Unintended Pregnancy in the United States

Of all pregnancies in the United States in 1987 (5.4 million), 57 percent were unintended at the time of conception. This figure includes pregnancies that were aborted, as well as both mistimed and unwanted pregnancies that led to live births (IOM 1995) (Table 2-6). In other words, of the estimated pregnancies in that year, less than half—43 percent, to be exact—were actually intended at conception and resulted in live births. The breakdown of unintended pregnancies shows that, while the majority of births from unintended pregnancies were from mistimed rather than unwanted pregnancies, half of all unintended pregnancies ended in abortion in that year. Whether the pregnancy was mistimed or unwanted does not affect the proportion of pregnancies ending in abortion: 51 percent of mistimed pregnancies and 50 percent of unwanted pregnancies end in abortion (Forrest 1994).

Furthermore, the trend toward increase in unintendedness seems to be worsening. During the 1970s and early 1980s in the United States, a decreasing proportion of births were unintended at the time of conception. Between 1982 and 1988, this trend reversed and there was an overall increase in the proportion of unintended pregnancies among both unmarried and married women, and particularly among poor women (IOM 1995; Williams and Pratt 1990).

Stratified analysis of these data upsets a number of preconceptions. First of all, women of all socioeconomic, marital-status, and age groups contribute to the pool of unintended pregnancies; adults as well as teenagers are having difficulty planning and preventing pregnancy. Second, although marital status, which is highly correlated with age, is also strongly related to whether a pregnancy is unintended, 4 out of 10 pregnancies among currently married women were either

TABLE 2-6 Estimated Proportions of Pregnancies (excluding miscarriages) by Outcome and Intention, Percentage of Pregnancies Unintended, and Percentage of Unintended Pregnancies Ending in Abortion, United States, 1987, by Marital Status, Age at Outcome, and Poverty Status at Interview

| Demographic Characteristics | Total Pregnancies | All Pregnancies (miscarriages excluded) | | | Percentage of Pregnancies Unintended | Percentage of Unintended Pregnancies Ending in Abortion |
		Intended Pregnancies Ending in Births	Unintended Pregnancies Ending in Births	Abortions		
Total	100.1	42.8	28.4	28.9	57.3	50.4
Marital status						
Currently married	100.0	59.9	29.7	10.4	40.1	25.9
Formerly married	100.0	31.5	32.4	36.1	68.5	52.7
Never married	100.0	11.8	22.0	66.2	88.2	75.1
Age						
15–19	100.0	18.3	40.0	41.7	81.7	51.0
20–24	100.0	39.4	29.7	30.9	60.6	51.0
25–29	100.0	54.8	23.8	21.4	45.2	47.3
30–34	100.0	57.9	21.0	21.1	42.1	50.1
35–39	100.0	44.1	25.1	39.7	55.9	55.1
40–44	100.0	23.1	31.3	45.6	76.9	59.3
Poverty Status						
<100%	100.0	24.6	35.6	39.8	75.4	52.8
100–199%	100.0	36.0	26.8	37.2	64.0	58.1
>200%	100.0	55.0	25.7	19.3	45.0	42.9

SOURCE: Institute of Medicine, The Best Intentions: Unintended Pregnancy and the Well-Being of Children and Families, S Brown, L Eisenberg, eds., Washington, DC: National Academy Press, 1995, based on: Forrest JD, Epidemiology of unintended pregnancy and contraceptive use, American Journal of Obstetrics and Gynecology 170:1485–1488, 1994.

mistimed or unwanted. Third, the high rate of unintendedness in the United States is not explained by a higher incidence of abortion among minority women; it is simply that the total U.S. pregnancy rate, the total rate of unintended pregnancy, and the U.S. abortion rate are all higher than those rates in other Western nations, among all U.S. women (IOM 1995; Henshaw and Van Vort 1994). Fourth, although in 1987 82 percent of pregnancies in teenagers aged 15–19 were described as having been unintended, the same was true of 61 percent of pregnancies in women aged 20–24, 56 percent of pregnancies in women aged 35–39, and 77 percent of pregnancies in women over age 40; even among women aged 25–34, between 42 and 45 percent of all pregnancies were described as unintended (IOM 1995). Fifth, while unmarried status is the most important factor in determining whether an unintended pregnancy will end in abortion, it is still the case that 1 in 4 unintended conceptions is aborted by currently married women. Sixth, while adolescents as a group do have the highest rate of unintended pregnancies—82 percent of all adolescent pregnancies are unintended—the proportion of unintended pregnancies among adolescents that end in abortion is not substantially different from other age groups and actually lower than in the older age groups (Forrest 1994).

THE CONSEQUENCES OF UNINTENDED PREGNANCY

The consequences of unintended pregnancy are of various kinds—biological, social, economic, and emotional—and will also vary among regions, countries, and individuals. In addition, they will vary in their gravity from setting to setting, yet there is little evidence that unintended pregnancy is ever a truly trivial event. This section focuses on abortion and maternal mortality and morbidity as the principal biological consequences of unintended pregnancy. It also addresses the matter of the sexually transmitted diseases as a correlate of sexual activity that, more and more, must be taken into account in thinking about women's reproductive health in general and contraception in particular.

Abortion

Everywhere in the world, unintendedness in pregnancy is the antecedent of virtually all induced abortions (Chen 1995). The reasons for which women everywhere seek abortion reside in three fundamental causes: nonuse of contraception; contraceptive misuse or method failure; and lack of postovulatory or postcoital methods that a woman can use if she has been exposed to unprotected sex, in order to obviate the need to confront the dilemmas of abortion.

The 40 million to 60 million abortions that take place worldwide each year represent 20–30 percent of all the world's pregnancies, or from 30 to 45 abortions per 1,000 women of reproductive age annually (WHO 1991).[8] From 26 million to 31 million of these are legal; the remainder—somewhere around 20 million—

are nonlegal and mostly definable as "unsafe." This means that there is 1 unsafe abortion to every 10 of the world's pregnancies, or a ratio of one unsafe abortion to every seven births (WHO 1994). Of the total number of unsafe abortions, 17.6 million (88 percent) take place in the less developed countries, although there are significant variations among and within regions in terms of incidence of abortion and related mortality (WHO 1994) (see Table 2-7).

Important to note is that, owing to the lack of appropriate contraceptives and counseling services, abortion was, and remains, the principal means of fertility regulation in the countries of central and eastern Europe (CCEE) and the newly independent states of the former USSR (NIS), sometimes equaling the number of live births and even exceeding it by two or three times. As a possible consequence of the economic crisis in which these countries find themselves, women fear that bringing up children is simply not affordable. At the same time, these governments are concerned about rapid decline of fertility rates to levels under replacement (Brandrup-Lukanow 1995).

First-trimester abortion, performed with appropriate sterile technique by trained personnel, is a very safe surgical procedure and rates of complications have been decreasing in the United States (IOM 1995). However, unsafe abortions are characteristically performed by the woman herself, by nonmedical individuals, or by health workers in unhygienic conditions, and most occur where abortion is either illegal or, if it is legal, where service access and quality are limited (WHO 1994).

In developing countries, the risk of death following complications of unsafe abortion procedures may be between 100 and 500 times higher than the risk of an abortion performed professionally under safe conditions (WHO 1994). The number of deaths worldwide each year that result from an abortion complication is estimated to be at least 70,000,[9] but the margin of error in such statistics is so large that these numbers could be as low as 50,000 or as high as 100,000. Risk of death due to unsafe abortion is at least 15 times higher in developing countries than it is in developed countries and, in some regions, may be as much as 40 to 50 times higher. Looked at a bit differently, mortality from unsafe abortion in developing countries is around 55 per 100,000 live births; in developed countries, that figure is 4 per 100,000 (WHO 1994) (see Table 2-7). Not surprisingly, the complications of unsafe abortions are a leading cause of maternal deaths, over 98 percent of which occur in the developing world, where they account for around 13 percent (1 in 8) of all pregnancy-related deaths (WHO 1994). Urban rates in developing countries may be much higher: One well-designed study in the early 1980s in Addis Ababa, Ethiopia, found that 54 percent of maternal deaths in that city were due to illegal abortion (Kwast et al. 1986). Nonetheless, limitations in data-collection systems make it highly likely that rural abortion rates are underestimated.

While the evidence is patchy and always fragile, there does appear to have been some overall decline in mortality from unsafe abortion. This may be due to

TABLE 2-7 Global and Regional Estimates of Incidence of, and Mortality from, Unsafe Abortions

Region	Number of Unsafe Abortions (thousands)[a]	Unsafe Abortions per 1,000 Women Aged 15–49	Number of Deaths from Unsafe Abortions[a]	Mortality from Unsafe Abortions per 100,000 Live Births	Maternal Deaths
World Total	20,000	15	70,000	49	13
More Developed countries[b]	2,340	8	600	4	14
Less Developed countries	17,620	17	69,000	55	13
Africa	3,740	26	23,000	83	13
Eastern Africa	1,340	31	10,000	101	15
Middle Africa	180	12	2,000	77	11
Northern Africa	510	16	1,000	23	7
Southern Africa	230	22	500	36	13
Western Africa	1,480	34	10,000	104	14
Asia	9,230	12	40,000	47	12
Eastern Asia[c]					
Southeastern Asia	2,850	25	5,000	43	13
Southern Asia	6,000	21	33,000	81	14
Western Asia	380	13	1,000	22	8
Europe	260	2	100	2	10
Eastern Europe	110	5	<100	4	13
Northern Europe[c]					
Southern Europe	150	4	<100	2	16
Western Europe[c]					
Latin America	4,620	41	6,000	48	24
Caribbean	170	19	400	50	19
Central America	890	31	800	23	14
South America	3,560	47	5,000	58	26
Northern America[c]					
Oceania	20	17	<100	29	5
USSR (former)	2,080	30	500	10	23

NOTE: Figures may not add to totals owing to rounding.

[a]Based on 1990 U.N. projections of births.

[b]Japan, Australia, and New Zealand have been excluded from the regional estimates but are included in the total for developed countries.

[c]For regions where the incidence is negligible, no estimates have been made.

SOURCE: World Health Organization. Abortion: A Tabulation of Available Data on the Frequency and Mortality of Unsafe Abortion, 2nd ed. Geneva: Division of Family Health. 1994.

TABLE 2-8   Mortality Risks Associated with Pregnancy and Selected Health Procedures

	Deaths per 100,000 Cases	
Procedure	United States	Developing Countries[a]
Legal abortion	1	4–6
Female sterilization	4	10–100
Delivery of live birth	14	250–800
Cesarean section	41	160–220
Illegal abortion[b]	50	100–1,000
Hysterectomy	160	300–400

[a]Estimated.
[b]Performed by untrained practitioners or outside medical facilities.

SOURCE: Population Crisis Committee, World Abortion Trends, Briefing Paper No. 9, September 1982. Cited in: World Health Organization. Abortion: A Tabulation of Available Data on the Frequency and Mortality of Unsafe Abortion, 2nd ed. Geneva: Division of Family Health. 1994.

changes in abortion laws and increased access to safe medical abortions and menstrual regulation; increased fertility regulation through contraception; and increased provider skills both within and outside formal health systems. However, this overall picture of decline masks an increase among certain groups in all parts of the world, notably unmarried adolescents in urban areas, where they may represent the majority of all abortion seekers. At the same time, as we will see below in the case of the United States, the general, popular image of the woman who seeks abortion does not accord with statistical reality. In the developing world, many women who seek abortions are married or live in stable unions, already have several children, may be using abortion to limit family size or space births, or may be resorting to abortion as a consequence of contraceptive failure or lack of access to modern contraception (WHO 1994).

In addition to the hemorrhage so often associated with induced abortion, there are other primary and secondary complications which, if they do not produce fatality, may well produce serious and chronic disability. Infections may spread throughout the reproductive tract and produce acute pelvic inflammatory disease (PID), with tubal damage, secondary infertility, predisposition to ectopic pregnancy, chronic pain, and, in severe cases, formation of abdominopelvic abscess requiring emergency surgery and occasionally resulting in death (Meheus 1992). The procedure itself may cause mechanical damage to vagina, uterus, or adjoining structures; cervical lacerations may be responsible for subsequent miscarriage or premature births; and, where the procedure involves introduction of chemicals into the vagina, resulting tissue destruction may also contribute to infection. There may be additional sequelae in the form of negative effects on subsequent pregnancy outcomes, notably, low birth weight, midtrimester spontaneous abortion, and premature delivery.

Abortion in the United States

The majority of all pregnancies in the United States can be considered unintended and half of those are resolved by abortion. As indicated earlier, of all the pregnancies in the United States in 1987 (6.3 million), 57 percent (3.5 million) were unintended at the time of conception and, of those unintended pregnancies, 51 percent ended in abortion. Of the total number of pregnancies in 1987 in the United States, 29 percent were terminated by abortion (IOM 1995). The number of reported abortions in the United States increased substantially between 1972 and 1989 in the wake of the 1973 *Roe v. Wade* Supreme Court decision legalizing abortion. In 1972, approximately 600,000 legal abortions were reported; in 1978, 1.1 million were reported. However, through the 1980s, the annual number of abortions in the United States has remained more or less stable, with approximately a million and a half legal abortions each year during the 1980s; 1.6 million in 1990; and 1.5 million in 1991 and 1992, respectively (Henshaw and Van Vort 1993; Koonin et al. 1992).

Overall, women undergoing abortions tend to have had no previous live births and are having the procedure for the first time. The majority are unmarried, white, and young (24 percent under age 19, 33 percent between ages 20–24). About half of all abortions are performed before the eighth week of gestation, five out of six before the thirteenth week; younger women tend to obtain abortions later in pregnancy (Koonin et al. 1992).

From the perspective of proportion of unintended pregnancies that end in abortion, these patterns persist. The most powerful predictor remains marital status: 75 percent of all unintended pregnancies among unmarried women in the United States in 1987 terminated in abortion, compared to 53 and 26 percent among formerly married and currently married women, respectively.

Age is less consistently predictive. Fifty-one percent of unintended pregnancies among women aged 15–19 and women aged 20–24 end in abortion, then there is a slight decline to 47 and 50 percent in women aged 25–29 and 30–34, respectively. The rates jump to 55 percent in women aged 35–39 and to 59 percent in women aged 40–44; in other words, about 6 out of 10 women aged 40–44 who experience an unintended pregnancy seek abortion. Poverty status is the weakest predictor: The percentage of women obtaining an abortion to resolve an unintended pregnancy is only slightly lower among affluent women than it is among low-income women (IOM 1995) (refer back to Table 2-6).

There has been a slight diminution in the U.S. abortion rate since the early 1980s. However, it remains two to four times higher than rates in other comparable market economies,[10] of which very few have abortion rates even approaching those in the United States, even though access to abortion in those countries is often easier than it is in the United States (see Table 2-9). The high U.S. rate is not a function of a higher incidence of abortion among minority women, as is often thought to be the case; the U.S. abortion rate is higher overall than rates in other market economies, among whites as well as among all U.S. women. The high U.S. rate is due entirely to its higher total pregnancy rate (average number of pregnancies [births plus abortions]) and the high proportion of those pregnancies that are unintended (IOM 1995).

All in all, the popular image of the U.S. woman most likely to elect abortion to resolve an unintended pregnancy—the poor minority teenager—is inaccurate (Kaiser/Harris 1995). Substantial percentages of U.S. women in every age and socioeconomic category terminate unintended pregnancies with abortion; even among currently married women, that proportion is still 26 percent.

Maternal Mortality

Significant gains have been made in infant and child survival in developing countries over the past few decades; much less progress has been made in maternal survival (Rosenfield and Maine 1985). Recent recalculations by WHO and UNICEF indicate that maternal mortality is higher than previously estimated, with some 590,000 maternal deaths worldwide as of 1990, compared to the 509,000 figure calculated from an earlier model (WHO 1996; WHO 1991). The most significant differences between the old and new models are in Africa; estimates for Asia and Latin America changed little. In Africa, the overall revised maternal mortality ratio[11] for 1990 was 880 maternal deaths per 100,000 live births, compared to the earlier estimate of 630 per 100,000, with a range from 1,061 in Eastern Africa to 343 in Northern Africa. The ratio for the less developed regions as a group was 586 maternal deaths per 100,000 live births; the overall maternal mortality ratio for the more developed regions in 1990 was 27 (WHO 1996). Expressed somewhat differently, the chance of dying from pregnancy-related causes between 1975 and 1984 ranged from 1 in 9,850 in Western Europe to 1 in 19 in Western Africa (Herz and Measham 1987). Table 2-8 compares the mortality risks associated with pregnancy and selected health procedures—legal abortion, female sterilization, delivery of live birth, cesarean section, illegal abortion, and hysterectomy—in the United States and in the developing countries.

These are much greater discrepancies in maternal mortality rates between developed and developing countries than those observed in connection with infant mortality rates (Rosenfield 1989). Furthermore, there are many reasons for believing that these figures are gross underestimates. Even in the United States in the 1980s, official statistics on maternal mortality were thought to underestimate incidence by 20 to 30 percent, with underestimates in the developing world significantly higher (Rosenfield and Maine 1985). This overall picture is compli-

TABLE 2-9 Abortion Rates per 1,000 Women Aged 15–44, by Country, 1980 and 1985–1992

Country	1980	1985	1986	1987	1988	1989	1990	1991	1992
Australia	13.9	15.6	16.4	16.3	16.6	—	—	—	—
Belgium	—	7.5	—	—	—	—	—	—	—
Canada	12.6	11.3	11.2	11.3	11.6	12.6	14.6	14.7	14.9
Denmark	21.4	17.6	17.7	18.3	—	—	18.2	—	—
Finland	—	12.4	—	11.7	—	—	11.5	—	—
France[a]	15.3	14.6	13.9	13.3	13.2	—	—	—	—
Federal Republic of Germany (former)[a]	6.6	6.1	6.3	6.6	6.3	5.6	5.8	—	—
Ireland[b]	4.8	5.2	5.2	4.8	5.0	4.9	5.4	—	—
Italy[a]	18.7	16.8	16.0	15.3	15.3	—	12.7	—	—
The Netherlands[c]	6.2	5.1	5.3	5.1	5.1	5.1	5.2	—	—
New Zealand	8.5	9.3	10.5	11.3	12.8	12.9	14.0	14.4	—
Norway	16.3	16.3	17.1	16.8	17.1	17.9	16.7	—	—
United States	29.3	28.0	27.4	26.9	27.3	26.8	27.4	26.3	25.9
United States, whites[d]	24.3	22.6	21.8	21.2	21.2	20.9	21.5	20.3	—

[a]Statistics for France, Germany, and Italy may be incomplete.
[b]Abortion is illegal in Ireland and the reported rate is based on abortions obtained in England and Wales by women reporting Irish addresses.
[c]Data from the Netherlands are for residents only.
[d]Data for whites in the United States include most Hispanic women.

SOURCES: Alan Guttmacher Institute. Unpublished data, 1994. Henshaw S, E Morrow. Induced Abortion: A World Review, 1990 Supplement. New York: The Alan Guttmacher Institute, 1990. Henshaw S, J Van Vort. Abortion Services in the United States, 1991 and 1992. Family Planning Perspectives 26:100–106: Table 1, 1993. Canadian Center for Health Information. Therapeutic Abortions, 1991. Ottawa, Ontario: Statistics Canada, 1993. United Nations. Abortion Policies: A Global Review. Vol. II. New York: Department of Economic and Social Development, United Nations, 1993.

cated by the fact that rates in some population subgroups can be significantly higher. In terms of age, a very early first birth increases a woman's risk of dying from pregnancy-related causes, and adolescent first-births and births at the end of a woman's reproductive period generally are associated with a higher likelihood of pregnancy-related complications.[12] Residence also skews the numbers, since rural mortality rates are almost inevitably higher, as they are for very underserved urban slum peripheries. What is clear is that, in general, the likelihood that a woman will die in pregnancy or childbirth depends on how many times she is pregnant. This means that the *lifetime* risk of maternal mortality is many times greater than ratios indicate because the ratio ignores the effect of repeated pregnancies; each pregnancy adds to total lifetime risk (Walsh et al. 1993).

Sexually Transmitted Reproductive Tract Infections

Of all the health problems that women confront, infection of the reproductive tract is most closely connected with family planning programs. Reproductive tract infections (RTIs), notably the sexually transmitted reproductive tract infections,[13] are also positioned at the nexus between female health, safe motherhood, child survival, and HIV prevention, for each of which they have profound implications (Cates and Stone 1992; Wasserheit and Holmes 1992).

Reproductive tract infections, particularly those that are sexually transmitted, are hardly new and, until now, have been traditionally unrecognized in most developing countries as either a necessary or an appropriate component of health programs. What is new is the heightened attention accruing to them as a category of "emerging diseases" (IOM 1992). The recognition that sex is the primary mode of transmission of the HIV virus that results in AIDS, together with the size and flow of donor resources to combat that disease, have ratcheted up interest in RTIs in general and sexually transmitted diseases (STDs) in particular. Interest has also been heightened by recognition of STDs as implicated in cervical cancer and, possibly, hepatocellular cancer and, as diagnostic technology has improved, the sheer number—over 50—of STDs has been revealed. Finally, the momentum of demographic change, intra- and international mobility, relentless urbanization, and economic and political volatility have demonstrated that the burden of morbidity and mortality these diseases generate is a large and global matter (Brunham and Embree 1992; IOM 1992a; Over and Piot 1993).

Any complacency about having conquered the "first-generation" STDs—gonorrhea, syphilis, and chancroid—has been amply challenged both by their recent resurgence virtually worldwide, as well as by a "second generation" of sexually transmitted organisms. The essentially new syndromes associated with four major pathogens—chlamydia, herpes simplex virus (HSV), human papilloma virus (HPV), and the human immunodeficiency virus (HIV)—are more difficult to identify, treat, and control, and they impose a much larger burden of chronic morbidity, disability, and death.

TABLE 2-10 Sexually Transmitted Disease Microbial Agents and the Conditions They Produce in Women and Children

Etiologic Agent[a] Conditions	Acute Disease	Pregnancy-associated	Chronic
Bacteria			
Neisseria gonorrhoeae	Urethritis Cervicitis Salpingitis	Premature delivery Septic abortion Postpartum endometritis Conjunctivitis neonatorum	Infertility Ectopic pregnancy Disseminated gonococcal infection
Chlamydia trachomatis	Urethritis Cervicitis Salpingitis Reiter's syndrome	Conjunctivitis Infant pneumonia Postpartum endometritis	Trachoma Ectopic pregnancy Infertility
Treponema pallidum	Primary and secondary syphilis	Spontaneous abortion Stillbirth Congenital syphilis	Neurosyphilis Cardiovascular syphilis Gumma
Viruses			
Human immuno-deficiency virus (HIV)	Acute viral syndrome	Perinatal HIV Prematurity Stillbirth	AIDS and related conditions
Human papilloma-virus (HPV)	Genital warts	Laryngeal papilloma in infants	Squamous epithelial neoplasias of genitalia
Herpes simplex virus (HSV-2)	Genital ulcer	Spontaneous abortion Premature delivery	Primary and recurrent genital herpes
		Neonatal herpes and associated mortality Aseptic meningitis	Neurological sequelae
Hepatitis B virus (HBV)	Acute hepatitis	Perinatal HBV	Chronic hepatitis Cirrhosis Hepatoma Vasculitis

[a]Other bacterial STD agents include *Mycoplasma hominis, Ureaplasma urealyticum, Gardnerella vaginalis, Calymmatobacterium granulomatis*, and Group B β-hemolytic *streptococcus*. Other viral STD agents include cytomegalovirus, *molluscum contagiosum* virus, and human T-lymphotropic virus (HTLV-1). *Trichomonas vaginalis*, a protozoan, and *Candida albicans*, a fungus, are also STD agents.

SOURCES: Brunham RC, JE Embree. Sexually transmitted diseases: Current and future dimensions of the problem in the Third World. IN Reproductive Tract Infections: Global Impact and Priorities for Women's Reproductive Health, A Germain, KK Holmes, P Piot, JN Wasserheit, eds. New York: Plenum. 1992. Cates W Jr. Sexually transmitted diseases. IN Reproductive Health Care for Women and Babies: Analysis of Medical, Economic, Ethical, and Political Issues, BP Sachs, R Beard, et al., eds. New York: Oxford University Press. 1995. Over M, P Piot. HIV infection and sexually transmitted diseases. IN Disease Control Priorities in Developing Countries, DT Jamison, WH Mosley, AR Measham, JL Bobadilla, eds. New York: Oxford University Press, for the World Bank. 1993.

Sexually transmitted diseases generate a variety of acute and chronic sequelae, particularly for females[14] and children (see Table 2-10). In addition, there is an "epidemiological synergy" between HIV and other STDs, since a number of STDs act in various ways, some poorly understood, as pivotal cofactors in the transmission or acquisition of HIV (Alexander 1990; Laga 1992; Wasserheit 1992). HIV is, of course, incurable and almost inevitably lethal, and perinatal transmission occurs in about 20 to 30 percent of births in each pregnancy to infected mothers (Gwinn et al. 1991). However, a number of other STDs (HSV, HPV, and hepatitis B [HBV]) are also incurable, are transmissible perinatally, and produce high levels of morbidity in both mother and child. And, beyond their large biomedical and emotional burdens, the STDs as a group— particularly HIV/AIDS—produce sizable socioeconomic costs to societies and individuals everywhere; their dimensions are discussed in Chapter 5 (Over and Piot 1993). This is acutely distressing since, at least in theory, all RTIs are preventable or treatable and a number of nonviral infections are curable, although drug resistance is emerging in some strains (Chen et al. 1992; Germain et al. 1992; Stein 1990; Wasserheit and Holmes 1992).

Like unintended pregnancy, STDs display what has been called "biological sexism," since they discriminate biologically against women. Females and males alike are at risk of sexually transmitted disease. However, female physiology and symptomatology, as well as the behavior patterns associated with these diseases, put females at greater risk of (a) acquiring an STD, especially at an earlier age; (b) acquiring a sexually transmitted infection from any single sexual encounter; (c) more difficult diagnosis; (d) speedier progression of concurrent disease; (e) more severe, long-term, systemic sequelae, including PID, ectopic pregnancy, chronic pain, and cervical cancer; and (f) inappropriate or untimely medical care (Cates and Stone 1992; Hatcher et al. 1994).

Because both pregnancy and infection are "transmitted" through sexual intercourse, women need three types of effective protection, depending on their own reproductive desires and circumstances. If they do not wish to become pregnant, they require protection against both conception and infection simultaneously. If they have no reason to anticipate sexually transmitted infection, they still may require protection against conception. Finally, if women want to become pregnant but also require protection against infection, they need another kind of protection, usually labeled a microbicide. Women have a much higher risk of acquiring an STD from a single coital event—in the case of gonorrhea, risk of acquisition is 25 percent for men and 50 percent for females—so that every single coital event must be protected.

At the present time, only abstinence provides complete protection against sexually transmitted reproductive tract infections.[15] Male and female condoms, when used properly, also provide good protection, although many women encounter male resistance to using either type of condom. All other contraceptives

TABLE 2-11 Effects of Contraceptives on Bacterial and Viral Sexually Transmitted Diseases (STDs)

Contraceptive Methods	Bacterial STD	Viral STD
Condoms	Protective	Protective
Spermicides	Protective against cervical gonorrhea and chlamydia	Undetermined *in vivo*
Diaphragms	Protective against cervical infection; associated with vaginal anaerobic overgrowth	Protective against cervical infection
Hormonal	Associated with increased cervical chlamydia; protective against symptomatic pelvic inflammatory disease (PID)	Not protective
Intrauterine Device	Associated with PID in first 20 days after insertion	Not protective
Natural family planning	Not protective	Not protective

SOURCE: Cates W Jr, KM Stone. Family planning: The responsibility to prevent both pregnancy and reproductive tract infections. IN Reproductive Tract Infections: Global Impact and Priorities for Women's Reproductive Health, A Germain, KK Holmes, P Piot, JN Wasserheit, eds. New York: Plenum Press. 1992.

provide protection against only some STDs (see Table 2-11), although this is not trivial since other STDs are part of the susceptibility pattern for HIV/AIDS (Laga 1992). In sum, only one modern contraceptive is currently on the market that protects men and women against sexually transmitted disease: the condom, whose protective power depends heavily on perfect use.[16] In all cases, women must contend with the power imbalance between the sexes that favors men (Aral and Guinan 1984; Cates and Stone 1992; Larson 1989). Thus, there is a compelling need for safe and effective contraceptive and microbicidal methods that women can use without the cooperation, or consent, of their male partner (Claypool 1994; Stein 1990).

INVOLVEMENT OF MALES IN CONTRACEPTION

The Alan Guttmacher Institute recently commented that, since men's role in contraceptive use is so typically small, the question about what couples are doing to avoid unintended pregnancies should be, What are *women* doing? The 1995

TABLE 2-12   Percentage of Couples[a] Using Male Methods of Contraception[b]

Country	%	Country	%
Japan	54	Jordan	5
United States	22[c]	Pakistan	4
China	12	Cameroon	3
Philippines	9	Egypt	3
Colombia	8	Guatemala	3
Thailand	8	Indonesia	2
France	7	Kenya	2
Mexico	6	Nigeria	1

[a]In the countries of North Africa, the Middle East, and Asia, only currently married women aged 15–49 are included; data for all other countries are for married women and those in other sexual relationships.

[b]Male methods include withdrawal, condom, and vasectomy.

[c]Data for the United States are from special analyses of the 1988 National Survey of Family Growth, which surveyed 8,450 women of all marital statuses aged 15–44, supplemented by data from other national sources. This figure may be higher: Hatcher et al. give a figure of 25.7 percent for couples (women aged 15–44) in the United States using male methods (Hatcher RA, J Trussell, F Stewart, et al., Contraceptive Technology—16th Revised Edition, New York, Irvington Publishers, 1994, Table 5-1).

SOURCE: Alan Guttmacher Institute. Hope and Realities: The Gap Between Women's Aspirations and Their Reproductive Experiences. New York: The Alan Guttmacher Institute. 1995.

Guttmacher analysis of the latest data from the Demographic and Health Surveys (DHS) finds that the proportion of couples relying on male methods—the condom, withdrawal, or vasectomy—ranges from 1 to 12 percent in most countries. In Japan, where the condom is the leading contraceptive method in overall use, the proportion of couples who rely on male methods is 54 percent; in the United States, where the condom and vasectomy are both important, estimates of couple use of male methods range from 22 percent (Guttmacher Institute 1995a) to 27.5 percent (Hatcher et al. 1994)(see Table 2-12). The Guttmacher analysis also found that, in the limited number of countries where the DHS collected such information, even when husbands know of at least one contraceptive method, they do not commonly discuss family planning with their wives, at least as reported by women (see Table 2-13 and Table 2-14).

    In a slightly different set of countries, with only one exception (Burundi), women wanted a smaller family size than did their husbands, although in all the Sub-Saharan African countries women still desired rather large families (see Table 2-15). In this same sample, however, while smaller proportions of husbands than of wives said that they did not want any more children, the differences between husbands and wives in this respect were not very large, ranging from 4 to 9 percentage points (Guttmacher Institute 1995a).

The presumption has been that men's limited involvement in contraception is driven by the fundamental gestalt that, in virtually all societies, defines the roles, status, and power of females as inferior and subordinate to those of males. This presumption has, in turn, driven the historical emphasis placed by family planning programs on women, to the virtually *a priori* exclusion of men (Kabeer 1992; Sachs 1994; Sadik 1995). Except for the Population Council's intramural basic science research program, which has included attention to development of male contraceptives, that presumption has also driven the investment in contraceptive research and development, at least partly because of the view that male interest in being involved in contraceptive use was quite limited in most populations. As a consequence, men did not benefit from the first contraceptive revolution.

That view has been something of a self-fulfilling prophecy (Population Reports 1994) and has been tested in only a fragmentary way; most reports on male attitudes toward contraception have come from women. However, as some countries have gathered data on male perceptions of contraception in connection with the Demographic and Health Surveys, there appears to be more heterogeneity in male attitudes than might be expected, even in Africa, where high fertility has deep cultural and socioeconomic roots (UNFPA 1995). At the same time, there is no question that greater male involvement in contraception is a large and commanding need in terms of public health and the well-being of children and the family.

The need is no less in the United States, where one in 15 men fathers a child while he is a teenager (Marsiglio 1987) and where attention is now being given to the possibility of expanding family planning clinic services to men (Burt et al. 1994). The rationales include the need to include male partners in STD testing, treatment, and education; adding services for men as part of managed care marketing strategies; and the national emphasis on male responsibility in welfare and child support enforcement programs, an integral part of every welfare reform program currently under consideration by the U.S. Congress (Schulte and Sonenstein 1995). The topic of male participation in contraception is taken up in more detail in the next chapter in connection with the use of male methods and the market for contraceptives.

CONCLUDING COMMENT

At the outset of this chapter, "needs" were defined as "a state of felt depriva-

TABLE 2-13 Husbands' Involvement in Family Planning Decisions (selected countries)

Country and Survey Year	No. of Interviewees[a]	% Who Know of at Least One Method	% Approving of Family Planning (FP)	% Who Have Discussed FP with Their Wives in the Last Year[b]	% Who Have Ever Used Contraception		% Currently Using Contraception		% Family Member Deciding		
					Modern	Any	Modern	Any	W	H	J
Burundi, 1987	542	92	94	48	2	52	NA	NA	—	—	—
Cameroon, 1991	814	74	37	30	17	48	6	20	—	—	—
Egypt, 1988–1989	9,000 (women)	—	—	—	—	—	—	—	14	25	61
Cairo	469	100	92	61	78	81	65	70	—	—	—
Upper Egypt	1,053	96	84	47	52	56	40	44	4	59	36
Ghana, 1988	943	79	77	46	26	41	9	20	—	—	—
India, 1986 (rural)	250 (women)	—	—	—	—	—	—	—	4	24	38[d]
Kenya, 1989	1,170	95	91	65	35	65	25	49	—	—	—

Mali, 1987[c]	970	65	16	28	2	16	1	4	—	—	—	—
Morocco, 1992	—	—	—	47	—	—	—	—	—	—	—	—
Niger, 1992	—	—	—	11	—	—	—	—	—	—	—	—
Pakistan, 1990–91	1,354	79	56	14	18	25	10	15	—	—	—	—
Turkey, 1991 Semi-urban	366 (women)	—	—	—	—	—	—	—	62	8	25
Rural	358 (women)	—	—	—	—	—	—	—	29	23	46

NOTE: NA = not applicable; W = wife, H = husband, J = joint.

[a] Husbands, except where otherwise noted.
[b] Among those who knew at least one contraceptive method.
[c] Includes all men, regardless of marital status.
[d] 22 percent of the family planning decisions in rural India in this survey were made by the extended family.

SOURCES: Derived from tables in McCauley AP, B Robey, AK Blanc, JS Geller, Opportunities for women through reproductive choice, Population Reports, Series M, No.12, July 1994. Data for Morocco and Niger are from Hopes and Realities: Closing the Gap Between Women's Aspirations and Their Reproductive Experiences, New York, The Alan Guttmacher Institute, 1995.

TABLE 2-14   Women's Discussion of Family Planning with Their Husbands (selected countries)

Country and Survey Year	% Using Family Planning Among Those Who:	
	Discussed with Husband	Did Not Discuss with Husband
Botswana, 1988	40	18
Burundi, 1987	14	2
Ghana, 1988	24	7
Kenya, 1986	36	11
Senegal, 1986	23	9
Sudan, 1989–1990	19	3
Togo, 1988	39	31

SOURCE: Based on graphics in Hopes and Realities: Closing the Gap Between Women's Aspirations and Their Reproductive Experiences, New York, The Alan Guttmacher Institute, 1995 (based on data from Demographic and Health Survey country reports, with special tabulations of the data files for Pakistan).

tion of some basic satisfaction." We have spoken about the *general* areas of need that have to do with societal and individual health and options and that make contraception a commanding issue for societies and individuals who wish to use it. We have also indicated that, beyond these general areas of need, there are very *specific* needs for new technologies that are not now being satisfied adequately. A new approach to estimating the overall unmet need for contraception identifies somewhere around 228 million women worldwide (not men, whose needs must also be taken into separate account) who can fairly be said to be in need of contraception. Overwhelming majorities of women want to control their fertility, even in Sub-Saharan Africa with its traditionally high value accorded to large families. And very large numbers of women, even those who have not yet achieved their desired family size, nonetheless state that they failed in their intentions with regard to their last pregnancy, either because they did not mean to have it at all or because they meant to have it at some later date.

Another dimension of general need is the sheer number of years women require protection from unintended pregnancy since, somewhat ironically, as completed family size continues to fall worldwide, women's lifetime exposure increases; a woman who wants only two children will require 20 years of protec-

TABLE 2-15 Male Perspectives on Desired Family Size

Country	Desired Family Size		% Wanting No More Children	
	Husbands	Wives	Husbands	Wives
Niger	12.6	8.5	2	9
Cameroon	11.2	7.3	10	14
Tanzania	7.4	6.4	17	23
Burundi	5.5	5.5	—	—
Ghana	6.6	5.5	19	23
Pakistan	5.4	5.3	33	40
Morocco	4.1	3.9	43	52
Kenya	4.1	3.9	44	52
Egypt	3.3	2.8	61	67

SOURCE: Based on graphics in Hopes and Realities: Closing the Gap Between Women's Aspirations and Their Reproductive Experiences. New York: The Alan Guttmacher Institute. 1995 (based on data from Demographic and Health Survey country reports, with special tabulations of the data files for Pakistan).

tion from that exposure. This means that, for a number of reasons, the same contraceptive is unlikely to be appropriate for an ever-longer and more biologically various life span, thus requiring a more various set of contraceptive alternatives.

Ancillary analyses tell us about other aspects of the general need for contraception. These include the women all over the world, still in their teens, whose physical well-being and life chances are at special risk: young women spending longer periods of time before entering into formal union, with a greater amount of sexual activity than seems to have been the case in the past; young women following tradition and continuing to enter union very early; and those young women of whom one-quarter to one-half are having their first child before any formal union. These are not exclusively Third World phenomena: In 1987, 1.2 million pregnancies occurred in the United States among women under 20, almost all of which were resolved outside marriage, with about half of those terminating in abortion. This is, of course, part of a bigger picture: The 1995 projection for the number of abortions worldwide is 52 million—28 percent of the 139 million live births projected for this year—about 21 million of which will be performed in countries where they are illegal and, presumably, unsafe. If so many women are resolving their pregnancies in this fashion, one must assume they need contraceptive help.

In Chapter 5 we will focus on those *specific* areas that point to a need for *new* contraceptive technologies, not only because they expand the range of contraceptive options overall, in itself a compelling need, but because they fill needs that are not now being met adequately. These include the need for contraceptives suitable for women who have been exposed to unprotected sexual intercourse, contraceptives with anti-infective properties, and methods for men.

REFERENCES

Alan Guttmacher Institute. Hopes and Realities: The Gap Between Women's Aspirations and Their Reproductive Experiences. New York: The Alan Guttmacher Institute. 1995a.

Alan Guttmacher Institute. Women, Families, and the Future: Sexual Relationships and Marriage Worldwide (Fact Sheet). New York: The Alan Guttmacher Institute. 1995b.

Alexander, NJ. Sexual transmission of human immunodeficiency virus: Virus entry into the male and female genital tract. Fertility and Sterility 54(1):1–18, 1990.

Aral SO, ME Guinan. Women and sexually transmitted diseases. IN Sexually Transmitted Diseases. KK Holmes, P-A Mardh, PF Sparling, PJ Wiesner, eds. New York: McGraw-Hill. 1984.

Brandrup-Lukunow A. Family Planning and Reproductive Health in CCEE/NIS: Background Paper for ECO/UNFPA Conference on Women's Status and Health. Copenhagen: WHO-EURO. 1995.

Brunham RC, JE Embree. Sexually transmitted diseases: Current and future dimensions of the problem in the Third World. IN Reproductive Tract Infections: Global Impact and Priorities for Women's Reproductive Health. A Germain, KK Holmes, P Piot, JN Wasserheit, eds. New York: Plenum. 1992.

Burt MR, LY Aron, LR Schack. Family Planning Clinics: Current Status and Recent Changes in Services, Clients, Staffing, and Income Sources—Report to The Henry J. Kaiser Family Foundation. Washington, DC: The Urban Institute. 1994.

Cates W Jr, KM Stone. Family planning: The responsibility to prevent both pregnancy and reproductive tract infection. IN Reproductive Tract Infections: Global Impact and Priorities for Women's Reproductive Health. A Germain, KK Holmes, P Piot, JN Wasserheit, eds. New York: Plenum. 1992.

Chen L, J Sepulveda, S Segal, eds. AIDS and Women's Health: Science for Policy and Action. New York: Plenum. 1992.

Chen V. A new social norm: All pregnancies intended. Carnegie Quarterly, Fall 1994–Winter 1995:10–11, 1995.

Claypool LE. The challenges ahead: Implications of STDs/AIDS for contraceptive research. IN Contraceptive Research and Development 1954 to 1994: The Road from Mexico City to Cairo and Beyond. PFA Van Look, G Pérez-Palacios, eds. Delhi: Oxford University Press. 1994.

Dixon-Mueller R, A Germain. Unmet need from a woman's health perspective. Planned Parenthood Challenges 1:9–12, 1994.

Dixon-Mueller R, A Germain. Stalking the elusive "unmet need" for family planning. Studies in Family Planning 23(5):330–335, 1992.

Fathalla M. Reproductive health in the world: Two decades of progress and the challenge ahead. IN Reproductive Health: A Key to a Brighter Future, J Khanna et al., eds. Geneva: World Health Organization. 1992.

Forrest JD. Epidemiology of unintended pregnancy and contraceptive use. American Journal of Obstetrics and Gynecology 170(5, Part 2):1485–1489, 1994.

Forrest JD. Timing of reproductive life stages. Obstetrics and Gynecology 82(1):105–111, 1993.

Fortney JA. Contraception—A lifelong perspective. IN Dying for Love: New Perspectives on Human Reproduction. Washington, DC: National Council for International Health. 1989.

Freedman R. Family planning programs in the Third World. Annals of the American Academy of Political Science 510:41, 1990.

Gelijns AC, CO Pannenborg. The development of contraceptive technology: Case studies of incentives and disincentives to innovation. International Journal of Technology Assessment 9(2):210–232, 1993.

Germain A, KK Holmes, P Piot, JN Wasserheit, eds. Reproductive Tract Infections: Global Impact and Priorities for Women's Reproductive Health. New York: Plenum. 1992.

Geronimus AT. Teenage childbearing and social disadvantage—Unprotected discourse. Family Relations 41:244–248, 1992.

Geronimus AT, S Korenman. The socioeconomic costs of teenage childbearing: Evidence and interpretation. Demography 30(2):281–296, 1993.

Geronimus AT, S Korenman. The socioeconomic consequences of teen childbearing reconsidered. Quarterly Journal of Economics 107:1187–1214, 1992.

Guttmacher Institute. See Alan Guttmacher Institute.

Gwinn M, M Pappaioanou, JR George, et al. Prevalence of HIV infection in childbearing women in the United States. Journal of the American Medical Association 265(13):1704–1708, 1991.

Hatcher RA, J Trussell, F Stewart, et al. Contraceptive Technology: 16th Revised Edition. New York: Irvington Publishers. 1994.

Henshaw SK. Induced abortion: A world view, 1990. Family Planning Perspectives 22:76–89, 1990.

Henshaw SK, JD Forrest. Women at Risk of Unintended Pregnancy, 1990 Estimates: The Need for Family Planning Services, Each State and County. New York: The Alan Guttmacher Instiute, 1993.

Henshaw SK, J Van Vort. Abortion services in the United States, 1991 and 1992. Family Planning Perspectives 26:100–106, 1993.

Herz B, AR Measham. The Safe Motherhood Initiative: Proposals for Action. Discussion Paper No. 9. Washington, DC: World Bank. 1987.

Hoffman SD, EM Foster, FF Furstenberg Jr. Revaluating the costs of teenage childbearing: Response to Geronimus and Korenman. Demography 30:291–296, 1993.

Institute of Medicine (IOM). In Her Lifetime: Female Morbidity and Mortality in Sub-Saharan Africa. M Law, CP Howson, PF Harrison, D Hotra, eds. Washington, DC: National Academy Press. 1996.

IOM. The Best Intentions: Unintended Pregnancy and the Well-Being of Children and Families. S Brown and L Eisenberg, eds. Washington, DC: National Academy Press. 1995.

IOM. Emerging Infections: Microbial Threats to Health in the United States. J Lederberg, RE Shope, SC Oaks Jr, eds. Washington, DC: National Academy Press. 1992.

Kabeer N. From Fertility Reduction to Reproductive Choice: Gender Perspectives on Family Planning. Institute of Development Studies Discussion Paper 299. Brighton, UK: University of Sussex. 1992.

Kaiser/Harris. National Survey Results on Public Knowledge of Abortion Rates. Menlo Park, CA: The Henry J. Kaiser Family Foundation. January 1995.

Ketting E. Global unmet need: Present and future. Planned Parenthood Challenges 1:31–34, 1994b.

King TM, JB Smith. From menarche to menopause: The contraceptive transition. IN Contraceptive Research and Development 1984 to 1994: The Road from Mexico City to Cairo and Beyond. PFA Van Look, G Pérez-Palacios, eds. Geneva: World Health Organization. 1994.

Koonin LM, JC Smith, et al. Abortion surveillance—United States. Mortality and Morbidity Weekly Report 1 (SS-5):1–33, 1992.

Kotler P. Marketing Management. Englewood Cliffs, NJ: Prentice Hall. 1988.

Kubicka I, Z Matejcek et al. Prague children from unwanted pregnancies revisited at age thirty. Submitted for publication, 1994, cited in The Best Intentions: Unintended Pregnancy and the Well-Being of Children and Families. S Brown, L Eisenberg, eds. Washington, DC: National Academy Press. 1995.

Kwast BE, RW Rochat, W Kidane-Mariam. Maternal mortality in Addis Ababa, Ethiopia. Studies in Family Planning 17:288-301, 1986.

Laga M. Human immunodeficiency virus infection prevention: The need for complementary STD control. IN Reproductive Tract Infections: Global Impact and Priorities for Women's Reproductive Health. A Germain, KK Holmes, P Piot, JN Wasserheit, eds. New York: Plenum. 1992.

Larson A. Social context of human immunodeficiency virus transmission in Africa: Historical and cultural bases of East and Central African sexual relations. Review of Infectious Diseases 11:716–724, 1989.

Lee PR, FH Stewart. Failing to prevent unintended pregnancy is costly. (Editorial). American Journal of Public Health 85(4):479–480, 1995.

Lotz P. Demand as a driving force in medical innovation. International Journal of Technology Assessment 9(2):174–188, 1993.

Luker K. Dubious conceptions: The controversy over teen pregnancy. American Prospective, 1991: 73–83, 1991.

Marsiglio W. Adolescent fathers in the United States: Their initial living arrangements, marital experience, and educational outcomes. Family Planning Perspectives 19(6):240–251, 1987.

McCauley AP, B Robey, AK Blanc, JS Geller. Opportunities for women through reproductive choice. Population Reports, Series M, No. 12 (Special topics), July 1994.

Meheus A. Women's health: Importance of reproductive tract infections, pelvic inflammatory disease and cervical cancer. IN Reproductive Tract Infections: Global Impact and Priorities for Women's Reproductive Health. A Germain, KK Holmes, P Piot, JN Wasserheit, eds. New York: Plenum. 1992.

Mosley WH, JL Bobadilla, DT Jamison. The health transition: Implications for health policy in developing countries. IN Disease Control Priorities in the Developing World. DT Jamison, WH Mosley, AR Measham, JL Bobadilla, eds. New York: Oxford University Press. 1993.

Mowery DC, N Rosenberg. The influence of market demand upon innovation: A critical review of some recent empirical studies. IN Inside the Black Box: Technology and Economics. N Rosenberg, ed. Cambridge, MA: Cambridge University Press. 1982.

Nelson RR, SG Winger. In search of a useful theory of innovation. Research Policy 6:36–76, 1977.

Over M, P Piot. HIV infection and sexually transmitted diseases. IN Disease Control Priorities in the Developing World. DT Jamison, WH Mosley, AR Measham, JL Bobadilla, eds. New York: Oxford University Press. 1993.

Population Reports. Opportunities for Women Through Reproductive Choice. Series M, No. 12, July 1994.

Robey B, SO Rutstein, L Morris, R Blackburn. The reproductive revolution: New survey findings. Population Reports, Series M. No. 11. Baltimore: Johns Hopkins School of Public Health, Population Information Program. 1992.

Rosenfield A. Maternal mortality in developing countries: An ongoing but neglected epidemic. Journal of the American Medical Association 262(3):376-379, 1989.

Rosenfield A, D Maine. Maternal mortality—A neglected tragedy: Where is the M in MCH? Lancet, 13 July: 83–85, 1985.

Sachs A. Men, sex, and parenthood. World Watch, March–April: 12–19, 1994.

Sadik N. The State of World Population 1995—Decisions for Development: Women, Empowerment and Reproductive Health. New York: United Nations Population Fund. 1995.

Stein Z. HIV prevention: The need for methods women can use. American Journal of Public Health 80:460–462, 1990.

Teubal M, N Arnon, M Trachtenberg. Performance in innovation in the Israeli electronics industry: A case study of biomedical electronics instrumentation. Research Policy 5:354–379, 1976.

Tinker A, P Daly, C Green, et al. Women's Health and Nutrition: Making a Difference. Discussion Paper 246. Washington, DC: World Bank. 1994.

Trussell J, J Koenig, C Ellertson, F Stewart. Emergency Contraception: A Cost-Effective Approach to Preventing Unintended Pregnancy. Unpublished manuscript. Princeton, NJ: Office of Population Research. November 1995.

United Nations Population Fund (UNFPA). Programme Advisory Note: Male Involvement in Reproductive Health. New York: UNFPA. 1995.

UNFPA. Programme of Action of the United Nations International Conference on Population and Development. Cairo and New York: UNFPA. 1994.

Walsh JA, CM Feifer, et al. Maternal and perinatal health. IN Disease Control Priorities in Developing Countries. DT Jamison, WH Mosley et al., eds. New York: Oxford Unviersity Press. 1993.

Wasserheit, JN. Epidemiological synergy: Interrelationships between human immunodeficiency virus infection and other sexually transmitted diseases. IN AIDS and Women's Health: Science for Policy and Action. L Chen, J Sepulveda, S Segal, eds. New York: Plenum. 1992.

Wasserheit JN, KK Holmes. Reproductive tract infections: Challenges for international health policy, programs, and research. IN Reproductive Tract Infections: Global Impact and Priorities for Women's Reproductive Health. A Germain, KK Holmes, P Piot, JN Wasserheit, eds. New York: Plenum. 1992.

Westoff CF. Reproductive Preferences: A Comparative View. Demographic and Health Surveys, Comparative Studies, No. 3. Columbia, MD: Institute for Resource Development. 1991.

Westoff CF, LH Ochoa. Unmet Need and the Demand for Family Planning. Demographic and Health Surveys, Comparative Studies, No. 5. Columbia, MD: Institute for Resource Development. 1991.

Williams LB, WF Pratt. Wanted and unwanted childbearing in the United States: 1973–1988. Advance data from Vital and Health Statistics, No. 189. Hyattsville, MD: National Center for Health Statistics. 1990.

World Bank. A New Agenda for Women's Health and Nutrition. Washington, DC: World Bank. 1994.

World Bank. World Development Report 1993: Investing in Health. New York: Oxford University Press. 1993.

World Health Organization (WHO). Maternal mortality and morbidity. IN 1996 World Population Monitoring Report (draft version). New York: United Nations Population Fund, Population Division. 1996.

WHO. Abortion: A Tabulation of Available Data on the Frequency and Mortality of Unsafe Abortion, 2nd ed. Geneva: Division of Family Health, World Health Organization. 1994.

WHO. Maternal Mortality: A Global Factbook. Geneva: World Health Organization. 1991.

WHO. Prevention of Maternal Mortality: Report of a WHO Interregional Meeting, Geneva, 11–15 November 1985. Mimeo. Geneva: World Health Organization. 1986.

Wulf D. The Unmet Demand for Family Planning. Unpublished manuscript. New York: The Rockefeller Foundation. 1995.

NOTES

1. The term "married" as used in this report includes marriages approved by civil, religious, or other customary practices; cohabiting and consensual unions that are socially recognized; and visiting unions where those are recognized.

2. The "KAP-gap" is defined as an inconsistency between a woman's stated childbearing preference and her practice of birth control as ascertained from surveys of her knowledge, attitudes, and practices (KAP) such as the World Fertility, Contraceptive Prevalence, and the Demographic and Health Surveys. Dixon-Mueller and Germain (1992) distinguish between a "conventional" KAP-gap which refers to women who say they want no more children but are not practicing contraception, and an "instantaneous" KAP-gap, which refers to women who say they want no more children or who want to postpone the next pregnancy, are exposed to the risk of pregnancy, and are not practicing contraception.

3. "Presumed" refers to the fact that it is not absolutely guaranteed that no unintended pregnancy will not occur.

4. Some analysts (Geronimus 1992; Luker 1991) argue that the negative effects of early childbearing may reflect the disadvantaged backgrounds of those adolescents who become parents rather than the timing of the birth itself. Recent analyses of large U.S. national data sets do, in fact, suggest that the negative socioeconomic effects of teenage childbearing are diminished when the mother's prepregnancy characteristics and within- and across-family heterogeneity are taken into account (Hoffman et al. 1993; Geronimus and Korenman 1992 and 1993). Still, so far at least, most researchers using varied approaches and data sets conclude that early childbearing is causally associated with negative outcomes over and above the effects of background (IOM 1995), an association that is much more powerfully true in the developing world (IOM 1996).

5. The National Survey of Family Growth (NSFG) is the most comprehensive source of information available on pregnancy and contraceptive use among reproductive-age women (15–44 years) in the United States. Conducted by the National Center for Health Statistics (NCHS), the survey is federally funded. Surveys were carried out in 1973, 1976, 1982, and 1988; respondents from the 1988 survey were briefly re-interviewed by telephone. The 1973 and 1976 samples were restricted to ever-married women, among whom most childbearing in the country had occurred. In 1982 and 1988, women of all marital statuses were included. The next round of the NSFG was conducted in 1995 and the data are being processed and analyzed. It has been designed to improve abortion reporting, clarify questions on unwanted and mistimed pregnancies, measure women's ambivalent feelings about becoming pregnant, and improve understanding of unplanned pregnancies through better measures of contraceptive use.

6. Women "at risk" of unintended pregnancy are defined as those who (a) have had sexual intercourse; (b) are fertile, that is, neither they nor their partners have been contraceptively sterilized and they do not believe that they are infertile for any other reason; and (c) are neither intentionally pregnant nor have they been trying to become pregnant during any part of the year (Henshaw and Forrest 1993).

7. The sections of this report dealing with unintended pregnancy have relied heavily on the exhaustive analysis of the Demographic and Health Surveys and other national surveys by The Alan Guttmacher Institute, partly in preparation for its recently released study, *Hopes and Realities: Closing the Gap Between Women's Aspirations and Their Reproductive Experiences* (1995). Where this is not the case or where a different analytic approach is taken to the Appendix Tables in that report, that is so indicated.

8. According to the World Health Organization, "Data on abortion in general and unsafe abortion in particular are scarce and inevitably unreliable because of legal and ethical/moral constraints which hinder data collection. Under-reporting and mis-reporting are common because women may be reluctant to admit to an induced abortion, especially when it is illegal. Few studies have achieved higher than 75 percent accuracy of reporting and, in some cases, only a quarter of abortions known to have been performed have been admitted to by respondents. In a rare follow-up study of 118 women

admitting only to spontaneous abortion in Mérida, Mexico, in 1979, 77 percent later admitted that the abortion had been induced" (WHO 1994). Nevertheless, the WHO document from which this citation was taken is as thorough and recent a compendium as exists anywhere and should be considered definitive at this point in time. Still, as the document itself indicates, the numbers provided, especially the numbers of unsafe abortions, should be considered undercounts. This is so even in the United States.

9. This figure supersedes a prior estimate of 200,000 generated from projections based on hospital records. Three factors should be taken into account in interpreting this number: The possibility of a concomitant underestimate in rural areas owing to under-reporting; the difficulty of distinguishing primary from secondary causes of death; and, most importantly, its direct relation with the total number of annual maternal deaths (WHO/FHE, personal communication, November 1995).

10. The term "comparable market economies" refers to selected European countries and Canada. China, the former Soviet Union and newly independent states of central Europe, and most developing countries report ratios to live births that are significantly higher than those in either the United States or other economically comparable countries (Institute of Medicine 1995).

11. The term "rate" has been traditionally used for this figure; it is, however, really a ratio and measures obstetric risk .

12. However, the largest absolute number of maternal deaths actually occur among low-risk women, since there are so many more low-risk pregnancies altogether, and because the complications of pregnancy, which also occur among low-risk women, cannot be predicted in advance.

13. The reproductive tract infections (RTIs) have been broadly defined to include sexually transmitted infections and infections that are nonsexually transmitted, and comprise three types of infection: (1) sexually transmitted diseases (STDs), such as chlamydial infection, gonorrhea, trichomoniasis (which may or may not be sexually transmissible), syphilis, chancroid, genital herpes, genital warts, and human immunodeficiency virus (HIV) infection; (2) endogenous infections, caused by overgrowth of organisms that can be present in the genital tract of a healthy woman, such as bacterial vaginosis and vulvovaginal candidiasis; and (3) iatrogenic infections, associated with medical procedures, such as female genital mutilation, poor delivery practices, cesarean section, unsafe abortion, and improperly performed pelvic examinations and IUD insertions (Brunham and Embree 1992; Meheus 1992). Of the three types of reproductive tract infections—sexually transmitted, endogenous, and iatrogenic—the majority are sexually transmitted in direct fashion (Brunham and Embree 1992). However, the iatrogenic infections are also important because they are linked to contraception, or the lack of contraception, through sepsis during the medical procedures cited above. Of the eight major STD pathogens producing RTIs, four are bacterial (chancroid, chlamydia, gonorrhea, and syphilis) and four are viral (HIV, human papilloma virus/HPV, herpes simplex type 2/HSV-2, and hepatitis B/HBV).

14. In the context of the sexually transmitted reproductive tract infections, it is unfortunately necessary at times to use the term "females" rather than "women." Normally, one would expect only women of fertile age to be at risk of such infection. However, rape and other sexual abuse of prepubescent females, as well as female genital mutilation where that is practiced, mean that it is sometimes the case that females—not women—come to bear a burden of sexually transmitted disease.

15. It is important to note in this context the behaviorally and biomedically significant distinction between abstinence for pregnancy prevention and abstinence for STD prevention: While the former implies only avoiding penis-in-vagina intercourse, the latter implies avoiding vaginal, anal, and oral intercourse.

16. Clinical trials of the protection provided by the female condom against sexually transmitted infections are now in progress, under the aegis of the National Institute of Child Health and Human Development of the U.S. National Institutes of Health.

3

Contraceptive Technology and the State of the Science: Current and Near-future Methods

INTRODUCTION

This chapter first speaks briefly about those contraceptive options that are available today. It then turns to options that are—all things being equal—likely to be developed or become available sometime during the decade that is beginning now, that is, between 1996 and the year 2006. The term "all things being equal" refers to the fact that the entry into the market of any new contraceptive method is not just a function of scientific innovation. It is also a function of the contextual dynamics addressed in other chapters in this report. Those dynamics encompass the character of the need and demand for contraception; the various economic and political factors that may prevail as a product advances from bench to shelf; and the social, cultural, religious, and personal variables that, in market terms, shape the need and demand for contraceptives and the extent to which they are, or are not, supplied. Chapter 4 deals with the science landscape in a more distant future, and with the concepts and mechanisms that are the most probable antecedents of very new and innovative contraceptive alternatives, for women and for men. These new possibilities are affected by some of the same dynamics that affect today's contraceptive methods; those are discussed in Chapter 6 and Chapter 7.

Because of the varying states of development of the technologies under consideration, Chapters 3 and 4 are organized differently. Chapter 3 is based on presentations made at the December 1994 Institute of Medicine workshop on Contraceptive Research and Development and the Frontiers of Contemporary Science, conducted as part of this study activity (Institute of Medicine [IOM] 1995). It consists of two parts, as follows:

94

• Current Options: This section sets the stage for discussion of new approaches to reversible contraception over the next decade and beyond. The section is organized by categories of *methods* that are presently available, that is, existing, named formulations that work through a variety of mechanisms and delivery systems. Table 3-1 summarizes these methods, their mechanisms of action, failure rates under typical and perfect use, advantages, disadvantages, side effects, and potential complications.

• Contraceptive Options in the Next Decade, 1995–2005: This section focuses on approaches that are at least in phase I of trials. For the most part, these are either improvements or novel applications of approaches that are already well known. These, too, are considered as *methods* and are organized in the same way as current options, in order to point more clearly to where improvements are under way. We recognize that, in some categorical instances, the boundary between prospects for the next decade and prospects for the years beyond is often blurred. This is a function of technology and of the degree of advance. In the first instance, a technology that seems promising disappoints in trials. In the second, there may be one or two advances that have become "available methods," but the contraceptive category to which it belongs is otherwise largely empty; good examples are barrier and postcoital methods and contraceptives for men.

Chapter 4 and its appendixes constitute the committee's efforts to respond to its charge to review the state of the relevant basic science and identify a range of potential areas and targets that would provide a foundation for fresh endeavor in contraceptive research and development. The chapter is based not only on the December 1994 workshop but on a set of authored papers found in the appendixes to this report. The chapter has three sections: (1) areas of inquiry or specific targets in the development of contraceptive methods for women, that is, "female methods"; (2) areas of inquiry or specific targets in the development of contraceptive methods for men, that is, "male methods"; and (3) an area that holds promise for the development of various contraceptive methods for both females and males, "immunocontraception," which subsumes the topic of "mucosal immunity" and its potential for generating new anti-infective and/or contraceptive barrier methods. The internal organization of each of these categories was determined by physiology and by the stage of scientific understanding. Because the stages of the female reproductive cycle are critical from both the technologic and policy perspectives, this particular section is organized according to that cycle. Because of the diversity in the levels of scientific advance, the sections of Chapter 4 that deal with methods for males and with immunocontraception are, necessarily, a mix of specific molecular targets and modes of action.

CURRENT OPTIONS

The reversible contraceptive options that are available today, almost all of

TABLE 3-1 Current Reversible Contraceptive Options, Mode of Action, Rates of Failure,[a] Advantages and Disadvantages

Method	Mode of Action	Unintended Pregnancy Rate		Disadvantages and Advantages	Side Effects	Dangers
		Typical Use	Perfect Use			
Female Hormonal Methods						
Oral Contraceptives						
Combined	Suppression of ovulation, changes in cervical mucus and endometrium	3%	0.1%	Protection against ovarian/endometrial cancer, pelvic inflammatory disease (PID), fibrocystic breast disease, ovarian cysts, iron-deficiency anemia, dysmenorrhea	Nausea, headaches, dizziness, spotting, weight gain, breast tenderness, chloasma	Cardiovascular (stroke, heart attack, blood clots, hypertension), depression, hepatic adenomas
Progestin-only	Changes in cervical mucus and endometrium, possible ovulation suppression	4%	0.5%	Protection against PID, iron-deficiency anemia, dysmenorrhea	Menstrual irregularities	Unknown
Implants Levonorgestrel subdermal implants (Norplant)	Similar to progestin-only	0.09%	0.09%	Effective for 5 years	Site tenderness, removal problems, menstrual irregularities, headache, weight gain, acne	Infection at implant site

	Mechanism of action			Benefits	Side effects	Risks
Injectables Depo-medroxyprogesterone acetate (Depo-Provera)	Suppression of ovulation, changes in cervical mucus and endometrium	0.3%	0.3%	Effective for 3 months Reduced risk of endometrial cancer, PID	Menstrual irregularities, headache, weight gain, delayed return to fertility	None proven
Intrauterine Devices (IUD): Progesterone T (Progestasert)	Inhibition of sperm migration, fertilization and ovum transport (progesterone is responsible for primary mode of action)	2%	1.5%	Diminished menstrual blood loss and relief of dysmenorrhea	Requirement for removal and reinsertion on an annual basis; increased cramping and menstrual flow	Ectopic pregnancy
Copper T 380A (ParaGard)	Copper is responsible for primary mode of action	0.8%	0.6%	Protection against ectopic pregnancy; 10-year useful approved life; decreased menstrual blood flow, possible decrease in fibroids	Increased menstrual blood loss, cramping, spotting, dysmenorrhea	Uterine perforation (rare), PID limited to 20–30 days post-insertion, anemia
Levonorgestrel T (Mirena)	Development of an endometrium with lessened sensitivity to circulating estradiol as result of high tissue concentration of progestin inhibiting synthesis of estradiol receptor	0.1%	0.1%	Reduced incidence of myomas, arrested development of endometriosis, prevention of progression of STDs to endometritis and PID		STD risks

TABLE 3-1 Continued

Method	Mode of Action	Unintended Pregnancy Rate		Disadvantages and Advantages	Side Effects	Dangers
		Typical Use	Perfect Use			
Barrier Methods:						
Spermicide alone	Inactivation of sperm	21%	6%	May protect against bacterial STDs	Vaginal irritation	None proven
Cervical cap with Spermicide	Mechanical barrier; inactivation of sperm	18%	11.5%	Protection against STDs	Cervical irritation, vaginal discharge, pelvic pressure, Pap smear abnormalities	Toxic shock syndrome
Diaphragm with Spermicide	Mechanical barrier; inactivation of sperm	18%	6%	Protection against STDs	Cervical irritation	Toxic shock syndrome, urinary tract infections
Condom	Mechanical barrier					
Male		12%	3%	Protection against STDs	Latex allergies	None
Female		21%	5%	Protection against STDs, including external genitalia	Difficult to insert	None

Non-Commodity-Based Methods				
Lactational Amenorrhea Method (LAM)	Based on enhancement of lactational physiology and identification of period of lactational infertility using three criteria	1–2% (6-mo. rate) 0–1%	No commodities necessary; enhances breastfeeding practices. Only applicable during the first 6 months postpartum	Side effects are a result of the enhanced breastfeeding behaviors, including improved maternal and child health	Provides no protection against STDs
Periodic Abstinence Methods:	Avoidance of coitus during days when fertilization might occur using a mathematical method (CM), a cervical mucus-based method (OM), or a combination of temperature shift and other signs (STM)	20% 0–1%	No commodities necessary; enhances breastfeeding practices. Another method should be started whenever any of the three criteria are no longer met		Provides no protection against STDs
Calendar Method (CM)		9%			
Ovulation Method (OM)		3%			
Symptothermal Method (STM)		2%	No commodities necessary, except a thermometer with STM; said to enhance couple communication; periods of abstinence required; provides no protection against STDs; requires daily observation and interpretation of fertility signs		

TABLE 3-1 Continued

Method	Mode of Action	Unintended Pregnancy Rate		Disadvantages and Advantages	Side Effects	Dangers
		Typical Use	Perfect Use			
Fertility Awareness Methods (FAM)	Avoidance of coitus and/or use of a barrier method during days when fertilization might occur	10%[b]	10%[b]	Combines understanding of fertility with use of barrier methods, potentially increasing efficacy	Those associated with the barrier method only	Provides limited protection against STDs
Coitus Interruptus	Withdrawal of the penis from the vagina prior to ejaculation	18%	4%	No commodity necessary, no advance planning or charting		Provides no protection against STDs
Emergency Contraception						
Emergency Contraceptive Pills (ECPs) (combined oral contraceptive pills containing combination of estrogen and progestin)	2 Ovral pills initially, 2 more 12 hours later; or 4 Lo/Ovral, Nordette, or Levlen initially, 4 more 12 hours later; or		75%	Relatively easy to obtain	Nausea, vomiting	Side effects may be severe

	4 Triphasil or Tri-Levlen (yellow only) initially, 4 more 12 hours later		
Minipills (progestin-only oral contraceptive pills)	20 Ovrette pills (.75 mg) initially, 20 more 12 hours later	75%	Contains no estrogen so can be used by women who cannot tolerate combined OCs
Mifepristone (a drug, also known as RU 486, that can function as an emergency contraceptive before pregnancy begins)	1 dose (NOTE: not yet available)	~99%	Less nausea and vomiting than ECP, and is more effective
IUD	Clinician inserts a copper T-shaped intrauterine device into the uterus	~99%	Can serve as a long-term contraceptive after the "emergency"; greater window of time than with ECPs and is most effective

[a]Rates are for U.S. women and were determined from: C Ellerton, Expanding access to emergency contraception in developing countries, Studies in Family Planning 26(5):251–262, 1995, and J Trussell, C Ellerton, Efficacy of emergency contraception, Fertility Control Reviews 4(2):8–11, 1995.

[b]D Rogow et al. A year's experience with a fertility awareness program: A report. Advances in Planned Parenthood 15(1):27–33, 1980. Other studies in Germany have shown FAM to be more efficacious than PAM, while other studies are equivocal.

which are for women, fall into the following broad categories: oral contraceptives, including emergency contraception; implants; and injectables; intrauterine devices; barrier methods; and non-commodity-based methods.

Although the past decade has seen the introduction of levonorgestrel subdermal implants (Norplant) and depo-medroxyprogesterone acetate (Depo-Provera or DMPA), these are technical variations of existing hormonal methods; they have new and/or different advantages and disadvantages, but they do not represent truly new physiologic concepts. The same can be said for some of the new female barrier methods, which, while their configurations are novel and represent a great deal of research, are still not manifestations of completely new ways of thinking about contraceptive technology. Currently available methods of emergency contraception, while receiving fresh attention, use existing products, although expansion of their availability and utilization would be, in itself, an important novelty.

Oral Contraceptives

Combination Oral Contraceptives

Beyond new delivery systems and minor modifications in active ingredients, hormonal methods of contraception have changed little since the birth control pill was first introduced, although research on lower-dose formulations has been a steady theme in the field. Today's hormonal contraceptives—consisting of various combinations of estrogens and progestins—can be delivered in the following ways: as pills taken orally, as implants, and as injectables.

Hormonal contraceptive methods work through a variety of mechanisms. The dual action of estrogen and progestin in combined oral contraceptives (COCs) serves both to suppress ovulation and change the nature of cervical mucus, making it less permeable to sperm. A fact that is very imperfectly recognized is that COCs have definite non-contraceptive advantages, including protection against ovarian and endometrial cancer, fibrocystic breast disease, benign ovarian cysts, ectopic pregnancies, and symptomatic pelvic inflammatory disease. And, with lower doses of estrogen, their disadvantages are infrequent.

Because of their established and good record of safety and efficacy, particularly in the modern formulations, there would seem to be scant incentive to improve OCs (Hatcher et al. 1994). However, the appearance of the injectable methods spurred competitive response in the market, as did the perception of needs in special subpopulations (e.g., older women) for whom some reformulation might be attractive (Hatcher et al. 1994). Taken conscientiously, oral contraceptives seldom fail.

Progestin-only Pills (POPs)

The marketing of progestin-only pills (POPs, often referred to as minipills[1]) began about 10 years after combined oral contraceptives were introduced. Although there are now a number of these preparations employing a variety of progestins, they account for a small portion of the OC market (Hatcher et al. 1994).

Progestin-only products are members of a family of progestin-only contraceptives which, in addition to being administered orally, may be administered by injection, implants, intrauterine devices, and vaginal rings. They prevent pregnancy through several modes of action: by inhibiting ovulation; thickening and decreasing the amount of cervical mucus (making it more difficult for sperm to penetrate; creating a thin, atrophic endometrium; and/or premature luteolysis (McCann and Potter 1994). Like regular oral contraceptives, progestin-only methods provide little or no protection against sexually transmitted infections, including HIV. Given perfect use, progestin-only pills have slightly higher rates of unintended pregnancy than combined OCs and cause sporadic bleeding in some women (Hatcher et al. 1994).

Implants

The first implant introduced onto the world market was Norplant, developed through a long process of intersectoral collaboration. When initially introduced, Norplant was remarkably successful. This long-acting contraceptive slowly and steadily diffuses a small amount of progestin through six slim, flexible rods inserted subcutaneously in a woman's upper arm and produces in most women the same cessation of ovulation and other physiologic changes that are associated with all progestin-based methods. Despite the somewhat cumbersome need to insert the rods, the method's long-term convenience (five years of protection in its present formulation) and low unintended pregnancy rates led initially to its quick adoption by many women in many countries, including the United States.

As with all contraceptives, Norplant has side effects for some women, primarily menstrual irregularities and, in some instances, weight gain. Experience of these sequelae led some women to request discontinuation within the first year of use. However, if not inserted properly, removal of the implants can be difficult in some instances, so that there were cases of difficult removals. As a consequence of adverse publicity about those experiences, as well as an alleged (but totally unproven) effect from the silicone in the rods, there was a widely publicized series of class action suits. Choice of this method dropped precipitously and requests for removal mounted, even in women who had been satisfied with the method (White 1995). These issues are discussed in Chapter 7 in the context of legal and regulatory issues.

Injectables

The underlying mechanism for the injectable contraceptive, Depo-Provera, is similar to that of progestin-only hormonal methods. It does not, however, have to be taken every day, but is effective for three months. For women who may wish to change their minds, this time commitment may or may not be a disadvantage, depending on the urgency with which they wish to reestablish fertility. For women who wish to continue with an injectable method, the need for quarterly injections can also be a problem if there are constraints on access to an appropriate health provider, although the method is somewhat forgiving since it has a variable grace period. Its contraceptive efficacy is very high and, again, like all progestin-only methods, Depo-Provera can be used by lactating women. The method is approved for use in over 90 countries, including the United States where it was finally approved in late 1992, its approval having been delayed because of its effect on dogs (Hatcher et al. 1994) (see Chapter 7). Several other injectables are available outside the United States, for example, Noristerat and Cyclofem.

Intrauterine Devices (IUDs)

Two intrauterine devices are currently available in the United States, the progesterone T (Progestasert System), which must be inserted and removed annually, and the Copper T 380A (CU T380, or ParaGard), which is effective for at least 10 years.[2] The levonorgesterol IUD (LNg IUD), not yet licensed in the United States, has a manufacturer-recommended duration rate of five years. There are also other IUDs available outside the United States, for example, Multiload and Nova-T.

All newer IUDs have very low failure rates (1 percent or less, equal to sterilization), and fewer side effects (bleeding and pain) than earlier devices. Although the exact mechanism of action of the IUD has been uncertain until quite recently, it now seems that fertilization and implantation rates are both decreased. All IUDs that have been tested experimentally or clinically induce a local inflammatory reaction in the endometrium that changes the cellular and humoral components of the fluid contents of the uterine cavity; in humans, the entire genital tract then appears to be affected by the inflammatory fluids from the uterine lumen. This in turn affects the function and viability of gametes, thus decreasing the rate of fertilization, either in the altered tubal milieu or in the uterine cavity (Bardin 1996).[3]

Barrier Methods

Chemical Barriers

Barrier methods of contraception fall into two, sometimes overlapping, categories: (1) *physical barriers* (male and female condoms, and diaphragms and cervical caps for women), which differentially prevent the passage of sperm and other constituents of semen to the partner's genital tract; and (2) *chemical barriers*, a more varied class of products and delivery systems. Chemical barrier methods contain a spermicide, which kills or immobilizes sperm (and other cells). The delivery vehicle can be a cream, gel, foam, film, or other formulation. A combined barrier approach involves using a physical barrier with a spermicide; the diaphragm and cervical cap are examples of this combination. The spermicidal agent in most products sold in the United States is nonoxynol-9, a nonionic detergent or surfactant.

There is renewed public interest in barrier methods, since they constitute the only category of contraceptives now available that can reduce the risk of transmission of sexually transmitted diseases (STDs). However, because they are coitally dependent, their effectiveness depends upon consistent and correct use. And, since cultural and motivational factors influence that use, their efficacy varies widely. Prevalence of use of most barrier methods has been increasing in recent years; still, they are used by less than half of all sexually active couples engaging in behaviors that put them at risk of transmitting or acquiring an STD.

Mechanical Barriers

The principal barrier method currently in use is the male condom, whose utilization has increased steadily since the late 1980s in response to growing consumer concern about sexually transmitted infection. That same concern has provoked interest in developing new condoms for males that are impermeable to virus and thinner but stronger, and to place control of self-protection in women's hands by developing a female condom, called Reality in the United States and Femidom elsewhere. The concern has also generated a tension in approval processes at the U.S. Food and Drug Administration (FDA) which must weigh the urgency of the public health and individual need for protection from sexually transmitted disease, on the one hand, and the need to assure that new products are safe as barriers against conception and infection, on the other. In addition, the ethical and physiologic challenges of product testing are large and complex. Studies of spermicides and drugs to protect against HIV infection are particularly difficult, since failure could result in either unwanted pregnancy, the transmission of a potentially life-threatening sexually transmitted disease, or both (Russell 1996b).

Some of these problems have already affected the availability on the market of both Reality and Avanti, a new male condom. Avanti is the first condom available for use by individuals allergic to latex (the material used for the overwhelming majority of currently available male condoms) and the first male polyurethane condom to be approved by the FDA. Avanti went onto the U.S. market in a limited number of western states in the fall of 1994, approved by the FDA before the agency began requiring manufacturers of medical devices to perform extensive clinical testing prior to marketing. Although it is actually made of a synthetic material that is similar to the material used for Reality, the FDA determined that Avanti was "substantially equivalent" to the latex condom instead. The effect of this ruling was to exempt Avanti from the more rigorous clinical testing that had been required for Reality. However, the thinness of the material used for the first Avanti to go on the market produced breakage rates judged to be unacceptable. A thicker material is now being tested in clinical trials under the aegis of the National Institute of Child Health and Human Development (NICHD) (American Health Consultants 1995; Contraceptive Technology Update June 1995).

Other plastic condoms for males that are not polyurethane have also been developed. Carter-Wallace is bringing one to market and SmartPractice has developed the Tactylon condom. Core issues for any male condom are not only concerns about breakage, but concerns about the viral permeability of any material of which they are made.

The female condom has been on the market too short a time to assess its acceptability. Recent focus group research shows a positive response at about the 50–60 percent level; it is quite novel and will require familiarity with its use, on the part of men and women. Cost will continue to be an issue for many women, especially since reuse is not advised. While Reality is not without its limitations, it provides women with much more autonomy than other available methods, although it still requires some discussion with the male partner (WHO 1995b). A washable, reusable female condom would seem to be a useful area of improvement.

Non-commodity-based Methods

There are several approaches to contraception, often grouped as "traditional methods," that have undergone scientific scrutiny in recent decades, resulting in newly rediscovered, reliable, and efficacious methods of family planning that do not require dependence on the contraceptive technologies of the type described above. These methods rely on time-based barriers to conception, behavioral-based barriers to conception, or both. Time-based barriers to conception are methods that allow coitus at times when a conception cannot occur, while behavioral barriers are actions that prohibit semen from entering the vagina. Both are receiving more attention as a result of greater interest in reducing human exposure to drugs and artificial materials.

The Lactational Amenorrhea Method (LAM)

LAM, the newest method in this category, is an effective postpartum introductory family planning method based on breastfeeding's effect on a woman's fertility. LAM's efficacy depends on three parameters: a woman's menstrual period has not returned postpartum; she breastfeeds frequently, day and night; she gives her baby no other food or liquid regularly; and her baby is less than six months old. A change in any of these requries initiation of another method. LAM has shown up to 99.6 percent efficacy in clinical trtials (Pérez et al. 1992); other clinical studies have found only 1 to 2 pregnancies per 100 women in the first six months after delivery, by life table analysis (Labbok et al. 1994).

LAM's mechanism of action is based on the hypothalamic-pituitary-ovarian axis and its response to the suckling stimulus. Suckling sends neural signals to the hypothalamus. This mediates the level and rhythm of gonadotropin releasing hormone (GnRH) secretion. Early postpartum breastfeeding also affects pituitary responsiveness to GnRH. Since GnRH influences pituitary release of follicle stimulating hormone (FSH) and luteinizing hormone (LH), the hormones responsible for stimulating follicle development and ovulation in the ovary, frequent breastfeeding suppresses adequate ovulation and follicle development. In this manner, the woman's body is kept from producing eggs and becoming fertile in the early months after childbirth.

Periodic Abstinence Methods (PAM): Calendar Rhythm, Cervical Mucus/ Ovulation, and Symptothermal Methods

These methods provide instruction about the timing of ovulation during the ovulatory cycle and the days of potential fertilization of the ovum, and require abstinence at those times (Queenan and Labbok 1992). In recent decades several techniques have been developed, often referred to as "natural family planning (NFP) methods"; they have been comprehensively defined by the WHO as "methods for planning or preventing pregnancies by observation of naturally occurring signs and symptoms of the fertile and infertile phases of the menstrual cycle" and the practice of abstinence at those times.

Calendar Rhythm Although, worldwide, calendar rhythm remains the best known and most commonly used periodic abstinence method, new methods have been developed which allow abstinence decisions to be made in closer relationship to the actual physiology of the cycle in question. The two most widely taught methods are (1) ovulation (or cervical mucus) method, based on observations of changes in cervical mucus; and (2) the symptothermal method, which uses primarily basal body temperature changes in addition to calendar or observations of changes in cervical mucus. An estimated 2–5 percent of married American women exposed to the risk of pregnancy currently rely on these methods. Theoretically, these methods should provide reasonable efficacy; however, published figures on efficacy vary widely. Calendar rhythm generally is not prescribed today but may serve as an effective adjunct to newer methods.

Cervical Mucus, or Ovulation Method   This method relies on the sensation and/ or observation of mucus, observed vaginally or at the vulva, to identify its characteristics over time. The scientific basis for these signs and symptoms is clear: The changes in the mucus reflect normal physiological reaction to the dynamic estrogen and progesterone levels of the menstrual cycle which can be used to approximate the time of ovulation. Use of this method generally includes maintenance of a daily record, often in a monthly format, to aid in assessment of the phase of the cycle; charts have been developed using colored tabs or symbols to indicate different signs and symptoms.

The Symptothermal Method   The symptothermal method provides a multiple index approach and is based on the use of at least two indicators to identify the fertile period: the basal body temperature (BBT) shift, and either cervical mucus or calendar rhythm. The relationship between temperature and ovulation was identified as early as the 1920s: BBT, reflected in the temperature registered orally, rectally, or vaginally before rising in the morning, will rise slightly (about 0.2°–0.4°C, or about 0.4°–0.8°F) in concert with the increasing progesterone levels of the early luteal phase of the menstrual cycle. Generally, the shift is said to occur when the BBT reading is more than 0.05°C (0.1°F) higher than the highest of the previous six postmenstrual readings, although there are other acceptable approaches; a slight drop in temperature (about 0.1°F) may be noted around the time of ovulation. Interpretation of BBT charts may demand considerable education.

Fertility Awareness Methods   "Fertility awareness" is a term used when signs and symptoms are taught as part of general reproductive health and family planning or family life education. The term "fertility awareness method," on the other hand, generally applies when either periodic abstinence or a barrier method is used only for pregnancy avoidance during the fertile phase, as that is identified using any of the three periodic abstinence methods listed above. Thus, periodic abstinence may be a part of practicing a fertility awareness method or of natural family planning, but the philosophies behind the two approaches are different.

Postcoital Methods

Emergency Contraception

Interest in methods for emergency contraception is gaining momentum in the United States, although they have been available in Europe and the United Kingdom for over a decade. These methods are used after an act of unprotected intercourse, either because of method failure or failure to use a method. Emergency contraceptive approaches include the use of standard combination oral contraceptives (COCs) containing estrogen and progestin in a postcoital regimen to prevent pregnancy, a regimen of progestin-only minipills, or insertion of a copper-T intrauterine device. Mifepristone (RU 486) has been used as an emergency contraceptive in research trials but is not yet available for that purpose in any country.

When standard COCs are used for emergency contraception, they are called ECPs (emergency contraceptive pills). Though commonly known as the "morning after" pill, ECPs may actually be taken immediately after unprotected intercourse and up to 72 hours beyond; dosage and timing of administration vary according to formulation. Minipills are contraceptive pills that contain only progestin (and not estrogen). Their side effects (nausea and vomiting) are far less common than with COCs, but the window of use is narrower: The time limit for postcoital administration is 48 hours. The copper-T IUD can be inserted up to seven days after unprotected intercourse, is significantly more effective than either ECPs or minipills, and can be left in place to provide continuous effective contraception for up to 10 years. However, like any IUD, it requires skilled insertion using antiseptic practice and is not ideal for women at risk of sexually transmitted diseases (Hatcher et al. 1995).

In Europe, the main hormonal method used is the "Yuzpe Regimen," the sequential administration of higher-than-usual doses of estrogen and progestogen, marketed by Schering AG under the brand name PC4 and licensed in the United Kingdom and some European countries. The Hungarian company, Gedeon Richter, markets the progestogen-only product "Postinor" as a postcoital contraceptive in eastern Europe and some countries of the Far East (Hughes 1995).[4]

Each of the three methods that are available in the United States requires a prescription and all are currently marketed as regular methods of ongoing contraception; none is marketed as an emergency contraceptive, primarily because no pharmaceutical company has applied to the FDA to market emergency contraceptives (Kaiser/Harris 1995). Without FDA approval, manufacturers cannot market or advertise these products for postcoital use, so the normal educational function of drug promotion is absent (Hatcher et al. 1995). As a consequence, most women and many clinicians do not know about emergency contraception, even though a clinician may legally prescribe an approved drug for an unlabeled purpose ("off-label use") and even though considerable research demonstrates that emergency contraceptives are safe and effective (Grossman and Grossman 1994; Trussell and Ellertson 1995).

CONTRACEPTIVE OPTIONS FOR
THE NEXT DECADE, 1995–2005

While dramatically new approaches to contraception may take decades to develop (see Chapter 4), some areas of research and development have advanced and, all things being equal, could produce new contraceptive formulations within the next 10 years (PATH March 1993, June 1993, 1995). It takes a tremendous amount of time—a minimum of 15 years—to develop and market any new pharmaceutical from start to finish. For that reason, approaches considered here include only products that are already in some stage of the drug development process, even if that stage is relatively early.

Thus, this section is about transition, from the universe of existing contraceptive methods to the universe of shifting emphases indicated by the women's agenda and new targets that might permit response to those emphases and to the general public health need for a fuller range of contraceptive options for women and for men. The categories reviewed are: (1) improved methods for women, including improved oral contraceptives, new delivery systems, postcoital methods, and better barrier methods; and (2) more methods for men.

Improved Oral Contraceptives

Throughout the period during which oral contraceptives have been used—nearly 40 years—continually better formulations have been introduced, with improvements focusing on development of new progestins and lower levels of hormone content, both estrogen and progestin. Work continues in areas of further refinement.

One line of current OC research and development focuses on designing new regimens for taking the drug. These include shortening the pill-free interval and changing the sequence of administering estrogen and progestin (the so-called priming regimen). The purpose of these changes is to reduce the dose of the drugs without sacrificing what has been achieved in efficacy and cycle control.

Incorporating new estrogens into OCs—either natural estrogens or, further down the road, synthetic ones—is another area of current research. The goal is to reduce some of the drug's current undesirable side effects. These include, in some women, weight gain, mood swings, unfavorable bone and lipid effects, and increased blood coagulability, which occasionally can lead to thromboembolism and stroke.

New progestogens also offer hope for reducing the current liabilities of OCs. Moreover, they may allow researchers to develop contraceptives targeted specifically to a subset of the general pill-taking population, for example, OCs designed specifically for smokers, overweight women, or teenagers who are prone to acne.

While not as advanced, there is considerable research being conducted on the development of tissue-selective steroid hormones. The hope in this area is to come up with a steroid that specifically targets key reproductive tissues. Researchers may also be able to develop nonsteroid molecules that interact only with specific estrogen or progesterone receptors. Both of these advances could reduce the occurrence of unwanted side effects elsewhere in the body.

Because many women taking progestin-only formulations experience bleeding problems, a high priority in OC research today has become the mechanism of uterine bleeding. If it were better understood and these problems were prevented, women might more often choose and continue with this effective method of contraception. This is an area where basic science still has work to do.

Another area of work is predicated on the hormone responsible for seasonal breeding cycles in most mammalian species, melatonin, which has been found to combine with ovarian hormones to shut off the hypothalamic center directing ovulation. This line of inquiry has been pursued by a small pharmaceutical company, Applied Medical Research, which has developed "B-Oval," a new generation estrogen-free oral contraceptive containing a patented formulation of 75 mg melatonin and 0.5 mg norethindrone, the most widely used progestogen over the last 20 years. The product is in the preliminary stages of phase III clinical trials in the United States (Executive Briefing 1995).

Research into the areas mentioned above could provide significant improvements in a relatively short period of time. The consideration of recent scientific advances supports this notion. Our increasing understanding of the molecular mechanisms through which steroid hormones function, the development of molecular models for some of these mechanisms as well as effective screens for steroid receptors, and the recent identification of steroid receptor subtypes and their associated proteins provide a broad knowledge base. New developments in combinatorial chemistry and high-throughput screening allow researchers to make, and screen, enormous numbers of new chemical compounds in a very short period of time. The combination of this new knowledge with these relatively new techniques could make for a relatively short development period.

For many years, clinicians have recognized the additional benefits to reproductive health that OCs can provide, although women themselves have not (American College of Obstetricians and Gynecologists 1994 and 1985; Russell 1996b). As indicated earlier in this chapter, depending on a woman's age and health status, these benefits can include protection against ovarian and endometrial cancer, pelvic inflammatory disease, fibrocystic breast disease, ovarian cysts, ectopic pregnancy, iron-deficiency anemia, dysmenorrhea, and osteoporosis. As today's mandate for combining effective contraception with methods to improve women's health grows, this aspect of OCs should be considered in all future research and development decisions.

From a market perspective, there are two sets of arguments for the continued investment in improvements in oral contraceptives. One is that the pharmaceutical industry has an enormous amount of money and expertise already invested in this product line. In addition, with some exceptions, for instance, China, where IUD use is more common, and Japan, where the marketing of oral contraceptives is prohibited, oral contraceptives are the most frequently used method of reversible contraception in the world and thus constitute a large and established market. Furthermore, many of the liability issues that affected oral contraceptives in the past are now resolved, so that future risk is attenuated although, at least in the highly litigious climate in the United States, that risk is ever-present.

An alternative perspective is that there are enough highly effective oral contraceptives already on the market and improvements are likely to be quite marginal, so that further work in this field has low priority compared to the need for new products to meet new priorities. This leaves the question of whether, if funding were to be removed from OC research and development, it would then be shifted into other areas of contraception. Absent positive incentives, some companies currently in the field might dismantle their contraceptive research teams and devote the freed-up resources to other, less risky areas of research and development. There is also the matter of negative stimuli, one of which is the fact that the USFDA considers all oral contraceptives as belonging to a single class of drugs. Such "class labeling" prevents manufacturers from differentiating among products so that they can charge more for some formulations than others.

New Drug Delivery Systems

The principal focus of innovation in drug delivery systems for contraceptives has been on implants and injectables, a focus that includes not only attempts to improve the mechanisms of delivery but the pharmacological content of what they deliver. Implants and injectable contraceptives offer a number of advantages over other methods of contraception. Perhaps the most important is that they have a high degree of efficacy, combined with narrow margins for failure. Furthermore, the fact that they are, almost by definition, long-lasting—the most commonly used formulations range from three months (Depo-Provera) to five years (Norplant) in duration of efficacy—is seen as attractive by a number of women. Others, who do not want to be dependent on having to see a clinician, do not find these methods appropriate.

Current implants and injectables for women all contain progestins which, as noted earlier in this chapter, work by blocking ovulation and increasing the thickness of cervical mucus so that sperm have difficulty moving through the system. The pioneer in this area was Norplant; its successor, Norplant II, releases the same amount of levonorgestrel as the present Norplant formulation but through two rather than six implants, making insertion and removal easier. It is worth noting that the two-rod presentation might well have superseded the six-rod system that came onto the market, except for the fact that production of the original elastomer for the Silastic tubing was halted, requiring a shift to another elastomer and thereby slowing the approval process in the United States.

Other new implant systems are in various stages of development, again with emphasis focused on reducing the number of capsules, varying the length of effectiveness, and offering biodegradability. Considerable work is being done on single-rod implants, including Implanon, Uniplant, and a device using the progestin Nestorone (ST-1435). By reducing the number of rods implanted, the new products should make this long-lasting form of contraception more appealing to users. Now in phase III clinical trials, Norplant II and Implanon are the most advanced of the new possibilities (Coutinho 1993; Singh et al. 1985 and 1989).

Implant manufacturers are engaged in development of single-rod implants and, probably further into the future, biodegradable implants that will eventually dissolve in the body but will be removable, and hence reversible, for a while (Alexander 1995). Primate studies conducted by researchers under the aegis of NICHD suggest that the possibility is not far-fetched and that a levonorgestrel-containing biodegradable implant (Capronor) can provide adequate contraception for up to two years; however, the biodegradability aspect of this method remains challenging (Darney 1994) and we are still speaking of animal models. Other biodegradable formulations under study include norethindrone pellets (implants [e.g., Annuelle, Endocon]) and norethindrone microspheres (injectable).

Another product that should be available relatively soon is the vaginal ring, a doughnut-shaped ring that fits in the vagina and releases either progestin alone or a combination of estrogen and progestin. The progestin-only rings can be worn continuously; the combination rings would be removed for one week in every four to allow for menses. While less long-lasting than implants, these products offer advantages over daily pill-taking or insertion of another contraceptive product; at the same time, they are under the immediate control of the user, an important feature for many women. Researchers are also working on development of a vaginal ring for lactating women that would last for three months; efficacy and acceptability have been demonstrated in large multicenter trials (Landgren 1994; Mishell 1993).

Also well advanced is a new IUD that releases a progestin for up to five years. Already available in some European countries, this new device seems to have fewer side effects—for instance, cramping, blood loss, and increased risk of pelvic inflammatory disease—than traditional IUDs and has a very low pregnancy rate (WHO 1994b). The expectation is that new implants for women that are more easily inserted and removed, as well as a hormone-releasing vaginal ring, will be available by the year 2000; the progestin-releasing IUD should be available in the United States by the year 2005 (Alexander 1995; WHO 1995a).

The only contraceptive injectable for women on the U.S. market so far is Depo-Provera (although others are available elsewhere in the world). A number of institutions are working to develop new injectable contraceptives such as levonorgestrel butanoate (WHO 1995a) and, as mentioned above, norethisterone microspheres. Some of these products do contain estrogen as well as progestin, thereby overcoming the bleeding side effect.

While ranking high in efficacy, one problem with all implants on the market and most that are under development today is that they contain only progestin (as opposed to a combination of estrogen and progestin). In many users, progestin-only products cause irregular uterine bleeding as a side effect (particularly in the early stages of use), which limits their acceptability.

Although research on implants and injectables has focused on developing products for women (as has most contraceptive research), there are a few products that fall into this category that are now under development for men. These are discussed below in the context of new contraceptive methods for males.

Better Barrier Methods

Mechanical Barriers

The barrier methods of contraception that are now available are either mechanical (male and female condoms, diaphragms, and cervical caps), chemical (spermicides and other formulations), or some combination of both, all of which are inadequate to needs. Recognition of this inadequacy has motivated movement toward research to correct it, involving efforts by a number of public sector entities, including the World Health Organization's Special Programme of Research, Development and Research Training in Human Reproduction (WHO/HRP) and the Human Immunodeficiency Network (HIV/NET); the NICHD's Center for Population Research; and Family Health International and the Contraceptive Research and Development (CONRAD) Program, both supported by the U.S. Agency for International Development (USAID). The driving objectives of these efforts are to improve product safety and efficacy, formulations, and configurations; to widen the spectrum of barrier methods that women can control and use discreetly (Mauck et al. 1994, Stewart 1994); and to determine acceptability prior to decisions about market launch.

One especially active area of research is in efforts to combine contraceptives with effective mechanical barriers to sexually transmitted diseases (STDs). Included in this category are methods developed for contraception, some of which *may* provide protection against STDs. These include Lea's Shield and FemCap. Lea's Shield is a "one size fits all" device that blocks the cervix but has a valve that allows passage of cervical secretions and facilitates insertion. FemCap is a new cervical cap with a design that increases apposition to the cervix and vaginal wall and is sized based on parity. Both devices could become available within a few years. Their efficacy against pregnancy or infection is still unknown and their present costs would be prohibitive for many women. The usefulness in much of the developing world of any such coitus-dependent method that is both costly and dependent on access to privacy and clean water remains questionable.

In addition, manufacturers have developed a new vaginal sponge, Protectaid, which incorporates three spermicides that have a synergistic spermicidal and microbicidal effect and is designed to provide STD protection without irritating the vaginal epithelium (Psychoyos et al. 1994). The sponge contains a compound spermicide, microbicide, and virucide that, in laboratory studies, has inactivated HIV as well as chlamydia and trichomonas. With the withdrawal from the market of the Today sponge in 1995, there is no other comparable product available in any market.

Chemical Barriers

The spermicides that are now on the market are not very effective against either sperm or pathogenic organisms. This may be due to weaknesses in certain characteristics of these products. Due to their short period of activity and messiness, many of these formulations are not seen by users as particularly desirable. While some spermicides, specifically nonoxynol-9, can kill HIV and bacteria in laboratory studies, there is concern that, as a detergent, it may also kill cells and irritate the vaginal epithelium, thereby possibly elevating susceptibility to HIV transmission. This has led many researchers to suggest that research should now focus on noncytotoxic rather than cytotoxic methods of stopping sexually transmitted pathogens.

Any potential new barrier method should not compromise natural defenses and, if possible, should strengthen them. Defense mechanisms include a thick epithelial lining and mucus secretion during certain stages of the menstrual cycle, both of which provide a physical barrier. The vagina and cervix are also equipped to mount antibody and cell-mediated immune responses against pathogens, and secretions from these areas contain several nonspecific antibacterial and antiviral defense agents, including lysozyme, polyamines, zinc, hydrogen peroxide, lactoferrin, and B-defensins. Finally, the natural flora of the vagina, that is, lactobacilli, keep the vaginal pH low (Larsen 1993), creating yet another deterrent to microbes. Current research focuses on developing a chemical barrier that would be nontoxic and nonirritating to these beneficial microbes and at the same time capable of killing or disabling invading pathogens.

Researchers at Johns Hopkins University are working with the support of the NICHD and the National Institute of Allergy and Infectious Disease and, most recently, with the HIV/NET component of the Global Programme on AIDS, on development of buffer gels[5] that can maintain vaginal acidity even in the presence of semen and cervical mucus. The gels are created with nonmetabolizable polymers that should produce only minimal perturbation of the normal vaginal flora. Because the cell membranes and the vaginal epithelium are not permeable to polymers, they can provide high buffer capacity without producing the toxicity or irritation caused by high concentrations of membrane-permeable weak acids (e.g., lactic and acetic acids). Indeed, the gel simply increases the buffer capacity of vaginal fluids sufficiently to overcome the neutralizing action of semen and cervical mucus. Furthermore, compared with other broad-spectrum microbicides, an acidic buffer is less likely to irritate or disturb normal vaginal microflora.

This combination of characteristics suggests that the gels can be used to create new methods for vaginal protection against pregnancy and STDs and could also serve as drug-delivery vehicles for vaginal therapy (e.g., during menses and menopause, for vaginal bacteriosis). They may also help prevent the onset or relapse of vaginal and urinary tract infections. More specifically, the ReProtect gel formulation also has excellent qualities as a sexual lubricant; is inexpensive, colorless, and odorless; and its constituents are in products already approved by the FDA for vaginal use or that are generally recognized as safe. Pilot experiments using the mouse/HSV-2 model demonstrate that the gel's acidic-buffer action blocks vaginal and genital skin transmission of genital herpes infections, which suggests that it might also be effective against HIV infections. The gel will go into phase I trials in Boston, Malawi, India, Zimbabwe, and Thailand in 1996 (K Whaley, personal communication, February 1996). Another vaginal gel formulation, PC 213, comprised of sulphated polysaccharides, has completed Phase I vaginal irritation studies, under the aegis of the Population Council (Stein 1995).

Another possibility is a vaginal product containing squalamine, a natural substance that appears to be spermicidal as well as microbicidal. Isolated from animals, squalamine is thought to protect them from a wide range of diseases. Further animal studies are being conducted prior to doing safety studies in women, under a Cooperative Research and Development Agreement between NICHD and Magainin Pharmaceuticals (N Alexander, personal communication, 1995; Russell 1996a).

There is other research that builds on compounds derived from plants that have exhibited spermicidal and virucidal properties. The National Institute of Immunology in India has isolated oils from the neem tree (*Azadirachta indica*). One formulation, Praneem polyherbal cream, combines neem seed extract with soapnut extract (*Sapindus mukerossi*), and is said to induce local cell-mediated immunity. Phase II trials are reported to be under way in India. Other plant extracts being studied for their potential ability to kill sperm, bacteria, and viruses include papain from papaya and gossypol from cottonseed oil.

One unresolved and quite urgent issue concerning combination contraceptive *cum* anti-STD agents in the United States is how they will fare in the FDA approval processes. Guidelines from the agency will be utterly essential for research and development in this area if new methods are to make their way into a very needy market. At the time of this writing, there are no FDA guidelines for research and development activities with respect to products in this combined category.

New Postcoital Methods

Antiprogestins

A rich and novel area of work in recent years has been around the anti-progestins (sometimes referred to as antiprogestogens), steroid antihormones with a unique ability to block the action of progesterone at the cellular level through binding to the progesterone receptor in target tissues (Van Look and von Hertzen 1993). Progesterone exerts well-documented effects throughout the reproductive system (including the uterus, cervix, breast, and pituitary-hypothalamic system) and plays a key role in both establishing and maintaining pregnancy. It also exerts less well-defined actions on tissues outside the reproductive system (e.g., brain, vascular endothelial cells) and on lipid metabolism (Baulieu 1993; IOM 1993).

The first antiprogestin was discovered fortuitously by scientists searching for an antiglucocorticoid, a compound that would interfere with the action of adrenal gland hormones, glucocorticoids, that are involved in the physiologic regulation of virtually all tissues in the body (IOM 1993). While several hundred anti-progestins have been synthesized, only three have been given to humans (mife-pristone, lilopristone, and onapristone). Just one of those, mifepristone—RU 486—has been extensively studied in humans, most widely as a means of nonsur-gical termination of early pregnancy (Van Look and von Hertzen 1993).[6] The compound has been licensed for that purpose in France, Sweden, and the United Kingdom, and is being manufactured in China. In the United States, RU 486 is in phase III clinical trials under the aegis of the Population Council (IOM 1993).

One of the most promising potential uses of antiprogestins is as a postcoital emergency contraceptive that would reduce the chance of undesired pregnancy after unprotected intercourse around the time of ovulation. Because of the critical role progesterone plays in early transformation of the endometrium (and its pos-sible role in follicular maturation and ovulation), researchers hypothesized that mifepristone might act as an effective postcoital contraceptive. Studies in En-gland and Scotland have supported this hypothesis (Baird et al.1988).

Researchers have also experimented with antiprogestins as expected menses inducers (EMIs, taken regularly just before the onset of expected menstruation) and missed menses inducers (MMIs, taken only when the menstrual period does not occur). Perhaps most promising has been work combining an antiprogestin (mifepristone) with a prostaglandin (gemeprost). In a recent study, researchers working in six countries demonstrated that a combination of mifepristone fol-lowed two days later by gemeprost-induced menstruation in 98 percent of a group of women who were up to 10 days late getting their periods (Van Look and von Hertzen 1993).

The potential of the antiprogestins goes well beyond emergency contraception. Their role in human health and disease could be large, given their applicability to a variety of reproductive and nonreproductive conditions. Research has suggested that antiprogestins may have clinical value in treating endometriosis, uterine leiomyomas (fibroid tumors), and endometrial and breast cancers. They also appear to offer value for obstetrics and fertility regulation. The antiprogestins also have potential for use as antifertility agents by inhibiting ovulation, preventing or disrupting implantation, and/or inducing luteal regression. During the early luteal phase, mifepristone may prove to be not only an effective postcoital agent used under circumstances of emergency but as a once-a-month pill or menses-inducer. The role of antiprogestins as ovulation inhibitors could be particularly attractive, since this is already a widely accepted category of contraceptive. Antiprogestins may also have clinical utility for the treatment of several other conditions, most importantly including meningioma (tumors arising from membranes surrounding the brain) and, because of their antiglucocorticoid effects, in palliative treatment of hypercortisolism due to Cushing's syndrome, some forms of depression and glycoma, and wound healing (Baird 1993; Croxatto et al. 1993; IOM 1993; Van Look and von Hertzen 1993).

There is much research to be done in all these areas and, from this broader perspective, the antiprogestin compounds should be highly attractive to industry. However, perhaps the most striking aspect of the antiprogestins, as seen in the history of RU 486, is the extent to which medical and economic decisions about their development, clinical testing, marketing, and use are being shaped by social and political forces, centering on strongly held, powerful secular and religious values either favoring or opposing abortion (Swazey 1992). The core issue in the controversy is the use of RU 486 or future antiprogestins as abortifacients (Banwell and Paxman 1992; Swazey 1992). The range of actions of the antiprogestins, together with incomplete understanding of their mechanisms (IOM 1993), can blur distinctions between contraception and abortion, conception and pregnancy, and become entangled in the sometimes vague legislative language used to describe events in the reproductive process (Banwell and Paxman 1992; Cook 1989; Swazey 1992). Roussel-Uclaf, the developer of mifepristone, assigned the rights for production and distribution of RU 486 in the United States to the Population Council, citing a "hostile political climate in the United States" (Roussel-Uclaf press release, cited in US Department of State 1993; Tanouye 1994) and is said to have closed its research laboratories in this area. In such a climate, it seems unlikely that any large pharmaceutical company would work in this product category, even were the financial gain to be large (Swazey 1992). Two European companies (Organon and Schering AG) have also developed effective antiprogestins, but have decided *not* to bring them to market.

Methods for Males

Other than modifications of the male condom, work on alternative contraceptive methods for men has been limited largely to techniques to permit reversal of sterilization, primarily different methods for occluding the vas deferens and use of no-scalpel vasectomy. A mechanical intervention that is nearing completion in India involves injecting into the vas deferens a non-toxic polymer (styrene maleic anhydride) that blocks the passage of sperm. Unlike a vasectomy, this method is intended to be reversible. Another substance, dimethyl sulphoxide (DMSO), can be injected to dissolve the first. While early animal toxicity studies suggested that DMSO might be carcinogenic, later studies proved those fears unfounded. The product is now being tested in clinical trials with humans.

The other area of work has centered on administration of hormones to inhibit spermatogenesis, the process of sperm production that is regulated by luteinizing hormone (LH) and follicle stimulating hormone (FSH). One hormonal method for men being investigated by the Population Council is a system of two implants which could provide a convenient one-year contraceptive method for men. One implant delivers an agonist of luteinizing hormone releasing hormone (LHRH) that suppresses sperm production; the other implant, required to compensate for resulting diminution of testosterone, the androgen that governs sexual function, supplies a synthetic androgen (MENT) (Waites 1992). This system is in phase I clinical trials in two countries, and entering human trials under the Population Council (WHO 1995a).

Antifertility vaccines that neutralize hormones required for sperm production or sperm maturation are also in the early stages of development, again under the aegis of the Population Council and the National Institute of Immunology (New Delhi). Phase I clinical trials were expanded in 1993 and, as of June 1995, 12 men had been immunized. The vaccine would be combined with the MENT implant to provide androgen replacement needed for normal sex drive and behavior.

In addition to the challenge of affecting spermatogenesis without impact on sexual function, there is the challenge of achieving infertility in all subjects. International multicenter studies by the WHO and CONRAD/USAID have been struggling with this dilemma and have produced considerable understanding but no product yet. Another challenge has been finding a delivery mechanism that can provide more than a week's worth of protection and there have been international collaborative efforts over the past 15 years to develop longer-acting steroid formulations. This research has focused on methods of administering testosterone, either as testosterone enanthate (TE) or testosterone buciclate, alone or in combination with a progestin such as DMPA or levonorgestrel, or anti-androgenic steroids (e.g., cyproterone acetate, CPA) to interfere with spermatogenesis (Contraceptive Technology Update, August 1995).

The problem with any method that is based on suppression of spermatogenesis is the two- to three-month delay between method initiation and infertility, requiring use of another contraceptive method during the initial months of use (PATH 1995). Researchers are evaluating and planning evaluations of the efficacy and acceptability of testosterone enanthate, levonorgestrel butanoate/testosterone buciclate (WHO/NICHD), 7-alpha-19-methyl-nortestosterone (MENT) (Population Council), levonorgestrel/testosterone enanthate, and desogestrel/testosterone enanthate (University of Washington/CONRAD). Work on the latter combination is particularly promising, since it exhibits faster suppression of spermatogenesis than any testosterone formulation alone. The level of suppression approaches complete azoospermia. When the drug is discontinued, sperm counts rapidly return to normal. Some analysts predict that such a product could be available by the year 2005 (Alexander 1995).

Because of the challenges of duration, lag times in return to fertility, and hormonal balance that have been the focus in work on male methods to date, there is something of a shift in research emphasis toward an emphasis on how to interfere with sperm maturation rather than sperm production (spermatogenesis), since that would avoid disruption of the hormonal balance needed for sexual function. Eventually, new knowledge on the basic biology of reproduction should allow researchers to interfere with spermatogenesis closer to the end of the process, that is, in the testes or epididymis rather than the brain or pituitary, thereby avoiding the wide range of systemic effects. The products of such research are unlikely to be available in the next decade and are, therefore, discussed in further detail in the following chapter.

A final avenue of research focuses on plant compounds that interfere with male fertility. The best known—and most controversial—of these compounds, gossypol, is derived from cottonseed oil. Studied now for over two decades, gossypol is known to effectively suppress sperm production, but has also caused hypokalemia and irreversible infertility in a significant number of subjects. *Tripterygium wilfordii*, a vine that grows in southern China, has also shown promise as a possible reversible male contraceptive. Researchers have thus far identified six components of the plant with antifertility activity. While toxicology studies have not been completed, these plant compounds show particular promise because they seem to work by interfering in sperm maturation in the epididymis, thus offering a potential contraceptive without side effects involving male sex hormones.

CONCLUDING COMMENT

At the outset of this chapter, we stated that there was reasonable probability that a number of improvements in existing contraceptive technologies could become available in the next decade. We also used the term "all things being equal." The case of RU 486, the tensions around the approvals of the Avanti and Reality condoms, and the still-pending fate of Norplant liability, make it clear that all things are not, in fact, equal. At the same time, the history of the oral contraceptive and the IUD, troubled in a variety of ways, suggests that the needs of individuals worldwide to plan their families somehow, sooner or later, wins out.

REFERENCES

Alexander NJ. Future contraceptives: Vaccines for men and women will eventually join new implants, better spermicides and stronger, thinner condoms. Scientific American 273(3):136–141, 1995.

American College of Obstetricians and Gynecologists (ACOG). Poll shows women still skeptical of contraceptive safety: ACOG News Release. Washington, DC: American College of Obstetricians and Gynecologists. 1994.

ACOG. Attitudes Toward Contraception. Princeton, NJ: The Gallup Organization. 1985.

American Health Consultants. AIDS Alert: Special Series on Avanti Condom 10(1):1–16, 1995; 10(2):17–32, 1995; 10(5)71–72, 1995.

Baird DR. Potential contraceptive effects of antigestogens. IN Clinical Applications of Mifepristone (RU 486) and Other Antiprogestins: Assessing the Science and Recommending a Research Agenda. MS Donaldson, L Dorflinger, SS Brown, LZ Benet, eds. Washington, DC: National Academy Press. 1993.

Baird DT, M Rodger, IT Cameron, et al. Prostaglandins and antiestrogens for the interruption of early pregnancy. Journal of Reproduction and Fertility 36:173–179, 1988.

Banwell SS, JM Paxman. The search for meaning: RU 486 and the law of abortion. American Journal of Public Health 82(10):1399–1406, October 1992.

Bardin CW. Mechanism of action of IUDs. Paper presented at: "IUDs—A State-of-the-Art Conference," National Institutes of Health, Bethesda, MD, 15–16 February 1996.

Baulieu EE. RU 486—A decade on today and tomorrow. IN Clinical Applications of Mifepristone (RU 486) and Other Antiprogestins: Assessing the Science and Recommending a Research Agenda. MS Donaldson, L Dorflinger, SS Brown, LZ Benet, eds. Washington, DC: National Academy Press. 1993.

Camp S. Emergency contraception in seven European countries. Reproductive Health Technologies Project 7:12, 1994.

Contraceptive Technology Update (untitled), August 1995.

Contraceptive Technology Update. Special Report: Studies Found Plastic Condom Unsafe, yet FDA Cleared It for Market, June 1995.

Cook RJ. Antiprogestin drugs: Medical and legal issues. Family Planning Perspectives 21(6):267–272, 1989.

Coutinho E. One year contraception with a single subdermal implant containing nomegestrol acetate (Uniplant). Contraception 47:97–105, 1993.

Croxatto HB, AM Salvatierra, HD Croxatto, et al. Effects of continuous treatment with low dose mifepristone throughout one menstrual cycle. Human Reproduction 8:201–207, 1993.

Darney PD. Hormonal implants: Contraception for a new century. American Journal of Obstetrics and Gynecology 170:1536–1543, 1994.

Executive Briefing. Melatonin—A New Approach to Contraception. October 1995.

Farley TMM, MS Rosenberg, PJ Rowe, et al. Intrauterine devices and pelvic inflammatory disease: An international perspective. Lancet 339(8796):785–788, 1992.

Grossman RA, BD Grossman. How frequently is emergency contraception prescribed? Family Planning Perspectives 26(6):270–271, 1994.

Hatcher RA, J Trussell, F Stewart, et al. Emergency Contraception: The Nation's Best Kept Secret. Decatur, GA: Bridging the Gap Communications. 1995.

Hatcher RA, J Trussell, F Stewart, et al. Contraceptive Technology, 16th Revised Edition. New York: Irvington Publishers. 1994.

Hughes S. Emergency contraception—A hard pill to swallow? Scrip Magazine, October 1995.

Institute of Medicine (IOM). Summary of Proceedings: Workshop on Contraceptive Research and Development and the Frontiers of Contemporary Science, 9–10 December 1994. Washington, DC: Division of Health Sciences Policy. Unpublished document. 1995.

IOM. Clinical Applications of Mifepristone (RU 486) and Other Antiprogestins: Assessing the Science and Recommending a Research Agenda. MS Donaldson, L Dorflinger, SS Brown, LZ Benet, eds. Washington, DC: National Academy Press. 1993.

Kaiser/Harris. Survey on Obstetricians/Gynecologists' Attitudes and Practices Related to Contraception and Family Planning, 1 February–21 March 1995. Menlo Park, CA: The Kaiser Family Foundation. 1995.

Labbok M, A Pérez, V Valdés, et al. The Lactational Amenorrhea Method: A new postpartum introductory family planning method with program and policy implications. Advances in Contraception 10:93–109, 1994.

Labbok M, V Jennings. Advances in fertility regulation through ovulation prediction during lactation and during menstrual cycles. IN Contraceptive Research and Development 1994: The Road from Mexico City to Cairo and Beyond. PFA Van Look, G Pérez-Palacios, eds. Delhi: Oxford University Press. 1994.

[The] Lancet. Editorial: After the morning after and the morning after that. Lancet 345(8962):1381–1382, 1995.

Landgren B-M, A-R Aedo, E Johannisson, et al. Studies on a vaginal ring releasing levonorgestrel when used alone or in combination with transdermal systems releasing estradiol. Contraception 50:87–100, 1994.

Larsen B. Vaginal flora in health and disease. Clinical Obstetrics and Gynecology 36:107–121, 1993.

Mauck CK, M Cordero, HL Gabelnick, JM Spieler, R Rivera, eds. Barrier Contraceptives: Current Status and Future Prospects. New York: Wiley-Liss. 1994.

McCann MF, LS Potter. Progestin-only oral contraception: A comprehensive review. Contraception 50(6):S13–S21, 1994.

Mishell DR Jr. Vaginal contraceptive rings. Annals of Medicine 25:191–197, 1993.

Pérez A, M Labbok, J Queenan. A clinical study of the lactational amenorrhea method for family planning. Lancet 339:968–970, 1992.

Program for Appropriate Technology in Health (PATH). Contraceptive research and development: Progress toward a woman-centered agenda. OutLook 13(2), 1995.

PATH. Contraceptive technologies in development: Many leads, progress slow. OutLook 11(2):1–8, June 1993.

PATH. Selected Contraceptive Technologies in Development. Seattle, WA. March 1993.

Psychoyos A, G Creatsas, E Hassan, et al. Spermicidal and antiviral properties of cholic acid: Contraceptive efficacy of a new vaginal sponge (Protectaid) containing sodium cholate. Human Reproduction 8(6):866–869, 1994.

Queenan JT, M Labbok. Periodic abstinence: The "natural family planning" methods. IN The Best of Dialogues in Contraception. D Mitchell, ed. Los Angeles: Health Learning Systems. 1992.

Russell C. From frogs and sharks, a better vaginal foam? Washington Post, Health section, p. 7, 20 February. 1996a.

Russell C. The pill is popular but not well understood: New survey shows many women overestimate the risks, underestimate the benefits. Washington Post, Health section, p. 9, 6 February. 1996b.

Singh M, BB Saxena, R Craver et al. Contraceptive efficacy of norethindrone encapsulated in injectable biodegradable poly-dl-lactide-coglycolide microspheres: Phase II clinical study. Fertility and Sterility 52:973–980, 1989.

Singh M, BB Saxena, R Landesman, et al. Contraceptive efficacy of bioabsorbable pellets of norethindrone (NET) as subcutaneous implants: Phase II clinical study. Advances in Contraception 1:131–149, 1985.

Stein Z. Barriers Women Can Use in Preventing STDs/HIV: Summary and Recommendations from the November 1995 Meeting of the American Public Health Association, San Diego, California (memorandum). New York: Columbia University. November 1995.

Stewart F. Vaginal barrier contraceptives and infection risk. IN Barrier Contraceptives: Current Status and Future Prospects, CK Mauck, M Cordero, H Gabelnick, et al., eds. New York: Wiley-Liss. 1994.

Swazey JP, ed. Conference on the Development and Use of Antiprogestin Drugs: Social, Political, Economic, and Legal Issues, 6–7 February 1992, Palm Beach, Florida. Boston, MA: Medicine in the Public Interest. 1992.

Tanouye E. Technology and health: U.S. companies targeted in protest of abortion pill. Wall Street Journal, 8 July 1994.

Trussell J, C Ellertson. Efficacy of emergency contraception. Fertility Control Reviews 4(2):8–11, 1995.

U.S. Department of State. French abortion pill to be marketed in the U.S. by an American company. Incoming Telegram (unclassified) from U.S. Embassy Paris, 29 April 1993.

Van Look PFA, G Pérez-Palacios, eds. Contraceptive Research and Development 1984 to 1994: The Road from Mexico City to Cairo and Beyond. Delhi: Oxford University Press. 1994.

Van Look PFA, H von Hertzen. Post-ovulatory methods of fertility regulation: The emergence of antiprogestogens. IN Institute of Medicine. Clinical Applications of Mifepristone (RU 486) and Other Antiprogestins. Washington, DC: National Academy Press. 1993.

Waites G. Methods for the regulation of male fertility. Annual Technical Report of the Task Force on Methods for the Regulation of Male Fertility. Geneva: World Health Organization. 1992.

White K. Contraceptive makers chilled by court challenges. Journal of Women's Health 4(3), 1995.

World Health Organization (WHO). The Role of the Programme in Technology Development and Assessment: A Discussion Paper. Geneva: UNDP/UNFPA/WHO/World Bank/WHO Special Programme of Research, Development and Research Training in Human Reproduction. 1995a.

WHO. International Consultation for Policy-Makers on Women and AIDS in Preparation for the Beijing Conference, 6–8 February 1995. Geneva: Global Programme on AIDS. 1995b.

WHO. Challenges in Reproductive Health Research: Biennial Report 1992–1993. Geneva: Special Programme of Research, Development and Research Training in Human Reproduction. 1994a.

WHO (Special Programme of Research, Development and Research Training in Human Reproduction, IUD Research Group. A randomized multicentre trial of the Multiload 375 and TCu380A IUDs in parous women: Three-year results. Contraception 49:543–549, 1994b.

WHO. Annual Technical Report 1992. Geneva: Special Programme of Research, Development and Research Training in Human Reproduction. Geneva: World Health Organization. 1993.

NOTES

1. A minipill is an oral contraceptive containing no estrogen and generally less than 1 mg of a progestational agent per pill (Hatcher et al. 1994).

2. The U.S. Food and Drug Administration (FDA) recently approved labeling changes extending the use of the Copper T380A from 8 to 10 years and made two additional labeling revisions. First, the FDA added data from studies by the WHO, Population Council, and the manufacturer indicating that the risk of PID is highest 20 days post-insertion, then declines, and remains low and constant thereafter (Farley et al. 1992). Second, a history of ectopic pregnancy is no longer a contraindication.

3. This refutes the usually held perception that the major mechanism of action of IUDs in

humans is to disrupt implantation of a fertilized ova. Thus, it would seem to be no longer tenable to propose that the major action of IUDs is to induce abortion (Bardin 1996).

4. Oral contraceptives are packaged specifically for emergency contraception use in Bulgaria, Finland, Germany, Hungary, Jamaica, Malaysia, the Netherlands, Nigeria, Pakistan, Poland, Singapore, states of the former Soviet Union, Sweden, Switzerland, the United Kingdom, Uruguay, and Zimbabwe (Camp 1994). They have been marketed for emergency contraception in England since 1984.

5. The gels are currently covered by a patent application assigned to ReProtect, LC.

6. Antiprogestins that have reached *in vivo* testing include onapristone, lilipristone, and ZK 98 734 (Schering AG); ORG 31710 and 31806 (Organon); and HRP 2000 (Research Triangle Institute)(Institute of Medicine 1993).

4

Contraceptive Technology and the State of the Science: New Horizons

Beyond those contraceptive technologies that are likely to be developed within the next decade (Chapter 3), several lines of scientific research offer the promise of new and innovative approaches to contraception in the longer term. This chapter looks at these approaches within three broad categories: (1) female methods, (2) male methods, and (3) immunocontraception, areas that offer promise for both males and females. Together, these sections constitute a summary of the longer, fully referenced authored papers that were specifically commissioned for this study and appear in this report as Appendixes A, B, C, and D. Each section of this chapter is also linked to a table which summarizes the mechanisms that this committee considers important candidates for contraceptive research and the development of new methods.

A STRATEGY FOR BASIC RESEARCH ON CONTRACEPTION

Identification of Targets Through Molecular Biology

In all organisms a small number of germ cells are set aside from somatic cells in early embryogenesis. Usually they remain in an undifferentiated quiescent state while somatic cells are dividing and forming recognizable tissues and organs. Germ cells begin to divide rather late in fetal life after they have settled in the germinal ridge.

This gonial stage is followed by cessation of mitotic cell division, differentiation, maturation, and meiosis. Every step of gamete formation is unique. In addition there are support organs that are partly or entirely devoted to conception (testis, ovary, epididymis, prostate, fallopian tubes, uterus, sperm duct, penis, vagina) and subsequently to the protection and nourishment of the embryo (uterus). There cannot be another bodily function that has so much unique and essential paraphernalia devoted to it. It is this fact that provides the opportunities for selectively interfering with reproduction without affecting any other biological function. *Drosophila* geneticists estimate that about 100 genes—or 1 percent of the genome—can cause male and female sterility, respectively.

While humans may dedicate less of the genome to conception than do fruit flies, the number of tissues, organs, hormones, and the like devoted to conception suggests that there must be many genes with no other function as well. Look, for example, at the number of sterile humans who are otherwise perfectly healthy. It is this fact that provides abundant opportunities for selectively interfering with reproduction—in both males and females—without affecting any other biological function.

The basic knowledge of reproduction that is needed to conduct rational research on contraception can be summarized by two questions. First, what are the gene products that are expressed specifically in the various cells, tissues, and organs involved in reproduction? Second, which of these products is required for conception?

If we were trying to devise contraceptives for *Drosophila*, there would be little doubt how to proceed. Both questions would be asked simultaneously by carrying out saturation mutagenesis and isolating all sterile males and females. Saturation mutagenesis is the mutation of all genes within a species. This is accomplished by mutating each gene in one individual until all the genes have been mutated in a separate individual of *Drosophila*. Then a genetic screen would be used to select for the mutated individuals that are sterile to determine which genes are needed for reproduction. Each of the mutant genes would be cloned and sequenced so that some idea of their function could be predicted from similarities to genes known in the published data base. We would then have in hand a list of many genes that affect conception. We would select for further study only those genes that, when mutated, do not affect any other biological process but conception. Genes that meet these two criteria are candidates for contraceptive agents. Stated another way, the products of these genes are candidates for interference.

Next we would determine in what tissue and at what time each candidate gene is expressed. From its sequence we could predict whether the gene's product is a secreted extracellular product, a protein bound to cell membranes, a transcription factor, a component of the extracellular matrix, a growth factor, or perhaps a key hormone in the feedback loop that is required for reproduction. Having gathered this information, the basic research phase of *Drosophila* contraceptive development would be concluded, because we would have found our targets for contraception. We would have identified a large number of genes and their products that deal specifically with conception. Furthermore, we would know enough about what many of their products do to consider the rational design of contraceptive agents and to select a few that seem promising.

To what extent can we apply this strategy to human contraception? What tools are available to accomplish in humans (or the closest model organism) the same results? The only higher vertebrate that currently can be mutated to saturation is the zebrafish. There are powerful genetic tools available in the mouse such as transgenesis; the introduction of a gene; "knockouts," that is, the inactivation of an existing gene; and even a large number of mutants that have been identified and maintained over the years. Nonetheless, saturation mutagenesis in the mouse is not now feasible.

However, an important truth that has emerged through decades of research is that gene sequences and functions have been remarkably preserved throughout evolution. This makes it logical to assume that genes affecting conception that are identified in a zebrafish screen could be shown to play a similar role in the mouse by selectively "knocking out" the homologous mouse gene and observing the results. If the gene turns out to play a similar role in mouse reproduction— and also has a human homologue with an expression pattern resembling that of the mouse and the zebrafish—then a potential human contraceptive target has also been identified. It is by no means far-fetched to assume that *Drosophila* genes that are involved in conception may have homologues with the same function in humans.

A purely molecular biological method for identifying gene products that are specific for conception would use the principle of subtractive hybridization or the differential display of DNA copies of the messenger RNAs in a particular cell or tissue. Suppose, for example, that we wish to identify genes that are expressed solely in the epididymis. We would collect mRNA from epididymis tissue as well as from many other tissues and organs and then compare the populations of mRNA in order to identify genes that are expressed exclusively in the epididymis. Several genome companies are now sequencing all mRNAs (cDNAs) in many different tissues and then finding differences by computer search. Alternatively, it might be desirable to identify just those epididymis-specific genes that are regulated by androgen. Then the mRNA from control and hormone-stimulated epididymides would be compared for differentially expressed genes. One can imagine a number of important collections of tissue-specific or hormone-induced genes from which one could then choose possible targets for interfering with conception. These include cell-specific proteins of eggs, sperm, prostate, epididymis, and uterus. We would want to identify the battery of genes that is regulated by androgen, estrogen, progesterone, gonadotropin-releasing hormone (GnRH, sometimes referred to as LHRH), follicle-stimulating hormone (FSH), and luteinizing hormone (LH) in their respective target reproductive tissues.

Once we have identified genes that are specific for the target tissues and have cloned and sequenced their full-length cDNA, it is time to assay the gene for function because this method which, unlike a genetic screen, does not reveal whether the gene is required for conception. We only know that a given gene is tissue-specific and/or regulated by a hormone. The gene sequence is critical because it gives the best clue to the gene's function. The gene can then be knocked out in the mouse and antibodies made against the gene's product to see if they neutralize its activity. There are a number of methods to test whether the gene really is essential for conception but, in each case, the best functional assay can be chosen only when the gene's product has been identified.

In summary, the fact that successful conception relies on many different, highly specific biological events and organs presents a rich array of targets for contraceptive research. What modern methods provide are new and powerful ways of identifying the molecules required for conception. In this field the basic research need not be far in advance of the practical applications.

This proposed strategy will provide an efficient means of identifying new and relevant targets. Some of these targets will be more amenable to attack than others, either because of accessibility for delivery of inhibitory agents or because of the length of the window of biological need for normal function. Thus, selection among such targets will have to be made using criteria related to successful product development and not solely scientific merit.

Identification of Targets Through Research in Reproductive Biology

In addition to any new targets identified by the strategy outlined above, there are also already available for exploitation various exciting new targets that have been identified by ongoing basic research in reproductive biology and other related fields. Figure 4-1 displays the areas of the male and female reproductive structures where today's science points to potential targets for potentially significant advances in making more contraceptive choices available to more individuals.

In both men and women, the hypothalymus secretes the gonatropin-releasing hormone (GnRH) which, in turn, stimulates the pituitary to release luteinizing hormone (LH) and follicle-stimulating hormone (FSH), both of which are needed for steroid hormone production as well as sperm and egg development. Since the primary structure of GnRH was identified two decades ago, researchers have been designing, synthesizing, and testing agents that may be able to block the hormone's action. Some of these show promise for the development of new contraceptive products, some of which could conceivably appear by the end of the next decade.

In addition to the neuron itself, there are targets throughout the GnRH neuronal network that might be activated or inhibited, providing a wealth of possible contraceptive agents. In fact, several peptidic agonists and antagonists of GnRH have already been identified. Each of these two classes has a different mode of action: While antagonists work by blocking a receptor, agonists operate by stimulating it so much that it is ultimately inhibited.

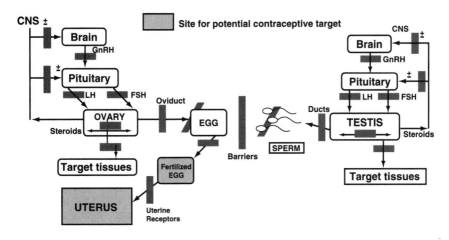

FIGURE 4-1 Potential targets for development of new contraceptive technologies. SOURCE: Prepared for this report by Neena Schwartz.

The GnRH agonists available today have proved useful in the treatment of certain conditions, including prostate cancer, endometriosis, polycystic ovarian disease, and the induction of ovulation for *in vitro* fertilization. So far, however, they have not been potent enough to be used as contraceptives. The best hope in this area lies in the development of nonpeptide GnRH antagonists which, because they are orally active, make better drug candidates than do peptides. While all GnRH antagonists reported to date are, in fact, peptides, new approaches that have permitted development of a nonpeptidic growth hormone analogue makes the possibility of a nonpeptidic GnRH analogue more likely.

Several GnRH agonists have also been developed. Current clinical applications of these compounds include the treatment of precocious puberty and restoration of fertility in GnRH-deficient men and women, the treatment of prostate cancer in men, and the treatment of uterine fibroids, endometriosis, and polycystic ovarian disease in women. Higher doses of the agonists could be used to suppress spermatogenesis in males. While the reversibility and absence of toxicity of these analogues have been established, there are some potential problems. The most important is the need to replace testosterone, whose production is also stopped by blocking GnRH, in order to maintain libido. Also promising is current research that focuses on suppressing the production or action of FSH and LH, attractive targets because of the important role these hormones play in gametogenesis in both sexes. In males, researchers believe that FSH analogues will be able to selectively block spermatogenesis without affecting testosterone secretion. In females, the degree to which FSH affects estrogen production remains unclear. If an FSH inhibitor did decrease estrogen, the hormone would have to be replaced. Another approach would be to target agents such as inhibin and activin, growth factors which also affect FSH secretion.

Several industrial and academic programs are working to develop FSH agonists or antagonists and are taking advantage of the new availability of cloned human FSH receptors. They are also profiting from the new techniques of combinatorial chemistry, a chemistry-based technology platform that generates large arrays of screenable compounds for rapid drug discovery that are, in effect, libraries of small organic molecules, peptides, or oligonucleotides. Nonsteroidal agents in general offer good opportunities for innovative companies, particularly those specializing in design of small molecules, drug delivery systems for proteins or large molecules, and in combinatorial chemistry.

APPROACHES TO NEW CONTRACEPTIVES FOR FEMALES[*]

Recent advances in molecular and cellular biology have provided a better understanding of female reproductive processes—including oogenesis, follicular maturation, ovulation, fertilization, and implantation—than ever before. This knowledge will have major impact on the development of new contraceptives for women. The challenge now is to select from the many potential targets those that can be manipulated to achieve contraception with minimal or no impact on other organ systems; the more specific and more limited the systemic effects of a contraceptive are, the less likely they may be to produce the sorts of side effects that are troublesome in greater or lesser degree to many women. Table 4-1 summarizes those potential target areas the study committee identified as being particularly promising.

The cascade of events involving GnRH, LH, and FSH described above and depicted in Figure 4-1 is what regulates successful follicular development and ovulation. Recently, the GnRH receptors were cloned, an advance that will permit a wider range of possibilities for intervening in these processes. One possibility would be to suppress the receptor, either through agonists or antagonists, which would certainly halt follicular maturation and ovulation. However, this approach would also require steroid replacement to avoid unwanted effects elsewhere in the body. Another possibility would be to modify the intermittent or pulse-like rhythm of GnRH secretion in such a way as to exert a disproportionate effect on follicular development relative to steroid synthesis.

Another option would be to target FSH from the start. It is now considered likely that the growth factor activin plays a key role in maintaining FSH expression. Two activin inhibitors, inhibin and follistatin, have now been identified and shown to suppress both FSH production and follicular development following

---

*Please refer to Appendix A for the full text of the authored and fully referenced paper on which this section is based.

systemic administration in animals. This interference was specific to activin's role in the reproductive system (DePaolo et al. 1991; Vale et al. 1994, 1990).

Once FSH reaches the ovary, there are still many ways to interfere with follicular maturation. A unique organ, the ovary contains hundreds of thousands of follicles—the sacs containing developing ova—that die naturally during a female's lifetime. Of the 400,000 follicles found in human females at puberty, for example, only about 400 will ever make it to ovulation, a process of attrition that is depicted in Figure 4-1 (see Appendix A). A better understanding of this process could lead to new contraceptive approaches.

Most ovarian cell death is caused by apoptosis, or programmed cell death. Researchers have now identified several substances in the ovary that affect apoptosis by acting either as follicular survival factors or as mediators of cell death. These substances include gonadotropins, steroid hormones, interleukins, and cytokines such as IGF-1. Researchers have also have identified a number of transcription factors—factors controlling gene expression—that regulate apoptosis (Artini et al. 1994; Erickson and Danforth 1995; Hsueh et al. 1994).

Meiotic cell division, which allows for the combination of maternal and paternal DNA when two gametes meet, occurs only in male and female gonads. The process therefore provides a good target for contraception. One particularly promising point of intervention occurs when the ovary's primary oocytes are released from prophase I and allowed to progress to metaphase II (Grigorescu et al. 1994), an event regulated by a factor called maturation promoting factor (MPF). Further study could provide clues to new drugs that might interfere with follicular maturation (Dorce 1990).

Greater research into and understanding of the molecular and cellular events involved in oocyte maturation have provided some new and some unexpected targets. Among the unexpected are a class of "orphan receptors," some of which may have endogenous ligands yet to be discovered, while others appear not to be ligand-dependent and rather respond to other metabolic influences or synthetic molecules. Many of these "orphans" are nuclear receptors active in gametogenesis and further study may provide important new reproductive leads (Becker-Andre et al. 1994; Chen et al. 1994; Heyman et al. 1992; Ikeda et al. 1994; Lala et al. 1992; Luo et al. 1994; O'Malley 1991; Shen et al. 1994).

Specific Targets

Contraceptive Targets Between Oocyte Development and Ovulation

The final stage of follicular development, follicular rupture, presents yet another promising contraceptive target. One factor essential to the process, the PGS-2 gene, could provide an ideal way to inhibit this one specific event while otherwise leaving the reproductive system alone (Morris and Richards 1993, 1995).

TABLE 4-1 New Horizons for Contraceptive Research and the Development of New Female Methods

Mechanism	Description
I. Mechanisms underlying the pulsatile release of GnRH (gonadotropin releasing hormone) and the differential regulation of FSH and LH synthesis and secretion.	
GnRH	
Long-acting agonist analogues	Initial stimulation and eventual desensitization of the receptor and attenuation of receptor signal transduction. These agents inhibit fertility but also reduce steroid production and induce postmenopausal symptoms, and they therefore would require steroid replacement therapy.
Receptor antagonists	Immediate suppression of gonadotropin secretion, although higher doses are required than of the agonists. Potential for further optimization using high throughput GnRH receptor assays.
Antagonists of SF-1	SF-1 is a transcription factor that controls the development of the gonadotrope. Antagonists to it could suppress the pituitary-gonadal axis; however, unless it were highly selective for oogenesis/ovulation, replacement therapy would still be required.
FSH (follicle-stimulating hormone) Activin inhibitors Inhibin Follistatin	Activin is probably the key tropic factor maintaining expression of FSH. Inhibin provides a negative feedback signal that shuts off FSH secretion; follistatin serves to limit all effects of activin. Small molecules could interfere with these functions. Inhibin suppresses only a subset of activin effects, so that the drugs could be relatively specific to the suppression of reproduction.
II. Specific molecular events associated with maintenance of oocytes in prophase I and release of this block by the ovulatory stimulus only in mature follicles; determination of the suitability of these targets for pharmaceutical intervention.	
Meiosis MPF (maturation promoting factor) OMI (oocyte maturation inhibitor) GVB (germinal vesicle breakdown)	One potential point of intervention is the regulation of progression of primary oocytes from prophase I to metaphase II. Synthetic analogues may be efficient as agonists, as well as antagonists, for pharmacologic manipulation of the onset of meiosis. MPF has been identified as an intracellular factor that regulates this transition.

TABLE 4-1 Continued

Mechanism	Description

III. Apoptosis research, to include the developing follicle as a target. Apoptosis research in diverse areas, including this one, could be mutually informative. An important research objective is better understanding of the mechanism by which the dominant follicle progresses while other developing follicles undergo atresia.

| FSH blockers
Deglycosylated FSH antagonists

Extracellular fragment of FSH receptors | Blocking the continuing maturation of preovulatory follicles or causing their premature demise using apoptotic factors is one potential contraceptive target. Gonadotropins, estrogens, growth hormone, growth factors, a cytokine, and nitric oxide act to ensure preovulatory follicle survival, while androgens, interleukin-6, and gonadal GnRH-like peptides are apoptotic factors. FSH, a gonadotropin, acts as a survival factor preventing the demise of early antral follicles, one of which is selected for final maturation and ovulation. Blocking FSH using an antagonist or a neutralizing protein would act in an ovary-specific manner, preventing ovulation. This method would therefore require physiologic replacement therapy. |

IV. Examination of molecular and cellular aspects of follicular development and definition of the key players, their specific targets, and identification of endogenous and synthetic ligands should become major research objectives.

Melatonin	A hormone intimately involved in reproduction, its transcriptional effects are manifest through the orphan receptor RXR. A combination of melatonin and a synthetic progestin has been tested as a novel type of oral contraceptive preparation (see Chapter 3).
Orphan receptors	These receptors can be regulated by a synthetic pharmaceutical in a manner that impacts on relevant biological processes without knowing whether or not a given receptor has an endogenous ligand.
GCNF (germ cell nuclear factor)	A nuclear hormone restricted in expression to developing gametes and detectable in all stages of oocyte development.
SF-1 (steroidogenic factor 1)	May also play a key regulatory role in gametogenesis, in addition to being a positive transcriptional regulator of steroidogenic enzymes.

continued on next page

TABLE 4-1 Continued

Mechanism	Description

V. Elucidation of the factors that control follicular rupture: Inhibition of this process would be an ideal way to prevent fertilization and simulate a normal nonconception cycle with unaltered steroid patterns and levels and cycle length.

PGS-2 (COX II)	The LH surge induces the expression of the prostaglandin synthase 2 gene (PGS-2) that codes for an enzyme whose activity is essential for follicular rupture. If this enzyme were selectively inhibited, ovulation would be eliminated without the blocking of luteinization and the synthesis of steroid hormones.

VI. A reexamination of established targets, for example, the steroid hormone receptors, would seem merited, given the recent observation that tissue-selective compounds can be developed to control specific subsets of genes that are regulated by the natural hormone.

Estradiol and tamoxifen	Both are ligands for the estrogen receptor but induce distinct conformational changes within the receptor with distinct biological consequences *in vivo*.

VII. Expeditious examination of combinations of antiprogestins and other hormonal or antihormonal drugs should be undertaken, toward a method of emergency or once-a-month contraception. A more effective combination could be developed in a relatively short time frame.

Oxytocic agents	Drugs that stimulate uterine contractility alone or in combination with drugs that accelerate tubal transport and cause expulsion of the embryo from the uterus.
Delivery	Vaginal, instead of oral, administration of hormonal formulations based on single or combined steroids may increase efficacy and reduce gastrointestinal side effects of emergency contraception.
Mifepristone	An antiprogestin that can delay ovulation owing to temporary arrest of the growth of the dominant follicle, can offset the positive feedback of estrogen on the discharge of gonadotropin from the pituitary gland, and can disrupt the required secretory changes of the endometrium. This, in turn, could prevent either fertilization or implantation, depending on the stage of the menstrual cycle at which it is taken. Taken in combination with estrogen, it may be more effective and have fewer side effects. In addition, given in the time frame between ovulation and implantation, mifepristone prevents fertility.

TABLE 4-1 Continued

Mechanism	Description
Epostane and Azastene	These enzyme inhibitors act to prevent progesterone synthesis. Epostane has been shown to terminate pregnancy in about 80 percent of women up to the eighth week of pregnancy; however, nausea was a common side effect. This approach may affect synthesis of adrenal steroids and is therefore problematic.
Combinations	Combinations of progesterone synthesis inhibitors and progesterone receptor blockers (mifepristone) might be more effective than either alone. A combination of an anti-estrogen and an antiprogestin might also be effective, given the objective of putting endometrial development out of synchrony with or making it hostile to the embryo.

VIII. Studies should be carried out in nonhuman primates to develop the concept, and test the safety, of immunization against progesterone as a simple and easily reversible contraceptive method.

Progesterone antibodies	Active immunization against progesterone would result in exposure of the endometrium to unopposed estrogen. However, through administration of a synthetic progestin that does not cross-react with the antibody, during the last quarter of the cycle withdrawal bleeding would occur.

IX. The most promising of the adhesion molecules should be studied to determine how essential they are for initial blastocyst attachment to the endometrial epithelium.

Integrins Collagen, laminin, fibro-nectin, vitronectin integrin $\alpha_4\beta_1$	Changes in the expression of several integrins may define the putative period of uterine receptivity for blastocyst attachment. Blockade or disruption of this expression could provide a specific means of preventing implantation.
High-molecular-weight (MW) glycoprotein	A high MW glycoprotein involving N-acetyl-galactosamine and other determinants and secreted from the endometrial glands during the period of uterine sensitivity for implantation in humans, it is believed to be involved in the initial adhesion phase of implantation.
Muc-1 (episialin)	A member of the family of mucin glycoproteins and found in the endometrial epithelial cells of mouse uterus. Ways of decreasing it prematurely or delaying its down-regulation, necessary for implantation, could be the basis for a contraceptive approach.

continued on next page

TABLE 4-1 Continued

Mechanism	Description
HB-EGF (heparin-binding epidermal growth factor)	May be important for establishing uterine receptivity for implantation and causing stromal cell proliferation. Its appearance can be blocked by antiprogestins and thus may be a good contraceptive target.
Trophinin and tastin	Although the significance of these factors in implantation remains to be determined, they may also be useful new leads for a contraceptive acting to prevent blastocyst attachment.

X. Increased attention to research in growth factors and cytokines, particularly those shown to regulate endometrial functions and implantation.

IL-1 (interleukin-1)	Treatment of mice with IL-1R (receptor) antagonist during the preimplantation period prevented pregnancy. The importance of IL-1 remains to be seen, however, as attempts to repeat early trials have been unsuccessful.
CSF-1 (colony-stimulating factor)	May also be a critical factor for implantation. Breeding of homozygous mice lacking CSF-1 resulted in implantation failure.
TNF-α (tumor necrosis factor α)	Synthesis of this cytokine is induced through the gene regulatory action of CSF-1. TNF-α inhibits decidualization of human endometrial stromal cells *in vivo*; thus, the balance between CSF-1 and TNF-α may be critical for normal progression of the implantation process.
LIF (leukemia inhibitory factor)	If it can be shown that LIF is essential for implantation in species other than the mouse, then means to disrupt uterine LIF function for a short period should be sought. LIF secretion from human endometrial cell cultures peaks around the time of implantation in a conception cycle. LIF may provide an important lead in the development of specific anti-implantation agents. The most specific approach would appear to be through interference with binding of the specific LIFR α subunit to the LIF receptor complex.
IGF-1 (insulin-like growth factor)	IGF-1, its receptor, and the IGF-binding proteins 1–4 are all localized to the endometrial epithelial cells and highest at the early- to mid-secretory phase of the cycle. These changes may be modulated by the embryo and are essential for implantation.
FGFs (fibroblast growth factors)	Involved in angiogenesis, disruption of the gene for FGF-4 in mice causes severe inhibition of the growth of the blastocyst inner cell mass and failure of pregnancy just after implantation.

TABLE 4-1 Continued

Mechanism	Description
XI. Development of nonpeptide GnRH antagonists would have utility both before and after fertilization.	
	Nonpeptide antagonists are likely to be simpler and cheaper to produce and may be able to block the action of trophoblast GnRH in stimulating hCG secretion, which is necessary to support pregnancy. Other factors may also be involved in regulation of early hCG production and their identification and use to inhibit early hCG production could cause early pregnancy failure without disrupting menstrual cyclicity.

In the current enthusiasm about new ovarian targets, researchers should not forget about new ways of looking at old targets, notably steroid hormone receptors. Such a reexamination is justified by the fact that it is now possible to develop tissue-selective compounds that affect a specific subset of genes regulated by these hormones. Particularly promising for the contraceptive field would be discovery of the targets of progesterone and estrogen receptors in the ovary. Such results could possibly lead to the development of tissue-selective modulators of oocyte maturation (Allan et al. 1992; McDonnell et al. 1995; Tzukerman et al. 1994).

Postovulation Contraceptive Targets

After ovulation, an ovum enters the oviduct (or fallopian tube), where it may or may not be fertilized by a spermatozoon. If it is, the fertilized egg progresses through the oviduct for another 72 hours, where it undergoes more mitotic cycles over the next 3–4 days, eventually forming a blastocyst (Croxatto 1995). The blastocyst attaches to the uterine wall, then undergoes several more steps before finally completing implantation. Thus, the consensus of many national and international medical and legal entities is that pregnancy does not begin until the completion of implantation of the fertilized ovum in the woman's uterus[1] (Cook 1989). It is reasonable to believe, therefore, that agents that prevent that implantation would be more widely accepted than those that cause early pregnancy failure. From the perspective of current science, such agents are entering the realm of possibility with the discovery of new anti-implantation agents.

In many animals, administering hormones that cause embryos to be retained in the oviduct also blocks fertility. In humans, however, such interference can lead to life-threatening intratubal (ectopic) pregnancy and thus cannot be considered a contraceptive option. Another possibility may be speeding up the time it takes a zygote to pass through the oviduct. While animal studies had indicated that premature passage through the oviduct would impede pregnancy (Adams 1980; Ortiz et al. 1991), this has not been the case in humans. Any contraceptive based on accelerating oviductal transport would also have to cause expulsion of the embryo by stimulating uterine contractility.

Potential anti-implantation targets fall into one of three categories: hormones, cell-adhesion molecules, and cytokines/growth factors. While results of experiments testing the importance of estrogen to implantation in animal models (primates) have been mixed, an absence of progesterone has inevitably produced pregnancy failure. There are three ways to stop the action of progesterone: preventing its synthesis using enzyme inhibitors, intercepting the hormone in circulation with specific antibodies, and blocking its action at the receptor level using an antiprogestin. All these methods have their drawbacks, and it has been suggested that combining the first and third may offer the most promise. All these processes offer opportunities for interference, yet even if effective combinations were to be designed, they would still have the disadvantage of being relatively nonspecific, an attribute that runs counter to the thrust of this report. As indicated in the preceding section, targets for contraceptives must be highly specific. (For research results on such methods, see Birgerson et al. 1987; Crooij et al. 1988; Gemzell-Danielsson et al. 1993; Ghosh and Sengupta 1993; Ghosh et al. 1994; Greene et al. 1992; Harper 1972; Selinger et al. 1987; Swahn et al. 1990.)

One of the first events in the implantation process is the blastocyst's attachment to the uterine epithelial surface, an event carried out by cell-adhesion molecules. Researchers have studied one family of such molecules, called integrins, in the human endometrium and concluded that blocking these molecules could provide a specific way to prevent implantation (Ilesanmi et al. 1993; Lessey 1994; Lessey et al. 1992 and 1994; Schultz and Armant 1995). A number of other cell-adhesion molecules are under investigation for their role in implantation (see, for example, Fukuda et al. 1995; Jentoft 1990; Kliman et al. 1995; Strous and Dekker 1992; Zhang et al. 1994 a and b). A potential problem with all these agents is that, unless they have a long biological half-life, it will be hard to determine the optimum time in the cycle to administer them.

It is only recently that the third category of biological agents—endogenous proteins called cytokines and/or growth factors—has been found to play a key role in implantation. Researchers have studied several of these, including interleukin-1 (De et al. 1993; Frank et al. 1995; Tabibzadeh et al. 1990; Tackacs et al. 1988; Simón et al. 1993a, 1993b, 1994), colony-stimulating factor 1 (Pollard et al. 1991), and tumor necrosis factor α (Hunt et al. 1993; Inoue et al. 1994; Tartakovsky and Ben-Yair 1991). Perhaps the most promising work to date has been on leukemia inhibitory factor (LIF) (see, for example, Bhatt et al. 1991; Chen et al. 1995; Hilton et al. 1988; Stewart et al. 1992; Willson et al. 1992;

Yamamoto-Yamaguchi et al. 1986; Yang et al. 1994; Yang et al. 1995a, 1995b; Zhong et al. 1994).

In experiments where the gene for LIF was knocked out in mice, the animals, while fertile and otherwise healthy, could not maintain pregnancy because of implantation failure. While LIF's role in humans has not yet been established, there is preliminary evidence that, in rabbits, this cytokine is involved in implantation. In addition, LIF levels rise in human endometrial cells during the early and mid-luteal phase. If further research supports these results, LIF or its specific receptor subunit may make an excellent contraceptive target, although several concerns remain. These include significant structural similarities with other cytokines (suggesting a possible lack of specificity), uncertainty regarding the timing and frequency of administering the agent, and the impact on pregnancy should a LIF blocker be given too late.

Already developed for possible use before fertilization, agonists and antagonists of GnRH may also interfere with the hCG (human chorionic gonadotropin) secretion needed for luteal support and maintaining early pregnancy. While some animal studies have shown promise for agents causing luteolysis (premature demise of the corpus luteum, which interferes with progesterone secretion and thus maintenance of pregnancy), work with primates has so far produced no good leads. One alternative way to achieve the same effect would be by blocking progesterone synthesis by the corpus luteum. In rhesus monkeys, such functional luteolysis has been demonstrated following administration of either azastene or epostane during the luteal phase of the cycle (Schane et al. 1978; Snyder and Schane 1985); in pregnant monkeys, pregnancy was terminated (Schane et al. 1978).

In Chapter 3, dedicated to contraceptive technologies that have at least reached phase I in the research and development trajectory, we discussed the very small number of postcoital contraceptive options that are available on the current international market. We included in that group RU 486, the only member of the newly discovered[2] group of compounds called "antiprogestins" to have become available for human use. As their categorical name suggests, these compounds are antagonists of progesterone, a steroid hormone which originates in the corpus luteum and without which pregnancy cannot be initiated or maintained (Van Look 1994). Finally, we also noted the prospects these compounds offer for intervening at various points in the female reproductive cycle, to prevent pregnancy before ovulation by inhibiting initiation of the ovulatory processes and, as well, to prevent pregnancy after ovulation up until the time of expected menses. Contraceptives designed to have effect during the postovulatory portion of the cycle are known as once-a-month contraceptives or menses-inducers and, as noted at various points in this report, are highly ranked on the women's agenda. The many processes taking place between ovulation and menses—or between ovulation and implantation if fertilization has occurred—offer abundant possibilities for once-a-month treatments (see Figure 4-2).

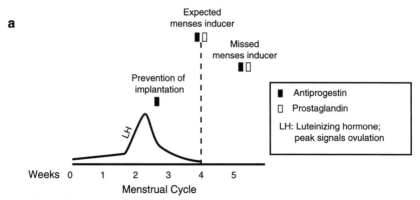

Expected Menses Inducer
• Desired regimen: once-a-month pill(s) administered shortly before expected menses
• Challenges: identifying correct mifepristone/prostaglandin dose and formulation, maintaining regular menstrual cycles

Missed Menses Inducer
• Desired regimen: occasional use when menses missed
• Challenges: identifying correct mifepristone/prostaglandin dose and formulation, maintaining regular menstrual cycles

Prevention of Implantation
• Desired regimen: once-a-month pill(s) administered shortly after ovulation
• Challenges: identifying ovulation, maintaining regular menstrual cycle

FIGURE 4-2   Possible regimens for using antiprogestins as menses inducers or as once-a-month pills. SOURCES: **a**—Adapted fromWorld Health Organization. Challenges in Reproductive Health Research: Biennial Report, 1992–1993. Geneva: World Health Organization, 1994. **b**—Reprinted from Institute of Medicine. Clinical Applications of Mifepristone (RU 486) and Other Antiprogestins: Assessing the Science and Recommending a Research Base. MS Donaldson, L Dorflinger, SS Brown, and LZ Benet, eds. Washington, DC: National Academy Press, 1994 (Figure B12.5, p. 272).

Menses-inducers can be divided into two categories: those that are used regularly just before the onset of expected menstruation (expected menses inducers, or EMIs) and those used only when the menstrual period does not occur (missed menses inducers, or MMIs). There are crucial differences between the two in terms of legal status, frequency and ease of use, and acceptability. In general, EMIs are more acceptable in more settings than are MMIs, though the acceptability of EMIs often depends on their mechanisms of action: Agents that prevent ovulation are far more acceptable than those which interfere with implantation or terminate early pregnancies. EMIs are obviously taken more frequently (and, perhaps, unnecessarily) than MMIs, which would be taken at most three or four times a year. Finally, owing to natural, month-to-month variability in menstrual cycling, EMIs are more difficult to use; at the same time, for some women

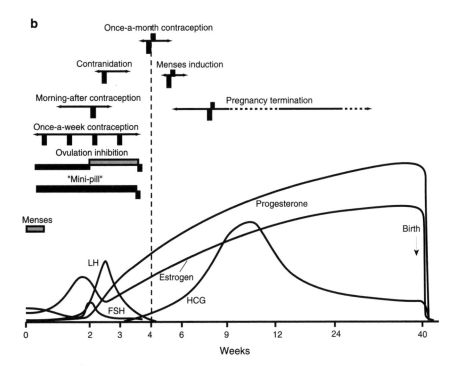

their inability to predict their next menstrual period precisely is a challenge for the use of MMIs (Van Look 1994).

Expected menses inducers work by ensuring the monthly sloughing of the endometrium at the time of expected menses, regardless of whether or not an embryo has implanted. Advance in developing such agents has been constrained by lack of understanding of the mechanisms that start and stop endometrial bleeding and by the political and religious unacceptability of the EMI approach in certain cultures and countries. Nevertheless, as indicated in Chapter 3, work with mifepristone as a possible component of an EMI has begun to produce further understanding. While the failure rate in initial studies was high (17 to 19 percent of women remained pregnant), more studies are under way combining mifepristone with the prostaglandin misoprostol. These results should be available in 1996 (WHO/HRP 1995). A related—and important—issue is the long-term safety of antiprogestin treatment. If these compounds are to be used over extended periods of time as oral contraceptives, answering the safety question will be as critical as establishing efficacy. Researchers should also consider whether novel delivery systems—such as transdermals or implants—would offer any special advantages for these compounds.

APPROACHES TO NEW CONTRACEPTIVES FOR MALES*

While the biology of the male reproductive system places certain limitations on contraceptive options for men, several recently discovered—and unique—cellular and molecular events within the system have opened up new possibilities (see Table 4-2). While there appears to be little or no research on the characteristics of what men would want in a contraceptive, objectively identified criteria for male contraceptives might not be unlike those objectively identified for female contraceptives: safe, effective, reversible, "user-controlled," and quickly effective. One criterion that appears frequently in the literature is that a contraceptive for men should have no impact on libido, a criterion that rarely if ever appears in the literature in connection with contraceptives for women.

Specific Targets

Long-loop Feedback System

Through a process that closely parallels oogenesis in the female, spermatogenesis is controlled from the brain with the production of gonadotropin-releasing hormone (GnRH) by the hypothalamus. GnRH in turn stimulates the anterior pituitary to secrete luteinizing hormone (LH) and follicle-stimulating hormone (FSH), both of which are required for normal sperm development in the testis and acquisition of fertilizing capacity.

Several studies have focused on the so-called long-loop feedback system as a contraceptive target (Wang et al. 1994) (see Table 4-2). The earliest, which tested the efficacy of androgen injections to disrupt the system (Handelsman et al. 1992), successfully achieved reversible azoospermia after a period of months. While researchers have attempted a similar strategy with GnRH agonists and antagonists, they have had to replace androgens to maintain the subjects' libido (Bagatell et al. 1993).

Targeting FSH alone should avoid this problem (Zirkin et al. 1994). Particularly promising is the hormone's β subunit, which, unlike its α subunit, is specific to FSH and thought to be responsible for receptor specificity. New research techniques have revealed many of the molecular details surrounding FSH's interaction with its receptor. This new understanding suggests several specific tactics for FSH interference.

Sperm Development in the Testis

Once spermatogenesis is initiated in the testis by reproductive hormones,

---

*Please refer to Appendix B for the full text of the authored and fully referenced paper on which this section is based.

there remain many potential ways to interfere before the process is complete. One attractive target is meiosis—which halves the number of chromosomes in a gamete's nucleus so it can combine with another gamete at fertilization—a process that occurs only in male and female gonads. A particularly promising possibility would rely on c-mos, a unique germ cell protein known to be involved in meiotic arrest in females. While in males, unlike females, meiosis is ordinarily a continuous process (and c-mos is expressed too late to have an impact), getting the protein expressed early may be able to stop meiosis and therefore sperm development.

Another possibility would be to genetically manipulate sperm cells before they are fully mature. Feasible strategies for contraceptive attack using gene-therapy techniques include the disruption of normally functioning transcription factors, proteins that bind to DNA with the effect of switching genes on and off. While the field is still a new one, researchers have already identified several transcription factors that are specific to germ cells (Chen et al. 1994). Inappropriate expression of any of these factors (either absence when they are needed or presence when they are not) is likely to disrupt sperm differentiation.

As an alternative to transcription factors, classical genetics techniques may offer options for interfering with sperm development. Many of the most important processes in meiosis and gamete production are conserved throughout all animal phyla, and we may be able to use what we know about other species. Genetic studies of the well-known *Drosophila*, for example, show that mutations in any of 400 of the female's 4,000 genes cause sterility. Similar studies in the male *Drosophila* could identify a similar set of potential targets.

Postmeiotic cells, or spermatids, may provide the best contraceptive target in the testis. Several key events occur nowhere in the body but in these cells. One is the formation of the acrosome, a structure at the head of the sperm containing enzymes that will allow it to penetrate the egg membrane. Another is the formation of the flagellum, or tail, which allows the sperm to swim. As researchers learn more about the cellular and molecular processes underlying these unique events, specifically disrupting them to achieve contraception should become a very real possibility.

A final category of potential targets in the developing sperm arise from the plasma membranes on these cells' surfaces. Like the sperm cell itself, components of these membranes are highly compartmentalized, and at least some of them are thought to play a key functional role. Researchers have identified several sperm proteins thought to be important in fertilization and have begun to map the location of these on the sperm membrane. Because the absence of a particular sperm protein in a given region of the membrane would likely lead to dysfunctional sperm, this line of research has opened up some potential new contraceptive options (Eddy and O'Brien 1994).

TABLE 4-2   New Horizons for Contraceptive Research and the Development of New Male Methods

Target	Mechanism
I. Long-loop feedback mechanisms	Injection of androgens accomplished reversible azoospermia, as did injection of GnRH agonists and antagonists combined with androgen replacement.
II. Inhibition of FSH secretion and/or action	It is generally agreed that FSH is required for spermatogenesis along with testosterone; therefore, a method targeting FSH or its receptor could disrupt spermatogenesis without affecting steroid hormones. The β subunit of FSH is unique and apparently responsible for receptor specificity, as well; FSH binds only to a tetrameric form of FSH receptor and the interaction between the two is complicated. Possible approaches include:
FSH (follicle-stimulating hormone)	• Reducing or eliminating the secretion of FSH. This would, however, require development of improved stable androgens, GnRH analogues, or activin antagonists, and their appropriate delivery systems.
	• Targeting FSH-β for immunologic destruction or neutralization through antibody binding in circulation. Although this method would afford great selectivity, it could potentially destroy the anterior pituitary, the site of FSH synthesis by cell-mediated immunity. A potential solution is the use of a B-cell epitope as a target, if one exists.
FSH receptor	• Use of anti-FSH receptor antibodies or mimetopes. This method could potentially backfire were the anti-FSH agent itself to act as a receptor activator.
	• Prevention of proper intracellular assembly of the tetrameric form of the FSH receptor. It would be necessary to determine how to prevent such assembly; the field of protein trafficking offers some hope in this area.
III. Control of Meiosis	Meiosis in males is a continuous event, whereas in females, it is halted at two points: the end of prophase I and during metaphase II. The responsible mechanisms for these pauses could possibly be used to arrest meiosis in the male. The arrest at prophase I is dependent on cAMP-dependent protein kinase A, which has great importance throughout the human system and is, therefore, not a likely candidate. However,
c-mos	arrest of metaphase II appears to involve c-mos, which is a unique germ cell protein. In males, its DNA is transcribed during meiosis but not translated until spermiogenesis begins. Could this translation begin earlier, during meiosis, it could potentially be a very powerful approach to fertility regulation.

TABLE 4-2 Continued

Target	Mechanism
IV. Genetic manipulation of sperm	In standard gene therapy, a stem cell is targeted and new genes are inserted into these cells to overcome the effects of damaged genetic material; used contraceptively, this method could be used to insert a defect for genetic material responsible for sperm-surface components specific to spermatogonia. A certain complexity arises when considering the introduction of the new genetic material, however. Since the primary spermatocytes are protected by the blood-testis barrier, a two-stage delivery system using the Sertoli cells as an intermediary would be necessary. Potential inserts would include: • Agents that disturb the functioning of transcription factors. • Replacement of nuclear histones with protamines could be targeted, since this process is specific to developing sperm cells. • Other genes responsible for fertility or infertility, using *Drosophila* as a model. Genes that have been conserved throughout the phyla may be identified in *Drosophila* and located in humans.
V. Inhibition of acrosome and tail formation	These processes are unique to the developing sperm and are thought to occur independently from hormonal regulation. • The acrosome is a product of the Golgi apparatus and first appears morphologically in spermatids. It is essential for fertility. Further exploration into its origins and development is necessary to isolate potential contraceptive targets. • Centriole attachment and tail formation occur only in spermatids, although centrioles have the potential to germinate flagella or cilia in all cells. Isolation of the causes and mechanisms of this differential development could provide unique contraceptive options.
VI. Alteration of sperm-surface proteins	During spermatogenesis, sperm acquire a highly polarized morphology with a quadripartite structure in which lipids and proteins are organized into highly regionalized domains which first appear during spermiogenesis. While some fertilization-related proteins are restricted to certain membrane domains, others are uniformly distributed, such as fertilin and PH-20. • Since germ cells invest heavily in elaborating and maintaining the organization of proteins within and on the sperm

continued on next page

TABLE 4-2 Continued

Target	Mechanism
	membrane, it is likely that interference with this system in any way could lead to the development of dysfunctional sperm.
	• Disruption of the timing of protein expression could also disorder the intricate organization of the sperm membrane. This could include fertilin, but also any other fertilization-related protein, or even, potentially, nonfertilization-related proteins, since the entire cascade of expression seems to be so delicately balanced.
VII. Interruption of epididymal function	The one- to two-week period that sperm spend traveling through the epididymis is essential to ultimate fertility function. The functional changes that occur—vigorous motility and ability to interact with the zona pellucida and egg membrane—are androgen dependent; however, the epididymis itself does not appear to synthesize hormones, nor do its functions appear to be linked to other biological functions. In addition, sperm are fully genetically formed by the time they reach the epididymis. For these reasons, targeting the epididymis seems potentially powerful with little adverse side effects.
	• Several proteins are secreted into epididymal fluid and are subsequently taken up onto the sperm surface. If any of these are necessary for sperm maturation, they could be beneficial targets. The creation of knockout mice may provide a way to pursue this possibility.
	• Similar to the use of organ-specific anti-estrogens in females, it may be possible to create epididymis-specific anti-androgens that could block the necessary action of androgens in epididymal sperm development.
	• Immunoneutralize epididymal-specific proteins.
VIII. Regulation of the inhibition of immune reactions by sperm	In many species, sperm are endowed with proteins delivered by the seminal vesicle that are immunosuppressive and make the sperm essentially immunologically silent to the female's immune system. If this event occurs in humans and could be blocked, it could offer a contraceptive target.
IX. Induction of premature acrosome reaction	Delivery of a ZP3 mimic to the sperm at some point prior to ejaculation could induce the acrosome reaction prematurely and thus make the sperm ineffective at penetrating the egg's outermost layers. However, in nature, the acrosome reaction typically occurs after spermhead capacitation, so that this

TABLE 4-2 Continued

Target	Mechanism
	technique may not be effective. In addition, the quantity of ZP3 mimic would have to be quite large in order to affect the multitude of sperm cells in, or emerging from, the epididymis. However, a substance produced by a well-known mutation in the T-locus in mouse sperm, which results in the uneven success of t-bearing sperm versus T-bearing sperm, owing to the ability of the t-bearing sperm to cause a premature acrosome reaction in the T-bearing sperm, may offer a clue to the utilization of this potential contraceptive method.
X. Inhibition of gamete interaction	PH-20, fertilin, and ZRK (a ZP3 receptor), among other sperm-specific proteins required for gamete interaction, could be targeted for suppression or blockade via epididymal manipulation, "conditional knockout," or immunosuppression, ultimately resulting in the inability of the sperm to "communicate" and thereby fertilize the ovum.

Sperm Maturation in the Epididymis

When sperm leave the testis, they must undergo more morphologic and biochemical changes before they are capable of fertilization. These final developments take place in the epididymis, which also serves as a sperm storage reservoir. Because this organ is where sperm specifically acquire their ability to fertilize eggs, it makes a promising male contraceptive target. Two advantages of contraception aimed at the epididymis are that this organ does not synthesize hormones and sperm enter it genetically fully formed; contraception aimed here is therefore less likely to produce adverse hormonal or genetic side effects than those targeting the testis.

During maturation, much of the sperm surface appears to be remodeled. These changes are mediated by products secreted by the epithelium of the epididymis. Although the precise components of this epididymal fluid have not been fully identified, it is known that its complex composition changes dramatically along the length of the tubule.

There are several possible approaches to interfering with sperm maturation. One would be to modify the expression of epididymal proteins. Researchers have identified several proteins that are secreted into epididymal fluid and subsequently adsorbed onto the sperm surface in humans and other mammals. If it is determined that any of these proteins are essential to sperm maturation, blocking their expression would constitute an excellent approach. Only recently have techniques that make this approach feasible become available (Gu et al. 1994). One way this could be accomplished would be to specifically knock out the gene coding for the protein, a strategy that has been used successfully in mice for nonreproductive proteins.

Another way to block sperm maturation would be to administer epididymis-specific anti-androgens. Androgen is essential for the normal functioning of this organ; without it, the size of the epididymis decreases dramatically and sperm fail to mature. Recent progress in administering organ-specific antiestrogens makes this approach seem feasible today. If it works, the strategy could become one of the best options for reversible male contraception.

Finally, once epididymis-specific proteins critical to sperm maturation are identified, researchers should be able to target and neutralize these proteins using immunocontraceptive methods; a more detailed discussion of immunocontraception follows below and in Appendix B, which this section summarizes. Antibodies produced by such a method should have greater access to epididymal cells than testicular cells because of the lack of a blood-testis barrier.

Gamete Interaction

A final category of strategies to achieve male infertility would be to interfere with a sperm cell's ability to interact properly with the egg. A possible approach within this category—as yet untested—would be to block immunosuppressive proteins that attach to the sperm surface in many species (Hamilton 1993). While researchers do not yet know if similar events take place in humans, interfering with whatever mechanisms allow sperm to evade the female immune system would offer interesting contraceptive possibilities.

One of the most important determinants of successful fertilization after a sperm and egg meet is the proper timing of the acrosome reaction, the release of enzymes for the sperm's acrosome that allow it to penetrate the egg's protective coat, or zona pellucida. The early release of these enzymes, when sperm and egg are still some distance apart, results in infertility.

Recently, researchers have identified some of the sperm proteins that are important in triggering the acrosome reaction. One of these, called zona receptor kinase (ZRK), may be a receptor for the egg protein ZP3. If scientists could develop a ZP3 mimic and deliver it to the male reproductive tract, such an agent might be able to prematurely induce the acrosome reaction, resulting in infertility. If the agent could be delivered to the epididymis, it would have a long period of time to have effect.

There are two potential problems with this approach, however. One is that ZRK binds, in nature, to ZP3 after full sperm capacitation within the female reproductive tract—a poorly understood process that involves changes in the sperm cell membrane—and introducing a ZP3 mimic before this stage may not be sufficient to induce the acrosome reaction. Second, because sperm are present at such high concentrations in the epididymis, any agent that acts there would also have to be present at a high concentration. On a more positive note, researchers have long known that a mutation on the T-locus of mouse sperm provokes a premature acrosome reaction in that species (Brown et al. 1989). Further study of this phenomenon may provide clues to achieving the same effect in humans.

Beyond the acrosome reaction, there are several other events that must take place at the proper time in order for egg and sperm to fuse successfully. These include sperm penetration of the egg's cumulus layer, primary binding to the zona pellucida (both of which take place before the acrosome reaction), secondary binding to the zona pellucida, penetration through the zona pellucida, and fusion of the sperm and egg plasma membranes (which occurs after the acrosome reaction). Researchers have recently identified several sperm proteins, including ZRK, PH-20, and fertilin, that are involved in the successful completion of all these events. Because all these steps are essential for fertilization, blocking any of them through application of new technologies offers powerful contraceptive potential.

APPROACHES TO IMMUNOCONTRACEPTION FOR MALES AND FEMALES*

The immune system, which under normal circumstances does not interfere with normal function of reproductive tissues, can be directed to respond to some proteins found in the reproductive system and interrupt reproductive processes. Determination of the best molecules to use for this purpose and definition of the effective dose and best manner of delivery of these proteins is an active and promising area of contraceptive research.

Unlike vaccines against most diseases, an immunocontraceptive would have to be reversible. However, it would not necessarily be given by injection; in fact, oral and vaginal preparations have shown as much promise to date as injectables. Yet while research on contraceptive immunogens has produced a number of promising results, as of this writing no such product, for humans or animals, has yet appeared on the market.

A reversible form of immunocontraception would offer several advantages over existing contraceptive methods: low cost, ease of use, infrequent administration for a long period of effectiveness, confidentiality and, above all, specificity. For an undetermined number of women and men, some or all of these attributes would be distinct advantages. For others, an immunocontraceptive might be seen as unacceptably systemic, despite certifiable specificity, and there also might be concerns about the uncertainties and individual variations in the lag time to activation and in reinstatement of fertility.

---

*Please refer to Appendix C for the full text of the authored and fully referenced paper on which this section is based.

The pathway to developing an immunocontraceptive is similar to that followed in traditional vaccine development: (1) discovery and characterization of appropriate immunogens (the proteins against which the body will mount an immune response); (2) developing methods for reliably reproducing those immunogens; (3) producing and purifying the proteins in the lab; (4) formulating doses; (5) testing on small animals and primates for immunogenicity, safety, and efficacy; (6) evaluating mechanisms of action; (7) conducting human trials for immunogenicity, safety, and efficacy; and (8) developing diagnostics to monitor responses of recipients.

Of these eight steps, the first is perhaps the most complicated. It is also the stage where many research efforts on contraceptive immunogens stand today. Virtually all reproductive processes—including gamete production, gamete transport, gamete interaction, blastocyst transport, and implantation—can be accessible to immune intervention. After targeting one process, selecting the most promising immunogens from among all possibilities can be a grueling task.

Specific Immunogens

Several criteria can help with this selection process (Griffin 1990). To make a good candidate, an immunogen should be essential to the reproductive process, act only on desired tissues, be accessible to the immune system, stimulate a sufficient number of neutralizing antibodies, be present in transient or low concentrations, and be amenable to synthesis in large quantities in the laboratory. Researchers must also have homologous animal models on which to test the candidate immunogen.

Immunogens studied for their contraceptive potential to date fall into one of four categories: (1) immunogens of the early conceptus, (2) reproductive hormones, (3) egg-surface antigens, and (4) sperm-surface antigens (see Table 4-3). Of these, those that act to prevent pregnancy before an egg is fertilized (the last three categories) have the greatest potential for acceptability. While both the male and female systems offer abundant potential for immunocontraception, research efforts to date have focused largely, though not exclusively, on methods of immunizing women against fertility or early pregnancy.

Immunogens of the Early Conceptus

Some of the most advanced immunocontraceptive products are based on human chorionic gonadotrophin (hCG), a hormone released by the early embryo that is involved in several events crucial to maintaining early pregnancy, including maintenance of the corpus luteum, progesterone production and, perhaps, implantation. To avoid undesirable side effects, researchers have focused on the hormone's beta (β) chain (either the entire chain or portions of it) rather than on its alpha chain (α), which is shared by several other hormones (Alexander 1992; Kharat et al. 1990).

The hCG-based immunogens have come from both natural and synthetic sources. Natural hCG formulations (derived from pregnancy urine) are under intensive study at India's National Institute of Immunology (Talwar et al. 1981; Talwar et al. 1990). In phase II clinical trials, researchers there have demonstrated an adequate immune response in 80 percent of the women tested, a response that lasted for about a year (Talwar et al. 1992 and 1994). While this formulation appears safe so far, there is a lag time of about three months between its administration and contraceptive effect, leaving women unprotected during this period. Sponsored by the World Health Organization, research on synthetic hCG vaccine formulations have progressed to phase I clinical trials, and phase II trials are now planned. Human female subjects produced significant levels of antibodies to the synthetic hCG (Jones et al. 1988; Jones 1990; Stevens et al. 1981; Stevens et al. 1990).

Egg-surface Antigens

Researchers thus far have identified three proteins on the zona pellucida, or outer membrane of ovulated eggs. Called ZP1, ZP2, and ZP3, formulations of these proteins have been tested as contraceptive immunogens in mice, dogs, rabbits, and monkeys. In all four species, fertility was significantly inhibited (Mahi-Brown et al. 1988; Millar et al. 1989; Skinner et al. 1984; Sacco et al. 1990).

However, a serious drawback of all these formulations has been a severe autoimmune reaction leading to premature ovarian failure. While such an unacceptable outcome has considerably dampened enthusiasm for a zona pellucida-based immunogen, some research groups are trying to get around the problem by identifying epitopes of the egg proteins that would induce antibody production without inducing a T-cell response (East et al. 1985; Rhim et al. 1992; Taguchi and Nishizuka 1980; Tung et al. 1987).

Sperm-surface Antigens

Sperm antigens offer at least two theoretical advantages over egg antigens. First, as proteins found only in sperm, they would have no chance of causing autoimmune reactions in women. Second, it may be possible to use the same antigen as a contraceptive immunogen for both men and women.

A woman's immune system could attack and incapacitate sperm at several points as they progress through the reproductive tract, including the vagina, cervix, uterus, and oviduct. Researchers have thus far identified and begun to study a number of different sperm antigens (see Table 5-6). Among the most advanced studies are on PH-20 (Phelps and Myles 1987; Phelps et al. 1988;

TABLE 4-3 Identified Candidate Immunogens for Contraceptive Formulations

Immunogen	Development and Specifications

I. Reproductive Hormones as Antigens

GnRH	Rise in anti-GnRH antibodies would reduce the levels of GnRH, LH, and FSH; steroid production would decline; and spermatogenesis would cease. The decline in androgens would result in a negative effect on libido and secondary sexual characteristics, and so this method would require supplementation with testosterone. The effects of GnRH immunogens in rats appear to be reversible. Because the immunogen causes shrinkage of male sex accessory glands, it offers a possible treatment for prostatic carcinoma or benign prostatic hyperplasia.
GnRH-DT	Potential prolongation of the anovulatory period occurring during postpartum amenorrhea induced by lactation. A phase I human immunogenicity trial is under way in two centers in India in postpartum women.
FSH Sheep FSH	Causes acute oligospermia, with the sperm that are produced being reduced in numbers, immature, and of poor quality, rather than complete azoospermia. This immunogen would require no exogenous androgen supplementation, has shown no toxicity in rats and monkeys, and is reversible. One of the more promising reversible male contraceptive options, the formula is likely to be based on recombinant proteins or synthetic peptides based on human or primate FSH, rather than the sheep hormone formulas currently in use.

II. Egg-surface Antigens

ZP1, -2, and -3	ZP3 has been shown to be an effective immunocontraceptive in rabbits and marmosets. However, ovarian pathology occurs and might lead to premature ovarian failure in humans, or even induce menopause. Tests in mice with a synthetic peptide corresponding to amino acids 328-342 of ZP3 have been shown to induce autoimmune oophoritis. Further research could produce a zona-based immunogen that could inhibit sperm-zona interaction but not cause ovarian disease (B cell epitopes rather than those which elicit T cell responses).

TABLE 4-3   Continued

Immunogen	Development and Specifications

III. Sperm-surface Antigens

PH-20		Immunization in female guinea pigs against this integral membrane protein of both the plasma and inner acrosomal membranes of guinea pig sperm has resulted in 100% contraceptive efficacy in early trials. PH-20 is likely a zona pellucida binding protein. Primate testing of a PH-20 immunogen derived from cDNA cloning is likely in the coming year.
LDH-C4 (LDH-X)		This protein is found in the mature sperm associated with the midpiece cytoplasm and, according to some reports, on the plasma membrane. Three baboon trials (of native mouse LDH-C4 or synthetic peptides from human LDH-C4) have been conducted and shown contraceptive efficacy of 75-80%. Deleterious side effects have not been noted and the contraceptive effect is reversed within one year after the last immunization. This antigen is a likely candidate for inclusion in a multideterminant formulation.
RSA-1	Hspa18 hSp17 mSp17	RSA-1 fulfills several criteria of a zona binding protein. Hspa18, the human homologue, has been localized on both the human sperm head and tail. Trials with recombinant forms of this antigen from the human (hSp17) and mouse (mSp17) have demonstrated a significant effect on reducing fertility.
Tcte-1	sp56	Egg-binding protein that interacts with ZP3. Tcte-1 and sp56 have the same molecular mass and sp56 was previously identified as an egg binding protein. Sufficient antibodies produced in the oviduct might block sperm binding or induce lysis.
SP-10		Human sperm protein associated with the acrosomal matrix and membranes of mature sperm. Sufficient titers of anti-SP-10 antibody must be generated in the oviductal fluids to agglutinate or lyse the relatively few acrosome-reacted sperm, thus inhibiting sperm/egg interaction. It is not clear yet if this is possible.
Acrosin		Antigen restricted in the mature sperm to the acrosmal membrane.
Others		99 other sperm or sperm proteins have been assigned immunocontraceptive candidacy, based on sperm surface labeling.

continued on next page

TABLE 4-3 Continued

Immunogen		Development and Specifications

IV. Immunogens of the Early Conceptus

hCG	hCG-tt (tetanus toxoid carrier)	Immunogen would induce formation of antibodies that inactivate the biological activity of hCG and thereby interrupt corpus luteum maintenance, endometrial receptivity, and thereby disrupt implantation.
hCGβ subunit vaccines		Beta-subunit-based vaccines offer the possibility of necessary specificity. In trials, menstrual regularity is maintained and ovulation is undisturbed.
HSD	βLH-DT (heterospecies dimer-ovine LH α subunit and human hCG β subunit)	In trials with HSD, protective levels are only reached in 80 percent of women and 3 months is required for protection to be conferred. Potential delivery methods such as slow release biodegradable microspheres or administration of recombinant antigen through vaccinia viruses may increase levels of protection. This approach is important conceptually: it shows that if sufficient antibodies to a contraceptive antigen are reached, infertility results.
Synthetic hCG Peptide		Synthetic oligonucleotide corresponding to the amino acid sequence 109–145 of the C terminus of β hCG. Conjugated to diphtheria toxoid. Similar mode of action as above, producing antibody to hCG.

Primakoff et al. 1985 and 1988), LDH-C4 (Goldberg 1975 and 1977; Hogrefe et al. 1987 and 1989; Lee et al. 1982; Wheat and Goldberg 1983 and 1985), RSA-1 (Lea et al. 1993; O'Rand et al. 1993a, 1993b; O'Rand and Widgren 1994; Yamasaki et al. 1995), and SP-10 (Anderson et al. 1987; Herr et al. 1990a, 1990b; Kurth et al. 1991). Each of these antigens acts at a different point or in a different manner on those sperm-egg interactions. PH-20, for example, functions at two stages: first, helping sperm penetrate the cumulus cells that surround the egg and, second, binding to the zona pellucida. In guinea pig studies, PH-20 immunizations have induced reversible infertility in both males and females. Recently, researchers sequenced PH-20 and found that the protein is the same in guinea pigs, mice, monkeys, and humans. They have now cloned and sequenced the monkey protein and are beginning studies to test its efficacy as a contraceptive in primates.

Ideally, a sperm immunogen would induce an immune reaction against all sperm-surface domains: the tail, midpiece, head, and perhaps even the inner-acrosomal membrane, which forms a major part of the head's anterior surface after the acrosome reaction. While inner-acrosomal antigens alone would offer the advantage of a highly specific, precisely timed target, they would also have to stimulate antibodies at a high enough level to affect the antigens within a narrow window of time. For that reason, focusing on surface antigens may make more sense at present. Because no single antigen may provoke a strong enough immune response, researchers working on different proteins may ultimately combine their efforts to produce one formulation containing several sperm immunogens.

Multideterminant Immunogens

In research less advanced than in the case of hCG, the reproductive hormone gonadotrophin-releasing hormone (GnRH) has shown promise as the base of contraceptive immunogens for both men and women. In research with male rats, these formulations resulted in a significant suppression of spermatogenesis that proved to be reversible. One drawback in the male is that it also affects libido and secondary sexual characteristics and would therefore have to be supplemented with testosterone (Ladd et al. 1988 and 1989). In females, these formulations have been tested in primates, with mixed results (Talwar et al. 1993), and phase I human trials are currently under way in India.

More promising as a male contraceptive are immunogens based on the hormone FSH. In trials with male monkeys, FSH immunizations caused significant oligospermia (70 percent reduction in sperm count), which resulted in virtually zero fertility (Moudgal et al. 1988a, 1988b, 1992; Moudgal and Aravindan 1993). This effect was reversible, and toxicity studies in both monkeys and rats have shown no complications. A clear advantage of the FSH immunogen is that, unlike GnRH, it does not require androgen supplements to maintain libido and secondary sexual characteristics.

In immunocontraceptive research to date, the best efficacy results have been at the level of 80 percent (for the hCG-based immunogen) and 75 percent (for the LDH-C4-based formulation). Because both these percentages are well below the 95 percent efficacy of today's oral contraceptives, no formulation so far has provided a significant improvement over current contraceptive methodologies.

These results have led many researchers to believe that the ultimate contraceptive immunogen may turn out to be a combination of different immunogens, possibly hCG and one of the sperm proteins. The chances of developing such a multideterminant formulation could be enhanced by changes in current FDA requirements to test individually for safety and efficacy each component of any new drug containing several different compounds.

Several recent areas of research should contribute significantly to the development of an effective immunogen. In the area of antigen delivery, for example, researchers have inserted the sperm antigen SP-10 into live, attenuated salmo-nella bacteria. When administered through the gut to female mice, this novel formulation induced an effective gamete-specific immune response (Curtiss 1990; Srinivasan et al. 1995).

Another interesting possibility comes from recent research on the direct injection of DNA rather than of an antigen. While not yet attempted with DNA encoding reproductive molecules, this work on so-called "naked DNA immuni-zation" has spawned a paradigm shift in the broader field of vaccine research that may yet have a major impact on the field of immunocontraception (Wolff et al. 1990).

Mucosal Immunity*

In females, the vaginal and cervical mucosa are the first line of defense against invasion by foreign molecules. Given proper reinforcements, this natural barrier could be used to block the successful entry of both microbial pathogens and sperm. The mucosal membranes of the body include the respiratory tract, conjunctiva (inner surface of the eyelids), intestinal tract, mammary glands, and the urogenital tracts of the male and female. The surface area of this complex system is nearly 400 square meters and, within it, nearly 80 percent of all immu-noglobulin-producing plasma cells reside in the intestinal mucosa, making this organ the largest reservoir of immune cells in the body. Because stimulation of the mucosal immune system at one site could elicit an immune response at a distant site, researchers believe that oral administration of immunogens could lead to effective localized immunity in the urogenital tract (Haneberg et al. 1994; Lehner et al. 1992 and 1993; Ogra and Karzon 1969; Ogra and Ogra 1973). The most promising achievement would be a vaccine that produces both a local as well as a systemic immune response that would in turn supplement the mucosal immunity.

An example of where early work is going on at this interface is Reprogen's attempt to define the molecular mechanisms involved in fertility and the mucosal immune function of the urogenital tract, toward development of interventions that are both immunocontraceptive and anti-infective. One foundation concept is that, in about five percent of infertile couples, at least one member of the couple produces an antibody that binds to the male's sperm cells and blocks activity; antibodies are found in both the cervical and male urogenital mucosa. Thus the developmental effort is toward formulating sperm head and tail proteins that can induce both a strong IgA secretory and a systemic antibody response, for use in contraception. The other piece of the foundation is identification of antigens on

---

*Please refer to Appendix D for the full text of the authored and fully referenced paper on which this section is based.

gonorrhea and chlamydia organisms that will generate both IgA and serum antibodies to block bacterial attachment and infection (Robbins-Roth 1994).

Three general requirements exist for successful oral immunization: (1) a formulation that achieves survival in the mucosal environment, (2) an adequate delivery of antigen to inductive sites, and (3) stimulation of an appropriate protective immune response. Researchers face several challenges to developing an oral immunization (e.g., Challacombe and Tomasi 1980; Mowat 1987). These include low absolute absorption of antigen via oral administration (meaning that a large initial dose is required) and the possibility that the systemic immune system may not respond to oral immunization. Nevertheless, because orally administered immunogens could have fewer adverse side effects than those delivered systemically, research in this area is considered important. Isolation of appropriate immunogens is a critical step in the overall process but, as with vaginal formulations, the delivery system can play a key role in the effectiveness of a mucosal vaccine, just as it does in the case of vaginal formulations. Mucosally active adjuvants, or "helpers," administered with immunogen, increase the immune response to the immunogen and decrease the quantity needed (Grun and Maurer 1989). The candidate most likely to succeed will be some combination of adjuvants or a "hybrid" mucosal immunogen.

The site of immunization may also play an important role in efficacy. Vaginal immunization has a relatively low success rate when compared with injection into the pelvic presacral space, via the intraperitoneal route, or via rectal administration. The vaginal epithelium provides a significant barrier to antigen uptake. Relatively little is known about the male urogenital mucosal system, but it would appear that rectal immunization could be effective in inducing certain mucosal immune reactions in the male as well.

Because the lower female urogenital tract already has a strong defense system in place, it makes sense to take advantage of this natural characteristic to block the entry of both sperm and pathogens. Primary oral immunization followed by repeated local boosting (vaginal or rectal) may be particularly effective. By combining the body's general natural defense mechanisms with the specificity possible through immunology, such an approach offers promise for development of a highly effective, user controlled, and reversible contraceptive as well as an anti-STD agent.

CONCLUDING COMMENT

This chapter was prepared as a summary of the individually authored technical papers that constitute the appendixes to this report, to which the reader is referred. It is intended as a bridge among what the committee believes to be the pressing public health and individual needs for new contraceptive technologies; the market that will or will not respond to those needs; and the regulatory, legal, and sociopolitical climate that will or will not make that response fall into some zone of reasonable possibility.

REFERENCES

Adams CE. Retention and development of eggs transferred to the uterus at various times after ovulation in the rabbit. Journal of Reproduction and Fertility 60:309–315, 1980.

Alexander NJ. Contraceptive Vaccine Development. IN Vaccine Research and Developments. W Koff, H Six, eds. New York: Marcel Dekker. 1992.

Allan GF, X Leng, SY Tsai, et al. Hormone and antihormone induce distinct conformational changes which are central to steroid receptor activation. Journal of Biological Chemistry 267:19513–19520, 1992.

Anderson DJ, PM Johnson, WR Jones, et al. Monoclonal antibodies to human trophoblast and sperm antigens: Report of two WHO-sponsored workshops, 30 June 1986, Toronto, Canada. Journal of Reproductive Immunology 10:231–257, 1987.

Artini PG, C Battaglia, G D'Ambrogio, et al. Relationship between human oocyte maturity, fertilization and follicular fluid growth factors. Human Reproduction 9:902–906, 1994.

Bagatell CJ, AM Matsumoto, RB Christensen et al. Comparison of a gonadotropin-releasing hormone antagonist plus testosterone (T) versus T alone as potential male contraceptive regimens. Journal of Clinical Endocrinology and Metabolism 77(2):427–432, 1993.

Becker-Andre M, I Wisenberg, N Schaeren-Wiemers, et al. Pineal gland hormone melatonin binds and activates an orphan of the nuclear receptor superfamily. Journal of Biological Chemistry 269:28531–28534, 1994.

Bhatt H, LJ Brunet, CA Stewart. Uterine expression of leukemia inhibitory factor coincides with the onset of blastocyst implantation. Proceedings of the National Academy of Sciences, USA 88:11408–11412, 1991.

Birgerson L, A Lund, V Odlind, et al. Termination of early human pregnancy with epostane. Contraception 35:11–120, 1987.

Brown J, JA Cebra-Thomas, JD Bleil, et al. A premature acrosome reaction is programmed by mouse t haplotypes during sperm differentiation and could play a role in transmission ratio distortion. Development 106:769–773, 1989.

Challacombe SJ, TB Tomasi. Systemic tolerance and secretory immunity after oral immunization. Journal of Experimental Medicine 152:1459–1472, 1980.

Chen DB, R Hilsenrath, ZM Yang, et al. Leukemia inhibitory factor in human endometrium during the menstrual cycle: Cellular origin and action on production of glandular epithelial cell prostaglandin *in vitro*. Human Reproduction 10:911–918, 1995.

Chen F, AJ Cooney, Y Wang, et al. Cloning of a novel orphan receptor (GCNF) expressed during germ cell development. Molecular Endocrinology 8:1434–1444, 1994.

Cook RJ. Antiprogestin drugs: Medical and legal issues. Family Planning Perspectives 21(6):267–272, 1989.

Crooij MJ, CC deNooyer, BR Rao, et al. Termination of early pregnancy by the 3β hydroxysteroid dehydrogenase inhibitor epostane. New England Journal of Medicine 319:813–817, 1988.

Croxatto HB. Gamete transport. IN Reproductive Endocrinology, Surgery, and Technology. E Adashi, JA Rock, Z Rosenwaks, eds. Philadelphia: Lippincott-Raven. 1995.

Curtiss R III. Attenuated *Salmonella* strains as live vectors for the expression of foreign antigens. IN New Generation Vaccines, GC Woodrow, MM Levine, eds. New York: Marcel Dekker. 1990.

De M, TR Sandford, GW Wood. Expression of interleukin 1, interleukin 6 and tumor necrosis factor α in mouse uterus during the peri-implantation period of pregnancy. Journal of Reproduction and Fertility 97:83–89, 1993.

DePaolo LV, M Shimonaka, RH Schwall, et al. *In vivo* comparison of the follicle-stimulating hormone-suppressing activity of follistatin and inhibin in ovariectomized rats. Endocrinology 128:668–674, 1991.

Dorce M. Control of M-Phase by maturation-promoting factor. Journal of Reproduction anf Fertility 97:83–89, 1993.

East IJ, BJ Gulyas, J Dean. Monoclonal antibodies to the murine zona pellucida protein with sperm receptor activity: Effects on fertilization and early development. Developmental Biology 109:268–273, 1985.

Eddy EM, DA O'Brien. The Spermatozoon. IN The Physiology of Reproduction, 2nd ed., Vol. 1. E Knobil, JD Neill, eds. New York: Raven Press. 1994.

Erickson GF, DR Danforth. Ovarian control of follicle development. American Journal of Obstetrics and Gynecology 172:736–747, 1995.

Frank GR, AK Brar, H Jikihara, et al. Interleukin-1β and the endometrium: An inhibitor of stromal cell differentiation and possible autoregulator of decidualization in humans. Biology of Reproduction 52:184–191, 1995.

Fukuda MN, T Sato, J Nakayama, et al. Trophinin and tastin, a novel cell adhesion molecule complex with potential involvement in embryo implantation. Genes and Development 9:1199–1210, 1995.

Gemzell-Danielsson K, M-L Swahn, et al. Early luteal phase treatment with mifepristone (RU 486) for fertility regulation. Human Reproduction 8:870–873, 1993.

Ghosh D, P De, J Sengupta. Luteal phase estrogen is not essential for implantation and maintenance of pregnancy from surrogate embryo transfer in the rhesus monkey. Human Reproduction 9:629–637, 1994.

Ghosh D, J Sengupta. Anti-nidatory effect of a single, early post-ovulatory administration of mifepristone (RU 486) in the rhesus monkey. Human Reproduction 8:552–558, 1993.

Goldberg E. Isozymes in testes and spermatozoa. IN Isozymes: Current Topics in Biological and Medical Research. MC Rattazzi, JG Scandalios, GS Whitt, eds. New York: Alan R. Liss. 1977.

Goldberg E. Lactate dehydrogenase-X (crystalline) from mouse testes. IN Methods in Enzymology: Carbohydrate metabolism, Part B, Vol. XLI. New York: Academic Press. 1975.

Greene KE, LM Kettel, SS Yen. Interruption of endometrial maturation without hormonal changes by an antiprogesterone during the first half of the luteal phase of the menstrual cycle: A contraceptive potential. Fertility and Sterility 58:338–343, 1992.

Griffin D. Strategy of vaccine development. IN Gamete Interaction: Prospects for Immunocontraception. NJ Alexander, PD Griffin, NM Spieler, GMH Waites, eds. New York: Wiley-Liss. 1990.

Grigorescu F, MT Baccara, et al. Insulin and IGF-1 signaling in oocyte maturation. Hormone Research 42:55–61, 1994.

Grun JL, PH Maurer. T helper cell subsets elicited in mice utilizing two different adjuvant vehicles: The role of endogenous interleukin I in proliferative responses. Cellular Immunology 121:134–145, 1989.

Gu H, JD Marth, PC Orban, et al. Deletion of a DNA polymerase beta gene segment in T cells using cell type-specific gene targeting. Science 265:103–106, 1994.

Hamilton DW. Local immunity and sperm processing in the male reproductive tract. IN Local Immunity in Reproductive Tract Tissues. PD Griffin, PM Johnson, eds. New York: Oxford University Press. 1993.

Handelsman DJ, AJ Conway, LM Boylan. Suppression of human spermatogenesis by testosterone implants. Journal of Clinical Endocrinology and Metabolism 75(5):1326–1332, 1992.

Haneberg B, D Kendall, HM Amerongen, et al. Induction of specific immunoglobulin A in small intestine, colon-rectum, and vagina measured with a new method for collection of secretions from local mucosal surfaces. Infectious Immunology 62:15–23, 1994.

Harper MJK. Agents with antifertility effects during preimplantation stages of pregnancy. IN Biology of Mammalian Reproduction. KS Moghissi, ESE Hafez, eds. Springfield, IL: C.C. Thomas. 1972.

Herr JC, CJ Flickinger, M Homyk, et al. Biochemical and morphological characterization of the intra-acrosomal antigen SP-10 from human sperm. Biology of Reproduction 42:181–193, 1990a.

Herr JC, RM Wright, E John, et al. Identification of human acrosomal antigen SP-10 in primates and pigs. Biology of Reproduction 42:377–382. 1990b.

Herrmann W, R Wyss, A Riondel, et al. Effet d'un stéroide anti-progestérone chez la femme: Interruption du cycle menstruel et de la grossesse au début. Comptes Rendu de l'Académie des Sciences 294:933–938, 1982.

Heyman RA, DJ Mangelsdorf, JA Dyck, et al. 9-cis retinoic acid is a high affinity ligand for the retinoid X receptor. Cell 68:397–406, 1992.

Hilton DJ, NA Nicola, D Metcalf. Specific binding of murine leukemia inhibitory factor to normal and leukemic monocytic cells. Proceedings of the National Academy of Sciences, USA 85:5971–5975, 1988.

Hogrefe HH, JP Griffith, MG Rossmann, et al. Characterization of antigenic sites on the refined 3-A structure of mouse testicular lactate dehydrogenase-C4. Journal of Biological Chemistry 262:13155–13162, 1987.

Hogrefe HH, PTP Kaumaya, E Goldberg. Immunogenicity of synthetic peptides corresponding to flexible and antibody-accessible segments of mouse lactate dehydrogenase (LDH)-C_4. Journal of Biological Chemistry 264:10513–10519, 1989.

Hsueh AJ, H Billig, A Tsafriri. Ovarian follicle atresia: Hormonally controlled apoptotic process. Endocrine Reviews 15:707–724, 1994.

Hunt JS, HL Chen, et al. Normal distribution of tumor necrosis factor-a messenger ribonucleic acid and protein in the uteri, placentas, and embryos of osteopetrotic *(op/op)* mice lacking colon-stimulating factor-1. Biology of Reproduction 49:441–452, 1993.

Ikeda Y, WH Shen, et al. Developmental expression of mouse steroidogenic factor-1, an essential regulator of the steroid hydroxylases. Molecular Endocrinology 8:654–662, 1994.

Ilesanmi AO, DA Hawkins, BA Lessey. Immunohistochemical markers of uterine receptivity in the human endometrium. Microscopic Research Technique 25:208–222, 1993.

Inoue T, H Kanzaki, M Iwai, et al. Tumor necrosis factor α inhibits *in vitro* decidualization of human endometrial stromal cells. Human Reproduction 9:2411–2417, 1994.

Jentoft N. Why are proteins O-glycosylated? Trends in Biochemical Science 15:291–294, 1990.

Jones WR. Lessons from an anti-human chorionic gonadotropin contraceptive vaccine trial. IN Gamete Interaction: Prospects for Immunocontraception. NJ Alexander, PD Griffin, JM Spieler, GMH Waites, eds. New York: Wiley Liss. 1990.

Jones WR, J Bradley, SJ Judd, et al. Phase I clinical trials of a World Health Organization birth control vaccine. Lancet 1:1295, 1988.

Kharat E, NS Nair, K Dhall, et al. Analysis of menstrual records of women immunized with anti-hCG vaccines inducing antibodies partially cross-reactive with hLH. Contraception 41:293–299, 1990.

Kliman HJ, RF Feinberg, LB Schwartz, et al. A mucin-like glycoprotein identified by MAG (mouse ascites golgi) antibodies: Menstrual cycle-dependent localization in human endometrium. American Journal of Pathology 146:166–181, 1995.

Kurth BE, K Klotz, CJ Flickinger, et al. Localization of sperm antigen SP-10 during the six stages of the cycle of the seminiferous epithelium. Biology of Reproduction 44:814–821, 1991.

Ladd A, G Prabhu, YY Tsong, T Probst, et al. Active immunization against gonadotrophin-releasing hormone combined with androgen supplementation is a promising antifertility vaccine for males. American Journal of Reproductive Immunology 17:121, 1988.

Ladd A, YY Tsong, G Prabhu, et al. Effects of long-term immunization against LHRH and androgen treatment on gonadal function. Journal of Reproductive Immunology 15:85–101, 1989.

Lala DS, DR Rice, KL Parker. Steroidogenic factor 1, a key regulator of steroidogenic enzyme expression, is the mouse homolog of fushi tarazu-factor 1. Molecular Endocrinology 6:1248–1258, 1992.

Lea I, RT Richardson, EE Widgren, et al. Cloning and sequencing of human Sp17, a sperm zona binding protein. Molecular Biology of the Cell 4:248a, 1993.

Lee CY, JH Huan, E Goldberg. Lactate dehydrogenase from the mouse. IN Carbohydrate Metabolism: Part D, Methods in Enzymology. WA Wood, ed. New York: Academic Press. 1982.

Lehner T, LA Bergmeier, C Panagiotidi et al. Induction of mucosal and systemic immunity to a recombinant simian immunodeficiency viral protein. Science 258:1365–1369, 1992.

Lehner T, R Brookes, C Panagiotidi et al. T- and B-cell functions and epitope expression in nonhuman primates immunized with simian immunodeficiency virus antigen by the rectal route. Proceedings of the National Academy of Sciences, USA 90:8638–8642, 1993.

Lessey BA. The use of integrins for the assessment of uterine receptivity. Fertility and Sterility 61:812–814, 1994.

Lessey BA, AJ Castelbaum, CA Buck, et al. Further characterization of endometrial integrins during the menstrual cycle and in pregnancy. Fertility and Sterility 62:497–506, 1994.

Lessey BA, L Damjanovich, C Coutifaris, et al. Integrin adhesion molecules in the human endometrium: Correlation with the normal and abnormal menstrual cycle. Journal of Clinical Investigation 90:188–195, 1992.

Luo X, Y Ikeda, KL Parker. A cell-specific nuclear receptor is essential for adrenal and gonadal development and sexual differentiation. Cell 77:481–490, 1994.

Mahi-Brown CA, R Yanagimachi, ML Nelson, et al. Ovarian histopathology of bitches immunized with porcine zonae pellucidae. American Journal of Reproductive Immunology and Microbiology 18:94–103, 1988.

McDonnell DP, DL Clemm, T Herman, et al. Analysis of estrogen receptor function *in vitro* reveals three distinct classes of antiestrogens. Molecular Endocrinology 9:659–669, 1995.

Millar SE, SM Chamow, AW Baur, et al. Vaccination with a synthetic zona pellucida peptide produces long-term contraception in female mice. Science 246:935–938, 1989.

Morris JK, JS Richards. Luteinizing hormone induces prostaglandin endoperoxide synthase-2 and luteinization *in vitro* by A-kinase and C-kinase pathways. Endocrinology 136:1549–1558, 1995.

Morris JK, JS Richards. Hormone induction of luteinization and prostaglandin endoperoxide synthase-2 involves multiple cellular signaling pathways. Endocrinology 133:770–779, 1993.

Moudgal NR, GR Aravindan. Induction of infertility in the male by blocking follicle-stimulating hormone action. IN Immunology of Reproduction. R Naz, ed. Boca Raton, FL: CRC Press. 1993.

Moudgal NR, GS Murthy, N Ravindranath, et al. Contraception through regulation of endogenous FSH secretion: Prospects for the male. IN Human Reproduction and Contraception. S Takagi, GI Zatuchni, eds. Tokyo: Professional Postgraduate Services. 1988a.

Moudgal NR, GS Murthy, N Ravindranath, et al. Development of a contraceptive vaccine for use by the human male: Results of a feasibility study carried out in adult male bonnet monkeys (*Macaca radiata*). IN Contraceptive Research for Today and the Nineties. GP Talwar, ed. New York: Springer Verlag. 1988b.

Moudgal NR, N Ravindranath, GS Murthy, et al. Long-term contraceptive efficacy of vaccine of ovine follicle-stimulating hormone in male bonnet monkeys (*Macaca radiata*). Journal of Reproduction and Fertility 96:91–102, 1992.

Mowat AM. The regulation of immune responses to dietary protein antigens. Immunology Today 8:93–98, 1987.

Ogra PL, DT Karzon. Distribution of poliovirus antibody in serum, nasopharynx and alimentary tract following segmental immunization of lower alimentary tract with poliovirus. Journal of Immunology 102:1423–1427, 1969.

Ogra PL, SS Ogra. Local antibody response to polio vaccine in the human genital tract. Journal of Immunology 110:1307–1311, 1973.

O'Malley BW. Steroid hormone receptors as transactivators of gene expression. Breast Cancer Research and Treatment 18:67–71, 1991.

O'Rand MG, J Beavers, EE Widgren, et al. Inhibition of fertility in female mice by immunization with a B-cell epitope, the synthetic sperm peptide, P10G. Journal of Reproductive Immunology 25:89–102, 1993a.

O'Rand MG, RT Richardson, N Yamasaki. Zona pellucida binding of mammalian spermatozoa. Journal of Reproduction, Fertility, and Development 39(Suppl.):43–44, 1993b.

O'Rand MG, EE Widgren. Identification of sperm antigen targets for immunocontraception: B-cell epitope analysis of Sp17. Reproduction, Fertility, and Development 6:289–296, 1994.

Ortiz ME, G Bastias, O Darrigrande, H Croxatto. Importance of uterine expulsion of embryos in the interceptive mechanism of postcoital oestradiol in rats. Reproduction, Fertility, and Development 3:333–337, 1991.

Phelps BM, P Primakoff, DE Koppel, et al. Restricted lateral diffusion of PH-20, a pi-anchored sperm membrane protein. Science 240:1780–1782, 1988.

Phelps B, DG Myles. The guinea pig sperm plasma membrane protein, PH-20, reaches the surface via two transport pathways and becomes localized to a domain after an initial uniform distribution. Developmental Biology 123:63–72, 1987.

Pollard JW, JS Hunt, W Wiktor-Jedrzejczak, et al. A pregnancy defect in the osteopetrotic *(op/op)* mouse demonstrates the requirement for CSF-1 in female fertility. Developmental Biology 148:273–283, 1991.

Primakoff P, H Hyatt, DG Myles. A role for the migrating sperm surface antigen PH-20 in guinea pig sperm binding to the egg zona pellucida. Journal of Cell Biology 101:2239–2244, 1985.

Primakoff P, W Lathrop, L Woodman, et al. Fully effective contraception in female guinea pigs immunized with the sperm protein PH-20. Nature 335:543–546, 1988.

Rhim SH, SE Millar, F Robey, et al. Autoimmune disease of the ovary induced by a ZP3 peptide from the mouse zona pellucida. Journal of Clinical Investigation 89:28–35, 1992.

Robbins-Roth C, ed. Highlights of the Annual National Conference on Biotechnology Ventures: Reprogen, Inc.—On the Trail of Mechanisms. Bioventure View 9(11), December 1994.

Sacco AG, EC Yurewicz, MG Subramanian, et al. Analysis of the porcine zona pellucida M_r=55,000 antigen for contraceptive use. IN Reproductive Immunology 1989, L Mettler, D Billington, eds. Amsterdam: Elsevier. 1990.

Schane HP, JE Creange, AJ Anzalone, et al. Interceptive activity of azastene in rhesus monkeys. Fertility and Sterility 30:343–347, 1978.

Schultz JF, DR Armant. β_1 and β_3 -class integrins mediate fibronectin binding activity at the surface of developing mouse peri-implantation blastocysts. Journal of Biological Chemistry 270:11522–11531, 1995.

Selinger M, IZ Mackenzie, MD Gillmer, et al. Progesterone inhibition in mid-trimester termination of pregnancy: Physiological and clinical effects. British Journal of Obstetrics and Gynaecology 94:1218–1222, 1987.

Shen WH, CC Moore, Y Ikeda, et al. Nuclear receptor steroididogenic factor 1 regulates the Mullerian inhibiting substance gene: A link to the sex determination cascade. Cell 77:651–661, 1994.

Simón C, A Frances, GN Piquette, et al. Embryonic implantation in mice is blocked by interleukin-1 receptor antagonist. Endocrinology 134:521–528, 1994.

Simón C, GN Piquette, A Frances, et al. Interleukin-1 type I receptor messenger ribonucleic acid (mRNA) expression in human endometrium throughout the menstrual cycle. Fertility and Sterility 59:791–796, 1993a.

Simón C, GN Piquette, A Frances, et al. Localization of interleukin-1 type I receptor and interleukin-1β in human endometrium throughout the menstrual cycle. Journal of Clinical Endocrinology and Metabolism 77:549–555, 1993b.

Skinner SM, T Mills, HJ Kirchick, et al. Immunization with zona pellucida proteins results in abnormal ovarian follicular differentiation and inhibition of gonadotropin-induced steroid secretion. Endocrinology 115:2418–2432, 1984.

Snyder BW, HP Schane. Inhibition of luteal phase progesterone levels in the rhesus monkey by epostane. Contraception 31:479–486, 1985.

Srinivasan J, S Tinge, R Wright, et al. Oral immunization with attenuated Salmonella expressing human sperm antigen induces antibodies in serum and the reproductive tract. Biology of Reproduction 53:462–471, 1995.

Stevens VC, B Cinader, JE Powell, et al. Preparation and formulation of an hCG antifertility vaccine: Selection of an adjuvant and vehicle. American Journal of Reproductive Immunology 6:315–321, 1981.

Stevens VC, JE Powell, M Rickey, et al. Studies of various delivery systems for a human chorionic gonadotropin vaccine. IN Gamete Interaction: Prospects for Immunocontraception. NJ Alexander, PD Griffin, JM Spieler, GMH Waites, eds. New York: Wiley-Liss. 1990.

Stewart CC, P Kasper, LJ Brunet, et al. Blastocyst implantation depends on maternal expression of leukemia inhibitory factor. Nature 369:76–79, 1992.

Strous GJ, J Dekker. Mucin-type glycoproteins. Critical Reviews in Biochemical and Molecular Biology 27:57–92, 1992.

Swahn ML, M Bygdeman, S Cekan, et al. The effect of RU 486 administered during the early luteal phase on bleeding pattern, hormonal parameters and endometrium. Human Reproduction 5:402–408, 1990.

Tabibzadeh S, KL Kaffka, PG Satyaswaroop, et al. Interleukin-1 (IL-1) regulation of human endometrial function: Presence of IL-1 receptor correlates with IL-1-stimulated prostaglandin E_2 production. Journal of Clinical Endocrinology and Metabolism 70:1000–1006, 1990.

Tackacs L, EJ Kavacs, MR Smith, et al. Detection of IL-1α and IL-1β gene expression by *in situ* hybridization: Tissue localization of IL-1 mRNA in the normal C57BL/6 mouse. Journal of Immunology 141:3081–3094, 1988.

Taguchi O, Y Nishizuka. Autoimmune oophoritis in thymectomized mice: T cell requirement in adoptive transfer. Clinical Experiments in Immunology 42:324–331, 1980.

Talwar GP, SK Gupta, AK Tandon. Immunologic interruption of pregnancy. IN Reproductive Immunology. N Gleicher, ed. New York: Alan R. Liss. 1981.

Talwar GP, OM Singh, R Pal, et al. A vaccine that prevents pregnancy in women. Proceedings of the National Academy of Sciences, USA 91:8532–8536, 1994.

Talwar GP, O Singh, R Pal, et al. Vaccines against LHRH and HCG. IN Immunology of Reproduction. R Naz, ed. Boca Raton, FL: CRC Press. 1993.

Talwar GP, O Singh, R Pal, et al. Anti-hCG vaccines are in clinical trials. Scandinavian Journal of Immunology 36(Suppl. 11):123, 1992.

Talwar GP, O Singh, R Pal, et al. Experiences of the anti-hCG vaccine of relevance to development of other birth control vaccines. IN Gamete Interaction: Prospects for Immunocontraception. NJ Alexander, PD Griffin, JM Spieler, GMH Waites, eds. New York: Wiley-Liss. 1990.

Tartakovsky B, E Ben-Yair. Cytokines modulate preimplantation development and pregnancy. Developmental Biology 146:345–352, 1991.

Tung KSK, S Smith, C Teuscher, et al. Murine autoimmune oophoritis, epididymoorchitis, and gastritis induced by day 3 thymectomy. American Journal of Pathology 126:293–302, 1987.

Tzukerman MT, A Esty, D Santioso-Mere, et al. Human estrogen receptor transcriptional capacity is determined by both cellular and promoter context and mediated by two functionally distinct intramolecular regions. Molecular Endocrinology 8:21–30, 1994.

Vale W, L Bilezikjian, C Rivier. Reproductive and other roles of inhibins and activins. IN The Physiology of Reproduction. E Knobil, JD Neill, eds. New York: Raven Press. 1994.

Vale W, A Hsueh, C Rivier. The inhibin/activin family of hormones and growth factors. IN Handbook of Experimental Pharmacology, Vol. 95/11: Peptide Growth Factors and Their Receptors, II. New York: Springer-Verlag. 1990.

Van Look PFA. Presentation on menses-inducers at an Institute of Medicine Workshop on Contraceptive Research and Development and the Frontiers of Contemporary Science, Washington, DC, Institute of Medicine, 9–10 December 1994.

Wang C, R Swerdloff, GMH Waites. Male contraception: 1993 and beyond. IN Contraceptive Research and Development 1984 to 1994. PFA Van Look, G Pérez-Palacios, eds. New York: Oxford University Press. 1994.

Wheat TE, E Goldberg. Antigenic domains of the sperm-specific lactate dehydrogenase C_4 isozyme. Molecular Immunology 22:643–649, 1985.

Wheat TE, E Goldberg. Sperm-specific lactate dehydrogenase C_4: Antigenic structure and immunosuppression of fertility. IN Isozymes: Current Topics in Biological and Medical Research, Vol. 7. MC Retezzi, JG Scandalios, GS Whitt, eds. New York: Alan R. Liss. 1983.

World Health Organization, Special Programme of Research, Development and Research Training in Human Reproduction, Task Force on Post-ovulatory Methods of Fertility Regulation. Menstrual regulation by mifepristone plus prostaglandin: Results from a multicentre trial. Human Reproduction 10:308–314, 1995.

Willson TA, D Metcalf, NM Gough. Cross-species comparison of the sequence of the leukemia inhibitory factor gene and its protein. European Journal of Biochemistry 204:21–30, 1992.

Wolff JA, RW Malone, P Williams, et al. Direct gene transfer into mouse muscle *in vivo*. Science 247:1465–1468, 1990.

Yamamoto-Yamaguchi Y, M Tomida, M Hozumi. Specific binding of a factor inducing differentiation to mouse myeloid leukemic M1 cells. Experimental Cell Research 164:97–102, 1986.

Yamasaki N, RT Richardson, MG O'Rand. Expression of the rabbit sperm protein Sp17 in COS cells and interaction of recombinant Sp17 with the rabbit zona pellucida. Molecular Reproduction and Development 40:48–55, 1995.

Yang Z-M, S-P Le, D-B Chen, MJK Harper. Temporal and spatial expression of leukemia inhibitory factor in rabbit uterus during early pregnancy. Molecular Reproduction and Development 38:148–152, 1994.

Yang Z-M, S-P Le, D-B Chen, et al. Expression patterns of leukemia inhibitory factor receptor (LIFR) and the gp130 receptor component in rabbit uterus during early pregnancy. Journal of Reproduction and Fertility 103:249–255, 1995a.

Yang Z-M, S-P Le, D-B Chen, et al. Leukemia inhibitory factor (LIF), LIF receptor and gp130 in the mouse uterus during early pregnancy. Molecular Reproduction and Development 42:407–414, 1995b.

Zhang Z, C Funk, SR Glasser, et al. Progesterone regulation of heparin-binding epidermal growth factor-like factor gene expression during sensitization and decidualization in the rat uterus: Effects of the antiprogestin ZK 98.299. Endocrinology 135:1256–1263, 1994a.

Zhang Z, C Funk, D Roy, et al. Heparin-binding epidermal growth factor-like growth factor is differentially regulated by progesterone and estradiol in rat uterine epithelial and stromal cells. Endocrinology 134:1089–1094, 1994b.

Zhong Z, Z Wen, JE Darnell Jr. STAT3: A STAT family member activated by tyrosine phosphorylation in response to epidermal growth factor and interleukin-6. Science 264:95–98, 1994.

Zirkin BR, C Awoniyi, MD Griswold, et al. Is FSH required for adult spermatogenesis? Journal of Andrology 15:273–276. 1994.

NOTES

1. During the first 14 days of its development, the product of the fertilized egg is variously termed the conceptus, the zygote, the blastocyst, or the "preembryo." It is after implantation that what is properly termed the embryo forms in the center of the conceptus; the remaining 99 percent of the tissue gives rise to the placenta and other extraembryonic membranes. The embryo develops into a fetus at about 8 weeks after fertilization or 10 weeks after the last menstrual period (Cook 1989).

2. The first laboratory and clinical data on RU 486 were presented by Herrman et al. in 1982.

5

The Market for New Contraceptives: Translating Unmet Need into Market Demand

Chapter 2 documents the existence of a considerable unmet need for contraception in both the industrial and developing economies of the world. The argument is made that there is a compelling public health[1] case for broadening the portfolio of contraception options, for women and men everywhere. Chapters 3 and 4—most particularly the latter—offer rich evidence for new paths in contemporary science that could expand those options and answer specific and highly critical needs for which there are now no adequate or appropriate solutions.

Yet, as irrefutable as the need may be and as promising the science, response from pharmaceutical firms in the United States and western Europe will be conditioned by the difficulties of translating need and promise into a profitable market. The high costs and risks of committing to the development of any medical technology are such that no firm will undertake commercialization without at least a strong belief in the existence of a substantial market of consumers able and willing to pay, in other words, the existence of market demand. In the case of new contraceptives, that belief is qualified by factors whose effects are economic and whose causes are several and complex. This is a major dilemma.

The present chapter explores this dilemma from several perspectives. The first is a qualitative look at present market demand as expressed in overall patterns of contraceptive use, worldwide and in the United States.

The second focus is on specific areas of contraceptive need that seem most readily translatable into market demand, that is, "niches" that are either empty or quite inadequately filled. The indicators of these niches include the various limitations in the current array of contraceptives as expressed in the side effects experienced by users, failure and discontinuation rates reflecting side effects and other constraints to adoption and continued use, and sterilization as a contraceptive option that is not always appropriate. This focus also encompasses the implications of the sexually transmitted diseases for contraceptive technology and their relevance for the contraceptive market.

The third perspective has to do with consumer preferences, with particular attention to the content and character of the "woman-centered agenda" and the issues it raises.

The fourth perspective is quantitative: a look at today's market for contraceptives in terms of numbers of actual and potential users and dollar values; lessons to be learned from the world vaccine market, with which the contraceptives market is in some ways analogous; and subsidized procurement as a market factor.

The chapter closes with a discussion of the cost-effectiveness of contraception and what that might mean as an incentive to investment in contraceptive R&D and the intimate and necessary relationship of that investment with the market for contraceptive technologies.

CURRENT CONTRACEPTIVE USE

Contraceptive Use Worldwide

Contraceptive prevalence[2] among women currently married or in union (a group designated by the abbreviation MWRA, or "married women of reproductive age") increased worldwide from 30 percent during 1960–1965 to 57 percent in 1990. The increase was much more dramatic in the developing countries, where prevalence rose from 9 percent to 53 percent in that same period (UN 1994, cited in WHO/HRP 1995). The increase was especially dramatic in eastern Asia and Latin America, slightly less so in other parts of Asia and in North Africa, least of all in Sub-Saharan Africa. The range is wide: Contraceptive use prevalence in Africa is currently estimated at 17 percent, quite a difference from Latin America, for example, where prevalence is almost 65 percent (see Table 5-1 and Table 5-2 for data for developing countries).

There is also great variability within regions. While overall prevalence in the Arab States and Europe averages 44 percent, the range is from almost zero in some Persian Gulf countries to 68 percent in Turkey. And, in Asia, where the overall prevalence is 62.5 percent, the range is from 10 percent in Afghanistan to a use prevalence of 80 percent or more in China. Variability in contraceptive use prevalence among the industrial countries is much narrower (Guttmacher Institute 1995a; WHO/HRP 1995).

The overwhelming majority—90 percent—of women using contraception in the developing countries are using modern methods. Globally, the most used method is female sterilization (tubectomy or tubal ligation). Thirty percent of all contracepting couples worldwide relied on female sterilization as of 1990; in the

TABLE 5-1 Basic Data, Total Population, and Contraceptive Use, World and Developing Countries, 1994 and Projected for 2005 (in thousands)

	1994	2005
World		
Total population	5,646,200	6,665,120
Total female population	2,803,790	3,307,980
Women of reproductive age (aged 15–49)	1,415,810	1,681,040
Women of reproductive age, married or in union (MWRA)[a]	976,728	1,145,490
Contraceptive users among all women	595,103	755,817
Developing Countries		
Total population	4,418,180	5,364,550
Total female population	2,172,230	2,642,990
Women of reproductive age (aged 15–49)	1,106,570	1,368,950
Women of reproductive age, married or in union (MWRA)[a]	784,897	953,815
Contraceptive users among all women	457,759	625,521
Contraceptive users among married/in union women	445,692	602,417

[a]MWRA = married women of reproductive age, defined as "married or living with a man," vis-à-vis "now widowed, divorced, or no longer living together."

SOURCE: United Nations Population Fund. Contraceptive Use and Commodity Costs in Developing Countries, 1994–2005. New York, 1995. Data for total population are from the United Nations 1992 estimates and projections. User data are derived from sample surveys carried out in 69 developing countries in the 1980s and 1990s; these countries contained 90 percent of the population and 94 percent of contraceptive users of all developing countries in 1990. Contraceptive prevalence for the period of analysis was projected using a demographic approach that takes the level of contraceptive prevalence as estimated from the latest national survey and then projects increases in contraceptive prevalence as a function of estimated changes in total fertility rates. The basis is the United Nations medium population projection. These rates are then applied to the number of MWRA *and* unmarried women who use contraception; the fact that there are now data from 34 countries for this second population group makes its inclusion in global calculations of contraceptive prevalence possible for the first time.

TABLE 5-2 Number of Contraceptive Users, by Method, World and Developing Countries, 1994 and Projected for 2005 (in thousands)

	Sterilization			Pill	Injectable	IUD	Condom	Other	Total Users
	All	Female	Male						
				World					
1994	233,597	183,323	50,274	92,060	11,879	127,156	51,451	78,960	595,103
2005	290,599	232,514	58,085	120,097	9,375	152,325	58,965	4,456	755,817
				Developing Countries					
1994	200,149	161,107	39,042	51,352	10,461	112,115	24,778	46,837	445,692
2005	258,847	210,031	48,816	76,603	17,058	137,079	35,702	77,128	602,417

SOURCE: United Nations Population Fund. Contraceptive Use and Commodity Costs in Developing Countries, 1994–2005. New York, 1995. Data are derived from sample surveys carried out in 69 developing countries in the 1980s and 1990s; these countries contained 90 percent of the population and 94 percent of contraceptive users of all developing countries in 1990. Contraceptive prevalence for the period of analysis was projected using a demographic approach that takes the level of contraceptive prevalence as estimated from the latest national survey and then projects increases in contraceptive prevalence as a function of estimated changes in total fertility rates. The basis is the United Nations medium population projection. These rates are subsequently applied both to the number of MWRA (married women of reproductive age) *and* to the number of unmarried women who use contraception; the fact that there are now data from 34 countries for this second population group makes its inclusion in global calculations of contraceptive prevalence possible for the first time.

developing countries, that figure was 38 percent (UNFPA 1994; WHO/HRP 1995). As for reversible methods, the IUD is the second most used method in the developing countries, primarily because of its extensive use in the People's Republic of China; it ranks fourth in the industrial economies, a ranking that might be higher were it not for the unavailability of the IUD in most of eastern Europe and its very limited use in the United States. The pill ranks third in the developing countries and is the most prevalent method in the industrial countries. The condom fails to even approach the levels of utilization in the developing countries that it has achieved elsewhere. In fact, all coitus-related methods (condoms, vaginal methods, withdrawal) are far less likely to be used in most developing countries than in the industrial countries. Because Norplant is so new and available in very few developing countries, use prevalence data are not included in the tables below. As of 1993, there were an estimated 1.5 million users of that method in developing countries (of whom 1.3 million were in Indonesia), with an admittedly arbitrary estimate of 6.8 million by 2005 (UNFPA 1994). It is important to remember that any ranking of method utilization reflects only what people *do*, not necessarily what they *prefer*; in much of the developing world, the full "mix" of methods that would permit individuals to truly express preference by choosing among real options is not generally available (WHO/HRP 1995) (see Table 5-3 and Table 5-4).

Contraceptive Use in the United States

In 1988, over two-thirds of women of reproductive age in the United States were at risk of unintended pregnancy, that is, they were sexually active and did not want to become pregnant but would be physically able to become pregnant if they or their partner used no contraceptive method (Forrest 1994b). Of those 39 million women, 35 million (9 in 10) were using a contraceptive and 4 million were not (Forrest 1994b).

Key problems in the use of reversible contraception in the United States and elsewhere are the high rates of discontinuation of use by 12 months after initiation and the number of unintended pregnancies among women who state that they or their partners were regularly using a method of contraception.

There is also evidence of unrealistic expectations regarding contraceptive use. This, in very small part, is due to side effects unidentified in premarketing clinical trials. In addition, known side effects are not taken into account appropriately in prescribing practice or the product information materials are so fully detailed that they are not read or fully understood (Carpenter 1989; Forrest 1994a). Further, the fact that contraceptives are used by theoretically healthy individuals who are not seeking prevention or cure, as those are medically understood, conditions the extent to which users are willing to make trade-offs, even when the costs of a potential pregnancy may be very high. The combination of all these factors with the unfettered litigiousness that characterizes the contemporary

American scene results in a distinctive and difficult environment in the United States.

Figure 5-1 presents the proportionate use of each principal contraceptive method in the United States in 1955, 1965, and 1988. Figure 5-2 presents a more detailed picture of shifts in that trajectory between 1960 and 1988. Figure 5-2 makes clear what is sometimes forgotten, that is, that the picture in 1955 in the United States was far from being a blank slate: Among currently married white women aged 18–39 in that year, 70 percent had used contraception at some point and 34 percent had used a method before their first pregnancy. Nonetheless, what was available for use was quite limited, in variety and efficacy, and either coitus-dependent (condom, diaphragm, douche, withdrawal, spermicides) or linked to the timing of coitus (periodic abstinence); only 4 percent of U.S. women had been sterilized for contraceptive purposes.

The broad pattern changes since the availability of oral contraceptives beginning in 1960 have been:

- Increase in total contraceptive use and pill use between 1955 and 1965 and decreased use of the diaphragm, condom, and periodic abstinence.
- Steep increase in interest in coitus-independent methods and in method efficacy.
- Increased reliance on female-controlled methods, especially in the 1960s.
- Steady growth in resort to contraceptive sterilization since the mid-1960s.
- Increased IUD use from the early 1960s till the early 1970s, then a sharp decrease to a stable but low plateau in the late 1980s.
- Decline in condom use in the early 1960s and 1970s, then increase in the 1980s.
- Rapid adoption of new methods—pill, Today sponge, injections, Norplant—as each appeared, with diminished utilization as side effects were experienced.

In addition to these larger patterns, there have been smaller patterns in contraceptive method use that have been dictated by differences and changes in the circumstances of women's lives. The result is a profile of how various female subpopulations tend to adopt or reject certain methods over time (see Table 5-5).

SPECIFIC NEEDS AND MARKET OPPORTUNITIES: THE LIMITATIONS OF AVAILABLE CONTRACEPTIVES

Side Effects

Like any medical intervention, all contraceptive methods have side effects. Some of those can be life threatening when a method is prescribed inappropriately for women for whom it is medically contraindicated or when an infection

TABLE 5-3 Contraceptive Use Among Married/in Union Women, by Method, and Region, 1994 (in thousands)

Method	Africa		Arab States and Europe		Asia and Pacific	
	No.	%	No.	%	No.	%
Sterilization	1,625	11.8	1,057	5.3	179,318	49.2
Female	1,541	11.2	1,030	5.2	140,905	38.7
Male	84	0.6	27	0.1	38,413	10.5
Pill	3,507	25.5	6,081	30.7	28,579	7.8
Injectable	1,748	12.7	146	0.7	7,559	2.1
IUD	1,145	8.3	5,461	27.6	100,205	27.5
Condom	512	3.7	1,225	6.2	21,076	5.8
Other[a]	5,240	38.0	5,818	29.4	27,545	7.6
Other[c]	—	—	—	—	—	—
Total	13,777	100.0	19,791	100.0	364,282	100.0

NOTE: — = no data available.

[a]Data for Africa designate as "Other" vaginal methods, Norplant, and traditional methods. In the U.S. National Survey of Family Growth, "Other" included jellies and creams, suppositories and inserts, the Today sponge, douche, diaphragm, foam, periodic abstinence, and withdrawal.

[b]No implants were available in the United States at the time these data were gathered.

[c]This category includes data on users as follows: diaphragm, 2 million/5.7 percent; periodic abstinence, 0.8 million/2.3 percent; withdrawal, 0.8 million/2.2 percent; spermicides, 0.6 million/1.8 percent; sponge, 0.4 million/1.1 percent.

results from an associated surgical intervention (Carpenter 1989; Hatcher et al. 1994). Nonetheless, while not negligible, the mortality attributable to contraceptive use is very small. For the most part, women's concerns about the contraceptive technologies that are currently available have to do with side effects that are distressing or annoying in themselves or that lead women to conclude that something bad may be going on in their bodies. These side effects include nausea, headaches, and weight gain due to the pill; increased bleeding, dysmenorrhea, and expulsion associated with the IUD; menstrual changes from implants and injectables; and the irreversibility of sterilization. These will vary among individuals according to severity, cultural meaning, and the extent to which they impinge on the ability to live life. Other health-related considerations have to do

Latin America and Caribbean		Total Developing Countries		USA (1988)	
No.	%	No.	%	No.	%
18,148	37.9	200,149	44.9	13,686	39.2
17,631	36.9	161,107	36.1	9,617	27.5
517	1.1	39,042	8.8	4,069	11.7
13,183	27.6	51,352	11.5	10,734	30.7
1,008	2.1	10,461	2.3	—[b]	—
5,303	11.1	112,115	25.2	703	2.0
1,965	4.1	24,778	5.6	5,093	14.6
8,233	17.2	46,837	10.5	76[b]	0.6[a]
—	—	—	—	4,620	13.1
47,840	100.0	445,692	100.0	34,912	100.0

SOURCE: For all data except for the United States, United Nations Population Fund. Contraceptive Use and Commodity Costs in Developing Countries, 1994–2005 (Technical Report No. 18). New York, 1994. For the U.S. data, National Center for Health Statistics, 1988 National Survey of Family Growth, cited in Alan Guttmacher Institute, Facts in Brief: Contraceptive Use. New York, March 1993.

with method qualities that produce difficulty, such as manipulation of the genitals; associated physical exams; fear of surgery, loss of potency, or diminution of libido; and random myths (Bongaarts and Bruce 1995). Table 5-6 presents the risks and side effects of currently available contraceptive methods; it also presents their noncontraceptive benefits.

Developing Countries

An extensive review of published and unpublished studies of contraceptive utilization in the developing world indicates that one in every five women with an unmet need for contraception is not using a modern contraceptive method, owing

TABLE 5-4 Contraceptive Usage, Method Rankings, Selected Regions and Countries

Total Developing World (1994)	Africa	Arab States and Europe	Asian and Pacific	Latin America and Caribbean	More Developed Regions[a]	USA (1988)	USA (1995)
Tubectomy	Other	Pill	Tubectomy	Tubectomy	Pill	Pill	Pill
IUD	Pill	Other	IUD	Pill	Condom	Tubectomy	Tubectomy
Pill	Injectable	IUD	Vasectomy	Other	Tubectomy	Condom	Condom
Other[b]	Tubectomy	Condom	Pill	IUD	IUD	Vasectomy	Periodic abstinence
Vasectomy	IUD	Tubectomy	Other[c]	Condom		Other[c]	Injectable[d]
Condom	Condom	Injectable	Condom	Injectable		Diaphragm	Diaphragm
Injectable	Vasectomy	Vasectomy	Injectable	Vasectomy		IUD	IUD

NOTE: Tubectomy = tubal litigation.

[a]Northern America, Japan, Europe, Australia/New Zealand, former USSR.
[b]"Other" here includes vaginal methods, Norplant, and traditional methods.
[c]"Other" includes vaginal methods, periodic abstinence, and withdrawal.
[d]Depo-Provera.

SOURCES: United Nations Population Fund. Contraceptive Use and Community Costs in Developing Countries 1991–2005. Technical Report No. 18. New York, 1994. Ortho Pharmaceutical Corporation. 1995, 1993, and 1991 Annual Birth Control Studies. Raritan, NJ, 1995. Shah IH. The advance of the contraceptive revolution. Health Statistics Quarterly 47(1):9–15. 1994.

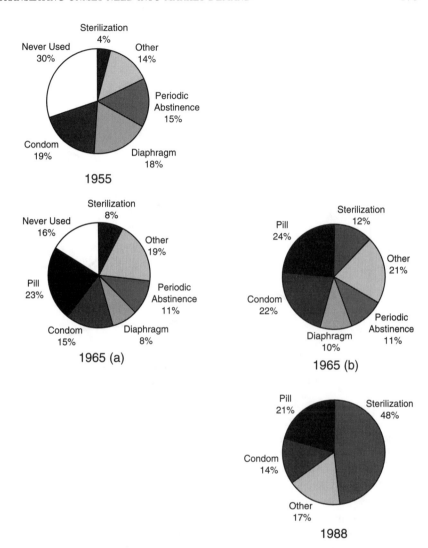

FIGURE 5-1 Contraceptive use, United States, 1955, 1965, and 1988, percentages of users. SOURCE: JD Forrest. Contraceptive use in the United States: Past, present, and future. Advances in Population 2:29–48, 1994. NOTE: (a) = currently married white women 18–39; (b) = married women under 45.

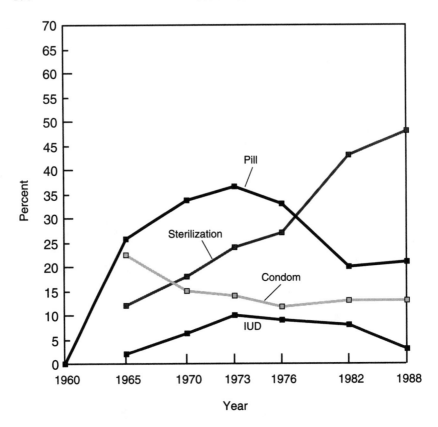

FIGURE 5-2 Trajectory of change in method use, United States, 1960–1988.
SOURCE: Adapted from JD Forrest. Contraceptive Use in the United States: Past,
present, and future. Advances in Population 2:29–48, 1994.

to poor or absent access to services, perception of side effects, or health concerns
associated with modern contraceptives (WHO/HRP 1995). Health concerns,
sometimes deriving from lack of clear understanding about the method and its
side effects—are by far the most important single reason for nonadoption and, in
most countries, are more frequently reported than all other concerns combined.
Access in many rural settings is also a major problem. The principal foci of
concern are the pill, the IUD, and sterilization. Among women with health
concerns, contraceptive prevalence is reduced by an average of 86 percent for the
IUD, 71 percent for the pill, and 52 percent for sterilization (Bongaarts and Bruce
1995).

   This does not mean that other factors do not matter, only that they may be
somehow qualified or cannot be documented as quantitatively significant. For

TABLE 5-5 Contraceptive User Characteristics, U.S. Women, 1988 and 1995, by Method

Method	User Characteristics (1988)	User Characteristics (1995)
Tubal ligation	Women 30–44; increased use among formerly married, black and Hispanic women, less educated and lowest-income women	More married women between 35 and 50 with 2 or more children and higher incomes
Vasectomy	Currently married women, white women relying on partner	No change identified.
Pill	Women under 25, unmarried women, women who intend to have children; increased use among better educated women, among whites, and among those with higher incomes; declines only among teenagers	Increasing use of low-dose pills by women in their 30s and, to lesser extent, by women over 40
Condom	Somewhat increased use, sharp increase among teenagers, unmarried and never-married women	Increasing use by women over 40
Diaphragm	White, college educated, and never-married women who intend to have children; slight decline overall, sharp decline among unmarried women and women under age 30	Use now highest between ages 25 and 40 (mainly between ages 30 and 35), women with college and postgraduate degrees; longer use
IUD	Women who intend to have no more children, previously married women, Hispanic women, those with less education; overall decline, especially among women 25–34, formerly married and less educated, sharpest decline among Hispanic women.	More women in 30s and 40s with at least one child, in married/mutually monogamous relationship

SOURCES: For 1988, Alan Guttmacher Institute. Facts in Brief: Contraceptive Use. New York: The Alan Guttmacher Institute, March 1993. For 1995, Ortho Pharmaceutical Corporation, Executive Summary: 1995 Ortho Annual Birth Control Study. Raritan, NJ, 1995.

TABLE 5-6 Risks, Side Effects, and Noncontraceptive Benefits of Contraceptive Methods

Method	Noncontraceptive Benefits	Risks	Side Effects
Implantable contraceptives	May protect against acute PID, ovarian and endometrial cancers; lactation undisturbed; may decrease menstrual blood loss and pain; suppression of pain associated with ovulation	Infection at implant site; difficult removal; not protective against viral STDs, including HIV/AIDS	Tenderness at implant site, menstrual cycle disturbance (amenorrhea becomes less common over time), weight gain, breast tenderness, headaches, ovarian enlargement, dizziness, nausea, acne, dermatitis, hair loss
Injectable contraceptives	May protect against PID, ovarian cancer, and endometrial cancers; decreased menstrual blood loss and risk of anemia; decreased menstrual pain; suppression of pain associated with ovulation; decreased frequency of seizures	Decreased bone density; not protective against viral STDs, including HIV/AIDS	Menstrual cycle disturbance (amenorrhea becomes more common over time), weight gain, breast tenderness, depression, delay in return of fertility, decreased HDL cholesterol levels, headaches
IUDs	None known; progestin-releasing IUDs may decrease menstrual blood loss and pain	Slight increase in risk of PID in first 20 days after insertion; perforation of the uterus, anemia; not protective against viral STDs, including HIV/AIDS	Menstrual cramping, spotting, increased bleeding
Oral contraceptives	Protects against acute infection of the fallopian tubes (PID), ovarian and endometrial cancers, benign breast masses, ovarian cysts; decreased ectopic pregnancy; decreased menstrual blood loss and risk of anemia; decreased menstrual pain, suppression of pain associated with ovulation	Estrogen-associated: slight increase in blood clot complications, stroke, liver tumors, hypertension, heart attacks, cervical erosion or ectopia, cervical chlamydia Progestin-associated: diabetes-related changes, hypertension, heart attacks	Estrogen-associated: nausea, headaches, fluid retention, weight gain, increased breast size, breast tenderness, stimulation of breast tumors, watery vaginal discharge, rise in cholesterol concentration in gallbladder bile, uterine fibroids

Method			
		Associated with increased cervical chlamydia; not protective against viral STDs, including HIV/AIDS	Progestin-associated: weight gain, depression, fatigue, headaches, decreased libido, acne, increased breast size, breast tenderness, increased LDL cholesterol level, decreased HDL cholesterol level, chronic itch
Male condoms	Protects against bacterial and viral STDs, including HIV/AIDS; delays premature ejaculation; erection enhancement; prevention of sperm allergy	None known	Decreased sensation during intercourse, allergy to latex, possible interference with erection, loss of spontaneity
Female condoms	Protects against STDs, including HIV/AIDS, including on the vulva	None known	Decreased sensation during intercourse, allergy to polyurethane; aesthetically unappealing and awkward to use for some
Barrier methods (diaphragm, cervical cap, sponge)	Protects against bacterial STDs, prevention against HIV/AIDS not proven; diaphragm protects against cervical infection and neoplasia	Vaginal trauma, toxic shock syndrome (rare), cervical erosion	Vaginal and urinary tract infection (anaerobic overgrowth); vaginal discharge if not removed appropriately; allergy to spermicide, rubber, or latex; pelvic pressure, bladder or rectal pain; penile pain

TABLE 5-6 Continued

Method	Noncontraceptive Benefits	Risks	Side Effects
Spermicides	Spermicides with nonoxynol-9 protect against gonorrhea and chlamydia; prevention against viral STDs, including HIV/AIDS, undetermined	None proven; however, tissue irritation may enhance susceptibility to HIV infection	Tissue irritation, yeast vaginitis, allergy to spermicidal agents

NOTE: STDs = sexually transmitted diseases; PID = pelvic inflammatory disease.

SOURCES: Institute of Medicine. The Best Intentions: Unintended Pregnancy and the Well-Being of Children and Families. S Brown, L Eisenberg, eds. Washington, DC: National Academy Press. 1995. Ehrhardt AA, JN Wasserheit. Age, gender, and sexual risk behaviors for sexually transmitted diseases in the United States. IN Research Issues in Human Behavior and Sexually Transmitted Diseases in the AIDS Era. JN Wasserheit, SO Aral, KK Holmes, PJ Hitchcock, eds. Washington, DC: American Society for Microbiology. 1991. Hatcher RA, J Trussell, F Stewart, et al. Contraceptive Technology, 16th Revised Edition. New York: Irvington Publishers, 1994.

example, even in areas where high fertility norms persist, birth spacing is considered highly desirable; the quintessential case is Sub-Saharan Africa. Another example is the weight of male disapproval of family planning. Evidence from Demographic and Health Surveys (DHS) and studies of fertility decision making suggests that this may either be changing in some settings or may be overstated. Women often assume the existence of male opposition simply because they are afraid to raise the topic with their partners, a reflection of very fundamental issues of power and control (Bongaarts and Bruce 1995; WHO/HRP 1995).

The United States

Research in the United States consistently reports significant lack of the kind of information among adults and adolescents that would allow them to perhaps more fully appraise the relative risks and benefits of contraception. As in the developing world, that limitation affects method adoption and continuation (Forrest 1994b; Institute of Medicine 1995).

The example of oral contraceptives (OCs), on the market for more than 35 years and used by 10 million American women, is informative. A 1993 poll commissioned by the Association for Obstetrics and Gynecology (ACOG) found that 54 percent of their sample of American women believed that there were "substantial risks" (mainly cancer) associated with oral contraceptives (Gallup Organization 1994). Relatively few women knew the several noncontraceptive benefits of the pill and 42 percent believed there to be no health benefits from pill use other than pregnancy prevention. Only 6 percent were aware that the pill is actually protective against cancer; in fact, in the 1993 survey and an earlier ACOG survey in 1985, the same proportions of women—one-third—cited cancer as the chief risk of using oral contraceptives (Gallup Organization 1994). In both the 1985 and 1993 surveys, better than two-thirds of the sample incorrectly believed that OC use was more risky or as risky as childbirth, even though the opposite is true (Gallup Organization 1994).

A telephone poll of 1,000 American women, conducted for the Kaiser Family Foundation in 1995, found that only one-quarter of women of reproductive age are confident that oral contraceptives are "very safe" for the user; others expressed a spectrum of concern, with 43 percent considering them "somewhat safe," 18 percent "somewhat unsafe," and 11 percent "very unsafe." Six out of 10 of these women cited worries about potential health risks, while many others expressed concern that the pill does not protect against sexually transmitted diseases or that it is ineffective in preventing pregnancy. One-third incorrectly thought that oral contraceptives increased the risk of ovarian cancer and 40 percent said there was no effect; only 16 percent correctly said that the pill actually reduces that particular risk (Russell 1996).

Part of the problem is the likelihood of inadequate provider–client communication. For instance, a random-sample, telephone survey by the Kaiser Family Foundation and Louis Harris & Associates in October–November 1994 found that most American women with the potential of experiencing an unplanned pregnancy are uninformed or misinformed about the "morning-after" pill, an emergency contraceptive option currently available off label in the United States that can prevent a potential pregnancy up to 72 hours after unprotected sex (Kaiser/Harris 1995).[3] A separate survey found that while 78 percent of U.S. obstetrician-gynecologists in the United States are very familiar with emergency contraceptive pills (ECPs), another 22 percent are somewhat familiar with them, and 72 percent of the entire sample consider the method both safe and effective, most have prescribed it only for a handful of their patients within the last year (Kaiser/Fact Finders 1994). Thus, only one-third of women polled indicated that they knew that anything could be done after unprotected sex to prevent pregnancy and half of those who do know are misinformed about proper timing. The difficulty seems to be that, in general, clinicians make their female patients aware of ECPs in response to an emergency situation rather than during routine contraceptive counseling; when women do call in, they may well encounter receptionists who do not know about emergency contraception (Kaiser/Harris 1995).

Many clinicians also retain negative perceptions of the IUD dating back to the Dalkon Shield disaster, even though new configurations and formulations make IUDs excellent options for many women (Westoff et al. 1992). Adolescents are especially compromised by their low level of information about contraceptives, tied up as it is in their substantial ignorance about sexuality, fertility, and sexual health. This, in turn, impinges negatively on health-seeking and family planning behavior, though lack of information is far from the only factor (Zabin et al. 1991). Nevertheless, the disposition of some U.S. media to overstate modest risks and understate the major health and social benefits of contraception does little to enhance thoughtful decision making about contraceptive use. The adverse and unbalanced media coverage of Norplant motivated women who were experiencing no problems to seek removal and, in undetermined degree, fueled a litigation "explosion" noted in the media themselves (Economist 1995; Herman 1994; Kolata 1995).

At the same time, there are unresolved uncertainties that make the use of certain methods inappropriate for some women and, in some cases, for rather large groups of women. The IUD for women with an active, recent, or recurrent pelvic infection or for women at high risk for a sexually transmitted disease is inappropriate. The jury is still out in connection with a slight increase in breast cancer risk among younger users of oral contraceptives, even though lifetime increased risk is close to zero. Nor are oral contraceptives or Norplant advisable for women with significant cardiovascular risk profiles, particularly in women over 35 (Hatcher et al. 1994). In a discussion later in this report of "informed choice," the point is made that prescribing any contraceptive method to women for whom it is contraindicated is patently a great disservice to them; it is also a great disservice to the reputation of the technologies themselves. However, overall, modern hormonal and intrauterine contraceptives are extremely safe in comparison to the risks of pregnancy, a fact that is poorly understood.

Contraceptive Failure and Discontinuation

Contraceptive effectiveness, failure, continuation, and discontinuation are intimately linked since they are, in important respects, functions of one another. The likelihood that a contraceptive will fail to protect the user depends primarily on two factors. The first is the inherent efficacy of the method itself when used properly (perfect use); this includes technical attributes that make a method easy or difficult to use. The second factor has to do with the characteristics of the user: how often the method is used correctly and consistently, frequency of intercourse, and age (Hatcher et al. 1994).

An example: Although combination oral contraceptives have a perfect-use pregnancy rate of 0.1 percent during the first year of use, the typical-use pregnancy rate is closer to 3 percent (Hatcher et al. 1994) because, as with many medications, compliance with daily pill use is difficult for many women. A far more extreme example is the ovulation method of periodic abstinence, with first-year probabilities of failure of 3 percent during perfect use but as high as 86 percent during imperfect use (Trussell and Grummer-Strawn 1990).

In thinking about the need for new contraceptives, it is important to remember that the majority of today's reversible methods are hard to use perfectly all the time. How consistently the method is used correctly reflects both the user's skill and determination—or lack of them—as well as the inherent complexity and limitations of the methods themselves (Institute of Medicine 1995). It is also important to remember that the components of "determination" reflect some sort of internal balancing of benefits and burdens (Bulatao and Lee 1983), some personal calculus of choice (Zabin 1994), that is, in most individuals in varying measure, a labile blend of immediate and more distant circumstances and pressures, personality, attitudes, feelings, beliefs, motivation, and ambivalence that may well defy the individual's own explanatory powers (Maynard 1994). The complexity of this subject is reflected in a rich literature covering at least two decades of attempts at understanding; it is also reflected in the incompleteness of that literature, which leaves major age groups and populations almost unexamined (Institute of Medicine 1995). Nonetheless, whatever the determinants, the costs of contraceptive failure are the high rates of abortion and unintended and unwanted pregnancy among women using some reversible methods, particularly those that are coitus-related.

Developing Countries

Analysis of DHS data from 11 developing countries[4] found high discon-

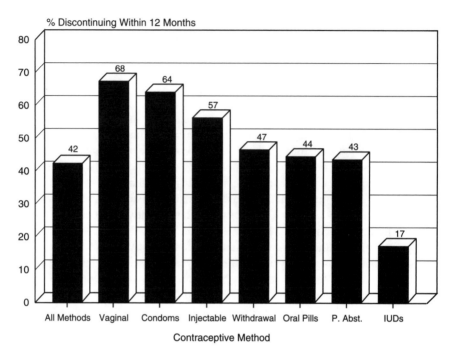

% Discontinuing Within 12 Months

FIGURE 5-3 Cumulative percentage discontinuing a contraceptive method by 12 months, average for 11 developing countries. P. Abst. = periodic abstinence. SOURCE: WHO. Perspectives on Methods of Fertility Regulation: Setting a Research Agenda (Background Paper). Geneva: UNDP/UNFPA/WHO/World Bank/HRP. 1995.

tinuation rates for all reversible contraceptive methods over the five-year period prior to survey. Rates reflected either dissatisfaction with the method itself or with the service providing it. In the countries studied, average use of any method other than the IUD was under 15 months. Forty-two percent of all contraceptive use was terminated by the twelfth month after adoption, 11 percent because of contraceptive failure (unintended pregnancy), and 11 percent for health concerns and side effects. Overall, 68 percent of users of vaginal methods[5] and 64 percent of condom users discontinued their use by the end of the first year (see Figure 5-3). Discontinuation rates varied by country and method, from a low of 25 percent in Indonesia to a high of 65 percent in the Dominican Republic (a country where 70 percent of users are, in fact, sterilized). Failure rates for condoms and periodic abstinence were similar to typical-use rates estimated for the United States (Trussell and Kost 1987), and failure associated with the IUD was even lower in the 11 developing countries than in the United States; failure rates for the pill, vaginal methods, and withdrawal were significantly higher, however. Not surprisingly, method failures, particularly the failure of traditional methods, resulted

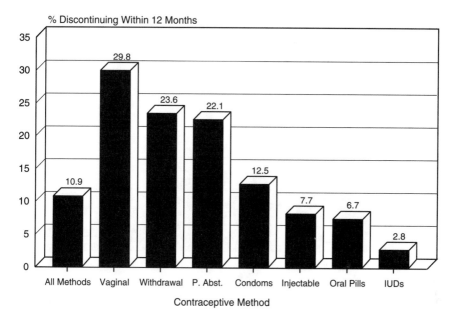

% Discontinuing Within 12 Months

FIGURE 5-4 Cumulative percentage discontinuing by 12 months due to contraceptive failure, average for 11 developing countries. P. Abst. = periodic abstinence. SOURCE: WHO. Perspectives on Methods of Fertility Regulation: Setting a Research Agenda (Background Paper). Geneva: UNDP/UNFPA/WHO/World Bank/HRP. 1995.

in high rates of unintended pregnancy, often leading to induced abortions (WHO/HRP 1995). This is, nonetheless, somewhat misleading: These are method-specific termination rates and many women may, in fact, change to another method, so that the more important figures have to do with continuation to *some* method.

As for causes of discontinuance, 1 out of 5 users of vaginal methods, periodic abstinence, and withdrawal discontinued the method before the end of the first year because of contraceptive failure; the comparable figure for the pill and injectable was 1 in 14 users (see Figure 5-4). Health concerns were the reason for discontinuance for about 1 in 5 users of the pill and injectable, but were of little consequence for users of vaginal methods, periodic abstinence, and withdrawal (see Figure 5-5). Figure 5-6 summarizes these two factors and their contribution to method discontinuance.

In the first month after discontinuation, of the 58 percent of women who discontinued contraceptive use in the four Latin American countries[6] in the sample, 16 percent became pregnant or wanted to do so, 15 percent changed to another modern method, 8 percent changed to a traditional method, and 19 percent abandoned contraception altogether even though they did not want to be-

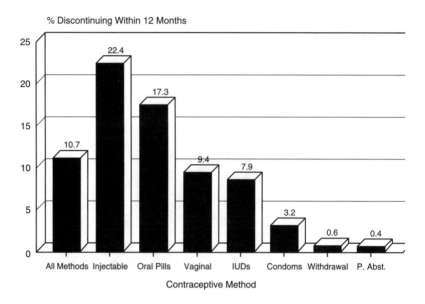

FIGURE 5-5 Cumulative percentage discontinuing by 12 months due to side effects and health concerns, average for 11 developing countries. P. Abst. = periodic abstinence. SOURCE: WHO. Perspectives on Methods of Fertility Regulation: Setting a Research Agenda (Background Paper). Geneva: UNDP/UNFPA/WHO/World Bank/HRP. 1995.

come pregnant. The IUD had the lowest discontinuation rate (17 percent) and was judged favorably with regard to both method failure and health concerns compared to other modern reversible methods. In general, there is much variability in contraceptive behavior following method discontinuation, by method and by country. In fact, there is so much variability in terms of preferences relating to future contraceptive use that it is impossible to identify a single method or set of methods as the globally preferred choice of most women. In most countries, while oral contraceptives are the preferred "next method," there is little basis for certainty that any supposedly preferred method would actually be chosen when the decision to adopt it materialized (WHO/HRP 1995).

In sum, perceived or real side effects and health concerns are major factors in the decision to use contraception; for choosing a specific method; for switching; and for abandoning use of modern methods, especially hormonal methods, entirely (WHO/HRP 1995). The totality of these findings is highly relevant to appraising the need for new contraceptive methods. The analysis by the World Health Organization's Human Reproduction Programme (WHO/HRP) concludes:

> It is obvious that a substantial number of women will need to switch methods before finding one that suits them, or will need to discontinue use in order to have a pregnancy that they have only been delaying, or will need to switch methods as they make the life course transition from delaying a birth to pre-

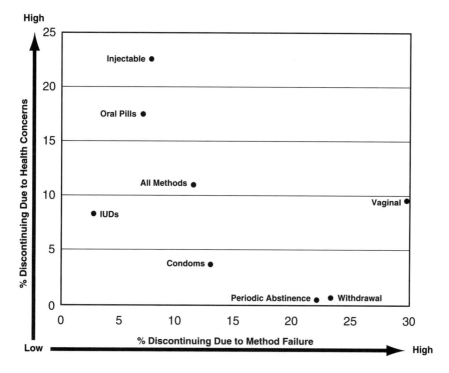

FIGURE 5-6 Summary scattergram of contraceptive methods by percent discontinuing their use within 12 months because of method failure or health concerns. SOURCE: WHO. Perspectives on Methods of Fertility Regulation: Setting a Research Agenda (Background Paper). Geneva: UNDP/UNFPA/WHO/World Bank/HRP. 1995.

venting a birth. However, they also discontinue or switch because the current state of the available contraceptive methods, especially of hormonal methods, is far from satisfactory. Side-effects and health concerns, [perceived or real], remain major factors in discontinuing the use of hormonal methods, while barrier methods and especially vaginal and traditional methods often lead to accidental pregnancy. For these different reasons, hormonal methods and traditional methods have discontinuation rates that are high and broadly similar. Both the expansion in method mix and the improvement in contraceptive technology appear necessary to increase the satisfaction with the method use and to reduce the incidence of unintended pregnancies because of method failure or abandonment of use by the dissatisfied users (WHO 1995:45).

The United States

Table 5-7 presents failure rates and continuation rates associated with all contraceptive methods under both perfect and typical use for the U.S. population

(Hatcher et al. 1994). As common sense would predict, just as in the 11 developing countries discussed above, method failure is associated with low-efficacy reversible methods, while there are real and imagined health concerns concerning high-efficacy reversible methods, especially those that are least susceptible to user error: implants, IUDs, and injectables. There is also variability within some method categories. For instance, today's oral contraceptives contain much lower doses of estrogen and therefore produce significantly fewer side effects and implications; they also are less forgiving of human error. Failure is also significant in cumulative terms: Current U.S. estimates indicate that the typical woman in the United States will experience one contraceptive failure for every 2.25 live births (Trussell and Vaughn 1989).

As in almost everything else having to do with contraception, there is variation in cause and consequence from subpopulation to subpopulation. Formerly married (separated, divorced, widowed) women have the highest rates of failure in the use of reversible contraceptive methods; married women have the lowest. Women whose incomes are 200 percent or less of the poverty level are twice as likely as higher-income women to have a contraceptive failure, a major contributor to the high concentration of unintended pregnancy in these same groups (Forrest 1994b; Institute of Medicine 1995).

Error rates in pill taking are high and the costs of those error rates are also high. Of the 3.5 million annual unintended pregnancies in the United States, over 1 million are related to OC use, misuse, or discontinuation, with 61 percent of these occurring in women who discontinue OCs. Of that group, 67 percent did not immediately substitute other contraceptives and 33 percent adopted less reliable methods. This is a particularly important consideration for the approximately 3.7 million U.S. women who initiate OC use each year since that group commonly experiences side effects and has a high discontinuation rate. It is also an important consideration in terms of cost: The costs incurred owing to unintended pregnancies in women who discontinue OCs are close to $2.6 billion annually (Rosenberg et al. 1995).[7] European women do better yet, even there, 20 percent do not maintain their regimens (Waugh 1994). There was also more failure associated with the less reliable methods; the failure of periodic abstinence rose from 16 to 25 percent during the 1980s and there were slight increases in failure rates for the condom and diaphragm as well (Institute of Medicine 1995).

Another, partially related, source of concern is the high contraceptive failure rate among females under age 20, more than one-quarter of whom experience contraceptive failure during the first 12 months of use, with the lowest-income teens having the highest failure rates. Teens have very poor success with periodic abstinence: 52 percent of low-income teens experience failure, as do 28 percent of higher-income teens (Moore et al. 1995). Younger teens appear to have a

TABLE 5-7 First-year Contraceptive Failures and Continuation Rates, United States

Method	% of U.S. Women Experiencing Accidental Pregnancy Within the First Year of Use		% of U.S. Women Continuing Use at One Year
	Typical Use	Perfect Use	
Chance	85	85	
Spermicides	21	6	43
Periodic abstinence	20		67
Calendar method		9	
Ovulation method		3	
Symptothermal method		2	
Postovulation method		1	
Withdrawal	19	4	
Cap			
Parous women	36	26	45
Nulliparous women	18	9	58
Diaphragm	18	6	58
Condom			
Female (Reality®)	21	5	56
Male	12	3	63
Pill	3		72
Progestin only		0.5	
Combined		0.1	
IUD			
Progesterone T	2.0	1.5	81
Copper T 380A	0.8	0.6	78
LNg 20	0.1	0.1	81
Depo-Provera	0.3	0.3	70
Norplant (6 capsules)	0.09	0.09	85
Female sterilization	0.4	0.4	100
Male sterilization	0.15	0.10	100

SOURCE: Hatcher RA, J Trussell, F Stewart et al. Contraceptive Technology (16th Revised Edition). New York: Irvington Publishers. 1994.

particularly hard time taking pills properly, though older teens do almost as well as older women in contraceptive use (Guttmacher Institute 1994).

Overall continuation rates in the United States are highest for the high-efficacy, provider-controlled methods (implant, IUD, injectable), followed by the pill. Periodic abstinence and the male condom follow at some distance, with the poorest continuation rates for the low-efficacy, coitus-dependent vaginal methods (diaphragm, spermicides, cervical cap, sponge). There are a number of resemblances between these continuation rates and those in the developing countries analyzed above: When continuation rates are ranked, patterns of use of the IUD, periodic abstinence, pill, condom, and vaginal methods are similar. The major and quite striking difference is continuation with injectables, in this case Depo-Provera (depo-medroxyprogesterone acetate, or DMPA). While the continuation rate for DMPA in the United States is very high, it is low in some developing countries, overwhelmingly because of menstrual-related side effects. The IUD is also interesting in this connection. IUD use rates in the United States, while stable since 1988, are still very low; even prior to the negative sequelae and media coverage of the Dalkon Shield experience, IUD prevalence never surpassed 8 percent, well below the prevalence of the pill or tubal sterilization (Ortho 1991). Nonetheless, while IUD use in the United States is far below that in the developing countries, U.S. women continue to report high satisfaction with the method (Ortho Surveys 1991–1995), just like women in the developing countries.

If there is any global "rule" that can be derived from these reasonably definitive analyses of contraceptive use in developing countries and in the United States, it is that, overall, methods that perform better on the efficacy scale measure poorly on the health concerns scale, and vice versa, at the same time that both safety and efficacy are, in most circumstances, equally valued (WHO/HRP 1995). This rule is consistently expressed despite variation in patterns of contraceptive use, nonuse, and discontinuation; despite the remarkable safety of hormonal contraceptives; and despite such subjective criteria as preferences regarding ease of use, mode and duration of action, and willingness to tolerate the shortcomings inevitably associated with any contraceptive method. On its face, this would seem to be a profound contradiction and what might be called the "contraceptive technology predicament." However, its more subtle meaning may be that, for some women, the more mediated methods (pills and implants, for example) simply arouse greater generic concern than do less mediated ones (barrier methods, for example), even though the latter may be recognized as generally less effective. From this perspective, safety commands first priority, while efficacy may occupy a position further down the scale where "effective enough" is located. The tension between such valuations and the tradeoffs for unobtrusiveness, security, and separation from coitus that are associated with long-acting, provider-dependent methods, is substantial.

Sterilization as a Contraceptive Option

About one in three contraceptive users in the developing world has looked to sterilization as a way of terminating childbearing. There is anecdotal material that reflects user lack of knowledge about the risks and consequences of sterilization and a certain amount of prospective anxiety. While there is evidence of some regret, particularly among women sterilized at younger ages (e.g., in their 20s), there is also satisfaction among many women who have had a tubal sterilization, satisfaction primarily related to the permanence of the method and the problems associated with reversible methods. The method is rightly seen as highly effective and not difficult to "use"; its safety, as measured in side effects, is defined as "medium," comparable to the IUD, safer than the pill and injectables, but less safe than the low-efficacy vaginal methods and periodic abstinence (WHO/HRP 1995). In considering the primary problems reported for the major contraceptive methods in the Demographic and Health Surveys, 19 percent of the problems reported for sterilization had to do with health concerns, compared to 42 percent for the pill and 35 percent for the IUD (Bongaarts and Bruce 1995).

It is reasonable to view sterilization rates, particularly among younger women and men, as an indicator that other, reversible alternatives are unavailable or unsatisfactory. Nevertheless, as noted earlier, it is only possible to reach this conclusion where options actually exist. In many countries, sterilization is a popular choice; in others, it reflects the fact that there are no other options or that the options that do exist are unappealing because they are difficult to use, because they are unreliable at a time when having no more children has transcendent importance, because users do not like the side effects or because users are simply weary of dealing with them. In countries where a range of options is available (e.g., Colombia, Costa Rica, Iran, Malaysia, Singapore, South Africa, Thailand, and Tunisia in the developing world, and Austria, Canada, and the United States in the developed world), sterilization does reflect choice. In some countries, for example, China and India, sterilization is a preferred method in national or local government programs and rates reflect that emphasis.

Despite an apparently wide range of reversible contraceptive options in the United States, sterilization is nonetheless the most common form of contraception for all racial and income groups (Ingrassia et al. 1995). One reason is that the range of choice is actually narrower than it seems. The typical woman in the United States choosing sterilization is about 30 years old and has two to three children, with 10 to 15 years of fecund life left during which she could become pregnant but does not wish to. When several IUDs were withdrawn from the U.S. market during 1985–1986, leaving only the Progestasert IUD, which had a small group of users, the remaining options for women who could not or would not use the pill formulations then available but wanted a coitus-independent, unobtrusive, and very effective method, were female or male sterilization (Mosher 1990). As noted above, although two IUDs are now available in the United States,[8] the method has a distance to go before it even regains its mid-1970s market share of around 9.5 percent.[9]

Finally, the promise of Norplant as a most effective alternative (FDA 1995) for women uncertain about terminating fecundity has been checked by adverse press coverage and litigation largely deriving from problems related to implant removal seen only in a small percentage of women. The fact that sterilization is often covered by public or private health insurance is a further incentive for its utilization, especially since insurance coverage for reversible methods is scanty and uneven (Kaeser and Richards 1994).

The core issue in sterilization is its suitability to the stage in the life span when it is—or is not—clear that more children are wanted. Some understandings that are relevant to sterilization appropriateness are emerging from the Collaborative Review of Sterilization, a prospective multicenter study in the United States which has followed 10,000 women undergoing tubal sterilization, each for a minimum of five years, some as long as 10–14 years. Early findings from that study indicate that failure and regret rates are higher than previously thought: 6.9 percent of women sterilized had reported regret during at least one follow-up period and 6.2 percent indicated that they had sought reanastomosis (sterilization reversal) or talked with a health professional about reversal (Wilcox et al. 1990 and 1991). Age at time of sterilization had the most pronounced effect on regret: Women under age 30 were two to three times more likely to report regret than were women aged 30–35, irrespective of parity, marital status, or education. Participants with a history of abortion and those undergoing sterilization concurrent with cesarean section were also at greater risk of regret, as were women receiving public economic assistance (Wilcox et al. 1991).[10]

Prevalence of Sexually Transmitted Disease, Including HIV/AIDS

There already seems to be a rather loud demand signal in the market "asking" for an industry response to the mounting risk of sexually transmitted disease (STD): Use of dual contraceptive methods, a reasonable indicator of such demand, is on the rise, at least in the United States. In 1979, just 3 percent of respondents reported dual method use; by 1988, respondents in another study reported 16 percent dual use (Plech et al. 1993; Zelnick and Kantner 1980). In the 1988 National Survey of Family Growth, women were asked which methods they used to protect themselves or their partners from infection. Responses to the question revealed that 4.24 million women reported use of the condom as an STD prophylaxis, but did not report use of the condom as a contraceptive. Altogether 10.4 million women of a total of 57.9 women aged 15–44 reported use of condoms for prevention of pregnancy or STDs or both. By the late 1980s, women seeking safer sex were buying 30 to 40 percent of all condoms in the United States (Rinzler 1987).

Since then, tracking of dual use through the annual Ortho Birth Control

Surveys has recorded a steady increase in such use. In 1991, 23 percent of all women and almost 31 percent of unmarried women in the Ortho sample reported altered practices related to STD concerns; in 1994, 46 percent of all surveyed women reported using condoms in addition to their primary contraceptive; by 1995, that figure was 52 percent (Ortho Birth Control Studies 1991, 1993, 1995). Half of those using dual methods reported doing so for STD protection. This would suggest that the other half may have been double-protecting itself against conception; if so, this may reflect perceptions of limited method efficacy and a strong commitment to not becoming pregnant. Whatever the objective, it seems clear that women in the United States are vigorously interested in methods that will protect them against sexually transmitted disease and that there is enough dual use to indicate that many are also vigorously interested in simultaneously protecting themselves from conception. There are a few clues that this is not easy to do: In the couple of instances in the United States where it has been examined, contraceptive decision making and utilization around dual method use appear to be complex and difficult (Kost and Forrest 1992; Landry and Camelo 1994). At the same time, the importance of preventing the sexually transmitted diseases, particularly the viral infections, cannot be overstated, if for no other reason than the fact that once an individual is infected with a viral STD, he or she will henceforth always be infected.

The public health aspects of the resurgence of STDs are addressed in Chapter 2. The purpose of this section is to more precisely quantify that resurgence. A very recent worldwide study by the World Health Organization's Global Programme on AIDS, done in collaboration with the Rockefeller Foundation, discovered the following sobering facts.

Sexually Transmitted Disease Worldwide

At least 333 million new cases of curable sexually transmitted diseases were predicted to occur in the world in 1995. This includes 12 million new cases of syphilis, 62 million new cases of gonorrhea, 89 million new cases of chlamydial infection, and 170 million new cases of trichomoniasis (WHO/GPA 1995). In 1990, using a modified Delphi technique, the WHO estimated that, in that year, there were over 250 million new cases of *all* sexually transmitted diseases (WHO/GPA 1995). Thus, this new estimate of 333 million new cases of just four of the STDs—chancroid and the major viral STDs (e.g., herpes, human papillomavirus, and hepatitis B) were not included because of data deficiencies—is a huge increase. Table 5-8 summarizes the prevalence and incidence data for all four diseases for all of the world's regions.

Results of several large studies of human papillomavirus (HPV) and its relation to cervical cancer are also worrisome. It is clear that most, if not all, of the 500,000 cases of cervical cancer worldwide each year are caused by HPV. A 22-country study of HPV prevalence in cervical cancer patients found an overall

TABLE 5-8 Estimated New Cases of the Curable Sexually Transmitted Diseases, All Regions, 1995

Region	Syphilis	Gonorrhea	Chlamydia[a]	Trichomoniasis	Total by Region	[Chancroid][b]
North America	140,000	1.8 million	4 million	8 million	14 million	
Western Europe	200,000	1.2 million	5 million	10 million	16 million	
Australasia	10,000	0.13 million	300,000	1 million	1 million	
Latin America and the Caribbean	1.3 million	7.1 million	10 million	18 million	36 million	
Sub-Saharan Africa	3.5 million	16 million	15 million	30 million	65 million	
Northern Africa and the Middle East	620,000	1.5 million	2.9 million	4.6 million	10 million	
Eastern Europe and Central Asia	100,000	2.3 million	5 million	10 million	18 million	
East Asia and Pacific	330,000	3 million	6.2 million	13 million	23 million	
South and Southeast Asia	5.8 million	29 million	40 million	75 million	150 million	
Global Totals	12 million	62 million	89 million	170 million	333 million	[7 million]

[a]This refers to *chlamydia trachomatis* in adults.

[b]No estimates could be made for chancroid using the same methodology developed for the other four diseases, since understanding of the epidemiology and natural history of the disease is poor and there is yet no good diagnostic for estimating prevalence and duration of infection. The estimate given here for chancroid is based on the ratio of syphilis to chancroid in the previous WHO (Delphi) estimates for those two diseases and the 1995 estimate for syphilis.

SOURCE: World Health Organization. An Overview of Selected Curable Sexually Transmitted Diseases (WHO/GPA/STD/95.1). Geneva: WHO/Global Programme on AIDS, August 1995.

rate of 93 percent; it also found that just 4 of the 70 different types of HPV cause 80 percent of all cervical cancer cases, as identified in over 1,000 cervical cancer tumor specimens through use of new DNA techniques (American Health Consultants 1995; Bosch et al. 1995).

Sexually Transmitted Disease in the United States

For the four diseases analyzed by the WHO, the U.S. incidence of 14 million new cases in 1995, with an estimated prevalence of 52 million for 1995, ranks fifth among the nine WHO regions. U.S. prevalence rates are the same as those in Australasia but higher than rates in Western Europe, North Africa, the Middle East, and South and Southeast Asia. The U.S. incidence figure is also considerably higher than the estimate of 12 million new cases annually for *all* STDs in the United States that is commonly used (CDC 1990, cited in Rosenberg et al. 1992). The 1988 data indicated that three-quarters of all STDs in the United States were accounted for by three diseases: chlamydia (4 million cases), trichomoniasis (3 million), and gonorrhea (1.8 million).

Rates of infection in the United States vary by age and ethnicity. Among women attending family planning clinics from 1989 to 1993, chlamydia infection rates were 4.5 percent (whites), 5.5 percent (Hispanics), and 8.5 percent (African-Americans) (WHO/GPA 1995). Most worrisome is the fact that, in the United States, STD incidence increased rapidly during the 1960s and 1970s and has stayed at those high levels (Cates 1991). At present, 86 percent of all STDs occur among individuals 15 to 29 years old (NARHP 1995), two-thirds among individuals under age 25 (CDC 1992). The Maternal and Child Health Bureau reports that about 3 million U.S. adolescents contract an STD annually. Studies by the Alan Guttmacher Institute have found 15 percent of active teenage women to be infected with HPV; 15- to 19-year-olds also have a 1-in-8 chance of developing pelvic inflammatory disease (PID) and sexually active 10- to 14-year-olds are 7 times more likely to have a PID than 20- to 24-year-olds (Guttmacher Institute 1994). Nearly 200,000 cases of gonorrhea were reported among teens in 1989; visits by teenage women to fee-for-service practices for genital herpes infections grew from 15,000 in 1966 to 125,000 in 1989; and the number of visits for genital warts caused by HPV grew from 50,000 in 1966 to 300,000 in 1989, and perhaps three times as many women had asymptomatic cervical HPV infection (Hatcher et al. 1994).

CONSUMER PERSPECTIVES

Consumer Decision Making and Preferences

The market for any product is formed at the intersection of price, product availability, and consumer decisions. In a producer's ideal market, consumers "vote" for products by making at least an initial commitment through purchase and, best of all, by continued use; in other words, they are predictable and loyal consumers. In a less than ideal market, consumers may be so uninformed about their options, the range of their options may be so limited, and consumer motivations may be so intricate that it is hard to interpret the meaning of initial votes or to anticipate loyalty.

By these definitions, the market for contraceptives is not ideal. Contraceptive decision making is influenced by a welter of motivational factors: method safety[11] and effectiveness[12]; specific personal considerations; and availability, accessibility, and cost. Safety and effectiveness appear to be consistently important (WHO/HRP 1995) although, depending on the situation, there may be willingness to trade off efficacy against other method qualities, especially since side effects are tolerated differently by different women. For instance, in a setting where abortion is legal and safe, a woman's main concern may not be contraception, but she may be quite concerned about sexual disease transmission. A young woman who was recently divorced but who might want more children in a second marriage may be willing to put up with contraceptive side effects, for instance, changes in menstrual patterns, to avoid the sterilization she does not yet want to have.

In other words, the dominance assigned to each factor in contraceptive decision making will vary by age, relationship status, family size, culture, and circumstance; by perceptions and knowledge about individual methods; by ambivalence about childbearing; by interest in spontaneity and ease of use; and by issues of power and control. The notion of risk cuts across all these variables: risks to health, method failure, getting "caught" using a method when secrecy is desired, investment in a costly method that might not work out, resort to sterilization when one might have a change of heart. All this is projected against the complicated and changing nature of women's reproductive lives, their ability to exercise control over those lives, and by sometimes considerable forces in the larger political and social environment.

There is also the matter of access. In some developing countries and in the former socialist economies, contraceptive options are severely constrained and the information individuals receive is insufficient to making well-founded choices among those options that are available (Bongaarts and Bruce 1995; Bruce and Jain 1995). The latter is also true in the United States, where provider-client exchanges concerning reproductive choice are sometimes glaringly inadequate and contraceptive users may get much of their information from the media, often incorrectly (Institute of Medicine 1995; Moore et al. 1995; Tanfer 1995).

To come to conclusions about what is needed in the marketplace for contraceptive technology, we now depend on method utilization surveys which theoretically express how consumers vote by using, continuing, or discontinuing a given method. However, the meaning of those votes may be obscured both by whether they reflected real choice among real options and by who paid for the purchase. Thus, even though we are getting a better grasp on the specific attributes desired in contraceptive technologies by different populations in different circumstances, there is a true need for sophisticated market research in a range of settings (Snow 1994).

Perhaps the best evidence that consumers have long wanted something from the contraceptives market beyond its traditional offerings is the alacrity with which they have seized upon most new methods as they have come along. This has occurred despite the difficulty of "imagining" the new technology and seemingly without reference to anything but whether or not it might "work" (Forrest 1994a). Women are eagerly in search of something that is possibly better, only to be disappointed when they discover that no contraceptive is perfect for everybody; that there are still side effects for some users; that unexpected side effects or complications or inappropriate prescribing and patient management have contributed to litigable cases that muddy the picture of the method's utility; or that manufacturers have not adequately represented what remains unknown about their product.

The WHO/HRP review observes that users differ so markedly from one another in their criteria for selection of a contraceptive method that even people choosing a more or less similar product may be dissimilar in the relative importance they attach to the specific attributes of the product chosen. For instance, the IUD is chosen by women in India, Turkey, and the Republic of Korea primarily for its perceived effectiveness, but for its ease of use by postpartum women in the Philippines. Indian women chose the pill mainly for its ease of use, Korean women for its effectiveness. Indian women also chose the injectable DMPA for its ease of use, while Korean, Philippine, and Turkish women chose it for its convenient duration of action. For some, convenience and desire for spontaneity may determine method choice; others may care deeply about reversibility, discretion, duration of protection, no need for resupply visits, and so forth.

The review concludes that it is difficult—and probably inappropriate—to make large statements about product attributes that supposedly drive all consumer preferences; that there is really no consensus about some set of attributes that are invariable and intrinsic; and that, with the exception of safety and efficacy, all other contraceptive product attributes will vary in their meaning and priority for users according to situation (Snow 1994). In fact, some individuals in some circumstances may be willing to cede some efficacy for other, more valued or situationally appropriate attributes. This suggests that the point made in recent papers (e.g., Correa 1991; Germain 1993) that there has been, overall, undue R&D emphasis on effectiveness at the expense of safety or acceptability may also be situational. The current intent of the U.S. Food and Drug Administration to require efficacy trials of existing over-the-counter barrier methods is an example of where efficacy may, in fact, be an inappropriate emphasis. At the same time, any newly developed barrier method designed to protect against either conception or infection or both would be less attractive were its efficacy not assured at some reasonably safe level. The fact remains that the methods that have so far dominated the market for contraceptives have been those that do offer high efficacy (Ortho 1991, 1993, 1995; Snow 1994; WHO/HRP 1995). It is also true that it is the issue of safety, or the lack thereof, that is at the core of product liability.

All this raises further questions in connection with the ongoing debate about the relative merits of user control compared to provider control; reversibility compared to effectiveness; coitus-independence compared to coitus-dependence; and the need for concealment of contraceptive use compared to the desirability of partner involvement (Forrest 1994a). Some women are quite willing to trade off "having the doctor do it" for what they consider certainty and peace of mind. Some women not in a formalized relationship and whose sexual activity is sporadic are not necessarily opposed to coitus-dependence. Some women have partners with whom they can share contraceptive decision making; others do not. In sum, there appears to be a persistent divergence of opinion about the qualities that are wanted in contraceptives, who wants them, and what they mean to different groups and individuals[13] and it is this divergence that argues for the largest possible range of contraceptive options.

The "Woman-centered Agenda"

Over the past few years, importantly in connection with the International Conference on Population and Development held in Cairo in 1994, some ideas about what is missing in the contraceptives market have become clearer. There have been precise statements about specific technologies that are wanted which are so eminently desirable that they should be construed by industry as virtual instructions. These have become a core element of the "Contraception 21" Initiative launched by the Rockefeller Foundation and have come to be known as the "woman-centered agenda." As explained in Chapter 1, that agenda awards priority to the following contraceptive technologies:

- vaginal methods that protect against sexually transmitted reproductive tract infections, both in conjunction with contraception and independent from it;
- menses-inducers; and
- more methods for men.

Since current technologies are limited, and since a plausible case can be made that there is market demand for such products, these categories constitute market niches that would seem to merit new industrial investment.

Immunologic Contraception

Although it is not part of the Contraception 21 agenda, many researchers see immunologic contraception[14]—or what have most often been called "contraceptive vaccines"—as a potentially important new option for the next century, and several public research groups and some private companies are supporting research in that area. This research has evoked much controversy, and the Women's Global Network for Reproductive Rights (WGNRR), an advocacy group based in Amsterdam, coordinated a campaign which, by November 1994, had over 400 signatory groups from 38 countries. The WGNRR cites several concerns: (1) that these contraceptives would have a higher abuse potential than existing methods; (2) that, as presently designed, they would pose unique potential health risks to the autoimmune system; (3) that they would have cumbersome features interfering with efficacy,[15] and (4) that they would offer no real advantage over existing methods. More specific analysis lists the following potential disadvantages: (1) need for additional protection during the immunologic lag period and for ancillary testing to ascertain immune levels; (2) probable allergic responses to carrier proteins; (3) possible autoimmune-mediated pathologies and crossreactive immunity to other hormones; (4) difficulty in "switching off" immune response; (5) unlikely prospect of immediate surcease from side effects; and (6) unknown consequences to woman and fetus in the event of unknown pregnancy at the time of immunization and post-immunization pregnancy (Schrater 1995). These groups advocate that research funds be focused on more user-controlled methods, not more long-acting, provider-dependent immunologic methods that provide no protection from STDs and have the potential for coercive applications.

Not all women's health advocates agree (Ravindran and Berer 1994; IDRC 1994; Schrater 1994; Snow 1994), suggesting that immunologic contraception could possibly provide safe, effective, and acceptable methods. Researchers argue that such methods could be inexpensive and convenient for women; could be designed for regimens of different duration; might be made reversible; could offer a long-acting option for men as well; and provide a high degree of confidentiality for women who required it. They note that, because the immunization principle is now widely accepted in the large majority of cultures, contraceptive immunization could be incorporated into ongoing programs for communicable diseases (J Herr 1996, personal communication). Finally, the observation is made that the frontier area of mucosal immunity might eventually offer simultaneous protection against unintended pregnancy and infection (see Appendix D).

Attempts to encourage dialogue and understanding between advocates and researchers are ongoing, as part of a process that began with a meeting between representatives of women's health groups and scientists in Geneva in February 1991. Jointly organized by the WHO Special Programme of Research, Development and Research Training in Human Reproduction (WHO/HRP) and the International Women's Health Coalition, it bore the title "Creating Common Ground:

Women's Perspectives on the Selection and Introduction of Fertility Regulation Technologies." Since then there have been six meetings to continue that dialogue, including regional meetings (Manila 1992, Nairobi 1993, Yaoundé 1994), focused topics such as anti-fertility vaccine research (Geneva 1992), the ethics of contraceptive development (Geneva 1994), and participation in regional/national research needs assessments (Yaoundé 1994). The intention is to sustain and broaden the dialogue (WHO/HRP 1995).

The analysis of the contemporary science that was a major element in this committee's work suggests to some members of the committee that there are enough avenues being opened up by immunologic research to merit continuance. Even were no female "vaccine" to result from that research, worthy advances might have been made toward methods for men and toward vaginal methods which might be protective against conception and sexually transmitted infection. Regular review of the status of progress in these areas, as well as in the broader field of relevant immunologic research, could nourish the dialogue that has been initiated between concerned women's groups and scientific researchers, and perhaps shift investment out of areas that appear to be less productive in terms of the needs of women and their potential for the market.

THE DIMENSIONS OF THE MARKET FOR CONTRACEPTIVES

Potential demand in the market for contraceptives is composed of those who have already "voted" by using contraception and by some portion of those who are not using them. The fact that the market consists of users and nonusers implies that two kinds of market dynamics are of consequence. One is the overall size of the market and any increase or decrease in the total number of contraceptive users. The other has to do with shifts in what methods are being used or adopted. It is of interest to *all* producers of contraceptives that the market keep growing; it is of interest to *individual* producers that consumers remain loyal either to their product or, if they switch methods, to the firm.

Numbers of Contraceptive Users

The contraceptive market can be defined in terms of the number of actual and potential contraceptive purchasers or by the associated dollar value of the purchases themselves (PATH 1994b). In terms of numbers of actual and potential purchasers, the world's contraceptive user population has been growing steadily and presently stands at 57 percent of all married women of reproductive age (MWRA),[16] or 595 million theoretically possible purchasers. In addition, it is estimated that an additional 220 million women state that they do not wish to be pregnant but are not using any method. Of these, 446 million are in the developing countries. Applying a medium projection, the United Nations Population Fund (UNFPA) estimates that, by 2005, there will be 755 million MWRA worldwide using contraceptives. In the developing world, there will be 602 million MWRA using contraceptives; if unmarried women are added, that total becomes 625 million contraceptive users in the developing economies by the year 2005 (UNFPA 1994).

The Dollar Value of the Market for Contraceptives

All things being equal, a much larger population could mean a much larger potential market (even taking into account the fact that actual markets are always smaller than potential markets). That is not now the case for contraceptives. While the public sector has traditionally defined markets in terms of volume of doses, manufacturers evaluate markets in terms of revenues and profits (Mercer 1994).

As of 1992, the total world contraceptives market was somewhere around $2.5 billion annually. Oral contraceptives (OCs) are by far the biggest component of that market, accounting for around $2.0 billion in sales worldwide in 1992, up from $1.5 billion in 1988 (see Chapter 6, Table 6-8). This is a total percentage increase for the entire period of close to 40 percent, or around 10 percent annually. The United States accounted for around half of the market in 1992 with estimated sales of close to $1 billion. The next largest market is Europe ($738 million), followed at some distance by the Latin American market, where Brazil, Argentina, and Mexico accounted for $108 million in sales of oral contraceptives in 1992. The market consisting of Africa, Asia, and Australia accounted for $68 million in OC sales and undefined "others" for another $72 million (Frost and Sullivan 1993) (Table 5-9). These figures include large-volume procurements tendered in the United States by UNFPA for programmatic use in developing countries.

Nonetheless, the oral contraceptive market is perceived as essentially saturated (Reprogen 1995). There are now at least 36 different formulations of oral contraceptives sold in the United States alone; these are primarily combination products, with about a dozen progestin-only pills (Hatcher et al. 1994). To these formulations must be added products manufactured in Europe and in some developing economies. Oral contraceptives accounted for 84 percent of U.S. sales by U.S. manufacturers in 1989; that proportion is projected to drop to 80 percent by 1999 (Table 5-10). The expectation was that there would be displacement of some of the OC market by condoms, diaphragms, and Norplant. However, the sharp decline in Norplant use which began in 1993 and the role of injectables were not accounted for in those projections, so that percentages can be expected to shift, although at this point unpredictably.

Of the remaining market balance, condom sales account for about half and are growing, apparently in response to heightened concern about sexually transmitted diseases, including HIV. Sales in Europe in 1993 were close to $493

TABLE 5-9 Worldwide Oral Contraceptive Markets, by Region and By Country, 1992 Sales (in millions of U.S. dollars)

Region and Country	By Country 1992 Sales (US$)	% Total	By Region 1992 Sales (US$)	% Total
North America			$1,104	52.8
United States	$995	47.6		
Canada	109	5.2		
Europe			738	35.3
Germany	227	10.8		
France	125	6.0		
United Kingdom	93	4.4		
Italy	72	3.4		
Belgium	35	1.7		
Spain	21	1.0		
Latin America			108	5.2
Brazil	40	1.9		
Argentina	26	1.3		
Mexico	17	0.8		
Africa, Asia, and Australia			68	3.3
South Africa	6	0.3		
Australia	2	1.1		
Others	301	14.4	72	3.4
	—	—	—	—
	$2,090	100.0	$2,090	100.0

SOURCE: Frost and Sullivan. U.S. Market Intelligence Report: U.S. Contraceptive and Fertility Product Markets (Report #5021-54). New York, October 1993.

million, with a projection to $617 million by 1998 (see Table 5-11). In the United States, 1993 condom sales were $147 million, with a projection for 1998 of $193 million. The U.S. market currently produces over 100 different condoms (Hatcher et al. 1994), but the market is dominated by seven firms, of which just three are the primary producers of all condoms sold in the United States.

The rest of the market in 1992 consisted of spermicides, Norplant, IUDs, and diaphragms, with that descending order of importance in the U.S. market but a somewhat different order in Europe and the developing economies, where the IUD is better accepted and Norplant does not yet have widespread presence.

Between 1989 and 1994, sales by U.S contraceptives manufacturers grew at an average of 4 percent a year, with sales of oral contraceptives growing at the slowest pace (2.64 percent annually) and condoms and IUDs growing the fastest, at 6.9 and 5.5 percent, respectively (Frost and Sullivan 1993). Sales of Norplant, introduced onto the U.S. market in February 1991, went from zero to $35 million in the method's first year on the market. In its best year, 1992, Norplant accounted for $141 million of Wyeth's $7.9 billion in worldwide sales (Kolata 1995), with a compound annual growth rate (CAGR) of 13.4 percent as of 1993 (Frost and Sullivan 1993). By 1994 that figure was down to $51 million and, as of 1995, adverse publicity and negative word-of-mouth have driven sales down from 800 a day to about 60 (Kolata 1995).

These market patterns suggest the following. First, it appears that, together, the realities and perceptions of side effects and lack of appreciation of the benefits of reversible hormonal contraceptives will continue to constrain their more widespread and effective use, since it is unlikely that further modifications of these methods will significantly reduce the current array of side effects. Much industry research over the past years has focused on improving today's hormonal contraceptives, yet it is hard to foresee any major future value added in connection with these methods, at least one substantial enough to achieve a quantum leap in utilization.

Second, the market has demonstrated that it will respond to at least some public health needs when the consumer population signals a demand for such a response. The case in point is the effect on the market of concerns about sexually transmitted disease, as different kinds of populations became aware of that public health need and the possibility of dual method use. While condoms are not costly items, the increase in their sales volume has generated respectable growth in market share.

Third, all things being equal, a new product that patently responds to unmet needs can quickly command a sizable market share, even with much of its potential volume unrealized. The predicament in which Norplant has landed does not nullify the extent to which it struck a responsive chord in the marketplace. The popularity of the IUD in developing countries and the initial success with Norplant in those countries where it has been introduced suggest that many women do, in fact, have lively interest in very effective, long-lasting methods that can resolve contraceptive needs, delay sterilization, and protect fecundity. And, although attitudes toward Depo-Provera are a mix of enthusiasm and reserve, it too has been well received in a number of developing countries, where there are 15 million users; it continues to have high initial adoption rates in the United States, particularly among younger women seeking an alternative to the pill (Ortho 1995). Again, women send a signal to the market that they want other options.

The Market for Contraceptives in the Developing Economies

The emphasis in the preceding analysis on the U.S. and European markets corresponds to the fact that the dollar value of the contraceptive market in the

TABLE 5-10 U.S. Contraceptive Sales, U.S. Manufacturers, 1989 and
Projected to 1999 (in millions of U.S. dollars and product percentage of total
sales)

Year	Oral Contraceptives		Condoms		Diaphragms	
	U.S.$	%	U.S.$	%	U.S.$	%
1989	960.8	84.1	115.4	10.1	3.4	0.3
1990	989.3	83.8	122.8	10.1	3.5	0.3
1991	1,016.5	81.1	131.6	10.5	3.8	0.3
1992	1,041.5	80.5	138.4	10.7	3.9	0.3
1993	1,065.6	79.9	146.7	11.0	4.0	0.3
1994	1,087.7	79.2	155.2	11.3	4.1	0.3
1995	1,107.6	78.4	165.3	11.7	4.2	0.3
1996	1,127.1	77.6	174.3	12.9	4.4	0.3
1997	1,146.2	76.9	183.5	12.3	6.0	0.4
1998	1,161.2	75.8	193.0	12.6	6.1	0.4
1999	1,175.6	74.8	204.3	13.0	6.3	0.4

[a]Cumulative annual gross earnings.

developing economies is substantially less than that of the contraceptive market
in the industrial economies, even though the latter represents a much smaller
number of consumers. As of 1992, total annual contraceptive sales in developing
nations represented less than 16 percent of the global contraceptive market. In
contrast, the industrial economies, with less than one-third[17] of all the world's
users of contraceptives, generated approximately 84 percent of global contraceptive revenues (PATH 1994a) (see Figures 5-7a and b).

The market for reversible contraceptives is affected by the extent to which
sterilization is selected as a contraceptive option, which becomes meaningful for
the market when it is translated into absolute numbers. As of 1994, 200 million
individuals in the developing countries had opted for sterilization; at current
adoption rates of about 11 million women and 3 million men annually, the cumulative total of individuals who have opted for sterilization projected for 2005 will

IUDs		Spermicides		Norplant		Total Sales	Total CAGE[a]
U.S.$	%	U.S.$	%	U.S.$	%	U.S.$	(%)
19.4	1.7	43.4	3.8	0.0	0.0	1,143.4	—
20.2	1.7	44.9	3.8	0.0	0.0	1,180.6	3.3
21.3	1.7	46.4	3.7	35.1	2.8	1,253.4	6.2
23.3	1.8	47.9	3.7	40.1	3.1	1,293.8	3.2
24.0	1.8	48.0	3.6	45.3	3.4	1,065.6	3.1
24.7	1.8	49.4	3.6	50.8	3.7	1,373.4	3.0
26.8	1.9	50.9	3.6	57.9	4.1	1,412.7	2.9
27.6	1.9	52.3	3.6	65.4	4.5	1,452.4	2.8
29.8	2.0	52.2	3.5	74.6	5.0	1,491.8	2.7
30.6	2.0	53.6	3.5	85.8	5.6	1,531.9	2.7
33.0	2.1	55.0	3.5	97.4	6.2	1,571.6	2.6

SOURCE: Frost and Sullivan. U.S. Market Intelligence Report: U.S. Contraceptive and Fertility Product Markets (Report #5021-54). New York, October 1993.

be 262 million. Sterilization now accounts for almost half of all contraceptive use in Asia and 38 percent in Latin America (UNFPA 1994).

The weight of this phenomenon has already been felt in some markets. A survey of developing countries in the 1980s found that, first, the role of the private sector diminished as use of government-provided sterilization grew and, second, that this decrease occurred at the expense of private-sector sales of reversible methods (Cross et al. 1991). The other aspect of sterilization that is relevant to the market is that it is, with the IUD, the least expensive method of contraception per couple-year of protection (UNFPA 1994). The initial cost of sterilization is high—it is the second most expensive contraceptive commodity after the pill. However, it is a one-time cost and so becomes very cost-effective in terms of couple-years of protection, although any large up-front cost is very important in the decision-making processes of individual users. A country like

TABLE 5-11 Condom Retail Sales in Europe, 1993 and Projected for 1998 (in millions of U.S. dollars)

	1993	1998	CAGR[a]
Italy	193	213	2.0
Germany	112	136	4.0
Spain	74	99	6.0
United Kingdom	67	94	7.0
France	46	74	10.0
Total	493	617	4.6

[a]Compound annual growth rate.

SOURCE: Frost and Sullivan. U.S. Market Intelligence Report: U.S. Contraceptive and Fertility Product Markets (Report #5021-54). New York, October 1993.

India, with a large population and a growing economy which, all things being equal, might generate private-sector purchases of reversible contraceptives in considerable numbers, has a population policy that emphasizes sterilization and thus displaces potential purchases of other, reversible options. That policy is undergirded by important cultural reasons for choosing sterilization, such as lower expectations that there will be remarriage and second families, and gender roles.

There is a virtual pandemic at present of efforts at health care reform worldwide, with heavy emphasis on privatization of health care, cost containment, and cost recovery. In settings where the trend is toward privatization, it is not inconceivable that pricing structures might be adjusted in an upward direction; at least that could occur in the upper tiers of such structures where purchases are made by those not using public health services. In settings where the public sector continues to dominate contraceptive procurement, greater incentives to the market would have to come from increased volumes of users which, in turn, would have to be motivated by government policies.

Another contributor to the disproportionate values of the two markets is the markedly higher prices that can be charged in the industrial economies. In the developing economies, private-sector prices may be lower and, more critically, national public sectors or overseas development assistance agencies subsidize large contraceptive procurements for low-cost or free distribution. These distributions are made primarily through governments, which presently supply about 86 percent of all modern methods used in developing countries—95 percent of the clinical methods of sterilization and IUDs, 57 percent of pills, and 47 percent of condoms. This largely describes the picture in Asia, where the large majority of the population and contraceptive users live.

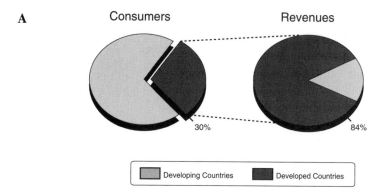

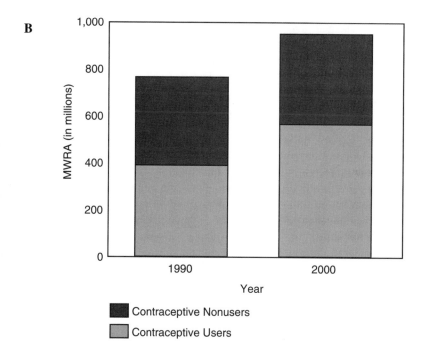

FIGURE 5-7 **A**: The contraceptive market in industrial and developing economies. **B**: The structure of the market in developing countries, 1994 and 2005. SOURCE: Program for Appropriate Technology in Health (PATH). Enhancing the private sector's role in contraceptive research and development. IN Contraceptive Research and Development 1984–1994: The Road from Mexico City to Cairo and Beyond. PFA Van Look, G Pérez-Palacios, eds. Delhi: Oxford University Press. 1994.

At the same time, public-sector dominance in the developing countries is not monolithic. In Sub-Saharan Africa, though the public sector may increasingly be the source of supply for modern methods of contraception, almost two-thirds of condom users are now supplied by the private sector. In the Arab States and Europe, the private sector supplies more contraceptives than do governments, except for sterilizations; the IUD and injectables are about equally divided between government and private sources. Finally, in Latin America, governments supply more sterilizations and IUDS than does the private sector in the ratio of 60/40, but the private sector supplies the bulk of each of the other methods (UNFPA 1994).

Lessons from the Vaccine Field

In 1993, the United Nations Children's Fund (UNICEF) and WHO commissioned Mercer Management Consulting to do a study of the commercial aspects of global vaccine supply, as a contribution to more effective implementation of the Children's Vaccine Initiative (CVI) and the Expanded Programme on Immunization (EPI).[18] Even though the vaccine and contraceptives market are not fully analogous, there are enough similarities so that some of the conclusions of the Mercer analysis may be illuminating.

Similarities and Differences Between Vaccines and Contraceptives

The world vaccine market, until recently valued at around $2 billion, has been reestimated by Mercer at close to $3 billion. Of this total, the basic pediatric vaccines account for approximately $1 billion, proprietary products (Haemophilus influenza type b [Hib], hepatitis A, and hepatitis B) for another $1 billion, and the adult vaccine market for most of the balance. Thus, in dollar value, the vaccine market, at least for the present, is not so very much larger than the current contraceptives market. However, as indicated above, the annual growth rate of the global contraceptives market is around 4 percent. The annual growth rate for the number of doses of pediatric vaccines for the EPI between 1982 and 1992 was 7 percent, fueled almost entirely by developing country demand.

After years of stagnating or diminishing revenues, the world vaccine market is now growing rapidly, spurred by a new generation of proprietary products such as Hib and the hepatitis vaccines. These products have revitalized the vaccine industry and motivated manufacturers not only to continue producing vaccine but even to invest to strengthen their competitive position. A series of agreements and acquisitions has provided manufacturers with broader product portfolios, increased geographic access, and stronger R&D capacity (Mercer Management Consulting 1994).

The reinvigoration of the global vaccines market over the past decade is attributable in considerable measure to advances in the field of immunology and the consequent launch of a few proprietary products that are of worldwide attractiveness. There are some analogies between the two markets. Both vaccines and contraceptives are what might be called "social products" that have a somewhat paradoxical value: The social returns to the development, availability, and widespread use of such products exceed the private returns, that is, what people are willing to pay for that social value. In the case of vaccines, the returns to private developers appear to be high enough (at least in industrial-economy markets) that they will invest in new products. The public sector is also willing to invest; for instance, the U.S. National Institutes of Health provides significant subsidies to vaccine development.

The cardinal difference between vaccines and contraceptives is that vaccine consumption has a commanding externality, or spillover benefit, in the form of "herd immunity," which is the protection that immunization affords nonimmune individuals by reducing the number of infected individuals in a given community below the critical level needed to sustain transmission. Within such a community, the likelihood of a susceptible individual coming into contact with someone who has a specific disease is thus diminished. This is why immunization against the major childhood diseases is compulsory and subsidized in all industrial economies and, increasingly, in many developing economies.

Contraception, at least as typically regarded, does not have an externality that is so clearly compelling. There is painfully ample justification for thinking about unwanted pregnancies as burdens on the health and well-being of societies, families, and individuals, and even as major factors in various social pathologies. It is possible to talk about "epidemics" of unintended pregnancy and unsafe abortion and to make demographic arguments about high fertility as a contributor to planetary "illness." There is also much wider societal recognition of the misery and poor prospects of the unwanted child. Yet, these analogies and arguments have not achieved the same appeal in the public mind that is attached to childhood immunization. That said, the Children's Vaccine Initiative is still searching for strategies that will engage the private sector more systematically in ways that can assure continued R&D investment and a stable level of supply.

Nonetheless, the social returns to contraception are sizable enough so that it has historically received some subsidy in the United States, as well as internationally. New analysis (Trussell et al. 1995b) now permits us to consider contraception from the standpoint of cost-effectiveness, a perspective that offers yet another rationale for investment. However, the savings that can be gotten from contraception generate benefits to industry only in the most indirect way. Thus, cost-effectiveness arguments for industrial investment are not yet persuasive, even though, as we shall see in Chapter 6, the pharmaceutical industry is, more and more, driven by considerations of cost-effectiveness.

In sum, in the case of vaccines, the science is newly productive and its results benefit a larger proportion of those able to pay a satisfactory price; subsidy is available for those who cannot pay and, at least in the United States, appears to be politically safe. In addition, the ill health that is prevented by immunization consists of diseases that are recognized as real and direct threats to children; while the concept of pregnancy as an illness is not unknown in many contexts, the concept of pregnancy as a disease is not appealing and simply does not have the same notional status as immunization. Furthermore, childhood immunizations do not have anything to do with sexuality, about which the U.S. population entertains a large and complex ambivalence, nor is it connected to the complex and profound personal and societal issues that surround pregnancy. Finally, although there have been adverse effects from vaccines (Institute of Medicine 1992), these are now well known and can be anticipated in connection with the development of new products; also, the National Vaccine Compensation Act has set parameters around the unpredictability of litigation, so that new "blockbuster" vaccine products have not met disaster in the marketplace. Yet, in spite of these differences, there are enough commonalities between vaccines and contraceptives so that the experience with vaccines offers ideas in areas pertinent to enhancing the environment for contraceptive research and development. One of these areas is subsidy.

The Role of Subsidy and High-Volume Procurement

One of the main charges of the Mercer vaccine study was to examine the role of subsidized procurements in the vaccine market. A standard question in this connection is whether such procurements are positive incentives in the marketplace or, on the contrary, act as disincentives. The Mercer analysis concluded that, in the case of vaccines, high-volume public-sector procurement does "move the market," that is, it influences manufacturers' behavior and thus can help or hinder the achievement of programmatic goals. The fact that UNICEF purchases roughly 40 percent of developing-country vaccines from 10–12 core suppliers, with the balance satisfied through direct procurement and local production, has been crucial to expanding demand for vaccine doses over the past eight years. UNICEF procurement is based on a strong tiered pricing system in which other customers, including industrial-country governments, pay a price for a given product that covers all production and overhead costs, provides research and development funds for new vaccines, and generates a reasonable return. Mercer finds this pricing structure to be a positive incentive to the market and beneficial to all parties, but notes that such positive effect requires continual reinforcement, in the form of improved country forecasting; more precise targeting of supply to countries most in need; sustained public-sector knowledge about the economic and technical issues faced by suppliers; ongoing, collaborative public/private-sector evaluation of procurement strategy; and evaluation of manufacturers not only on price but on supply security, R&D capacity, and access to new products (Mercer Management Consulting 1994).

Subsidized procurement is also a component of international family planning policy. The United Nations Population Fund (UNFPA) has managed such independent, centralized procurement for contraceptives since1983 and the pace of utilization has more than tripled over the last few years. Donors are increasingly using UNFPA procurement services because the Fund has developed the ability to manage competitive bidding for bulk purchases from manufacturers and suppliers in over 20 countries worldwide and can negotiate low prices while ensuring product quality. In 1988–1989, 47 and 59 countries, respectively, asked UNFPA to procure contraceptives using UNFPA or external resources;[19] currently, the Fund serves approximately 120 countries altogether. In 1994, UNFPA spent $104 million on procurement, of which $82 million was spent on contraceptives and a little over $1 million on raw materials (for example, hormonal steroids) for the manufacture of contraceptives. The Fund's reading of the current situation is that because contraceptive prevalence rates are increasing in most countries, because the absolute number of couples of reproductive age keeps growing, and because population groups such as single persons and adolescents are increasingly in need of contraceptive services, the commodity volumes required by individual countries can only rise. This expansion, together with the customary unpredictability in the number and timing of requests for UNFPA procurement assistance, have made it clear that much greater resource allocations for contraceptive commodities and a more efficient procurement system are needed if emergency funding gaps and stockouts are not to surge in size and frequency (UNFPA 1995).

As a consequence, a proposal was prepared at the request of the UNDP and UNFPA Executive Board for the establishment and management of a Global Contraceptive Procurement Program that will create a "revolving fund" for procurement of contraceptive commodities essential to reproductive health programs—including family planning and sexual health programs—in developing countries with economies in transition. Several multilateral (including the World Bank and the European Union) and bilateral agencies are expected to contribute to the fund, to be managed as a trust, for purchase of buffer stocks of commonly requested contraceptive commodities from established manufacturers. The program will procure contraceptives by pharmaceutical composition or generic description within pre-agreed (i.e., WHO-approved) specifications at the lowest available international price and the revolving fund principle will ensure that the buffer stock will be maintained at some predetermined level to compensate for volatility. Replenishment of the fund will be accomplished primarily by recovering funds from UNFPA country program allocations; an additional fee or premium will be put back into the program to increase the amount of available funds, offset overhead and such contingency costs as exchange rate fluctuations, as well as to help ensure that requests made to the program were truly of an emergency nature and not regular requirements. Support will also be provided through various mechanisms for improving country-level logistics and procurement capabilities.[20]

A major consequence of the Mercer study that is relevant to contraceptives is that UNICEF has changed its policies for donating vaccine so that, rather than giving vaccine to any nation that requests it, UNICEF now targets donations to the poorest countries. The hypothesis is that this reconstituted UNICEF customer list will force many more countries to begin buying vaccine; this may, in turn, provide a greater incentive for U.S. manufacturers to participate more fully in the developing-economy vaccine market (Institute of Medicine 1995b).

While a demographic argument for increased access to family planning options is insufficient, it is useful as another perspective on the potential market for contraceptives, including new contraceptives. UNFPA has defined the unmet need for contraceptive commodities on the basis of projected population figures from 1994 to the year 2005. The agency has calculated the numbers of contraceptive users and new acceptors that will be required to limit growth to a "medium" population projection of 950 million more people worldwide by that year. The conclusion is that, to not surpass that projection, there would have to be a modest increase—about one-half of a percentage point a year—in contraceptive prevalence in developing countries, an increase from the current rate of 57 percent to 63 percent by 2005. This small increase, combined with the large absolute growth expected in the number of married/in union women, would produce an increase of 157 million users over the period. While this sounds modest, 86 percent of that increase in users would have to come from regions with low current prevalence, primarily Sub-Saharan Africa, where most governments are severely constrained in what they can spend in the health sector and are greatly dependent on external assistance (World Bank 1993).

To achieve the level of contraceptive use needed to accomplish this demographic goal, large amounts of contraceptive commodities will be required between 1994 and 2005: 196 million sterilizations, 436 million IUD insertions, 898 million injections, over 12 billion cycles of pills, and 70.3 billion condoms (55.7 billion for family planning and 14.6 billion for STD/HIV prevention), signifying a cumulative total cost of $8.1 billion for the period 1993–2005. If another $587 million is added for the projected 6.8 million Norplant users, the grand total would be almost $9 billion over the 12-year period, an average annual cost of somewhere around $650 million (UNFPA 1994), considerably more than the current market share for these regions.

UNFPA has estimated that in 1994 governments, including multilateral and bilateral donors, would provide 75 percent of all modern contraceptive methods, albeit with widely varying proportions in the commodities supplied, a total cost to governments of $398 million. Donor contributions represent approximately $100 million (in 1992, USAID spent $39.9 million on contraceptive commodities and UNFPA, using its own resources, spent $17.1 million plus $33.9 million on behalf of others, a total of $90.0 million). UNFPA goes on to conclude that developing countries would provide 56.5 percent, or $298.4 million, of the costs of contraceptive commodities in 1994, much of which is accounted for by China and India. Thus, the private sector accounts for about 25 percent of the total, or $130 million, a large part of which is sales. Private-sector and pharmacy participation in the market is widely variable from region to region, ranging from highs of 62 and 33 percent in Latin America and the Caribbean, respectively, to lows of 7 and 0.3 percent in Asia and the Pacific, respectively (see Table 5-12).

One unknown variable in determining whether subsidy is either an incentive or disincentive to the market is the size of the subsidy and the extent to which it can be depended upon to continue. At present, direct donor subsidies account for about 25 percent of public-sector participation in the provision of contraceptive commodities to developing economies. This is smaller than the UNICEF participation in the vaccine market but it is not inconsequential. The U.S. portion of direct external donor assistance in 1993 was 16.3 percent of total donor funding for contraceptive commodities and there are currently questions about whether that level will be sustained. Funding for contraceptive purchase and distribution is just part of the total funding picture for the field as a whole and is addressed as such in Chapter 6.

THE COST-EFFECTIVENESS OF CONTRACEPTION

As both a public and a private good, contraceptive technologies have a double identity. Both public and private decisions are made to acquire those technologies, and each decision-making process employs different criteria. However, one criterion that is shared between public-sector and private-sector purchasers of contraceptive technologies is value for money, that is, the potential for maximum gain for expenditure.

An important source of guidance to achieving value for money in health-related spending is estimation of the cost-effectiveness of different health interventions and medical procedures (World Bank 1993). Because the application of cost-effectiveness analysis to health is difficult, relatively little has been done in a way that permits resource allocation across a broad range of options (World Bank 1993). This is especially true for developing countries where most health services have traditionally been provided by public sectors whose agendas have been ruled by forces other than cost-effectiveness. Where such analysis has been undertaken, the emphasis has been on the curative side of the health care equation, since costing out the effectiveness of prevention, with its long-term payoffs and multiple externalities, is particularly difficult.

Until recently, little cost-effectiveness analysis had been done in connection with family planning, despite the fact that failure to avert unintended pregnancies is patently very costly to the society (Lee and Stewart 1995). This may be due to the fact that contraception is a preventive intervention with payoffs too long-term, obvious, or various to quantify, or to a perception that cost-effectiveness is unimportant relative to the successful achievement of demographic objectives. Another possibility is that contraceptive commodities are a relatively small pro-

TABLE 5-12 Estimated Sources of Supply of Modern Methods of Contraception in Developing Countries, by Method and by Region, 1994 (in %)

Source	Modern	Sterilization	Pill	Injectable	IUD	Condom
Total						
Government	86.3	95.0	56.7	66.8	94.4	47.1
Private	13.7	5.0	43.3	33.2	5.6	52.9
Pharmacy	4.1	0.0	32.7	5.8	0.2	40.7
NGO	0.6	0.5	0.8	0.5	0.5	0.4
Other	9.1	4.5	9.8	26.9	5.0	11.8
Sub-Saharan Africa						
Government	65.0	53.2	67.4	81.3	62.9	35.5
Private	35.0	46.8	32.6	18.7	37.1	64.5
Pharmacy	4.3	0.0	7.1	0.3	0.0	18.6
NGO	3.2	0.6	3.4	2.0	5.5	3.4
Other	27.4	46.3	22.1	16.4	31.6	42.5
Arab States and Europe						
Government	42.5	82.3	32.6	47.9	49.8	22.2
Private	57.5	17.7	67.4	52.1	50.2	77.8
Pharmacy	31.6	0.0	62.3	6.8	2.7	72.9
NGO	0.7	0.0	0.9	2.7	0.9	0.1
Other	25.2	17.7	4.2	42.5	46.6	4.8

Latin America and the Caribbean

Government	38.2	58.7	12.6	17.1	58.3	18.4
Private	61.8	41.3	87.4	82.9	41.7	81.6
Pharmacy	33.3	0.0	82.7	71.6	1.3	71.7
NGO	5.4	6.6	1.5	1.1	11.1	2.4
Other	23.1	34.8	3.2	10.2	29.3	7.4

Asia and the Pacific

Government	93.0	98.4	79.0	68.9	98.3	50.7
Private	7.0	1.6	21.0	31.1	1.7	49.3
Pharmacy	0.3	0.0	8.6	0.2	0.0	37.3
NGO	0.1	0.0	0.2	0.1	0.0	0.2
Other	6.7	1.6	12.2	30.8	1.7	11.8

NOTE: NGO = nongovernmental organization.

SOURCE: United Nations Population Fund (UNFPA). Contraceptive Use and Commodity Costs in Developing Countries 1994–2005. Technical Report No. 18. New York. 1994.

portion of the costs of a family planning delivery system and, in many cases, are donated or bulk-procured at concessional prices, so that cost-effectiveness considerations seem irrelevant. For countries that construct their family planning programs around one or two methods, there is little reason for such analysis.

Now, however, as health care costs have risen everywhere and the need for sectoral reform looms large, the issue is forced. No system component is immune to the urge for savings. Family planning must compete with other interventions, curative and preventive, for its share of public-sector allocations and managed care packages and for its position in the portfolios of institutions providing external assistance to developing economies. In this competition, family planning will be found to have real competitive advantage: First, it is highly cost-effective and, second, a good proportion of the ensuing savings can be realized within a 12- to 18-month time horizon (Forrest and Singh 1990; Stewart 1995). And because, in the developing world, there is accumulating pressure for a greater array of contraceptive methods, most of which cannot be locally procured, there are foreign exchange implications which may require more complex and precise calculations than has been the case.

Under the rubrics of family planning and contraception, there are two major considerations. One is the cost-effectiveness of family planning *qua* family planning, as a set of services that subsumes the provision of contraceptive technologies. The other is the cost-effectiveness of each contraceptive method relative to others. Each consideration plays a different role in decisions about technology utilization and the mix of methods that will be offered, and each also plays a role in the structure of the market and industry's perception of that market's value.

The Cost-Effectiveness of Contraception in the United States

Table 5-13 presents a summary of costs of the major conditions against which contraception is in some way protective, the costs per relevant intervention, and estimated savings. It includes sexually transmitted diseases, since those are transmissible through the same process as conception, and since a method that could provide simultaneous protection against both conception and infection is very high on the list of women's priorities for new technologies. The data are limited to the United States, since data elsewhere do not seem to exist at comparable levels of detail.

Figures 5-8a and b summarize the conclusions from a recent, most meticulous analysis of the economic value of contraception from the perspectives of a private payer and a publicly funded program. The study compared 15 methods in terms of their direct medical costs (the direct costs of using each method, the likelihood and costs of potential side effects, and the likelihood and cost of pregnancies due to contraceptive failure). The main outcome measures included 1- and 5-year costs and the number of pregnancies avoided compared with use of no contraceptive method. Thus, the baseline was the cost of using no contraception, which resulted in 4.25 pregnancies per sexually active woman, an outcome that costs private insurers or patients themselves $14,663 (including the weighted costs of prenatal and delivery services, abortions, miscarriages, and ectopic pregnancies) and costs public-sector payers $6,490. The copper-T IUD proved most cost-effective and, because of its high efficacy, associated savings are correspondingly high: $14,122 for private payers and $6,269 for public payers. For those who want no more children, sterilization is also highly cost-effective but saves less since its (one-time) cost is more; implants and injectables are also very cost-effective but, again, take time to be amortized. The use of emergency contraceptive pills (ECP) following unanticipated, coerced, or unprotected intercourse, or after a method failure, also results in significant cost savings. These figures are, of course, sensitive to changes in commodity prices. For example, in 1991, one study discovered average increases in the prices charged for the most-used oral contraceptives of around 42 percent (Daley and Gold 1993), which have especially powerful impact on constrained state-level health budgets.

However, the methods that are most cost-effective in terms of preventing pregnancy do not reduce the risk of sexually transmitted infection, although oral contraceptives, implants, and injectables do reduce risk for pelvic inflammatory disease. Unfortunately, the contraceptive methods that are also risk-reducing are less effective as contraceptives, so that double method use becomes necessary; this in turn reduces cost-effectiveness. Methods that are efficaciously STD-protective and contraceptive could be highly cost-effective, since STD prevalence and corresponding costs continue to rise (Donovan 1993; Hellinger 1993).

The bottom-line message from these analyses is simple. As the authors point out, "regardless of payment mechanism or contraceptive method, contraception saves money" (Trussell et al. 1995b). Even the crudest summation of putative savings is compelling: total estimated annual savings from averting unintended pregnancies ($1.8 billion for associated medical costs alone); teenage pregnancy ($10 billion, a figure which duplicates some of the medical costs of "unintended pregnancies" but introduces some welfare costs); and at least part of the costs of chlamydial infection, gonorrhea, and herpes (over $5 billion). These are not small dollars.

Contraceptive Cost-Effectiveness in the Developing World

Cost-effectiveness studies in the developing world have focused primarily on the costs of "excess fertility" to the family or society, defined from several perspectives: from a health perspective (births to women too young, too old, of too high or too closely spaced parity); from a demographic perspective (fertility that pushes population growth rates above 2 percent); or from a household perspective (what women or couples view as excess fertility). From the demographic perspective, family planning is viewed as particularly "cost-effective"

TABLE 5-13 The Cost-Effectiveness of Family Planning and Contraception, United States

Costs			Intervention		Savings	
Event/Condition	Dollar Costs		Intervention	Dollar Costs	X Averted	Dollar Savings
Unprotected sex (85 pregnancies per 100 typical women); estimated at 5,726,412 events/ yr. – mutual intercourse w/o contraception, method failures, and rapes	$3,795, typical managed care setting; $1,680 in publicly funded program		Publicly funded contraceptive services	$412 million (1987)	3.1 million UIP/yr.[a] (1.3 million births) (1.4 million abortions) (0.4 million miscarriages) 20,000 fewer LBWs 106,900 fewer births w/ no or late prenatal care	$1.8 billion/yr., immediate and short-term; $4.40 per public dollar[b]
			Emergency contraception (I)[c]	Managed care: $59 for ECP, $392 for copper-T IUD; public-sector setting: $35 for ECP, $172 for copper-T IUD	53/100 women treated with ECPs; 71/100 women treated w/ postcoital insertion of copper-T IUD	ECP: $142 in managed care setting, $54 in public-sector setting; Copper-T IUD: $123 in managed care setting, $53 in public-sector setting (plus cost savings from 10 yrs. of high-efficacy contraception)
			Emergency contraception (II)[c]	$71 for ECP in a managed care setting, $49 in public-sector setting	As above	Per yr.: $90 for users of cervical cap, $101 male condom, $115 diaphragm, $136 spermicides, $140

Teen pregnancy	$25 billion/yr.[d] ($18,133 by child's 20th birthday for family begun by teenage mother in 1990)	All births to teenage mothers	withdrawal, $156 periodic abstinence, female condom. Variable by frequency and % of births calculated as unwanted vs. mistimed
			$10 billion (40% of calculated expenditures)
Abortion		Government pays for abortions for poor women	670,000 abortions (1982–1988)
			$4.00 per public dollar (state funds)[e] $340–$415 million net savings over 2 yrs. for nation as a whole
STDs: Chlamydia/ herpes Gonorrhea Chlamydia[f]	Over $5 billion/yr. $2.18 billion/yr. (1990 projected)		
Ectopic pregnancy	$1.1 billion/yr.		
HIV/AIDS	$64 billion (1991)		

TABLE 5-13 Continued

Costs		Intervention		Savings	
Event/Condition	Dollar Costs	Intervention	Dollar Costs	X Averted	Dollar Savings
Reproductive cancers:					
Cervix		Barrier + spermicide contraceptives		The longer used, the lower the risk	
Ovarian and Endometrial	50,000 hospitalizations per yr. (1982)	Oral contraceptives		40%–50% decreased risk; starts soon after starting use; protective effect stronger w/ greater duration, lasts at least 15 yrs. after use stops	

NOTES: UIP = unintended pregnancy; UWP = unwanted pregnancy; ECP = emergency contraceptive pills (ordinary birth control pills containing estrogen and progestin, administered immediately after unprotected intercourse and up to 72 hours beyond, per regimen); LBW = low birth weight.

[a]This number would be larger were there to be no publicly-funded family planning services; in their absence, the resulting additional unintended pregnancies would include 509,000 additional unintended births and 516,000 additional abortions.

[b]Savings vary by state, e.g., savings in the state of California would have been an average of $7.70 per public dollar by prevention of an estimated 136,800 unintended pregnancies each year.

[c]I and II refer to two scenarios for ECP use. I = the traditional one in which a woman seeks treatment from a clinician following unprotected intercourse. II = provision of ECPs during an annual visit to a clinician for later use should unprotected intercourse occur. Only costs associated with medical care are included in these calculations and are probably understated (Trussell et al. November 1995).

aThis estimate for 1990, which includes direct payments from Aid to Families with Dependent Children (AFDC), Medicaid, and Food Stamps, does not include other public costs such as job training; housing subsidies; the Women, Infants, and Children (WIC) supplemental food programs; subsidized school meals; special education; foster care; or day care.

eSince the Hyde Amendment went into effect in 1977, no federal Medicaid funds have been available for abortion unless the woman's life is endangered; only 13 states provided local Medicaid funds for poor women's abortions in most circumstances as of 1993. In 1987, 12 percent of all abortions in the United States were paid for with public funds, virtually all of which were state funds.

fIncludes costs of uncomplicated illness and PID and its sequelae, including ectopic pregnancy ($4,235 each), infertility, mortality, hospitalization, and outpatient treatment. Washington AE, RE Johnson, LL Sanders. *Chlamydia trachomatis* infections in the United States: What are they costing us? JAMA 257(15):2070–2072. April 17, 1987.

SOURCES: Holt R. Emergency Contraception: Working Paper on Pharmaceutical Company Involvement. Los Angeles, CA: Pacific Institute for Women's Health, Western Consortium for Public Health, August 1995. Peipert JF, J Gutmann. Oral contraceptive risk assessment: A survey of 247 educated women. Obstetrics and Gynecology 82(1), July 1993. Planned Parenthood Federation of America, Inc. Fact Sheet: The Cost-Effectiveness of Family Planning and Reproductive Health Care. New York, 1993. Planned Parenthood Federation of America, Inc. Fact Sheet: Abortion and Access to Abortion Services. New York, 1993. Trussell J, J Koenig, C Ellertson, F Stewart. The cost-effectiveness of emergency contraception. Unpublished manuscript. Princeton, NJ: November 1995.

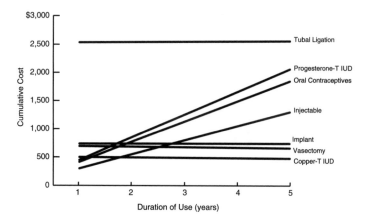

FIGURE 5-8a Cumulative costs associated with selected contraceptive methods in the managed payment model.

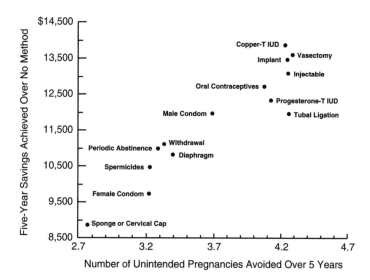

FIGURE 5-8b Cost savings and pregnancies avoided over 5 years for contraceptive methods compared with no method, managed payment model. SOURCE (Figures 5-8a and 5-8b): J Trussell, JA Leveque, JD Koenig et al. The economic value of contraception: A comparison of 15 methods. American Journal of Public Health 85(4):494–503, April 1995.

where fertility and mortality rates are high; savings are expected to be realized through reductions in maternal mortality and child deaths. More comprehensively, and as a very general rule, the higher the rates of fertility and mortality, the lower the costs per infant and child death averted, the higher the savings to government, and the greater the theoretical cost-effectiveness of family planning. As in industrialized countries, savings to government may include cost per pregnancy per mother, cost of care for a child in the first year of life, the benefits of preventing incomplete abortions and their subsequent treatment, and, more broadly, sectoral savings in education, health care, housing, infrastructure, and social services. These societal savings are also weighed against the costs of achieving fertility reduction, and these costs depend on the motivation of women to control their fertility (Birdsall et al. 1987; Cochrane and Sai 1993; Fauveau 1991; Figa-Talamanca et al. 1986; World Bank 1993) or, in more recent parlance, their reproductive intentions.

The costs of unrealized reproductive intentions, as expressed in unintended and unwanted pregnancy, may be very high indeed at the household level and even more complex to quantify than either demographic or societal costs. There is a sadly expanding body of testimony to those costs and, in many ways, they are alike in many developed and developing countries, particularly in urbanizing environments. These consequences and their costs can be severe and lasting: abortion, insufficient participation in prenatal care, greater tendency to take behavioral risks during pregnancy, low birth weight, infant mortality, poor child health and development, maternal deaths and reproductive complications, postpartum depression, domestic violence, and economic hardship for others in the family (Institute of Medicine 1995a). Virtually all studies focus on portions of these consequences and subsets of intervening variables, since any systematic, aggregated analysis of such a vast array is probably impossible.

What has not been done in developing-country contexts is the sort of method cost-effectiveness analysis described in the preceding section. Since family planning programs will remain part of the content of public health services and, in some cases, of managed care, such analysis may be timely. This dearth of analysis may be on its way to being repaired: The contraceptive cost-effectiveness model discussed above is being considered for application in Chile (personal communication, S. Díaz 1995).

The Costs of Sexually Transmitted Reproductive Tract Infections

As discussed earlier in this report, the burden of the sexually transmitted diseases in the developing world is enormous, as are its social and economic consequences. The U.S. Public Health Service has estimated the societal costs of the sexually transmitted diseases in the United States to be in excess of $3.5 billion annually (Public Health Service 1991; see also Washington et al. 1986, 1987). The quantification of those consequences remained largely uncharted terrain until the publication of the recent work by Trussell et al. (1995a) which, in addition to calculating the savings from currently available contraceptive methods, calculates the potential impact of each method on the incidence and cost of sexually transmitted diseases and the resulting total costs or savings for the method.[21] The rank ordering of contraceptives by total costs changed only slightly when the costs of sexually transmitted diseases were included. When those costs are factored in, savings for each contraceptive method compared with "no method" increased slightly for the barrier methods (male and female condoms, diaphragm, cervical cap, sponge, and spermi-cides), ranging from $283 to $183 saved per year, and actually decreased for IUDs. However, these calculations may be to some extent artifactual: First, the FDA allows only latex and plastic male condoms and the polyurethane female condom to be marketed as prophylactics against STDs and, second, the relatively small impact of STD costs on total savings from use of contraceptive methods really derives from the low incidence of sexually transmitted diseases when all women of reproductive age are considered as a group. Were the same analysis to be focused on those age cohorts among whom incidence of STDs is highest, that is, just the younger cohorts, the savings impacts would be much greater (Trussell et al. 1995a).

So far, only one published study (Over and Piot 1993) has attempted that quantification for the developing world, even though there are fragments of evidence that the economic costs associated with the sexually transmitted diseases and their complications and sequelae are substantial. The impression is that the direct costs of treating the consequences of these diseases are much greater in developing countries because of higher barriers to care and patterns of antibiotic resistance. However, the only quantification of this impression is based on proxy data such as hospital admission records from gynecology wards. These suggest that the opportunity costs of these complications are, indeed, considerable. The treatment of pelvic inflammatory disease in Sub-Saharan Africa accounts for anywhere from 17 to 44 percent of admissions to gynecology wards, and in Nigeria ectopic pregnancies alone account for 15 percent (Meheus 1992; Piot and Rowley 1992). There is also evidence of high STD-associated indirect costs, that is, the value of the labor lost from morbidity, debility, and premature mortality, as well as the value of any labor diverted from other productive uses to care for the ill (Piot and Rowley 1992). Two sets of calculations—one estimating the average annual number of discounted healthy (or productive) days of life lost by women with STDs in an urban area in Africa, the other estimating the incidence of STD complications in infants born to infected women—indicate that STDs are major contributors to adverse pregnancy outcomes and that preventing STDs produces considerable health gains.

Except for AIDS, there are few data on the effectiveness and costs of the currently available interventions against STDs in the developing world, on the benefits of averting a single case of STD, or on the cases averted because of arrested transmission. Use of condoms to prevent HIV transmission, at a cost of

$30 per Disability-adjusted Life Year (Cochrane and Sai 1993), ranks among the 10 most cost-effective interventions to improve adult health. Nonetheless, the cost of providing condoms in urban Africa alone surpasses present government per capita expenditures on all health interventions (Piot and Rowley 1992). UNFPA projects requirements for condoms for STD/AIDS prevention in developing countries between 1993 and 2005 at 14,635 million, at a total cost of about $406.5 million, around $31.3 million annually. This figure is based on use in high-risk, transient encounters, that is, outside marriage or stable union; thus, the costs of condoms for use with a regular partner would be additional (UNFPA 1994).

Paying for Contraception

The savings that can be realized from contraception are of such magnitude that it is hard to understand why they appear to be so unappreciated by virtually all providers of health insurance coverage. The probability is that there are two general health care markets that will grow dramatically: managed care for the employed and Medicaid managed care, with the latter becoming more and more a for-profit, competitive enterprise (Winslow 1995). As of July 1994, about 65 percent of all private payers, close to 115 million people, were enrolled in some form of managed care plan, an increase of about 10 percent from the preceding year, a rate that is expected to persist (Bailit 1995). As managed care plans "industrialize," expand their dominance, and consolidate in different ways, they can be expected to be increasingly capable of driving other components of the health market, including the market for pharmaceuticals. Thus, the extent to which they reimburse contraception as one strategic element in the preventive and cost-savings components of their portfolios could become more of an incentive and, perhaps, a stabilizing force in the marketplace, both of which can serve as stimuli to innovation.

At least one of the dimensions of that shift would not seem to have been predictable. In April 1995, the *Wall Street Journal* reported the new interest of health maintenance organizations (HMOs) in the poor. Once shunned by HMOs, those eligible for Medicaid are now seen as a major source of enrollment growth—and of profits. The logic is that by providing Medicaid patients with their own primary-care doctors, HMOs believe they can curb the use of high-cost emergency rooms for routine care, thereby reining in costs while vastly improving health care for the poor. Since family planning services are a logical part of primary care and apparently much desired by many plan participants, and since it is not hard to grasp the cost-effectiveness of contraceptives, it would not be implausible for managed care plans to incorporate those components into their service delivery packages. It may be that some states at least will seek to mandate such inclusion. As of August 1995, a landmark bill had been passed by the

California State Assembly and was pending in the State Senate, calling for all health insurance plans to include most contraceptives.

If this is to be the case, it would represent a major change in current patterns. Not surprisingly, given a tradition of covering surgical procedures but not prevention, laparoscopic tubal ligation is routinely covered by 86 percent of large-group plans, preferred provider organizations (PPOs), and HMOs, and 90 percent of point of service (POS) networks. Coverage of vasectomy is roughly the same. This may partly explain some of the high rates of surgical sterilization in the United States and the low rates of IUD use (Lee and Stewart 1995), yet another case in which availability shapes demand, rather than vice versa. Two-thirds or more of all plan types—including 66 percent of large-group fee-for-service plans, 67 percent of PPOs, 83 percent of POS networks, and 70 percent of HMOs—routinely cover induced abortions employing dilation and curettage-suction aspiration. However, almost one-fourth of all coverage of abortion by large-group plans is restricted in some way, for instance, by requiring the provider to certify the concurrent presence of a specific medical indication (Guttmacher Institute 1995c).

However, coverage of reversible contraception is, indeed, "unequal and uneven" (Guttmacher Institute 1995c). Half of typical fee-for-service plans written for large groups or PPOs cover no reversible contraception whatsoever. Less than 20 percent of large-group indemnity plans or PPOs, and less than 40 percent of POS networks and HMOs, routinely cover all five of the most effective reversible methods (IUD and Norplant insertion, Depo-Provera injection, and oral contraception) in their typical plans. What is particularly surprising is that 66 percent of large-group plans do not cover oral contraceptives, the most used reversible method in the United States, even though 97 percent of those same plans typically cover prescription drugs. Similarly, even though 92 percent of those plans cover medical devices generally, only 24 percent cover Norplant, 18 percent cover IUDS, and 15 percent cover diaphragms. Coverage of oral contraceptives is much higher in POS networks and HMOs. Only 7 percent of HMOs provide no contraceptive coverage at all, and 39 percent cover all five methods (Guttmacher Institute 1995c).

From a cost-effectiveness standpoint, these patterns are not logical. An increase of just 15 percent in new oral contraceptive users would produce enough savings in the costs of pregnancy care to cover oral contraceptives for all users in a given health insurance plan. Another instance: A 4 percent increase in copper-T IUD use continued over five years would pay for all IUD users in the plan; an 18 percent increase in one-year IUD users would produce the same result (Lee and Stewart 1995). In an environment that will see dramatic growth in managed care, expanded coverage that would offer a full array of all available contraceptive methods would produce savings to plans and to the society at large, as well as a potentially guaranteed market for both new and existing contraceptives. While these shifts are preeminently a U.S. phenomenon, they are not exclusively so, and their power to move a market that is so responsive to U.S. demand is highly relevant to the wider market that includes the developing countries.

Public-Sector Coverage of Contraception in the United States

Unlike private insurers and health maintenance organizations, all 50 states and the District of Columbia are required by law to provide reimbursement for contraceptive services, and one in three women who made a family planning visit in 1988 (the last year for which comprehensive data are available) reported going to a publicly funded family planning clinic (Guttmacher Institute 1995c).

The proportions of public funding for family planning through different channels have changed a great deal in recent years. The overall pattern has been that, since the late 1980s, Medicaid has assumed the role of lead public funder for contraceptive services, as provision of contraceptive services through other mechanisms, notably Title X, has declined (see Figure 5-9). As of 1990, Medicaid accounted for 58 percent of all federal family planning expenditures, at a level of approximately $270 million; by 1992, that amount was $319 million and amounted to 50 percent of all public funding (Guttmacher Institute 1995c).

Another overall pattern has been that, when inflation is taken into account, total public funding for contraceptive services fell by 27 percent between 1980 and 1992, with Title X funding falling by 72 percent over that same period, with a corresponding increase in unintended pregnancy. At the same time, the costs of providing those services, including costs of contraceptive commodities, have risen; for example, the average price for oral contraceptives to publicly funded family planning clinics rose 42 percent in just one year, between 1991 and 1992 (Daley and Gold 1993).

The third pattern of interest is that of the general distribution of payment source for family planning visits. A striking 41 percent of all women who received family planning services paid for their most recent visit out of their own pockets, 25 percent were completely covered by insurance, 17 percent used insurance with a copayment or deductible, and 7 percent of visits were covered by Medicaid (Kaeser and Richards 1994). The fact that women pay so much out of their own pockets for these services can be viewed in two ways: One is that they value the services and the commodities enough to pay for them; the other is that systems that could cover at least some of the costs of contraceptive services do not, for one reason or another, do so. Both possibilities can coexist and both have market implications. The first is the expression of market demand; the second is that there is a large institutional purchasing capacity that remains unused. This leaves unaddressed the economics of over-the-counter contraceptive purchases, a question that has been raised in the many discussions about the wisdom of making oral contraceptives available without prescription. The decision for the time being, at least in the United States, is that OCs will remain a prescription product, so that the economic issues are moot for now. Still, it is worth noting that such

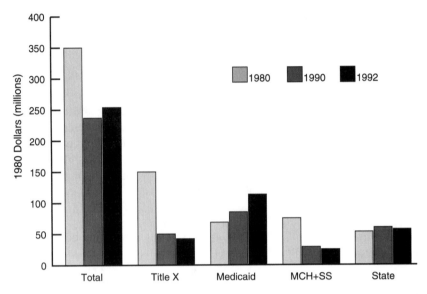

FIGURE 5-9   Public expenditure for contraceptive services, United States.   SOURCE: Alan Guttmacher Institute.   Uneven and Unequal: Insurance Coverage and Reproductive Health Services. New York and Washington: The Alan Guttmacher Institute. 1995.

purchases would not be covered by third-party payers but by individuals, who would assume the responsibility for purchase and for a greater share of physical risk.

CONCLUDING COMMENT

At the beginning of this chapter, we used the term "dilemma," one of whose meanings is "a difficult problem . . . seemingly incapable of a satisfactory conclusion" (Merriam-Webster's New International Dictionary 1986). The analysis reflected in this chapter persuades us that the problem of translating unmet need for new contraceptive options into market demand, though difficult, is not insoluble. While the existing array of contraceptive options represents a major contribution of science and industry to human well-being, it still fails to meet the needs of significant numbers of individuals in significant populations. Even if the general need is not seen as constituting attractive market demand (defined as need plus willingness and ability to pay), substantial components of that overall need do respond to such a definition. The epidemic of sexually transmitted infections; large gaps in an array of "menses-inducers" tailored to the wide range of women's practical, physiologic, and ideologic concerns; the paucity of methods for male participation in contraception; and the persistent importance of reducing method side effects; all are plausible indicators of commercially appreciable market demand.

A quantitative case can also be made. The numbers of contraceptive users has grown and continues to grow. While sterilization rates qualify those numbers, sterilization rates also represent an indeterminate number of consumers, particularly younger consumers, who might prefer a reversible method. Because availability shapes demand and because a full range of contraceptive options is often inaccessible, there is a potentially large population, importantly consisting of method-discontinuers and method-switchers, for new products. Availability of a good method mix has an independently positive effect on contraceptive use-prevalence, as well as on reduction in crude birth rates, and might be seen in itself as a market-driver. Finally, while it is true that inability to pay conditions profit margins in many instances, the cost-effectiveness of contraception is clear enough so that it should motivate expanded coverage where third-party payment is a factor, and subsidy for bulk purchases where that is required, again improving the level of demand and the size of the market for contraceptives, in the United States and abroad.

REFERENCES

Alan Guttmacher Institute. Hopes and Realities: Closing the Gap Between Women's Aspirations and Their Reproductive Experiences. New York: The Alan Guttmacher Institute. 1995a.

Alan Guttmacher Institute. Issues in Brief: The U.S. Family Planning Program Faces Challenges and Change. New York and Washington: The Alan Guttmacher Institute. 1995b.

Alan Guttmacher Institute. Uneven and Unequal: Insurance Coverage and Reproductive Health Services. New York: The Alan Guttmacher Institute. 1995c.

Alan Guttmacher Institute. Sex and America's Teenagers. New York: The Alan Guttmacher Institute. 1994.

American Health Consultants. Contraceptive Technology Update 16(9):105–120, 1995.

Ashford LS. New perspectives on population: Lessons from Cairo. Population Bulletin 5(1):22, 1995.

Bailit HL. Market strategies and the growth of managed care. IN Academic Health Centers in the Managed Care Environment. D Korn, CH McLaughlin, M Osterweis, eds. Washington, DC: Association of Academic Health Centers. 1995.

Birdsall N, SH Cochrane, J van der Gaag. The cost of children. IN Economics of Education: Research and Studies. George Psacharopolous, ed. New York: Pergamon Press. 1987.

Bongaarts J, J Bruce. The causes of unmet need for contraception and the social content of services. Studies in Family Planning 26(2): 57–75, 1995.

Bosch FX, MM Manos, N Muñóz, et al. Prevalence of human papillomavirus in cervical cancer: A worldwide perspective. Journal of the National Cancer Institute 87:796–802, 1995.

Bruce J, A Jain. A new family planning ethos. IN The Progress of Nations. New York: UNICEF. 1995.

Bulatao RA, RD Lee. An overview of fertility determinants in developing countries. IN Determinants of Fertility in Developing Countries, Vol. 2, RA Bulatao, RD Lee, eds. New York: Academic Press. 1983.

Carpenter PF. Innovation in patient information: The importance of facilitating informed choice. Infectious and Medical Disease Letters for Obstetrics and Gynecology XI(3), 1989.

Cates W. Teenagers and sexual risk taking: The best of times and the worst of times. Journal of Adolescent Health 12(2):84–94, 1991.

Centers for Disease Control and Prevention (CDC). Division of STD/HIV Prevention Annual Report, 1991. Atlanta: CDC, 1992.

Cochrane S, F Sai. Excess fertility. IN Disease Control Priorities in Developing Countries. DT Jamison, WH Mosley, AR Measham, JL Bobadilla, eds. New York: Oxford University Press. 1993.

Correa S. Population and Reproductive Rights Component: Platform Document, Preliminary Ideas. Paper prepared for the International Conference on Population and Development [Cairo 1994]. Development Alternative with Women for a New Era. February 1993.

Cross HE et al. Contraceptive Source and the For-Profit Private Sector in Third World Family Planning. Paper presented at the Annual Meeting of the Population Association of America, Washington, DC, March 21, 1991.

Daley D, RB Gold. Public funding of contraceptive, sterilization and abortion services, fiscal year 1992. Family Planning Perspectives 25(6):244–251, 1993.

Donovan P. Testing Positive: Sexually Transmitted Diseases and the Public Health Response. New York: The Alan Guttmacher Institute. 1993.

[The] Economist. On the needless hounding of a safe contraceptive. pp. 113–114, 2 September 1995.

Fauveau V. Matlab Maternity Care Program. Review paper prepared for the World Bank Department of Population and Human Resources. Washington, DC. 1991.

Figa-Talamanca I, TA Sinnathuray, K Yusof, et al. Illegal abortion: An attempt to assess its cost to the health services and its incidence in the community. International Journal of Health Services 16:375–389, 1986.

Food and Drug Administration. FDA Talk Paper: Norplant Update. Rockville, MD: U.S. Department of Health and Human Services, Public Health Service. 17 August 1995.

Forrest JD. Contraceptive use in the United States: Past, present and future. Advances in Population 2:29–48, 1994a.

Forrest JD. Epidemiology of unintended pregnancy and contraceptive use. American Journal of Obstetrics and Gynecology 170(5, Part 2):1485–1489, 1994b.

Forrest JD, S Singh. Public sector savings resulting from expenditures for contraceptive services. Family Planning Perspectives 22(6), 1990.

Frost and Sullivan. U.S. Market Intelligence Report: U.S. Contraceptive and Fertility Product Markets (Report #5021-54). New York: Frost and Sullivan. October 1993.

Gallup Organization. Women's Attitudes Towards Contraceptives and Other Forms of Birth Control (Poll conducted for the American College of Obsterics and Gynecology). Princeton, NJ. January 1994.

Germain A. Are we speaking the same language? Women's health advocates and scientists talk about contraceptive technology. IN Four Essays on Birth Control Needs and Risks. R Dixon-Mueller, A Germain, eds. New York: International Women's Health Coalition. 1993.

Guttmacher Institute. See Alan Guttmacher Institute.

Hatcher RA, J Trussell, F Stewart et al. Contraceptive Technology (16th Revised Edition). New York: Irvington Publishers. 1994.

Hellinger FJ. The lifetime cost of treating a person with HIV. Journal of the American Medical Association 270:474–478, 1993.

Herman R. Whatever happened to the contraceptive revolution? Washington Post, Health Section, 13 December 1994.

Hira SK, AB Spruyt, PJ Feldblum, et al. Spermicide acceptability among patients at a sexually transmitted disease clinic in Zambia. American Journal of Public Health 85(8):1098–1103, 1995.

Ingrassia M, K Springen, D Rosenberg. Still fumbling in the dark—Contraception: With all the condoms, pills and foams, why are so many women getting sterilized? Newsweek, 13 March 1995.

Institute of Medicine (IOM). The Children's Vaccine Initiative: Achieving the Vision. VS Mitchell, NM Philipose, JP Sanford, eds. Washington, DC: National Academy Press. 1993.

IOM. The Best Intentions: Unintended Pregnancy and the Well-Being of Children and Families, S Brown, L Eisenberg, eds. Washington, DC: National Academy Press. 1995a.

IOM. The Children's Vaccine Initiative: Continuing Activities—A Summary of Two Workshops Held September 12–13 and October 25–26, 1994. GW Pearson, ed. Washington, DC: National Academy Press, 1995b.

International Development Research Centre (IDRC). Position Paper on IDRC Support for Development of Immunological Contraceptives. Ottawa, Canada, June 1995.

Kaeser L, CL Richards. Barriers to Access to Reproductive Health Services. Paper submitted to the Institute of Medicine Committee on the Role of Planned Childbearing in the Health and Well-Being of Children, Women, and Families, Washington, DC. 1994.

Kaiser/Fact Finders. Survey on Obstetricians/Gynecologists' Attitudes and Practices Related to Contraception and Family Planning. Menlo Park, CA: The Henry J. Kaiser Family Foundation. 1994.

Kaiser/Harris. National Survey Results on Public Knowledge and Attitudes on Contraception and Unplanned Pregnancy. Menlo Park, CA: The Henry J. Kaiser Family Foundation. 1995.

Kolata G. Will the lawyers kill off Norplant? New York Times, section 3, p. 1. 28 May 1995.

Kost K, JD Forrest. American women's sexual behavior and exposure to risk of sexually transmitted diseases. Family Planning Perspectives 24:244–254, 1992.

Landry DJ, TM Camelo. Young unmarried men and women discuss men's role in contraceptive practice. Family Planning Perspectives 26:222–227, 1994.

Lee PR, FH Stewart. Editorial: Failing to prevent unintended pregnancy is costly. American Journal of Public Health 85(4):479–480, 1995.

Maynard R. The Effectiveness of Interventions on Repeat Pregnancy and Childbearing. Paper prepared for the Institute of Medicine Committee on Unintended Pregnancy. Washington, DC: Institute of Medicine. 1994.

Meheus A. Women's Health: Importance of reproductive tract infections, pelvic inflammatory disease and cervical cancer. IN Reproductive Tract Infections: Global Impact and Priorities for Women's Reproductive Health, A Germain, KK Holmes, P Piot, J Wasserheit, eds. New York: Plenum. 1992.

Mercer Management Consulting. Summary of UNICEF Study: A Commercial Perspective on Vaccine Supply. New York: Mercer Management Consulting. 1994.

Moore KA, BC Miller, D Glei, DR Morrison. Adolescent Sex, Contraception, and Childbearing: A Review of Recent Research. Washington, DC: Child Trends, Inc. June 1995.

Mosher WD, WF Pratt. Contraceptive use in the United States, 1973–88. Advance Data from Vital and Health Statistics of the National Center for Health Statistics 182:20, 1990.

Mosher WD. Contraceptive practice in the United States, 1982–1988. Family Planning Perspectives 22(5):198–205, 1990.

National Adolescent Reproductive Health Partnership. NARHP Update. Washington, DC: Association of Reproductive Health Professionals. 1995.

Ortho Pharmaceutical Corporation. Executive Summary: 1995 Ortho Annual Birth Control Study. Raritan, NJ. 1995.

Ortho Pharmaceutical Corporation. Highlights, 1993 Ortho Annual Birth Control Study. Raritan, NJ. 1993.

Ortho Pharmaceutical Corporation. Report on 1991 Ortho Annual Birth Control Study. Raritan, NJ. 1991.

Over M, P Piot. HIV infection and sexually transmitted diseases. IN Disease Control Priorities in Developing Countries, DT Jamison, WH Mosley, AR Measham, JL Bobadilla, eds. New York: Oxford University Press. 1993.

Piot P, J Rowley. Economic impact of reproductive tract infections and resources for their control. IN Reproductive Tract Infections: Global Impact and Priorities for Women's Reproductive Health. A Germain, KK Holmes, et al., eds. New York: Plenum Press. 1992.

Pleck JH, FL Sonenstein, L Ku. Changes in adolescent males' use of and attitudes toward condoms, 1988–1991. Family Planning Perspectives 25:106–110, 117, 1993.

Program for Appropriate Technology in Health (PATH). Contraceptive research and development update. Outlook (Special Issue) 13(20), 1995.

PATH. Enhancing the private sector's role in contraceptive research and development. IN Contraceptive Research and Development 1984–1994: The Road from Mexico City to Cairo and Beyond. PFA Van Look and G Pérez-Palacios, eds. Delhi: Oxford University Press. 1994a.

PATH. Market-Related Issues Affecting the Participation of the Private Sector in Contraceptive Development: A Final Report to the Rockefeller Foundation, 30 November 1994. Seattle, WA: 1994b.

Public Health Service, Department of Health and Human Services. Healthy People 2000: National Health Promotion and Disease Prevention Objectives. Washington, DC: U. S. Government Printing Office. 1991.

Ravindran TKS, M Berer. Contraceptive safety and effectiveness: Re-evaluating women's needs and professional criteria. Reproductive Health Matters 3:6–11, 1994.

Reprogen. Confidential Business Plan. Irvine, CA 1995.

Rinzler CA. The return of the condom. America's Health 6(6):97–107, 1987.

Rosenberg MJ, MS Waugh, S Long. Unintended pregnancies and use, misuse, and discontinuation of oral contraceptives. Journal of Reproductive Medicine 40(5):355–360, 1995.

Russell C. The pill is popular but not well understood: New survey shows many women overestimate the risks, underestimate the benefits. Washington Post, Health section, pg. 9, 6 February 1996.

Schrater AF. Immunization to regulate fertility: Biological and cultural frameworks. Social Science and Medicine 41(5):657–671, 1995.

Schrater AF. The pros and cons: Guarded optimism. Reproductive Health Matters 4, November 1994.

Snow R. Each to her own: Investigating women's response to contraception. IN Power and Decision: The Social Control of Reproduction. G Sen, R Snow, eds. Cambridge, MA: Harvard School of Public Health. 1994.

Stewart FH. Integrating essential public health services and managed care: Family planning and reproductive health as a case study. Western Journal of Medicine 163(Suppl.):75–77, 1995.

Tanfer K. Unpublished data on Norplant knowledge, use, and intentions, presented at National Institute of Child Health and Human Development conference on long-acting contraceptives, Bethesda, MD, September 1995.

Trussell J, L Grummer-Strawn. Contraceptive failure of the ovulation method of periodic abstinence. Family Planning Perspectives 22(2):65–75, 1990.

Trussell J, K Kost. Contraceptive failure in the United States: A critical review of the literature. Studies in Family Planning 18(5):237–283, 1987.

Trussell J, B Vaughan. Aggregate and lifetime contraceptive failure in the United States. Family Planning Perspectives 21(5):224–226, 1989.

Trussell J, J Koenig, C Ellertson, F Stewart. Emergency Contraception: A Cost-Effective Approach to Preventing Unintended Pregnancy. Unpublished manuscript. Princeton, NJ: Office of Population Research. November 1995.

Trussell J, JA Leveque, JDD Koenig, et al. Documenting the economic value of contraception: A comparison of 15 methods. Technical addendum to: The economic value of contraception: A comparison of 15 methods. American Journal of Public Health 85(4):494–503, 1995a.

Trussell J, JA Leveque, JDD Koenig, et al. The economic value of contraception: A comparison of 15 methods. American Journal of Public Health 85(4):494–503, 1995b.

United Nations Development Programme (UNDP), United Nations Population Fund (UNFPA), World Health Organization (WHO), and World Bank Special Programme of Research, Development and Research Training in Human Reproduction (HRP). Perspectives on Methods of Fertility Regulation: Setting a Research Agenda. Background Paper. Geneva: WHO/HRP. 1995.

UNFPA. Global Contraceptive Commodity Programme: Report of the Executive Director (DP/1996/3). Prepared for the First Regular Session of the UNDP and UNFPA Executive Board, 15–19 January 1996. New York: United Nations Population Fund. 1995.

UNFPA. Contraceptive Use and Commodity Costs in Developing Countries 1994–2005. Technical Report No. 18. New York: UNFPA. 1994.

Washington AE, RE Johnson, LL Sanders. *Chlamydia trachomatis* infections in the United States: What are they costing us? Journal of the American Medical Association 257(15):2070–2072, 1987.

Washington AE, PS Arno, MA Brooks. The economic cost of pelvic inflammatory disease. Journal of the American Medical Association 255:1732–1735, 1986.

Waugh MS. Report from European and U.S. surveys: OC compliance poorer among American women. Contraceptive Technology Update 15(12):157–172, 1994.

Westoff CL, F Marks, A Rosenfield. Physician factors limiting IUD use in the US. Paper presented at a conference on A New Look at IUDs—Advancing Contraceptive Choices, New York, 27–28 March 1992.

Wilcox LS, SY Chu, ED Eaker, et al. Risk factors for regret after tubal sterilization: 5 years of follow-up in a prospective study. Fertility and Sterility 55(5):927–933, 1991.

Wilcox LS, SY Chu, HB Peterson. Characteristics of women who considered or obtained tubal reanastomosis: Results from a prospective study of tubal sterilization. Obstetrics and Gynecology 75(4):661–665, 1990.

Winslow R. Medical upheaval: Welfare recipients are a hot commodity in managed care now. Wall Street Journal, 12 April 1995.

World Bank. World Development Report 1993: Investing in Health. New York: Oxford University Press. 1993.

World Health Organization (WHO). An Overview of Selected Curable Sexually Transmitted Diseases. (WHO/GPA/STD/95.1). Geneva: WHO/Global Programme on AIDS. 1995.

WHO. Perspectives on Methods of Fertility Regulations: Setting a Research Agenda (Background Paper). Geneva: UNDP/UNFPA/WHO/HRP. 1995.

Zabin LS. Addressing adolescent sexual behavior and childbearing: Self-esteem or social change. Women's Health Issues 4:93–97, 1994.

Zabin LS, HA Stark, MR Emerson. Reasons for delay in contraceptive clinic utilization: Adolescent clinic and nonclinic populations compared. Journal of Adolescent Health 12:225–232, 1991.

Zelnick M, JF Kantner. Sexual activity, contraceptive use and pregnancy among metropolitan-area teenagers: 1971–1979. Family Planning Perspectives 12:230–231, 233–237, 1980.

NOTES

1. For many reasons, all well beyond the purview of this study, the definition of "public health" has occupied the scholarly attention of many. For purposes of economy, we accept the following: "The application of scientific and medical knowledge to the protection and improvement of the health of the group" (F Brockington, cited in KL White, Healing the Schism: Medicine, Epidemiol-

ogy, and the Public's Health. New York: Springer-Verlag, 1991, p. 1). The ability to determine the number and spacing of births and the prevention of unwanted births is understood as central to the protection of the health of women, children, families, and communities.

2 . The contraceptive prevalence rate is defined in terms of the percentage of currently married (or in union) women aged 15–49 using a contraceptive method at the time of survey (WHO/HRP 1995).

3. Emergency contraceptive pills (ECPs) are high-dose oral contraceptives known for approximately 20 years to be effective in preventing pregnancy if taken within 72 hours after unprotected sex. Nausea and vomiting are common side effects and contraindications for oral contraceptives (OCs), such as history of stroke or heart attack, also apply to ECP users, though clinicians may make exceptions for some women for one-time use. Although OCs have not been approved by the Food and Drug Administration (FDA) for emergency contraception, doctors and other health providers who can write prescriptions may use any drug licensed by the FDA for unlabeled purposes.

4. Two data sets were used for this analysis. One included Ecuador, Egypt, Indonesia, Morocco, Thailand, and Tunisia; the other included Northeast Brazil, Colombia, Dominican Republic, Paraguay, and Peru. While the two sets of information are not exactly comparable, they provide useful insights with a reasonable degree of confidence (WHO/HRP 1995).

5. Diaphragm, jelly, douche, and foam tablets.

6. With the caveat that statements like the following are fraught with peril, this subset in the analytic sample—Northeast Brazil, Colombia, the Dominican Republic, and Peru—is quite representative geographically and, in a number of ways, culturally.

7. The figure is based on calculations of direct costs (medical services for abortions, pregnancy, and delivery) and indirect costs (work time that may be lost, costs resulting from complications of pregnancy) (Rosenberg et al. 1995).

8. The two are the CuT 380A (ParaGard), approved for 10 years of use, and the progesterone T (Progestasert System), approved for 1 year of use. The levonorgestrel-IUD (LNg IUD), developed by Leiras Oy in Finland, is not yet approved for use in the United States but may receive approval soon.

9. The acquisition in the summer of 1995 by Ortho of Gynopharma and its IUD and spermicide lines could be a noteworthy contributor to restoring the method to a greater share of the market.

10. The questions asked in the 1982 and 1988 National Survey of Family Growth permitted responses that indicated the following: Respondent had had all the children she wanted, or wanted none; her husband wanted no more; a pregnancy would have been dangerous to her health; she could not carry the pregnancy to term; she could not afford or take care of more children; or she did not like her previous method of birth control (Mosher and Pratt 1990).

11. "Safety" is defined by the Human Reproduction Programme of the World Health Organization as "fewer side-effects" (WHO/HRP 1995). The term also comprises the more general concept of "health concerns."

12. Strictly speaking, contraceptive effectiveness or efficacy is the proportionate reduction in the monthly probability of conception. In its loose everyday sense, the question of whether method X is effective is simply equivalent to: "Will it work?" (Hatcher et al. 1994).

13. There is, for example, a total dearth of knowledge about what male preferences for new contraceptives might be, simply because such questions have so rarely been asked. The authors of a recent study of spermicide acceptability in Zambia observe that, to their knowledge, theirs is the first prospective study of this sort to include male participants (Hira et al. 1995).

14. "Immunologic contraception" is the term that is increasingly being used to refer to immunologic applications whose purpose is to regulate fertility. They are directed against the immunologically accessible molecules involved in reproduction, either molecules on the surface of mature gametes (sperm and ova), or the hormones involved in the reproductive process, some of which play a role in the maturation of gametes, others regulating their release.

15. For example, a woman would be unable to determine whether or not her antibody levels were

providing a contraceptive effect without some sort of home diagnostic capability, for instance, a urine dipstick test.

16. MWRA, or "married women of reproductive age."

17. New population estimates suggest that, as of 1994, this figure is 25 percent.

18. The EPI vaccines target seven diseases: diphtheria, pertussis, tetanus, tuberculosis, polio, measles, and hepatitis B.

19. External funding sources for UNFPA procurement have included the World Bank, Germany, Canada, Finland, the Asian Development Bank, the United Nations Development Programme (UNDP), the United Kingdom's Overseas Development Agency (ODA), and the Government of Sri Lanka (UNFPA 1995).

20. UNFPA is not the only agency that procures contraceptives: In 1994, the United States Agency for International Development procured $46 million worth of contraceptives (down from $59 million in 1991); the International Planned Parenthood Federation procured a little over $6 million in contraceptives for its own affiliates and, during 1995, for some agencies and governments; and the World Health Organization spends $2.5 million of its $69 million budget for pharmaceuticals and medical supplies and equipment on contraceptives (UNFPA 1995).

21. The data sources for these calculations were as follows: Incidence rates from the Centers for Disease Control and Prevention, payment data from the literature and claims data, treatment protocols defined in Hatcher et al. (1994), and the private payer database and the 1993 edition of the Red Book to cost out each treatment. Cost per case was defined as the cost of treating each disease for as long as a person has it.

6

The Translators: Sectoral Roles in Contraceptive Research and Development

THE ROLE OF INDUSTRY IN CONTRACEPTIVE
RESEARCH AND DEVELOPMENT

The Pharmaceutical Industry

*Stage I: The First Contraceptive Revolution and the Primacy of Industry
(1951–1972)*

Since the 1950s, the involvement of the pharmaceutical industry in contraceptive research and development has passed through three stages, and it is now in a fourth stage whose future pace and direction are unpredictable. The character of that involvement has shifted in each phase in response to factors in the external environment that are peculiar to the field of contraceptive research and development and, perhaps, to the entire area of women's health. Although this chapter emphasizes the history and contemporary dynamics of the U.S. pharmaceutical industry, it incorporates information about firms outside the United States that are involved in some aspect of contraceptive research and development and raises issues deriving from the ongoing processes of industrial globalization.

Stage I, "the contraceptive revolution," can be said to have begun in 1951 more or less officially, when Carl Djerassi at Syntex filed a patent for norethindrone; it ended in the early 1970s. During this period, most contraceptive research and development was sponsored and carried out by large pharmaceutical companies, especially U.S. firms. The field was "pushed" by advances in steroid chemistry and the emergence of an array of complex plastics, neither of which had had human contraceptive uses as their original objectives. The developers of these first-phase contraceptives were well aware of cultural sensitivities about contraception and the consequent possibilities of corporate risk, but the perceived technological potential and market demand were overriding. A number of firms became engaged in the development and production of the new oral contraceptives (OCs). In the United States, those were Syntex, Searle, Upjohn, Wyeth, Merck Sharpe and Dohme, and the Syntex-Ortho partnership. Other U.S. firms were engaged in the development and production of the first modern intrauterine devices (IUDs): Ortho, Schmidt, American Caduceus Industries, Searle, and A.H. Robins. In Europe, the first firms to be involved in contraceptive research and development were Schering AG, Ciba, and Organon; British Drug House entered with two OC compounds in the early 1960s, and firms in Canada, Switzerland, and France with improved intrauterine devices in the early 1970s. Upjohn and Schering AG also presented the injectable contraceptives, Depo-Provera and Noristerat, for regulatory approval in this time period.

All this unfolded in a climate of general enthusiasm for the postwar "pharmaceutical revolution," and receptivity to effective, reversible, coitus-independent fertility regulation was rapid and enthusiastic. Regulatory requirements were fairly lenient, particularly for the IUD, and clinical studies were less sophisticated than they are today; thus, R&D time was shorter and effective patent life was longer. The taking of a daily pill over a goodly proportion of the reproductive life promised a large market, and the smaller size of the market for the long-acting IUD seemed not to be a problem (Gelijns and Pannenborg 1993). Only one firm abandoned the field during this time: Parke-Davis, whose management was worried about negative consumer reaction and conflict with company values.

Stage II: The Rise of the Public and Nonprofit Private Sectors and a Worldwide Orientation (1973–1987)

The second stage of contraceptive research and development began early in the 1970s, its onset marked by negative reports in the medical and lay press on OC side effects. Senate hearings in 1970 received some sensational press coverage and OC use declined noticeably. At roughly the same time, there were reports of side effects of the IUD, primarily the Dalkon Shield, and Robins took the device off the market in 1974.

The period also saw more stringent regulatory requirements, resulting in the extension of R&D time to between 10 and 17 years and, as a consequence, much greater R&D costs and reduction in effective patent life. The eruption of litigation against Robins spilled over onto other IUDs, as well as to oral contraceptives, and public perceptions of the pill and IUD became quite negative. Although oral contraceptives accounted for just under 4 percent of the prescription drug market as the 1980s began, there were more liability suits associated with that method each year of the new decade than for any other drug product (Djerassi

1989). As for the IUD, even though the copper-releasing and medicated devices were major improvements in safety, liability insurance had become essentially unavailable in the United States; even firms with FDA-approved IUDs left the market—and contraceptive research and development—altogether. Research indicating that IUD risks had been overestimated, together with improvements, motivated numbers of European and some developing-country women to return to the method. However, in the United States, only Alza's Progestasert was able to stay on the market and the IUD became virtually a nonoption for American women, never to regain its market share (Gelijns and Pannenborg 1993; NRC/IOM 1990). Contraceptive research and development became what it continues to be today: highly politicized, with consumer advocates and some women's groups arguing that developers and policy makers have been generically heedless of the needs and safety of women, and opponents of fertility control arguing against any contraceptive research and development whatsoever.

There was little mistaking the growing reluctance of U.S. industry to invest in contraceptive innovation; the barriers were everywhere. As something of a substitution effect, growing interest in family planning in developing countries drew the U.S. Agency for International Development (USAID) into the field, accompanied by funding that motivated research activity in universities and non-profit organizations, especially those with strong international networks. The Center for Population Research at the National Institute of Child Health and Human Development (NICHD), motivated by U.S. domestic concerns, also became a major source of funding for contraceptive research during this stage. In 1972, the World Health Organization's Special Programme of Research, Development, and Research Training in Human Reproduction was established. Among the nonprofit entities that were either created or that became more active during this stage were the Population Council's Biomedical Research Center, Family Health International (FHI), and the Program for Appropriate Technology in Health (PATH). There were also over two dozen university-based research programs, some of which also took on roles as intermediary funders of research at other universities, for example the Institute for International Studies in Natural Family Planning (IISNFP) at Georgetown University, the Program for Applied Research in Fertility Regulation (PARFR) at Northwestern University and its successor, the Contraceptive Research and Development (CONRAD) program at Eastern Virginia Medical School.

Wyeth, Schering AG, and Organon, recognizing the long-term profit potential of developing-country markets, set up manufacturing facilities in over 20 developing countries, including Bangladesh, Egypt, India, and Indonesia (PATH 1994). Second-generation lower-dose and multiphasic oral contraceptives, mini-pills, and more selective progestins reduced side effects and revived the reputation of oral contraceptives; when the secondary health benefits of the method also began to be appreciated, the structure of demand shifted back in their favor. And, owing to the sophistication, greater safety, and lower relative cost of endoscopic techniques, sterilization became by 1982 the most commonly used method in the United States. In the 1988 National Survey of Family Growth (NSFG), male and female sterilization together exceeded OC use and, in the 1990 telephone resurvey, sterilization by itself was the most commonly used method (Peterson 1990), even though, as a one-time permanent method with a limited pricing range and much subsidy, it did not offer industry a growing and profitable market niche. However, the profits that ensued from the other therapeutic and diagnostic uses of endoscopy were considerable so that the technology itself, overall, proved quite lucrative (Gelijns and Pannenborg 1993).

Yet the net result of the dynamics of Stage II was that, by the end of the 1980s, women in the United States had one effective reversible method, the pill, and one effective permanent method, sterilization.

Stage III: The Exodus of U.S. Industry and the Entry of Smaller Firms (1987–Present)

Beginning in the late 1970s, all but two of the U.S. pharmaceutical companies that had engaged in contraceptive research and development over the previous two decades had, to all intents and purposes, ceased any significant involvement in that field: Syntex, Searle, Upjohn, Mead Johnson, Parke-Davis, Merck Sharp and Dohme, Eli Lilly, and Wyeth all withdrew, although some remained involved in production. Of the nine large U.S. pharmaceutical firms that had entered contraceptive research and development in Stage I, all but two—Ortho, a subsidiary of Johnson and Johnson, and Wyeth-Ayerst—had exited by the end of Stage III, although Syntex, Searle, Upjohn, and Parke-Davis continued to produce and distribute the products their firms had developed. By the end of the 1980s, innovation in contraceptive research and development in the pharmaceutical industry resided largely in Europe, in the hands of Organon, Schering AG, and Roussel-Uclaf, a Hoechst subsidiary (Gelijns and Pannenborg 1993).

Another significant Stage III phenomenon was the entry into contraceptive research, development, production, and distribution by smaller companies. In Europe, this category has included firms like Gedeon Richter (Hungary), Alphatron (The Netherlands), Bioself (Switzerland), Cilag AG (Germany), Leiras (Finland), and Theramex (France) (see Table 6-9). In the United States a new pattern evolved, one of collaborative effort among public and private organizations: funding agencies, basic research facilities, university-based scientists, clinical trials organizations, nonprofit organizations, and smaller pharmaceutical companies, some of which were outside the U.S. (see Bronnenkant 1994). These organizational arrangements were unlike the standard model in the two preceding decades, that is, the single, large, integrated pharmaceutical company with, at most, one industry or nonprofit partner. In those years, basic research had been as likely to come out of industry as it was to emerge from the academic research community. In contrast, the multisectoral arrangements of the 1980s were flexible, opportunistic, varied, and complex, and the industry component was just one of several and as likely to be a smaller firm as a larger one. Almost all of these collaborations were focused on modifications of and new delivery systems for existing or improved compounds, namely:

- VLI (purchased by Whitehall Laboratories), National Institute of Child Health and Human Development (NICHD): vaginal sponge (Today)[1]
- Medisorb (formerly Stolle Research and Development Corporation), Ortho, World Health Organization (WHO), Contraceptive Research and Development Program (CONRAD), Family Health International (FHI): injectable microspheres
- Finishing Enterprises, Population Council, World Health Organization, Rockefeller Foundation, Ford Foundation: Copper T intrauterine device
- Wyeth-Ayerst, Leiras, Population Council, FHI, Program in Appropriate Technology in Health (PATH), individual clinical researchers worldwide: Norplant implants
- Ortho, Salk Institute, Medisorb (Stolle): LHRH analogues
- Alphatron, Vastech Medical Products, Population Council: nonsurgical vasectomy devices
- Upjohn, Dow Corning, Population Council, Battelle Institute, London International, Roussel UK: hormone-releasing vaginal rings
- London International, National Institute of Child Health and Human Development, Family Health International: polyurethane male condom (e.g., Avanti)
- Tactyl Technologies/SmartPractice, Contraceptive Research and Development (CONRAD) program: nonlatex (Tactylon) male condom
- Wisconsin Pharmacal, CONRAD, FHI, Reddy Health Care: female condom (Reality)
- YAMA, CONRAD, FHI: Lea's Shield.

Stage IV: The 1990s and the Biopharmaceutical Industry

The global pharmaceutical industry of the 1990s is composed of a great array of corporations devoted to the discovery, development, and commercialization of new pharmaceuticals. Over the years since the introduction of oral contraceptives, the industry has evolved and changed in response to a number of factors that are highly relevant to further advances in contraceptive research and development. Those factors include increases in the regulation of pharmaceuticals; a changing economic environment that has driven industry restructuring and stressed a global view of pharmaceutical markets; and—importantly—dramatic growth in the scientific tools and understanding of biology available to assist in the development of new pharmaceuticals. This understanding and these tools have spawned a whole new subset of the industry that is called the biotechnology sector and, in fact, suggest that the industry can be thought of as the "biopharmaceutical industry." The emergence of the biotechnology sector, together with what some analysts have referred to as a "structural revolution," are producing an ever-wider range of companies that differ greatly in size and organization; in the variety of their product development focus; and in the extent to which they either address the entire drug development process from basic research through to the marketing and sale of approved products or, instead, focus on one or more individual steps within that process.

The Demography of the Biopharmaceutical Industry

Numerous parameters can be used to define the companies that comprise the biopharmaceutical industry. One common metric is market capitalization, or the value that the market places on a company. Market capitalization is defined as the number of shares outstanding multiplied by the price per share. Clearly, since market capitalization varies with price per share, this metric is most easily determined for public companies whose shares trade on public securities exchanges. Figure 6-1 shows the market capitalization distribution of 232 pharmaceutical/biotechnology companies that are traded on U.S. exchanges. These companies range in market value from over $5 billion (e.g., Merck, Glaxo-Wellcome) to under $25 million (many small, public biotechnology companies). Absent from this chart is information on over 1,200 private small biopharmaceutical companies in the United States and Europe which tend to have market capitalizations of less than $100 million and most of which do not yet have any product revenues.

Figure 6-2 shows the annual net sales distributions of 244 pharmaceutical/biotechnology companies that trade on U.S. public exchanges. The bulk of revenues produced by these companies is generated by a minority of large corporations. To emphasize this point, the accounting firm of Ernst and Young has calculated the "Merck/Biotech Index," an assessment of the entire developing biotechnology industry as compared with Merck's ethical pharmaceutical business. According to the latest Ernst and Young survey in 1995, Merck had reported $15 billion in revenues, compared to $12.7 billion in revenues for the entire biotechnology industry for the 12-month period ending June 1995. During the same period, while Merck invested $1.2 billion in research and development and had a workforce of 47,500, the biotech industry invested $7.7 billion in research and development and had a work force of 108,000. In other words, R&D investment, while intense throughout the biopharmaceutical industry, is most heavily concentrated in the emerging company subsector. Industry estimates are that, despite the large investment of public funds in disease-specific areas, 92 percent of all drugs approved between 1981 and 1990 trace their origin to private-sector R&D programs. The growing importance of the R&D effort within young entrepreneurial companies is emphasized by statistics that show that even in R&D-intensive large companies such as Merck, 50 percent of all

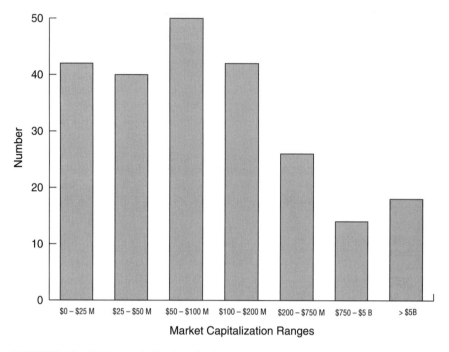

FIGURE 6-1   Market capitalization distributions of public pharmaceutical/biotechnology companies.   B = billion; M = million.   SOURCE: Disclosure Annual Industrial Database, 1995.

products presently in clinical trials were licensed from small companies and, to a lesser extent, universities.

Contemporary Industry Dynamics

There is little disagreement that the years since the late 1980s have brought profound transformations in the marketplace for human health products. The prospect of health reform accelerated a reorganization of the health care marketplace that was, in some respects, already under way. The precipitating factor was the relentless run-up in health care expenditures in the United States and the sense of urgency about the need to contain costs and shift from fee-for-service arrangements to managed care systems. The competitiveness and profitability of such systems depend on their cost-effectiveness. As a result, fixed-fee and capitation schedules, protocols, and guidelines have been implemented or recommended. In the same vein, there is growing interest in formularies and a consequent burgeoning of pharmacy benefit management organizations (PBMs) as

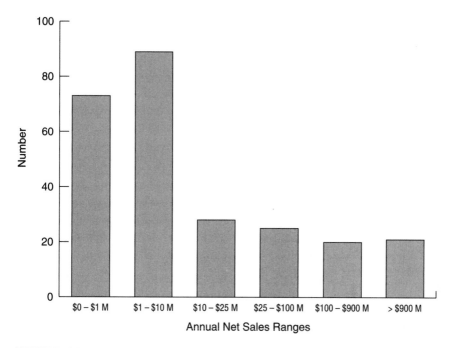

FIGURE 6-2   Annual net sales distributions of public pharmaceutical/biotechnology companies. M = million. SOURCE: Disclosure Annual Industrial Database, 1995.

ways to control the costs of pharmaceuticals. Health care purchasers in the 1980s, who were primarily physicians, tended to be generally cost-insensitive. Pharmaceutical profitability in the 1980s had exceeded all other industry sectors and drug companies had been able to grow almost entirely owing to price increases. It is now clear from different challenges to industry pricing that this strategy is no longer viable (Easton 1993; Pollard 1993).

The pharmaceutical industry has been adapting to these realities by essentially reconfiguring itself. Some firms are moving toward domination of a small number of specialty areas, some toward vertical expansion throughout the health value chain. Some are increasing their size in the belief that greater critical mass will drive success, others are aiming at being total disease-management companies in which drugs are just a part of total health care solutions.

The specter of shrinking profit margins has also motivated companies to view market share—that is, the percentage of sales within a particular market segment—as the most important determinant of near- and long-term success. The sense is that market share leaders will be the most cost-efficient players, whose cost-efficiency will yield them savings for reinvestment in research or for the sourcing of higher-value products (Easton 1993). Companies are attempting to retain market share for the drugs now coming off patent by converting them into over-the-counter (OTC) drugs; by building relationships with pharmacy benefit management organizations; by limiting price increases; or by responding to competition from generic drugs, either by building their own generic businesses, licensing out generic conversions of their drugs, or acquiring generic companies outright.

Some industry analysts argue that there will be an inevitable decline in the number of new drugs, for two reasons. One is that the science is more complicated; the other is that providers will increasingly depend on drug formularies to control costs. Furthermore, there is evidence that patients may have a much more powerful voice in determining managed care buying practices. Selection, addition, and substitution of formulary products will be based on product price and the amount of therapeutic or "user value" added, so that product improvements that are merely incremental are likely to be far less important than in the past. Yet, while "me too" and "incremental" products will be less attractive in the future, the opportunity for cost-effective "breakthrough" products for unmet medical needs remains. As a consequence, pharmaceutical companies will not just need to be more cost-efficient inventors, developers, and marketers to make more products pay off for shareholders; they will also have to be disciplined in focusing their research investment on a smaller, more select group of therapeutic categories. Speed to market, always important, will become more so. Established, experienced pharmaceutical companies will have an advantage because they have the best scientific understanding of what is needed in the field and the greatest resources to buy the innovative research required to develop the truly novel drugs that can break into formularies. Thus, despite pressure to cut prices and reduce profit margins, innovation and heavy R&D investment will continue to fuel the industry, with high rewards for novelty and being early to market with products that lower the cost of health care (Burrill and Lee 1993; Pollard 1993). For the large pharmaceutical companies ("big pharma") and for biotechnology firms, "pharmacoeconomics," or the linking of quality-of-life and outcome measures with efficacy data in the design and conduct of clinical trials, will be essential; it will be crucial in the development of products for "difficult audiences."

The need of the large pharmaceutical industry to purchase technology in some form is highly significant for the biotech industry and there is a sense that the redefinition of the pharmaceutical industry offers biotechnology a much wider set of opportunities to prove its value. As noted above, because biotechnology firms essentially invest all of their assets in research and development, they are far from losing their identity as the incubators of much of the progress in human health care (Lee and Burrill 1995). Table 6-1 depicts different dimensions of the way the pharmaceutical industry is being reshaped, its likely future directions, and the way innovative products might be expected to fit into that picture.

The Biotechnology Industry

Industry Structure

Most analysts trace the emergence of the "biotech industry" to the late 1970s/ early 1980s, with the foundation of a series of companies (Cetus, Genentech, Amgen, Biogen) that were started to exploit the commercial potential of recombinant DNA (rDNA) and monoclonal antibody (MAb) techniques. The former involves transferring genetic information from one organism to another, splicing and "gluing" it onto a vector molecule, and replicating or cloning it for a variety of purposes. MAb technology takes advantage of antigens on the surfaces of invading agents to trigger immune-system recognition and response in the form of antibodies, proteins that attach themselves only to the foreign antigen and nothing else, signaling subsequent processes that then destroy the invader. It is the specificity of MAbs, as well as the fact that they can be enlisted as transport mechanisms, that makes them so valuable in the development of diagnostics, therapies, and vaccines.

The techniques, once seen as arcane, have become commonplace. Yet the tradition of novel technology deployed to define and address problems in human health care, agriculture, and animal health remains the hallmark of biotech companies. Thus, new technology stories are often the hallmark of new companies, so that gene therapy, xenotransplantation, genomics, and the like have been fostered first in biotech companies and then been transferred to "big pharma" via partnership, acquisition, or adoption.

From its birth, the biotechnology industry has confronted a set of factors or "hurdles" whose confluence is seen as unique: massive breakthroughs in science and technology (but quite upstream in the R&D process); enormous capital needs with a long horizon to payback; financial markets and investor expectations that turn alternatively hot and cold; a regulatory hand that is seen as heavy; uncertainty about intellectual property rights; and a cost crisis in its primary market, which is health care (Burrill and Lee 1993). Financial analysts are unable to describe public biotech companies to their investment clients using standard financial parameters because the majority of these companies are essentially R&D operations without products, revenues, and earnings. The financial community has therefore adopted a categorization of companies that describes where they are in the product development and company development process. A jargon has emerged that divides companies into first-tier, second-tier, and third-tier. The first-tier companies have products and product revenues and can be judged using standard financial criteria (e.g., Chiron, Amgen, Genzyme). Second-tier companies have products that are new or close to the market and have established the business infrastructure needed to be a self-supporting entity (e.g., Cephalon, Matrix Pharmaceuticals). The third tier has the biggest population and generally consists of companies that went public in the last three years, with

TABLE 6-1 Trends, Worldwide Pharmaceutical Industry, 1970s and Beyond

Early 1970s–Mid-1980s	Mid-1980s–Mid-1990s	Mid-1990s and Beyond
Consolidation	**Further Consolidation**	
Many small companies	Fewer, larger corporations	Few, large corporations
		Small boutiques
Domestic focus	Global focus	Global reach
Technology driven	Technology dependent	Technology dependent
	Sales/service/distribution driven	Sales/service/distribution driven
	Competitive pricing	Competitive pricing
	Lower profitability	Potential to increase profits
	Increased government regulation	Increased government regulation
		Managed care

Managed Care and the Pharmaceutical Industry

Past	Future
Approvable products (safety/efficacy)	Marketable products (pharmacoeconomic outcomes)
Cost-based pricing	Positioning on value
Mega sales force	Multiple distribution techniques
Customer service	Customer alliances
	• Disease management
	• Outcomes studies
	• Education
	• Customized phase III and IV clinical trials
Science/sales driven	Customer/market driven

Evolution of Successful Products

Innovative products	Innovative products	Innovative products supported by global sales, service, and market infrastructure
	Competitive products supported by strong infrastructure	
Competitive niche products	Competitive niche products	Competitive niche products

SOURCES: Burrill GS, KB Lee Jr. Biotech 94: Long-Term Value, Short-Term Hurdles (The Industry Annual Report). San Francisco, CA: Ernst and Young US, 1993. Noonan KD. Trends in the *in vitro* diagnostics industry in the late 1990s. Clinica, Special Supplement, April 1994(1).

products still in preclinical animal testing or Phase I human clinical trials, with profits not expected till the end of the decade. Responses by several hundred industry CEOs to annual surveys by Ernst and Young continue to indicate that the largest, most mature, "top-tier" companies are mainly concerned about the complex regulatory environment, with some cyclical concerns about availability of capital. Mid-tier and small (lower-tier) companies worry most about inaccessibility and cost of capital. Unpredictability in the patent environment is significant for all biotechs, as it is for the large companies. The synergy between all these factors over the years has made the biotechnology subsector persistently volatile and its financing platform has generally been rocky.

Industry Strategies

As a result, the industry response has had to be one of very great ingenuity and flexibility, qualities that have been expressed in a plethora of strategic adaptations whose main objective was to somehow access costly resources to complete product development. A few firms tried to become fully integrated pharmaceutical companies, others to become vertically integrated firms in a niche area. A large number of firms sought to establish enough value to justify placing an initial public offering as a way of accessing capital; others worked to develop a blockbuster product as a route to acquisition by a larger company; and still others emphasized products that would require partnering with large companies in order to reach the market.

Virtual Integration Gradually, however, these strategies have been supplanted by other approaches that reflect adjustments to the realities of the changing marketplace, funding difficulties, and developmental disappointments. By 1994, the Ernst and Young annual industry analysis noted a paradigm shift to "virtual integration" and a proliferation of very pragmatic, selective, flexible relationships between biotechs and between biotechs and pharmaceutical companies (see Figure 6-3). These have included, but were hardly limited to, product swaps; development or acquisition of generic product lines; licensing in technologies, particularly late-stage technologies; partial acquisition of units or products; various combinations of different resources; and all manner of strategic partnerships (Lee and Burrill 1995).

Outsourcing Companies are also outsourcing, with high cost-effectiveness, to organizations that provide very narrowly defined services. A prime example is the "contract research organization" (CRO), an entity of possible practical interest in thinking about new strategies for revitalizing contraceptive research and development. CROs are basically third parties that provide research services on a contractual basis, focusing primarily on designing, conducting, and analyzing human clinical trials. Many CROs can also provide preclinical animal testing at

FUNCTION	OWN RESOURCES	POTENTIAL PARTNERS
Postmarketing sales support	Statisticians, record keeping	Specialty firms
Distribution	Warehousing, shipping Distribution	Drug wholesalers Generic companies Direct to buyers (e.g., HMOs, government, insurance companies)
Sales	Detailing	Customers Big pharmaceutical companies
Marketing	International and domestic coverage	• By market/indication • By geography Speciality marketers
Manufacturing	Manufacturing plant	Contract manufacturers Specialty-focused biotech intermediaries Big pharmaceutical companies' excess capacity
Clinical/regulatory development	Clinical expertise	Clinical research organizations Big pharmaceutical companies Other biotech companies Specialty consultants/ contractors
Development research	R&D spending	Academia R&D institutions Big pharmaceutical companies Government Other biotech companies

FIGURE 6-3 Virtual integration. SOURCE: Burrill GS, KB Lee Jr. Biotech 94: Long-Term Value, Short-Term Hurdles (The Industry Annual Report). San Francisco, CA: Ernest and Young US. 1993.

the front end of the development cycle and regulatory consulting services at the back end. While CROs have existed for more than two decades, a confluence of factors seems to be driving a resurgence. These factors include pricing pressure from organized buyers; a relative paucity of investment capital; staff cutbacks; lack of expertise in most biotechs in clinical development and in regulatory affairs; perceived increases in regulatory burdens; and buyers' demands for cost-efficiency data which add a whole new layer of complexity to clinical development strategies. (Examples of such companies are Quintiles Transnational, IBAH, and Clintrials.) The role of CROs is becoming more prominent as a feature in company strategies, particularly for those that can respond to the demands of drug companies for global capabilities so that products can be tested and filed simultaneously for approval worldwide. At one extreme, Abbott Pharmaceuticals contracts 80 percent of all its clinical development to CROs, other companies as little as 10–20 percent; industry trends are thought to be moving toward 50 percent. The volumes in dollar terms are not small: As of 1994, pharmaceutical and biotechnology companies were spending in aggregate roughly $26 billion annually. Of this amount, about two-thirds, or $17 billion, was spent on the kinds of services that CROs provide (Kreger 1994).

Alliances It is not surprising, then, that there has been steady growth in strategic alliances involving the biotech industry from the start of 1993 to mid-1995 (see Table 6-2). If the mid-1995 transaction rate is sustained, over the past three years there will have been close to 500 strategic alliances involving biotech companies, over 300 of those with large pharmaceutical companies and 150 with other biotechs. The number of mergers and biotech acquisitions is considerably less, a total of 123 projected for the same period (see Table 6-3). Table 6-3 shows the numbers of strategic alliances along with the numbers of financings, mergers and acquisitions, and downsizings as ways in which industry accesses capital, makes clear the relative importance of such alliances in overall industry strategy.

What may be surprising is that the biotech industry is not shrinking overall (see Table 6-4), despite the prevalent view among industry analysts who feel that there are too many biotechs and that some rationalization and compression will be necessary. The total number of companies, including those that have gone public, grew steadily over the same three-year period (1993–1995) and the industry's work force grew as well, even though an estimated 68 firms were seen as downsizing by the end of 1995 (see Table 6-4).

Globalization Another effect of the changes in the larger environment for "big pharma" and the biotech industry is that the industry has become increasingly

TABLE 6-2 Strategic Alliances in the Biopharmaceutical Industry, 1993 to Mid-1995

| | Number of Transactions | | |
	1993	1994	Year to Date 6/30/95
Large pharmaceutical company alliances with biotech company	69	117	73
Biotech-and-biotech alliances	43	52	26
Total	112	169	99

SOURCE: Vector Fund Management. BioWorld Financial Watch. Deerfield, IL 1995.

TABLE 6-3 How Biotechs Access Capital

	Number of Transactions		
	1993	1994	Year to Date, 6/30/95
Financings	190	174	105
Mergers and acquisitions	21	48	27
Downsizing	6	26	18
Strategic alliances	112	169	99

SOURCE: Data provided by Vector Fund Management, Deerfield, IL 1995.

global. Products are being developed with the intent that they will be made available to patients in many different countries. Consequently, many companies have operations in those countries; those that do not must develop extensive contractual relationships to allow their products to reach global markets. The implications of a global biopharmaceutical marketplace are profound. From the conception of a clinical program through development and launch, decisions must be made with an eye to entering markets governed by divergent rules. The globalization of business, coupled with the need to be more cost-efficient, is behind the movement to "harmonize" criteria for drug development and approval and has led to the creation of new companies that can expeditiously facilitate new drug development across borders; international CROs are an excellent example of this adaptation.

Furthermore, the biotech industry is growing in Europe, which as of 1994 had 386 biotech companies (Lee and Burrill 1995). In consequence, many European pharmaceutical and biotech companies are creating alliances with U.S. firms, providing capital as well as manufacturing and marketing support; and regulatory filings for foreign investment have increased dramatically. In addition, Europe's often less stringent regulatory requirements offer the opportunity for U.S. companies to initiate clinical trials more quickly and possibly gain market access sooner; other operational and tax advantages also add to the general offshore allure. Finally, the biotech industry has globalized to include countries in Latin America, Eastern Europe, China, India, and the Pacific Rim, which recognize the promise of biotechnology, offer new markets, and serve as sources of innovation. Corporate partnerships and sale or licensing of product rights are the strategies favored for penetrating the European and Japanese markets, with strategic partnerships also receiving significant emphasis in the United States. Going it alone in either terrain is difficult: International expansion inevitably requires additional infu-

TABLE 6-4 Biotechnology Industry Highlights ($ billions), 1992–1995

	Public Companies (Merck Index)[a]			Biotech Industry Total		
	This Year	Last Year	% Change	This Year	Last Year	% Change
1995						
Sales/revenues	$15	$10.5	47	$12.7	11.3	12
R&D expense	$1.2	$1.2	0	$7.7	$7.1	6.4
Net income (loss)	$3.0	$2.2	26	$(4.6)	($4.2)	10
Market capitalization	$73.0	$3.7	97	$52.0	$41.0	0.7
Employees	47,500	47,100	1	108,000	103,000	2.3
1994						
Sales	$5.2	$4.3	20	$7.7	$7.0	10
Revenues	$7.1	$6.0	17	$11.2	$10.0	12
R&D expense	$3.8	$3.0	27	$7.0	$5.7	23
Net loss	$2.1	$1.5	40	$4.1	$3.6	14
Market capitalization	$36.0	$39.0	(8)	$41.0	$45.0	(9)
No. of companies	265	235	13	1,311	1,272	3
Employees	53,000	48,000	10	103,000	97,000	6
1993						
Sales	$4.4	$3.3	35	$7.0	$6.0	17
Revenues	$6.1	$4.4	38	$10.0	$8.3	20
R&D expense	$2.9	$2.4	24	$5.7	$5.0	14
Net loss	$1.4	$1.4	0	$3.6	$3.4	6
Stockholders' equity	$10.5	$8.1	30	$15.9	$48.0	(6)
No. of companies	235	225	4	1,272	1,231	3
Employees	48,000	37,000	30	97,000	79,000	23
1992						
Sales	$3.4	$2.6	31	$5.9	$4.4	3.5
Revenues	$4.5	$4.5	29	$8.1	$6.3	28
R&D expense	$2.3	$1.5	54	$4.9	$3.4	42
Net loss	$1.4	$0.9	60	$3.4	$2.6	32
Stockholders' equity	$8.2	$4.5	83	$13.6	$10.7	27
No. of companies	225	194	16	1,231	1,107	115
Employees	37,000	33,000	12	79,000	70,000	13

[a]The MERCK Biotech Index is a measure devised by Ernst and Young, which assesses the entire developing biotech industry as compared with Merck's ethical pharmaceutical business.

SOURCES: Ernst and Young Biotech Industry Annual Reports: Biotech 93, 94, 95, 96.

sions of money, talent, and local know-how concerning regulatory approvals, product pricing and reimbursement, and marketing.

The theory has been advanced that an increasingly global market might be helpful in alleviating some of the constraints to contraceptive research and development that prevail in the United States, in terms of offering options for collaborative relationships (Rockefeller Foundation 1995a). Prominent among the arguments are that the regulatory environment might be less stringent elsewhere, that the pressures of liability would be less severe, that the political and ideologic environment might be less complex, and that clinical trials would be less costly. These are reasonable arguments to advance but each of them requires a complex and thoughtful examination, beyond what this study committee found feasible within its own constraints of time and resources. Another major—and persistent—constraint is the very real limitation of access to information, most importantly about prospective industrial relationships, information that is almost always well guarded. A brief retrospective glance at some partnership experiences, such as the efforts of some small U.S. firms to partner with European firms, Roussel-Uclaf's experience with RU 486, and the some of the experience with offshore production, have been too complex and the determining variables too diverse to permit easy, categorical conclusions. As just one example, the mutual perceptions of the United States and the European countries of the stringency of each other's regulatory processes appear to be quite discordant and efforts at harmonization move slowly.

The Risk-Benefit Assessment: Decisions by Private Firms to Invest

The General Process

The theme of financing has pervaded the present discussion because it lies at the heart of the complicated web of interdependence that is being woven among biotechnology and large pharmaceutical companies, in the United States and overseas. And, at the heart of the financing issue is the fact that the process of developing new pharmaceutical products is complex, long, and costly (see Figure 6-4). Estimates of the time and costs involved in developing new therapeutic ethical pharmaceutical products and taking them to market vary widely. A major source of variance is the product category itself; new chemical entities (NCEs) typically take more time and cost more money (OTA 1993). A 1989 industry survey estimated that 83 percent of total U.S. R&D dollars in that year were spent in the earliest stage of the process, that is, in advancing scientific knowledge and developing new products, as opposed to improving and/or modifying existing products though distinctions between these two categories of endeavor can be fuzzy (OTA 1993). This period of conceptual work and initial synthesis is also inherently risky; it may be that, out of every 10,000 new chemicals synthesized in the laboratory, FDA approval may be sought for only 1 (NRC/IOM 1990). And,

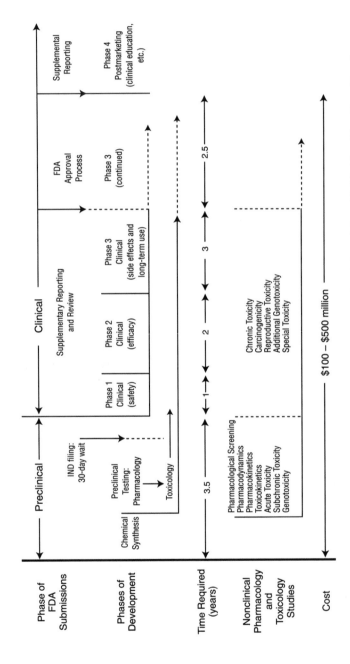

FIGURE 6-4 New drug development process, United States. SOURCE: Adapted from M. Mathieu, New Drug Development: A Regulatory Overview (3rd ed.). Waltham, MA: Parexel International Corporation, 1994, p. 17.

of 20 entities submitted to FDA for approval, only two may be approved and just one may actually be introduced as a new product (Harper 1983; NRC/IOM 1990; OTA 1993).

In 1993, the Office of Technology Assessment (OTA) reanalyzed earlier seminal studies of the costs of pharmaceutical R&D and calculated an average cost of developing a new drug at "no more than" $237 million (OTA 1993), with development time from identification of an NCE to market taking from 10 to 12 years. According to the Pharmaceutical Research and Manufacturers Association (PhRMA), the range can be from $100 million to $500 million and take a minimum of five to ten years from the time a decision is made to take a product into clinical development to the time it appears on the market. While this wide range in cost estimates may be related to product-specific needs, such as duration and number of patients in a series of clinical trials, they may also have to do with amortization of a large company's overhead vis-à-vis that of a "lean and mean" entrepreneurial biotechnology company. Still, it is simplistic to assume that product development will always be less expensive in biotech companies.

The Specific Case of Contraceptive Research and Development

One of the most important influences on the development of new contraceptives is the outcome of decisions by U.S. and European producers of pharmaceuticals and medical devices. Although governments and nonprofit organizations have made significant contributions to the funding of basic research and to the development of many contraceptive technologies, most of the currently available products were commercialized by U.S. and Western European firms.

A promising "reservoir" of basic biomedical research may be necessary, but it is by no means sufficient, to result in the introduction of new contraceptive technologies. Since basic scientific advances may have a number of possible pharmaceutical or medical device applications, choices about developing one or another of those will depend on assessment of a range of technologic, regulatory, and market factors. In addition, bringing a new contraceptive product to market takes years because of the long development cycle, numerous clinical trials, and complex regulatory approvals that are needed. Thus, today's dearth of new contraceptive products reflects decisions by pharmaceutical firms not to pursue research or development of new contraceptive products that were made 10–20 years ago.

It is tempting to seek single-factor explanations for what has or has not happened in the field of contraceptive research and development. The committee has struggled to do that and been confounded by the idiosyncracies of each "decision experience," since those respond to producer/product/provider/consumer characteristics, varying among themselves and according to time and circumstance. At the most fundamental level, these decisions are not controlled by any single factor but are the outcome of a comparison of the costs and returns (adjusted for risk, which is unusually significant in this product area) from investment in contraceptives, relative to alternative development programs and projects. In other words, a decline in development activities in contraceptives could have nothing to do with the economic or political conditions surrounding contraceptives but instead reflect significantly improved opportunities in some other product area. In fact, the situation with respect to contraceptives appears to reflect the operation of both forces—opportunities in other areas have improved, even as the risk-adjusted returns associated with new contraceptive products may have declined.

The decisions of firms, especially those previously active in contraceptive development, not to pursue development of new products, or to exit this product area altogether, also can negatively affect the stock of expertise needed to develop new products. Firms in the pharmaceuticals industry also typically specialize to some extent in specific types of products or therapies, which reflects the fact that they have accumulated considerable scientific, technical, and market-related knowledge that is specific to these areas and may not be relevant elsewhere. This type of knowledge often is not easily transferred between firms and cannot be purchased or otherwise acquired by a new firm without a long period of investment and learning. Because a number of firms formerly active in contraceptive technologies have exited this product area, much of this expertise has been lost and would-be entrants into the contraceptives field (e.g., biotechnology firms) cannot easily acquire it from incumbent firms or from other sources. Reversing the effects of firm exit on this stock of "know-how" thus may take considerable time.

The factors that must be considered when industry assesses a new biopharmaceutical program are:

- market
- management/human resources
- technology assessment
- competition
- regulatory requirements
- intellectual property position
- economics
  — cost to develop (time, money, people)
  — competitive position at launch
  — projected profitability
  — opportunity cost vis-à-vis other programs
- strategic reasons
  — synergy with other efforts
- other factors
  — e.g., political risk.

Simplifying the problem considerably, and abstracting from the issue of know-how, an individual firm's decision to pursue development of a new contraceptive technology (which may yield a family of products) is governed primarily by the expected returns to the large investment needed to commercialize this technology, i.e., the profits, relative to the costs of development (one way in which know-how enters this decision is in the confidence and reliability of a firm's judgments about costs and returns). There seems to be little evidence suggesting that the costs of developing a new contraceptive product *per se* are significantly higher than those involved in developing other pharmaceutical or medical products intended to be used for chronic administration: All of these products require lengthy development programs and large investments in clinical trials and regulatory approvals.

The differences between contraceptives and other pharmaceutical products appear to be more prominent, however, in the area of expected returns and the adjustments imposed by decision makers to adjust these returns for the risks associated with contraceptive products. Market success, especially for contraceptives, requires that a new product offer significant advantages in terms of factors like safety and convenience, as well as being reasonably competitive on price with existing products. Because existing contraceptive products (e.g., IUDs or oral contraceptives) are relatively inexpensive, they impose a "ceiling" on the feasible price in mass markets for new alternatives, and therefore depress projected returns from contraceptives relative to other pharmaceuticals or medical devices, whose delivery is more frequently covered by third-party reimbursement.

A rational decision maker will also adjust expected returns for risk, and this adjustment is likely to prove disadvantageous to contraceptives relative to other products. Riskier products demand a higher expected return in order to justify the investment in their development, and contraceptives appear to exhibit relatively high risks from two sources. The first is liability litigation, which is an unusually serious threat in contraceptives, just as it has been in vaccines (this factor is a serious risk mainly in the United States, but litigation risk appears to be increasing in several Western European markets as well). Like vaccines, contraceptives typically are administered to a huge market of individuals with normal health histories. As a result, the possibilities of side effects or unusual reactions, which may affect a very small fraction of the population, will yield a steady stream of claims. Moreover, many of these claims will be filed by healthy, often relatively young individuals and therefore may result in high damage awards. Thus, litigation risk in contraceptives appears to be unusually high relative to other pharmaceutical products.

The committee had entertained the idea of doing some comparative analysis of the costs of litigation for contraceptives compared to vaccines as a somewhat analogous category of products. However, considerable efforts to obtain hard data proved fruitless, since information about such costs is tightly held. The only information of this sort that appears in the public domain concerns the amounts of awards from cases that do go to court, a small tip of a large iceberg. Of the 2,063 suits filed against Searle over the past 20 years in connection with its intrauterine device, just 24 went to trial; approximately 800 were settled out of court for undisclosed amounts (Steyer 1995). It has been customary to think of litigation as a U.S. issue; however, 346 of the complaints against Searle were "foreign," primarily in Australia and the United Kingdom.

One must add to the financial risks associated with litigation the financial and other risks associated with the strong political opposition to many forms of contraceptive technology in the United States. These risks mean that the projected "hurdle rate" of return that a firm will require to undertake a contraceptive development project will be higher than the hurdle rate associated with other projects. When one combines this requirement for a higher hurdle rate of return with the low prices of the alternatives currently available, contraceptive development projects are likely to appear less attractive than alternative applications. Obviously, for firms with considerable expertise in this product field, this gap between the hurdle rate for contraceptives and other products will be lower, and this gap will be affected by many other influences as well. Nevertheless, these factors appear to depress the projected returns for commercial contraceptive development projects relative to those in other areas in which scientific advances may offer equally enticing product development possibilities.

If, as many analysts suggest, the biotech sector is the pharmaceutical industry's "R&D department," then one surrogate of the perceived commercial attractiveness of new products in women's health might be the number of biotech firms that report to be working in this area. A 1995 survey by Goldman Sachs of the product programs in 158 public biotech companies found that out of over 450 products undergoing clinical testing, only 5 described as "for women's health" had reached that stage (Goldman Sachs 1995). Still, in 1994 PhRMA reported that, among the large number of new drugs in development, there were "143 biotechnology medicines [and] 301 medicines for women" in pharmaceutical company pipelines. In terms of numbers, medicines for women were second only to the "327 medicines for older Americans" and well ahead of the 103 medicines for AIDS and AIDS-related diseases (PhRMA 1994). There seems to be growing attention to the area of women's health in the pharmaceutical industry: Ortho, Parke-Davis, Searle, and Wyeth-Ayerst all have what are considered more or less formally as "women's health programs." At the same time, only Ortho and Wyeth-Ayerst include contraceptives as part of that picture.

In conclusion, decisions of private firms to reduce their development efforts in contraceptives reflect the operation of a range of factors. No single factor dominates all others in the large majority of individual cases, and no single factor is inevitably the cause across all cases. Contraceptives are competing for scarce technical talent and funds with alternative product development programs, and the commercial attractiveness of other product development projects may shift for any one of a great variety of reasons. Moreover, because of the size and the duration of the private-firm investments necessary to bring a new contraceptive technology to market, one might see a decline in commercial development activity in the face of continued public support for the basic science underpinning contraceptive technologies. But when declines in public research support are combined with factors tending to depress the relative return on investment from contraceptive development projects, development activities are likely to be curtailed even more severely.

Current Industry Involvement in Contraceptive Research and Development

As of 1993, there were 57 manufacturers or "vendors" of contraceptive and fertility products in the United States (see Table 6-5).[2] Of those, 23 were manufacturers or vendors of contraceptive products. The committee identified over twice that number in the worldwide market (see Table 6-6).

One might expect contraceptives and fertility products to be areas of industrial interest with some affinity. In fact, there is surprisingly little crossover; firms active in both areas are usually subsidiaries or divisions of multinational pharmaceutical companies which have enough power and financial resources to develop products in several markets. Just five firms work in both product lines: Organon, Ortho, Syntex, Whitehall, and Wyeth-Ayerst. Ortho is a Johnson and Johnson subsidiary, Wyeth-Ayerst and Whitehall are part of American Home Products Corporation, and Organon is a subsidiary of Akzo NV. Only one, Ortho, which markets oral contraceptives, diaphragms, and spermicidal preparations is present in more than two product lines (Frost and Sullivan 1993). With its acquisition in summer of 1995 of GynoPharma, which dominated the U.S. market for IUDs and also had a line of spermicides, Ortho further increased its number of product lines and now has more product lines than any company worldwide.

The industrial profiles of the two product areas—contraception and fertility—are quite different. The fertility industry is less dominated by giants than is the contraceptives industry and is scattered among numerous, smaller competitors that tend to focus fairly narrowly, sometimes developing great expertise in a niche market and thereby becoming the dominant firm in that segment. The fertility products subgroup of the market is even more finely grained, counting many smaller participants, for example, those that develop and/or produce immunoassays and nonisotopic hormone tests and are attempting entry (Frost and Sullivan 1993).

The overall industrial picture in contraceptives is far more concentrated; in fact, it is described by at least one prominent industry analyst (Frost and Sullivan 1993) as pretty much an oligopoly, dominated by a few large and strong competitors who account for anywhere from 60 to 90 percent of total manufacturer revenues in this area. Table 6-7 shows revenues by product type and company

TABLE 6-5   Firms Manufacturing and/or Distributing Contraceptives, United States, 1993

Firm	OC[a]	Condom	Diaphragm	IUD	Spermicide	Implant[b]
Aladan		X				
Alza				X		
Ansell		X				
Berlex	X					
Carter-Wallace		X				
Finishing Enterprises				X		
GynoPharma[c]	X		X	X		
Mead Johnson	X					
Milex			X		X	
National Sanitary		X			X	
Okamoto		X				
Organon	X					
Ortho	X		X		X	
Parke-Davis	X					
Rugby Labs	X					
Schering Plough					X	
Schiaparelli-Searle	X					
Schmid		X			X	
Searle	X					
Syntex	X					
Thompson Medical				X		
Warner-Chilcott	X					
Whitehall					X	
Wyeth-Ayerst	X					X

[a]Oral contraceptives.
[b]Norplant.
[c]GynoPharma was sold in the summer of 1995 to Ortho Pharmaceuticals.

SOURCE: Frost and Sullivan. U.S. Contraceptives and Fertility Product Markets. New York, 1993.

TABLE 6-6 Firms Manufacturing and/or Distributing Contraceptives Worldwide, 1993 and 1994

Company	Product Manufactured or Distributed
Aladan	Condoms
Alza	IUDs (Progestasert)
Ansell	Condoms (including one with nonoxynol-9)
Berlex	Oral contraceptives (Tri-Levlen, Levlen)
Boehringer Ingelheim	Oral contraceptives
Bristol-Myers Squibb	Oral contraceptives
Carter-Wallace	Condoms (including one spermicidally lubricated)
CCC (Canada)*	IUDs
Cervical Cap Ltd.	Cervical cap (Prentif/manufactured by Lamberts/Dalston England)
Chartex (United Kingdom)	Female condom (Femidom)
Cilag (UK)*	Oral contraceptives
Dongkuk Trading (Korea)*	Condoms
Finishing Enterprises*	IUD
Gedeon Richter (Hungary)	Emergency postcoital contraceptive (Postinor)
Gruenenthal	Oral contraceptives
GynoPharma[a]	IUD (CuT380A [Paragard]) (distributor) Oral contraceptive (Norcept) Diaphragms (distributor for Schmid)
Hyosung (Korea)*	Condoms
Jenapharm (Germany)	Oral contraceptives
Kinsho Mataichi (Japan)*	Spermicides
Leiras Oy Pharmaceuticals (Finland)*	Progestin-releasing IUD (Mirena) Norplant (manufacture)
Lexis	Oral contraceptives (NEE)

TABLE 6-6 Continued

Company	Product Manufactured or Distributed
London Rubber	Condoms Diaphragms
Magnafarma	Oral contraceptives
Mayer	Condoms
Mead Johnson	Oral contraceptives (Ovcon)
Medimpex* (Hungary and USA)	Oral contraceptives/raw materials
Menarini	Oral contraceptives
Milex Products, Inc.	Diaphragms (Omniflex, Wide-seal) Jellies and creams (Shur Seal Jel has nonoxynol-9)
National Sanitary	Condoms
Okamoto, USA	Condoms
Organon (Akzo) (Netherlands)*	Oral contraceptives (Marvelon, Desogen, Jenest) IUD (Multiload) (manufacturing subsididary, Bangladesh)
Ortho Pharmaceutical* (Johnson & Johnson)	Oral contraceptives (Loestrin; Ortho-Cept, Ortho-Cyclen, Ortho Tri-Cyclen, Ortho-Novum, Modicon) Diaphragms (Allflex, Ortho Diaphragm) Spermicides* (Gynol) IUDs
Parke-Davis (Warner-Lambert)	Oral contraceptives
Polifarma	Oral contraceptives
Reddy Health Care	Condoms
RFSU of Sweden	Condoms
Roberts	Oral contraceptives
Rugby Labs	Oral contraceptives (Genora)
Safetex	Condoms

TABLE 6-6 Continued

Company	Product Manufactured or Distributed
Schering AG (Germany)*	Oral contraceptives* Injectables*
Schering Plough (USA)	Spermicides
Schmid	Condoms (including spermicidal condoms) Spermicides Diaphragms (distributed by GynoPharma)
Searle (Monsanto)	Oral contraceptives (Demulen)
Seohung (Korea)*	Condoms
Syntex	Oral contraceptives (Tri-Norinyl, Devcon, Norinyl, Brevicon)
Thompson Medical	Spermicides
Upjohn* (Upjohn Belgium)*	Injectable (Depo-Provera/DMPA)
Warner-Chilcott	Oral contraceptives (Nelova)
Whitehall	Sponge (Today)[b] Spermicides
Wisconsin Pharmacal	Female condom (Reality)
Wyeth-Ayerst (American Home Products)	Oral contraceptives (Lo-Ovral, Nordette, Triphasil) (joint venture, Egypt, production) Norplant (marketing, distribution)
Wyeth-Pharma (Germany)*	Oral contraceptives
Wyeth (France)*	Oral contraceptives

NOTE: An asterisk indicates that the firm supplies to UNFPA procurement. Where the firm is listed with more than one product line and is a UNFPA source, the product supplied is also marked with an asterisk.

[a]GynoPharma was sold to Ortho Pharmaceuticals in summer of 1995.
[b]Whitehall decided to discontinue the Today sponge because of the costs of bringing the plant up to U.S. Food and Drug Administration specifications.

SOURCES: Frost and Sullivan. U.S. Contraceptive and Fertility Product Markets. New York, 1993. United Nations Population Fund (UNFPA). 1993 Procurement Statistics. New York, 1993.

for 1990 and 1992. Of the 11 U.S. firms competing in the U.S. oral contraceptives market in 1992, Ortho and Wyeth-Ayerst controlled 70 percent of total revenues, followed by Berlex (a Schering subsidiary), Syntex, Parke-Davis, and Mead Johnson (a Bristol-Myers Squibb subsidiary), with roughly comparable shares running around 4 to 6 percent each. The remainder was shared among the five other competitors. There is no expectation that the concentration of this subsector of the industry will change, largely because of the extent of the investment needed to develop new oral contraceptives and labeling requirements that are perceived as benefiting larger companies. Ortho, Wyeth-Ayerst, Organon, and Berlex (Schering AG) are likely to continue their market dominance with the newer progestin-based formulations as well.

The rest of the industry is similarly oligopolistic. Even though there are over 100 different brands of condoms on the market (Hatcher et al. 1994), Carter-Wallace dominates with 60 percent of total revenues. There are just three competitors with diaphragm product lines and, again, Ortho got over half of 1992 revenues; Milex's share was around 40 percent. Ortho also gets half the revenues from the U.S. spermicidal preparations market, where there are six other competitors, one of which is Whitehall, like Ortho, part of American Home Products. Wyeth-Ayerst has the monopoly in the United States for the levonorgestrel contraceptive implant Norplant. Finally, the IUD line is very close to monopoly; until its sale to Ortho in summer 1995, GynoPharma was the market leader, with 94 percent of revenues. The IUD market is not likely to burgeon in terms of new entries since, as a very-long-term method that has been on the market for a long time, it generates a very modest margin of profit.

The international picture is also one of concentration. In the case of oral contraceptives, which account for the overwhelming bulk of all contraceptive revenues worldwide (over 80 percent in 1992), American Home Products and Johnson and Johnson still dominate but share the top of the worldwide OC market with the large European firms Schering AG and Organon, which increased their percentage share of sales between 1988 and 1992 (see Table 6-8). The four firms together accounted for 81 percent of all oral contraceptive sales worldwide in 1992, or $1.7 billion out of total worldwide sales of $2.1 billion. Four other large integrated firms—Searle (a Monsanto subsidiary), Syntex, Parke-Davis (a Warner-Lambert subsidiary), and Bristol-Myers Squibb—accounted for another $272 million, or 13 percent of sales. For all eight firms, oral contraceptive revenues were close to or well above the magic "$50 million-dollar market" figure; for seven other firms and miscellaneous "others," which shared the $133 million balance, that figure was much smaller and seems not to have constituted a major product line. There are, nevertheless, small firms which have evidenced commitment to engagement in new areas of contraceptive technology, notably Leiras of Finland, Gedeon Richter of Hungary, and Silesia of Brazil.

As noted at the outset of this chapter, the number of large pharmaceutical firms remaining in the research and development component of the contracep-

TABLE 6-7 Contraceptive Revenues (in millions of dollars), United States, 1990 and 1992, by Product Type and Company

Product	1990	1992
Oral Contraceptives		
Ortho	376.0	385.4
Wyeth-Ayerst	306.7	343.7
Syntex	69.3	62.5
Berlex	59.4	62.5
GD Searle	49.5	52.1
Parke-Davis	49.5	62.5
Mead Johnson	49.5	41.7
Others	29.7	31.2
Subtotal	989.6	1,041.6
Condoms		
Carter Wallace	70.0	81.7
Schmid	34.4	36.0
Ansell	14.7	16.6
Others	3.7	4.2
Subtotal	122.8	138.5
Spermicides		
Ortho	21.1	26.3
Whitehall	9.9	8.6
Schmidt	7.2	7.7
Others	6.7	5.3
Subtotal	44.9	47.9
Norplant	0.0	40.1
IUDs		
GynoPharma[a]	15.5	21.2
Alza	4.6	2.1
Subtotal	20.1	23.3
Diaphragms		
Ortho	2.1	2.0
Milex	1.2	1.7
GynoPharma[a]	0.2	0.2
Subtotal	3.5	3.9
Total (All product types)	1,180.9	1,295.3

[a]GynoPharma and its IUD and diaphragm lines were sold in summer 1995 to Ortho Pharmaceuticals.

SOURCE: Frost and Sullivan. U.S. Contraceptive and Fertility Product Markets. New York, 1993.

TABLE 6-8   Worldwide Oral Contraceptive Market, Sales 1988 and 1992 (in millions of U.S. dollars), by Company

	1988		1992	
Company	Sales	% Total	Sales	% Total
Wyeth (American Home Products)	452	30.2	610	29.2
Ortho (Johnson & Johnson)	392	26.2	458	21.9
Schering AG	244	16.3	372	17.8
Organon (Akzo)	129	8.6	245	11.7
Searle (Monsanto)	70	4.7	86	4.1
Syntex	90	6.0	71	3.4
Parke-Davis (Warner-Lambert)	42	2.8	69	3.3
Bristol-Myers Squibb	30	2.0	46	2.2
Boehringer Ingelheim	9	0.6	19	0.9
Menarini	3	0.2	13	0.6
Polifarma	0	0.0	13	0.6
Gruenenthal	6	0.4	13	0.6
Rugby Labs	4	0.3	10	0.5
Magnafarma BV	0	0.0	8	0.4
Upjohn	3	0.2	6	0.3
Others	22	1.5	52	2.5
TOTAL	1,496	98.5	2,090	97.5

SOURCE: Syntex data (I.M.S. data provided by Vector Fund Management, Deerfield, IL, 1995).

tives industry is very small: Ortho in the United States and Organon and Schering in Europe are the primary participants. Wyeth-Ayerst is engaged principally in R&D activities limited to modifications of implant technologies, and Merck, which has not been involved in contraceptives for decades, is sponsoring some research in immunologic contraception under a limited agreement with the University of Connecticut Medical Center.

The current picture of industry participation in contraceptive research and development is largely a continuance of the pattern of collaborative effort established in Stage III. These are typically with the public sector (primarily NIH/ NICHD [National Institute of Child Health and Development] and WHO/HRP [the World Health Organization's Human Reproduction Programme]); with a nonprofit entity which receives substantial infusions of public funds, for instance, the CONRAD program and Family Health International (FHI); or with a university partner. Partnerships between large and small firms are very few; at least, given information that is in the public domain, the big pharmaceutical firms remaining in contraceptive R&D appear to have no more than one or two such relationships (see Table 6-9). Furthermore, most of the products that are the

TABLE 6-9   Recent Industrial Involvement in Contraceptive Research and Development[a]

For-profit Companies	Product	Not-for-profit Partner(s)	Other For-profit Partner(s)
Advances in Health Technology	mifepristone		
Allendale Labs	Nonoxynol-9 film with benzalkonium chloride film	CONRAD	
Alphatron (previously Ovabloc Europe) (Netherlands)	Vas occlusion with silicone plug	WHO/HRP AVSC	
AM Resource	Bactericidal gel	NIH: NICHD	
Apex Medical Technologies	Nonlatex condoms	NIH: NICHD	London International Group
Apothecus	Vaginal film	WHO/HRP NIH: NIAID FHI	
Aphton	hCG immunocontraceptive	WHO/HRP	
Applied Medical Research, Ltd.	Estrogen-free minipill (B-Oval) containing melatonin and norethindrone (a progesterone)	Dutch government	
Baxter	Nonlatex condoms		
Bioself Distribution (Switzerland)	Basal body temperature thermometer		
Biosyn	Vaginal microbicides (spermicide C31G: protection from conception, STDs)	NIH: NICHD CONRAD University of Pennsylvania	
Biotech Australia	Work with inhibin as component of hormonal contraception for both men and women		

continued on the next page

TABLE 6-9　Continued

For-profit Companies	Product	Not-for-profit Partner(s)	Other For-profit Partner(s)
Biotechnology General (formerly Gynex)	Contraceptives, sublingual formulations		
Biotek	Long-acting spermicide suppository; new nonoxynol-9 formulations	NIH: NICHD Population Council CONRAD	
BKB Pharmaceuticals	Emergency contraceptive (CDB 2914)	NIH: NICHD RTI	
Cabot Medical	Silicone rubber ring (Fallope)		
Cilag AG (Germany)	Combined oral contraceptives		
Columbia Labs	Sustained release formulations of spermicides, natural progesterone	NIH: NICHD NIH: NIAID WHO	
Conceptus	Non-surgical fallopian tube sterilization	AVSC	
Curatek	Vaginal gel (bactericidal)		
Cygnus Therapeutics	Contraceptive patch 7-day contraceptive	FHI	Johnson & Johnson
Endocon	Biodegradable implant (Annuelle/NET)	CONRAD FHI	Wyeth-Ayerst
Female Health Company (formerly Wisconsin Pharmacal)	Female condom (Reality)	CONRAD FHI	
Femcap Inc.	Cervical cap	CONRAD FHI	
Gynetics	Combined oral contraceptives		
Integra	Spermicide with polymer barrier	CONRAD	

TABLE 6-9   Continued

For-profit Companies	Product	Not-for-profit Partner(s)	Other For-profit Partner(s)
Jenapharm (Germany)	Antiprogestins other than mifepristone	RTI	
Leiras Pharmaceuticals (Finland)	Progestin-releasing IUD (Levonova); levonorgestrel-IUD (Mirena); implants (Norplant)	WHO/HRP Population Council	
Lidak	n-Docosanol		
London International Group (UK)	Nonlatex condoms	NIH: NICHD	
Magainin	Spermicide/microbicide	NIH: NICHD (have CRADA)	
Medisorb (formerly Stolle Research)	New injectable formulations using biodegradables, microspheres	CONRAD FHI	Ortho
Merck	Immunocontraception	NIH: NICHD University of Connecticut Medical Center (3-yr. agreement with principal investigator)	
Novovax	Novel delivery systems	NIH: NICHD	
Organon (Akzo) (Netherlands)	Antiprogestins other than mifepristone, very potent and selective (Org 317-10, Org 33628); fixed-shape IUDs (CUSafe 300, Mark II, MLCu-375, Ombrelle-250); vaginal rings; combined oral contraceptives; zona pellucida (ZP) vaccine; 1-rod implant	University of Edinburgh Reproductive Biology Unit (licensing arrangement)	
Ortho (Johnson & Johnson)	Male method (steroid hormones); spermicides; combined oral contraceptives		Medisorb (see above)

continued on the next page

TABLE 6-9 Continued

For-profit Companies	Product	Not-for-profit Partner(s)	Other For-profit Partner(s)
Reprogen	Definition of molecular mechanisms in fertility/mucosal immune function of urogenital tract; vaccines against STDs/conception; endometriosis		Oxford Bioscience Partners
ReProtect	Buffer gel, monoclonal antibodies	NIH: NICHD, NIAID, FHI	Ultrafem
Roussel Labs (UK)	Levonorgestrel-releasing vaginal ring (Femring) (licensing agreement for Phase II clinical trials, manufacture, distribution)	NIH: NICHD, NIAID, WHO/HRP	
Schering AG (Germany)	Antiprogestins other than mifepristone; injectable (Mesigyna); male method, steroid hormones; contraceptive (ZP) vaccine; combined oral contraceptive	WHO/HRP Government of Indonesia	
Silesia (Chile)	Progesterone vaginal rings	CONRAD Population Council ICMER	
Tactyl Technologies	Nonlatex (Tactylon) condoms	NIH: NICHD CONRAD	
Theramex (France)	Minipill (NOMAC, Lutenyl), primarily for breast-feeding women; Uniplant	South-to-South	
Ultrafem	Virucide (BufferGel); feminine cups (GelCup, TherapyCup)		ReProtect
Upjohn	Injectable (Cyclofem)	WHO/HRP PATH (Concept Foundation)	

TABLE 6-9   Continued

For-profit Companies	Product	Not-for-profit Partner(s)	Other For-profit Partner(s)
VasTech Medical Products	No-scalpel male sterilization technique	Population Council	
Whitehall (American Home Products)	Spermicides		
Wyeth-Ayerst (American Home Products)	Biodegradable implant (Capronor-ll)	NIH: NICHD RTI FHI	
Yama	Lea's Shield	NIH: NICHD CONRAD FHI	
Zonagen	Zona pellucida (ZP-based) contraceptive vaccines	Baylor College of Medicine (rights to ZP proteins) CONRAD	Schering AG ($2.5 million for 7% company share) Triad Ventures Petrus Fund Woodlands Venture Reproductive Biotechnologies/Bangalore, India (collaborative agreements)

NOTES: AVSC = Association for Voluntary Sterilization; CONRAD = Contraceptive Research and Development Program; ICMER = Instituto Chileno para Medicina Reproductiva; NIH/NICHD = National Institute of Child Health and Human Development; FHI = Family Health International; RTI = Research Triangle Institute; PI = Principal Investigator; WHO/HRP = World Health Organization's Human Reproduction Programme; CRADA = Cooperative Research and Development Agreements; SBIR = Small Business Innovation Research (grants).

a This table is intended to illustrate the range of entities recently involved in the contraceptive development field and the range of activities in which they are engaged. Information was obtained from published materials and telephone conversations or written exchanges with staff in the entities listed. Some companies and/or contraceptive development projects may have been omitted inadvertently or have been omitted because the information was unavailable. This table is illustrative and is not meant to be an endorsement of any group or product by the National Academy of Sciences.

*b*Jenapharm was purchased by Schering AG in the summer of 1996.

focus of these partnerships have to do with new delivery systems or improvement of methods to enhance protectiveness against sexually transmitted infections. There is relatively little activity in radically new areas of research endeavor and truly pioneering work seems to be relatively unsupported through partnerships. Two European firms, Organon and Schering, have made considerable advances in the area of antiprogestins but have decided not to proceed, given the political dimensions of the release of RU-486, developed by Roussel-Uclaf. As for other frontier areas, Merck's involvement in immunocontraception is, for the present at least, limited. Of particular interest is the picture of some small start-up firms, for example, Applied Medical Research, Aphton, ContraVac, and Reprogen, all of which are struggling to find partnerships and support for entry with new technologies that are at varying stages of research and development.

Current Industry Involvement in Women's Reproductive Health

It may be illuminating to compare this picture with a recent picture of what is going on in the biopharmaceutical industry in connection with the larger field of women's reproductive health, excluding contraceptives, and anti-infectives for sexually transmitted diseases (see Table 6-10 and Table 6-11). In the area of women's reproductive health, emphasis is heavily on hormonal formulations, largely in connection with menopausal symptoms; work in anti-infectives consists of some work in vaccines, the balance in antiviral drugs. What is interesting about this picture is the nature of the partnerships through which a given research problem is being tackled and the ways in which these seem to differ from patterns in contraceptive research and development. The profile of relationships in both women's reproductive health and anti-infectives is one of partnerships between large pharmaceutical companies and small biotechnology companies and between biotechs. In the case of anti-infectives, the presence of venture capital seems more prominent, perhaps because larger firms that enter into partnership with small biotechs characteristically can muster up their own funds for such purposes. The committee was not able to identify any current investment in contraceptive research and development from the venture capital community.

This accords with what this committee was able to discern through its dialogues with pharmaceutical and venture capital firms in the course of the study period: That is, that the amount of partnering that is going on at present involves the large pharmaceutical industry in a relatively small way, displays no partnering between biotechnology or smaller pharmaceutical firms, and seems to enjoy very little presence of venture capital. That said, the committee readily admits that much of what goes on in the pharmaceutical industry in very new areas of research and development is—understandably—handled as highly privileged information.

ROLES OF THE PUBLIC AND NONPROFIT SECTORS IN CONTRACEPTIVE RESEARCH AND DEVELOPMENT

The public and nonprofit sectors have always played a role in contraceptive research and development, historically with their participation growing as industry has withdrawn. Table 6-12 describes the activities and functions of each of the principal participants. In general, their role can be summarized as comprising agenda-setting, motivating, and funding, the latter in research, development, production, and distribution, as well as in product evaluation and training support for investigators.

Funding for contraceptive research and development comes either from the public sector (i.e., governments or parastatal institutions established for the purpose of providing external development assistance) or from private sources (not-for-profit entities such as philanthropic organizations, individual philanthropists, nongovernmental organizations/NGOs, and the for-profit pharmaceutical industry).

Data on contraceptive R&D funding are difficult to gather and complex to analyze. The entities that provide or channel such funding all maintain their accounts differently and categorize expenditures in idiosyncratic ways, primarily because their program mandates or the larger mandates of their parent organizations require it. Furthermore, as institutional priorities shift for whatever reason, portfolio emphases shift accordingly and changes in allocations from one year to the next may be large. Nomenclature makes a difference, too: The accounting for "family planning" will not be the same as the accounting for "reproductive health," and "contraceptive research and development" will be subsumed under each of these rubrics in distinctive fashion. Also, the frontiers between basic research and everything else are sometimes hard to define; categorization of research in particular areas or further along the trajectory of development of individual methods may also be defined variously (Atkinson et al. 1985; NRC/IOM 1990).

This elusive funding picture is further complicated by variability in the ways funds circulate. A 1993 study of the structure of international research in reproductive health by the Rockefeller Foundation noted three levels in that structure: (1) the funding of research, (2) the conduct of research, and (3) provision of technical support, all of which overlap. Beyond those entities that are the primary sources of funding, there are intermediary entities that serve to channel funds from those primary sources to the actors in research all over the world and may be themselves engaged in the conduct of research. Both intermediaries and primary funders may also provide technical support to one another, which further muddles analysis. In general, however, funds generally move from government funding agencies and private foundations to university research centers, nonprofit research organizations, and small research firms (NRC/IOM 1990).

Private industry constitutes a special case, conducting some of its own in-

TABLE 6-10 U.S. Biopharmaceutical Industry Activities and Relationships in Research and Development in Women's Reproductive Health, Excluding Contraception

Company	Product	Indication	Partner
American Home Products	Estradiol 7-day	Menopausal symptoms	
Ares-Serono Group	Follicular stimulating hormone, recombinant (Gonal-F)	Infertility	
Atrix Laboratories	Luteinizing hormone releasing hormone, Atrigel delivery	Prostate cancer and endometriosis	Roche/Syntex
Cell Genesys	Follicle-stimulating hormone (FSH) produced by gene activation	Infertility	Akzo Nobel
ContraVac Diagnostics	Antibody test to quantitate/ characterize human sperm to measure male fertility; immunocontraception	Infertility (male)	Binax
Cygnus Therapeutics	Estrogen/progestin 7-day	Menopausal symptoms	American Home Products
Cygnus Therapeutics	Estrogen/progestin 3.5-day	Menopausal symptoms	American Home Products
Cygnus Therapeutics	Ethinyl estradiol 7-day	Menopausal symptoms	Warner-Lambert
Cygnus Therapeutics	Estradiol 7-day	Menopausal symptoms	Warner-Lambert, Sanofi

Company	Product	Indication	Partner
Cygnus Therapeutics	Estradiol 7-day	Menopausal symptoms	Johnson & Johnson
Ligand	Tissue-selective estrogen or progesterone agonists	Gynecological disease, cardiovascular disease	American Home Products
Ligand	Progesterone agonists replacement therapy	Breast cancer, hormone	American Home Products (option)
Noven Pharmaceuticals	Estrogen and progestogen, transdermal	Menopausal symptoms and osteoporosis	Rhône-Poulenc Rorer
Noven Pharmaceuticals	Estrogen (2nd generation transdermal)	Menopausal symptoms and osteoporosis	Ciba-Geigy, Rhône-Poulenc Rorer
Noven Pharmaceuticals	Progestogen transdermal	Menopausal symptoms and osteoporosis	Rhône-Poulenc Rorer
Pharmos	Estradiol-CDS	Post-menopausal	
TheraTech	Estradiol, transdermal	Menopausal symptoms	
TheraTech	Estradiol/progestin, transdermal	Menopausal symptoms	
TheraTech	Female hormone replacement therapy, transdermal	Oopherectomized women	Solvey

SOURCE: Goldman Sachs. U.S. Research: Biotechnology Products (2nd edition). New York, June 1995.

TABLE 6-11 Pharmaceutical Firms Currently Involved in Research and Development Relevant to Women's Reproductive Health, Excluding Contraception: Anti-infectives against Sexually Transmitted Diseases

Company	Indication/Product	Partner
3M Pharmaceuticals	Genital warts, antiviral (imiquimod)	n.d.
Aviron	Herpes vaccine	Venture-backed: Accel Advent Agingworth IVP
Biocine	Genital herpes vaccine (given postinfection as immunotherapy)	Joint venture: Chiron Ciba-Geigy
Biogen	Hepatitis B and C, antiviral (beta interferon)	n.d.
Burroughs Wellcome	Genital herpes, antiviral (Valtrex [valacyclovir])	n.d.
Glaxo	Hepatitis B, antiviral (lamivudine)	n.d.
Lidak	Genital herpes, labialis herpes, antiviral (Lidakol [n-docosanol])	n.d.
Hoffman-La Roche	Uncomplicated gonorrhea, antibiotic (Megalone [fleroxacin])	n.d.
Janssen Pharmaceutica	Candidiasis, antifungal (Sporanox [itra-conazole])	n.d.
North American Vaccine	Bacterial diseases	Affiliated with Biochem Pharma
Oclassen Pharmaceuticals	Genital warts, antiviral (Condylox Gel [podo-filox])	n.d.
Pfizer	Vaginal candidiasis, antifungal (Diflucan [(fluconazole])	n.d.

TABLE 6-11 Continued

Company	Indication/Product	Partner
Sandoz Pharmaceuticals	Candidiasis, antifungal (Lamisil [terbinafine])	n.d.
SmithKline Beecham	Herpes vaccine, hepatitis A/B combination vaccine	Acquired German flu vaccine producer in 1992
	Herpes infections, antiviral (pencyclovir, IV and topical)	n.d.
Virus Research Institute	Herpes therapies	Health Care Investments Harvard University
Warner-Lambert	PID, antibiotic (CI-990)	n.d.
Zeneca Pharmaceuticals	Gynecologic infections and PID, antibiotic (Merrem [meropenem]; intramuscular and intravenous])	n.d.

NOTE: n.d. = no data.

SOURCES: Pharmaceutical Research and Manufacturers of America. In Development: New Medicine for Infectious Diseases, 1994 Survey. Washington, DC. 1994. (Data current as of June 20, 1994.)

house research and funding external research at various points along the R&D pipeline (Rockefeller Foundation 1995b). An unknown (and apparently unknowable) amount of funding also flows from large pharmaceutical firms to universities and nonprofit research organizations and, what seems to be much less, to small R&D firms. Because industry must be attentive to the bottom line in ways that are somewhat different from the bottom-line concerns of nonprofit entities, its accounting for R&D expenditures is also distinctive. Most importantly in terms of getting a grasp on industry investment in contraceptive research and development, information about industry internal allocations is treated as proprietary and there are not the same pressures to disclose such information as those typically experienced by the public sector. In sum, there is a wide margin of error and ignorance in terms of tracking funding trends in contraceptive research and development and making comparisons within and between sectors.

TABLE 6-12 Participants Active in Contraceptive Research and Development, Public and Private Sectors, 1995[a]

U.S. Government Agencies

Contraceptive Development Branch and Contraceptive and Reproductive Evaluation Branch, Center for Population Research, National Institute of Child Health and Human Development, National Institutes of Health (CDB/CPR, CAREB/CPR, NICHD/NIH)	Established in 1968 as part of the National Institute of Child Health and Human Development of the U.S. National Institutes of Health, the Center for Population Research began its institutional life by supporting fundamental mission-oriented research; it expanded into CR&D in 1971. It does no research itself but manages research through contracts to universities, industry, and nonprofit institutions. The CPR is the world's principal funder of fundamental nondirected reproductive research and a major funder of research into the long-term safety and efficacy of marketed methods. The CDB currently supports research on male contraception (androgen replacement, peptide contraceptives, nonhormonal drugs, barrier methods) and female contraception (hormonal drugs, chemical barriers, immunocontraception). The CDB has established three Cooperative Contraceptive Centers, funded under congressional mandate, two of which focus on immune contraception, the other on vaginal methods. It also supports a biological testing facility, synthetic chemical and peptide facilities, and a primate testing facility, and has initiated a multicenter Clinical Trials Network to enable faster testing of promising products. It issues Requests for Proposals (RFPs) and for Applications (RFAs) and is developing its ability to enter more easily and quickly into Cooperative Research and Development Agreements (CRADAs) and Small Business Innovation Research (SBIR) grants. NICHD has also opened up a "Discretionary Funding Zone" as an alternative to RFAs that will channel support into High Priority Research Areas (HPRA), explicitly contemplated as a mechanism for accelerating contraceptive research and development.
U.S. Agency for International Development (USAID)	Of all U.S. agencies, only USAID and NICHD/NIH (q.v.) support contraceptive research and development, although the Department of Agriculture, the Department of Energy, and the National Science Foundation provide modest funding for reproductive biology. USAID conducts no research of its own but provides virtually all of FHI's and CONRAD's support through cooperative agreements. It is also the second largest bilateral funder of the WHO's Special Programme of Research, Development, and Research Training in Human Reproduction (WHO/HRP) and provides much of the funding for the Program for Appropriate Technology in Health (PATH) and for the work of the Population Council's International Center for Contraceptive Research (ICCR). USAID's major product accomplishments include development and/or evaluation of tubal bands and clips for female sterilization; evaluation and introduction of low-dose combined oral contraceptives and progestin-only pills; supporting the research that led to development of

the contraceptive vaginal sponge; evaluation and FDA approval of the Reality female condom; evaluation, introduction, and extension of lifetime effectiveness of the Copper-T-380A intrauterine device; evaluation and introduction of Norplant and Norplant II implants; and delineation and evaluation of the Lactational Amenorrhea Method (LAM) for child spacing. At present, USAID cooperating agencies (CAs) are involved with preclinical and clinical testing of two woman-controlled barrier methods, Lea's Shield and Femcap; testing of nonlatex male condoms; preclinical testing of compounds and formulations for spermicidal and virucidal activity; and clinical testing of vaginal contraceptive film preparations.

John E. Fogarty International Center National Institutes of Health

In October 1995, the Center announced the funding of initial awards under an International Training and Research in Population and Health Program jointly sponsored by Fogarty and NICHD. Seven awards have been made to U.S. universities to support programs for scientists and health professionals from developing countries concerned with population issues, including research and training in areas related to reproductive biology. These grants will be funded at a level of $1 million/year for 5 years.

U.S. Nonprofit Organizations

Nonspecialized Research Institutions

Research Triangle Institute (RTI)

Biodegradable polymers; delivery of contraceptive drugs, antiprogestins, male contraceptives, spermicides.

Salk Institute

Peptide antagonists of LHRH (GnRH) as ovulation inhibitors.

TABLE 6-12 Continued

Specialized Contraceptive Research Institutions

Contraceptive Research and Development (CONRAD) program, Eastern Virginia Medical School	Established in 1986 under a cooperative agreement with USAID, CONRAD's focus is on the improvement of existing contraceptives and development of new methods that are safe, effective, acceptable, and suitable for use in the United States and developing countries. CONRAD's mandate is to move contraceptive leads from the laboratory through phase I and II clinical trials. To this end, it supports timely and high-quality extramural subprojects conducted by collaborating investigators at universities, research institutes, and private companies worldwide. Current priority is assigned to methods that are controlled by the individual female user, are suitable for lactating women, are long-acting, interfere in the maturation/transportation/fertilization processes, and decrease transmission of HIV and other STDs, as well as to generic products for use by public-sector family planning programs at less cost than trade-name products. From January 1987 to November 1995, CONRAD managed approximately 175 extramural subprojects related to research, development, and testing of new contraceptive methods.
Family Health International (FHI)	FHI was founded in 1971 with funds from USAID, which continues its support. It has expanded its original mandate, which was to test and improve available contraceptive methods, to include development of new methods, the study of the impact of contraceptive use on the health of developing-country populations, and the strengthening of the research capacity of developing countries. As of 1995, around 15 percent of its overall budget was devoted to contraceptive development of new contraceptive methods, primarily in the clinical trials phase. Most recently, FHI conducted trials for the Reality female condom and Lea's Shield and has developed modified condoms for men.
Population Council	The Population Council's International Center for Contraceptive Research (ICCR) was established in 1971 to pursue scientific leads deemed ready for dosage formulation and clinical trials. It is the only R&D group that conducts extensive product formulation work in its own laboratories, under the aegis of its Center for Biomedical Research. Its present focus is on development and improvement of technology for unserved or underserved groups: methods under the user's control; methods for men, nursing and postmenopausal women, and teenagers; methods that do not alter women's menstrual cycles; compounds protective against STDs, including HIV; and methods of medical pregnancy termination. Under active investigation are contraceptive rings, levonorgestrel-releasing IUDs, improved implants and transdermal delivery systems for

women, microbicides, medical abortifacients, a two-implant system and immunocontraception for men, and "no-scalpel" vasectomy. The Council receives grants from foundations (Ford, Rockefeller, and Mellon), international organizations, and federal agencies (including NICHD and USAID), and also uses funds from its endowment to support some contraceptive research.

Program in Appropriate Technology in Health (PATH)	Founded in 1976, PATH's work in contraceptive R&D focuses on the production end of the R&D trajectory. The organization has worked with colleagues in 39 developing countries (including Bangladesh, Brazil, Egypt, India, Indonesia, Mexico, People's Republic of China, Philippines, Thailand, Turkey, Vietnam, and Zimbabwe) to conduct feasibility studies and provide technical assistance in technology transfer and good manufacturing practices in connection with the production of condoms, injectables, Copper-T IUDs, oral contraceptives, and spermicidal products. PATH also collaborated with the Population Council and other groups in introduction of the Copper-T-380A IUD and Norplant. Its support comes from a number of public- and private-sector sources, including USAID, foundations, UNFPA, World Bank, and WHO.
Program for the Topical Prevention of Conception and Disease (TOPCAD)	Established in October 1993, TOPCAD's mandate is to develop and evaluate new woman-controlled vaginal methods of preventing conception and/or STDs; foster international collaboration and training to test novel methods and train new investigators; and study consumer acceptance and use of vaginal topicals and the optimal delivery of newly developed methods. Funding comes from the Rockefeller Foundation, the CONRAD Program, and the Andrew W. Mellon Foundation; its headquarters are at Rush-Presbyterian-St. Luke's Medical Center, Chicago.
Consortium for Industrial Collaboration in Contraceptive Research (CICCR)	The CICCR was initiated in 1995 by the Rockefeller Foundation and the Andrew W. Mellon Foundation at the CONRAD Program, to foster research on new contraceptives, with emphasis on barrier methods, a range of monthly regimens for women, and methods for males. The CICCR will award grants for contraceptive R&D to not-for-profit research institutions working in collaboration with for-profit industrial partners, in the expectation that sharing cost and risk in the early stages of research will provide the momentum needed to drive the field.
Universities	Research and training in reproductive technology is ongoing at over two dozen U.S. universities.

TABLE 6-12 Continued

International Agencies

World Health Organization Special Programme of Research, Development, and Research Training in Human Reproduction (WHO/HRP)	Established by the WHO in 1971–1972, the "HRP" mobilizes and coordinates a worldwide effort to develop appropriate technologies and generate information in areas of reproductive health of high priority to developing countries. It works to strengthen human and material resources for research, to enable developing countries to address their own research needs and participate in global research efforts, and it supports collaborative research centers in 56 countries. Its present portfolio is organized around seven methods, including postovulatory, long-acting, and male methods, and immunocontraception. HRP is funded by voluntary contributions from member states in developed and developing regions and is cosponsored by the United Nations Development Programme (UNDP), United Nations Population Fund (UNFPA), and the World Bank. HRP's income for the 1994–1995 biennium came from a total of 23 funders worldwide, including 18 bilateral agencies, 3 multilateral organizations, and 2 foundations (Rockefeller and Ford). The United Kingdom is the largest contributor ($7.8 million for the 1994–1995 biennium), followed by the UNDP ($7.0 million), the United States ($5.5 million), the World Bank ($3.75 million), Norway ($2.38 million), Sweden ($2.0 million), Denmark ($1.9 million), and The Netherlands and Australia ($1.0 million each). The HRP's recently revised mission goals are to increase reproductive choices for women, expand male responsibility in reproductive health, respond to needs of developing countries, and coordinate and expand global research.
South to South Cooperation in Health	South to South is a network of contraceptive researchers from 14 countries, headquartered in Brazil. Research includes development of single-rod implants; a new progestin, ST 1435; menses inducers and emergency contraception, gossypol and Praneem polyherbal preparations; vaginal contraceptives; and immunocontraception.
United Nations Population Fund (UNFPA)	UNFPA provides support for contraceptive development activities, notably its support to WHO/HRP, as well as a major procurement activity for developing countries.
World Bank	Support for WHO/HRP.

Government Agencies (worldwide)

International Development Research Centre (IDRC) (Canada)	Support for contraceptive develoment activities.
Indian Council of Medical Research (ICMR)	Supported by the government of India at a level of $3.0 million in 1992.
Medical Research Council (MRC) (United Kingdom)	The British government provides support to its Medical Research Council (MRC) for work on fertility, contraception, and abortion ($5.8 million in 1992), as well as for basic research in molecular genetics ($17.7 million), fetal development and child health ($16 million), and infections and immunity (HIV) ($47 million).
Overseas Development Assistance (ODA)(United Kingdom)	The British government is also the leading bilateral supporter of the WHO/HRP and its contraceptive R&D activities.
Institut National de la Santé et de Recherche Médicale (INSERM/France)	Biomedical research; instrumental in development of RU 486.
National Research Institute for Family Planning (China)	The government of the People's Republic of China (GOPRC) has collaborated with the United Nations in the buildup of research capacities in human reproduction and family planning since early 1979 when agreement was reached for joint activities with the WHO/HRP. Between 1979 and 1994, UNFPA provided $13 million and WHO/HRP some $15 million to research institutes in Beijing, Chengdu, Guangzhou, Shanghai, and Tianjin for institutional strengthening and collaborative research activities. The GOPRC invested at least twice those amounts toward the same objectives. The Chinese National Research Programme for Family Planning has focused its priorities on development of new types and improvement of currently available IUDs, long-acting steroid contraceptives (once-a-month oral contraceptives, implants, vaginal rings, monthly injectables), male methods of fertility regulation (gossypol, long-acting testosterone esters), no-scalpel and reversible methods of sterilization, immunocontraception (antisperm antigen, ZP antibodies), medical abortion (herbal approaches, RU 486), and basic and applied research on reproductive physiology (implantation mechanism, testicular and epididymal function, ovarian function and regulation, IUD- and steroid-induced bleeding). There are 33 contraceptive manufacturers in China, producing over 40 varieties of oral contraceptives, injectables, spermicides, IUDs, and condoms.

TABLE 6-12 Continued

Nonprofit Private Sector

Foundations[b]

Rockefeller Foundation	The Rockefeller Foundation has been providing support for population research since 1963, when it declared population as a primary area of interest. In 1991, the Foundation began a collaboration with the WHO/HRP to support an initiative in Technical Cooperation Among Developing Countries (TCDC) to foster cooperation in research and research training in biomedical, social sciences, and public health research in reproductive health between two or more institutions in developing countries. In its 1995 Annual Report, the Foundation includes "Mobilization for Unmet Demand" among its nine core strategies, with a commitment of $14.75 million (the second largest allocation) toward mobilizing during the next decade "the resources to ensure availability of high-quality reproductive health and family planning services to all women in the developing world."
Andrew W. Mellon Foundation	The Andrew W. Mellon Foundation's interest in the population field dates from its beginning in 1969, when the Avalon and Old Dominion Foundations, which had a history of grants in the population field, were amalgamated to form the Andrew W. Mellon Foundation. Beginning in 1977, the Foundation has been providing grants to U.S. centers of reproductive biology, whose main purpose has been to provide support for postdoctoral fellows and junior faculty members working in areas relevant to contraceptive development. In 1995, Mellon joined Rockefeller in supporting the CICCR, described above.
Burroughs Wellcome Fund	Burroughs Wellcome has entered this arena with a 1995 funding level of $800,000 dedicated entirely to the training of researchers.
Howard Hughes Medical Institute (HHMI)	While HHMI does not support research in contraceptive research and development specifically, it does support fellowships in fundamental science of high relevance. As of 1994, the Institute was supporting 8 fellowships in the area of molecular and cell biology and genetics with particular relevance for contraceptive research and development.

^aThis table is intended to illustrate the range of organizations active in the contraceptive development field and the range of activities in which they are engaged. Information was obtained from annual reports, published materials on contraceptives, and telephone conversations or written exchanges with staff in the institutions and organizations listed. Some organizations and/or contraceptive development projects may have been omitted inadvertently or have been omitted because the information was unavailable. This table is illustrative and is not meant to be an endorsement of any group or product by the National Academy of Sciences.

^bThe following foundations all were providing support in the area of population and reproductive health in 1994, at the levels indicated in parentheses: the Carnegie Corporation of New York ($1 million), the Ford Foundation ($20 million), the John D. and Catherine T. MacArthur Foundation ($12.5 million), and the Pew Charitable Trusts ($1 million). However, none of the funds was for contraceptive research and development.

SOURCES: Bilian X, Advances of Contraception in China, Shanghai: National Research Institute for Family Planning, 1994. Contraceptive Development Branch, NICHD, Report to the National Advisory Child Health and Human Development (NACHHD) Council, Bethesda, MD, June 1995. Cook J, Tabular Material on Funding for International Health and Population, prepared for the Board on International Health, Institute of Medicine, Washington, DC, November 1995. Government of the People's Republic of China, Chinese Contraceptives, State Family Planning Commission of China, 1994. Government of the People's Republic of China, National Report of the People's Republic of China on Population and Development, formal submission to the International Conference on Population and Development, Cairo, 5–13 September 1994. Maguire ES, Meeting the Challenges: New Program Priorities and Initiatives for the Office of Population, US Agency for International Development, paper presented to Working Group on Reproductive Health and Family Planning of the Health and Development Policy Project, New York, 25 May 1994. National Research Council and Institute of Medicine, Developing New Contraceptives: Obstacles and Opportunities, L Mastroianni Jr, PJ Donaldson, TT Kane, eds., Washington, DC, National Academy Press, 1990. Program for Appropriate Technology in Health (PATH), Making a Difference in Women's and Children's Health, Seattle, WA, 1995. PATH, Contraceptive research and development: Progress toward a woman-centered agenda, Outlook 13(2), Seattle, WA, June 1995. Rockefeller Foundation, 1995 Annual Report, New York, 1996. WHO Special Programme of Research, Development, and Research Training in Human Reproduction, Research in Human Reproduction, Biennial Report 1993–1994, Geneva, 1994.

Funding Patterns Over Time: 1970–1990

Between 1973 and 1987, the pattern in federal funding was one of apparent overall increase. During that period, support for basic research in reproductive biology rose in current dollars from $30 million to $135 million, for contraceptive development from $7 million to $36 million. In constant dollars, the increases were 64 percent and 78 percent, respectively. However, that apparently positive trend conceals smaller, more significant, and less positive patterns that can be seen as predicting trends in the 1990s (NRC/IOM 1990).

First, foundation support for contraceptive research and development dropped dramatically in relative terms, from 22 percent of all federal and foundation funding for research in reproductive biology in FY1973 to around 3 percent by FY1987. Support for contraceptive development from the Ford, Rockefeller, and Mellon Foundations, and the Population Council, consistently much smaller than support for basic research, fell from about 18 percent to 10 percent in those same years (NRC/IOM 1990).

Second, while U.S. federal support for population research from FY1970 to FY1990 rose from $34.3 million to $231.2 million in current dollars, the trend in constant dollars was fairly flat. After 1982, the swings were less extreme than they had been in the 1970s: Increases and decreases in constant-dollar funding levels remained more or less in the low single digits except for a one-time 12 percent increase in 1987 to almost $74 million in U.S. federal funds for population research. However, each of the subsequent three years brought a decline in constant dollars, with each of the three successive years bringing a constant-dollar decline in federal support for population research. Federal support for population research totaled $232.2 million in 1990 current dollars, $6.4 million less than in 1989, a 3 percent drop; the drop from the 1989 constant-dollar level of $69.0 million to $63.5 million in 1990 was an 8 percent decrease. At the same time, the median cost of all population research projects rose by 4 percent; the median costs for contraceptive development and contraceptive evaluation projects exceeded that overall average considerably (USDHHS 1990).

Third, federal support for reproductive processes research fell from $141.6 million in 1989 to $134.5 million in 1990, the first time since 1977 that funds for this area declined. Contraceptive development also received less funding, dropping from the $26.9 million of 1989 to $25.6 million. Support for contraceptive evaluation decreased to $4.8 million in 1990, a far cry from its peak of $15.1 million in FY1980.

Fourth, as in the case of the foundations, federal funding for contraceptive development continues to be substantially less than the amount devoted to basic research. Since 1981, over 50 percent of all federal funding for population research has gone to basic research in reproductive biology, with studies of reproductive endocrinology dominating heavily. In 1990, 58 percent of all federal funding for population research went to reproductive processes, compared to

11 percent for contraceptive development and 2 percent for contraceptive evaluation.

Fifth, federal funding for research on reproductive processes has been heavily dominated by reproductive endocrinology, with 30 percent of all projects and 23 percent of the funds. Demography ranked second in funding, cell and molecular biology third. In terms of numbers of projects, cellular and molecular biology was second, demography third. The gaps between the disciplines in terms of funding were large: The dollar amount for reproductive endocrinology was twice that of demography and almost three times that of cell and molecular biology, which received only 15 percent of federal funds for research on reproductive processes. And, of all federal funding for population research, 22.5 percent was for research on the female reproductive system, 12.5 percent on the male reproductive system (USDHHS 1990).

Sixth, trends in worldwide funding, after peaking in 1972, fell sharply in 1975 (Lincoln and Kaeser 1987) and stayed relatively constant between 1977 and 1983. In the rest of the decade, a percentage increase of 138 percent in USAID support for contraceptive research and development and, subsequently, the onset of UNDP (United Nations Development Programme), UNFPA (United Nations Population Fund), and World Bank contributions to the World Health Organization's Human Reproduction Programme constituted the funding bulwark for the period.

Table 6-13 presents a compilation of funding trends in the public and private sectors between 1990 and 1995. The pattern was erratic over the five-year period but, overall, was one of modest increase in current dollars, but either flat or declining in constant dollars. The picture as this committee completes its work is mixed. At present, only four private foundations worldwide provide funding explicitly for contraceptive research and development: The Burroughs Wellcome Fund (U.S.A.), the Andrew W. Mellon Foundation, the Rockefeller Foundation, and the Wellcome Trust (United Kingdom). In 1995, all of these entities made some increase in the volume of funding in some way supportive of contraceptive research and development. The Burroughs Wellcome Fund, concerned about assuring maintenance of and fostering increase in the cadre of scientists for the field, made a first-year investment of $800,000 toward the training of scientists. The Rockefeller Foundation committed $14.75 million toward mobilizing during the next decade "the resources to ensure availability of high-quality reproductive health and family planning services to all women in the developing world" and, with Andrew W. Mellon, provided startup funds for the Consortium for Industrial Collaboration in Contraceptive Research (CICCR). The Wellcome Trust made a public commitment to invest £50 million in the area of population, including contraceptive research and development, primarily in the developing world.

Yet, as the Rockefeller Foundation notes in its related mission statement (Fathalla 1994),[3] foundation funds are small relative to the very large amounts required for the development of a new contraceptive method (see Figure 6-4), so

TABLE 6-13 Funding for Contraceptive Research and Development, Selected Institutions, Selected Years (in millions of U.S. dollars)

	Annual Average 1980–1983[a]	1990	1991	1992	1993	1994	1995
NIH/NICHD/CPR/CDB	8.4	11.5	13.5	15.25	17.0	15.2	18.7
USAID	8.0	6.7[b]	9.9	9.1	9.8	9.0	11.3
		10.9	20.5	16.9	22.4	19.0	21.1
WHO/HRP	6.7	6.7[c]	6.7	5.3	5.3	4.5[b]	4.5
		18.0	18.0	16.4	16.4	15.1	15.1
Andrew W. Mellon Foundation							
Reproductive biology	n.d.	1.4	1.7	1.3	1.9	1.5	1.5
Contraceptive development	n.d.	0.7	0.7	0.9	1.1	1.1	1.5
Total	n.d.	2.2	2.5	2.25	3.0	2.6	3.0
Rockefeller Foundation	n.d.	5.0	2.6	5.6	4.3	4.7	5.4

NOTES: USAID = United States Agency for International Development; NIH/NICHD/CDC/CPR = National Institutes of Health, National Institute for Child Health and Human Development, Center for Population Research, Contraceptive Development Branch; WHO/HRP = UNDP/UNFPA/WHO/World Bank Special Programme of Research Development and Research Training in Human Reproduction.

Information in this table was obtained from telephone conversations or written exchanges with the entities listed. Because of the complexity of funding flows and passthroughs, which can lead to misleading doublecounting, the table includes only the largest U.S. funders of contraceptive research and development, with the exception of the listing for the World Health Organization's Special Programme for Research, Development, and Research Training in Human Reproduction (WHO/HRP), whose funding represents support from 18 bilateral and 3 multilateral agencies and 2 foundations) (see Table 6-12 for detail). Owing to the proprietary nature of this type of information, the table does not include figures on pharmaceutical industry investment in contraceptive R&D. Older estimates of such investment (see Atkinson et al. 1985) and estimates calculated by the Program for Appropriate Technology in Health (PATH) in 1994, have ranged around $25 million a year, a figure said by some industry representatives to be considerably understated.

*a*SOURCE: LE Atkinson, R Lincoln, JD Forrest. Worldwide trends in funding for contraceptive research and evaluation. Family Planning Perspectives 17(5):196–207, 1985.

*b*The first row of figures presents the approximate values for contraceptive development research through FDA approval; the second row is that portion of USAID support for population that goes to biomedical research, which constitutes about 50 percent of all population research.

*c*The first row of figures refers to the line item for Technology Development and Assessment, which includes funding for long-acting agents, post-ovulatory methods, vaccines, male methods, natural methods, IUD research, and infertility, under the heading "Research and Development." The second row presents total expenditures on research and development and institutional strengthening for research, which also includes Technology Introduction and Transfer (some of which might be considered contraceptive R&D), Epidemiological Research, Social Science Research, and Regional Resources for Research. SOURCES: WHO/HRP. Financial Reports (1990–1991, 1992–1993, 1994–1995). Geneva. 1996.

that their value—and, in this sense, that value is substantial—is as a catalytic agent. There is other, related foundation investment: The Pew Charitable Trusts, Ford Foundation, John D. and Catherine T. MacArthur Foundation, the Hewlett Foundation, and the David and Lucile Packard Foundation all allocate some funding to population and reproductive health, but their funding streams are oriented toward policy, social scientific research, and family planning services.

A very large concern as this committee completes its work is the resurgence of political, judicial, and legislative controversy over family planning that is expressed in some measure in the November 1994 election of a new, more conservative U.S. Congress; ongoing attempts to reverse the Supreme Court's decision on abortion through adoption of a constitutional amendment (a prospect dormant since 1983); and the conceptual blurring of the lines of demarcation between contraception and abortion, not unrelated to the modes of action of certain types of fertility control (Rosoff 1995). All this, together with the prevailing lack of enthusiasm for U.S. foreign assistance and a climate of budgetary austerity unlikely to dissipate in the foreseeable future, are imposing a substantial chill on what has been a substantial funding flow—$550 million for all USAID population assistance program activity in FY 1995, cut by 35 percent for FY 1996. While this year's budget of the National Institutes of Health, of which the National Institute of Child Health and Human Development is a component, has not been affected by the austerities imposed on other government agencies, the future is always a question.

CONCLUDING COMMENT

Some of the tables in this chapter, though accurate, are misleading. The reader might gather the impression that much is happening in contraceptive research and development and ask why more is wanted.

There are two responses. The first is that, for the most part, current activity emphasizes enhancement of existing methods. This sort of "me-too" development can be important and is characteristically part of the development life of all technologies, few of which arrive on the human scene with no room for improvement. Yet, these modifications will still leave significant needs in significant populations unaddressed, needs that will require pharmaceutical pioneering.

Second, pioneering activity in contraceptive research and development will, in turn, require investment in basic research and in the early, highest-risk stages of the development process. Thus, funding to prime such activity, to share risk with academic researchers and corporate developers and, possibly, to leverage other infusions of funds, becomes key. The rationale is that, once a product completes phase II clinical trials, the chance of its getting into the marketplace is 50 percent, a notably brighter outlook for a corporation looking to develop new contraceptives (Harper 1996).

An increasingly frequent pattern of work in the contemporary pharmaceutical industry is a sequence of "virtual partnerships" and contract research arrangements at different junctures in the research and development processes. As noted above, this is not an unfamiliar pattern in contraceptive R&D; in fact, the willingness of small companies to risk engagement, and the willingness of the public and non-profit sectors to venture along with them, have been pivotal in advances in the field. It is now possible that the power and speed of combinatorial chemistry and high-speed computer modelling of compounds may make it more plausible for these sorts of collaborations to occur earlier in the research sequence. The partial nature of such early commitments might be attractive to biotechnology companies and might also mean that large pharmaceutical companies, wary of involvement in full product launch, would be willing to engage in different kinds of collaboration "closer to the bench."

The committee recognizes the difficulties international agencies face in obtaining additional funding for contraceptive research and development at a time of fiscal austerity. Still, the committee's scrutiny of funding for contraceptive research and development over the past 15 years indicates that it has, at best, remained flat in constant dollars and actually may have diminished. This means that cuts of any size have major implications. Targeted financial support from the public sector, notably by USAID and NICHD, has been critical in drawing U.S. university and not-for-profit institutional researchers into the field of reproductive biology and in catalyzing and sustaining the creative research partnerships that produced the advances in contraceptive research and development over the past two decades. The public sector also has particular strength and expertise in supporting the later stages of contraceptive research and development, for example, the clinical trials necessary to obtain the data required by the drug regulatory process. Any function that can expeditiously catalyze these sorts of ad hoc mechanisms across and within sectors could provide considerable value added. The reverse is also true; that is, any function impeding the healthy growth of such mechanisms is value lost.

REFERENCES

Atkinson LE, R Lincoln, JD Forrest. Worldwide trends in funding for contraceptive research and evaluation. Family Planning Perspectives 17(5):196–207, 1985.

Bronnenkant L. Panel discussion on vaccine development to meet U.S. and international needs. AIDS Research and Human Retroviruses 10:Supplement 2, 1994.

Burrill GS, KB Lee Jr. Biotech 94: Long-Term Value, Short-Term Hurdles (Industry Annual Report). San Francisco: Ernst and Young. 1993.

Burrill GS, KB Lee Jr. Biotech 93: Accelerating Commercialization (Industry Annual Report). San Francisco: Ernst and Young. 1992.

Djerassi C. The bitter pill. Science 245:354–361, 1989.

Easton R. Reform re-slices the market share pie. *In Vivo*: The Business and Medicine Report 11(7), 1993.

Fathalla MF. Mobilization of resources for a second contraceptive technology revolution. IN Contraceptive Research and Development 1984–1994: The Road from Mexico City to Cairo and Beyond. PFA Van Look, G Pérez-Palacios, eds. Delhi: Oxford University Press. 1994.

Frost and Sullivan. U.S. Contraceptives and Fertility Product Markets. New York, 1993.

Gelijns AC, CO Pannenborg. The development of contraceptive technology: Case studies of incentives and disincentives to innovation. International Journal of Technology Assessment in Health Care 9(2):210–22, 1993.

Goldman Sachs. U.S. Research: Biotechnology Products (2nd ed.). New York. June 1995.

Harper MJK. Funding For a New Partnership Between the Pharmaceutical Industry and Not-for-profit Research Institutions. Arlington, VA: Consortium for Industrial Collaboration in Contraceptive Research (CICCR). 1996.

Harper MJK. Birth Control Technologies: Prospects by the Year 2000. Austin: University of Texas Press. 1983.

Hatcher RA, J Trussell F Stewart, et al. Contraceptive Technology: 16th Revised Edition. New York: Irvington Publishers. 1994.

Kreger JC. Industry Overview: Contract Research Organizations (CROs)—A Clinically-Proven Route to Profits. Deerfield, IL. November 1994.

Lee KB Jr, GS Burrill. Biotech 96: Pursuing Sustainability: The Tenth Annual Industry Report. Palo Alto, CA: Ernst and Young LLP. 1995.

Lee KB Jr, GS Burrill. Biotech 95: Reform, Restructure, Renewal (9th Annual Industry Report). Palo Alto, CA: Ernst and Young LLP. 1994.

Lincoln R, L Kaeser. Whatever happened to the contraceptive revolution? Family Planning Perspectives 13(4):141–145, 1987.

National Research Council and the Institute of Medicine (NRC/IOM). Developing New Contraceptives: Obstacles and Opportunities. L Mastroianni Jr, PJ Donaldson, TT Kane, eds. Washington, DC: National Academy Press. 1990.

Office of Technology Assessment (OTA). Pharmaceutical R&D: Costs, Risks and Rewards. Washington, DC: Congress of the United States. 1993.

Peterson LS. Contraceptive Use in the United States: 1982–90—Advance Data from Vital and Health Statistics of the Centers for Disease Control and Prevention/National Center for Health Statistics No. 260. Hyattsville, MD: National Center for Health Statistics. 1995.

Pharmaceutical Research and Manufacturers of America (PhRMA). IN Development: New Medicines for Infectious Diseases. Washington, DC: 1994.

Pollard MR. Pharmaceutical innovation in the United States: Factors affecting future performance. International Journal of Technology Assessment in Health Care 9(2):167–173, 1993.

Program for Appropriate Technology in Health (PATH). Market-related Issues Affecting the Participation of the Private Sector in Contraceptive Development: A Final Report to the Rockefeller Foundation, 30 November 1994. Seattle, WA: 1994.

Rockefeller Foundation. Public/Private-Sector Collaboration in Contraceptive Research and Development: A Call for a New Partnership. Report from a Bellagio Conference, 10–14 April 1995. New York: Rockefeller Foundation. 1995a.

Rockefeller Foundation. International Research in Reproductive Health: A Guide to Agencies/Organizations. Paper prepared by World Health Organization Special Programme for Research, Development and Research Training in Human Reproduction. New York: The Rockefeller Foundation. 1995b.

Rosoff JI. The political storms over family planning: Supplement to chapters 1 and 7. IN The Best Intentions: Unintended Pregnancy and the Well-Being of Children and Families. S Brown, L Eisenberg, eds. Washington, DC: National Academy Press. 1995.

Steyer R. Searle nearing end of lawsuits over Copper 7 contraceptive. St. Louis Post-Dispatch P.1-E, 15 October 1995.

U.S. Department of Health and Human Services (USDHHS). Inventory and Analysis of Federal Population Research, Fiscal Year 1990. Bethesda, MD: Office of Science Policy and Analysis and Center for Population Research, National Institute of Child Health and Human Development, for the Interagency Committee on Population Research. 1990.

NOTES

1. In January 1995, Whitehall-Robbins Healthcare, the maker of the Today sponge, once the most popular over-the-counter contraceptive for women, announced that it would discontinue the product, saying that it could not assume the costs of bringing the plant up to FDA specifications. Whitehall is a division of American Home Products Corporation; when Today sales were at their peak in 1993, the method accounted for about $17 million out of American Home's $8 billion in sales.

2. The committee is grateful to the industry research firm Frost and Sullivan for giving the Institute of Medicine permission to use copyrighted information presented in this section.

3. In 1994, The Rockefeller Foundation stated its commitment to a strategy for resource mobilization in the field of population, including contraceptive research and development, noting that rather than adding its limited resources to an already impoverished field, it would invest in activities that would draw in more resources, help public sector programs to achieve their mission, and bring industry back. To accomplish this, the Foundation will use its convening power, commission authoritative studies, stimulate research, invest in human capital, and experiment with a challenge prize mechanism to stimulate innovation in the field (Fathalla 1994).

7

Issues of Law, Regulation, Information, and the Environment for Contraceptive Research and Development

The 1990 report on contraceptive development by the National Research Council and Institute of Medicine (NRC/IOM 1990) paid detailed attention to the magnitude of regulatory factors and product liability as obstacles to new advances in the field. The study committee did not find the U.S. Food and Drug Administration (FDA) and its regulatory authority over contraceptives to be major obstacles, owing to important legislative and procedural changes that had occurred in the decade of the 1980s. In fact, the committee voiced support for the FDA's rigorous review and approval processes and described its own limited recommendations as ways to make the evaluation of product safety more meaningful and more specific to different user populations.

In contrast, the study committee concluded that the impact of product liability litigation, particularly on the cost and availability of liability insurance, was a very large contributor to the climate of disincentives for the development of contraceptive products. The weightiest aspects of litigation were its unpredictability and the fact that evidence of compliance with FDA regulations was granted no special status in liability lawsuits in most states. Thus, the committee recommended that the U.S. Congress enact a product liability statute that would, first, establish uniform standards for lawsuits involving contraceptives and, second, give manufacturers of an FDA-reviewed contraceptive product a defense based on FDA's acceptance of that product.

This chapter is an update of the work of that 1990 committee, meant to respond to the following questions: What of note has happened since 1990 in the areas of regulation and product liability related to contraceptive research and development; has the weight of those two variables on the field increased or diminished; and what does that suggest, if anything, in the way of recommendations for action?

The first section of this chapter examines changes in the regulatory climate since 1990; the second section examines changes in the legal climate since that year, in each instance from the perspective of how those affect—or might affect—contraceptive research and development. The chapter then turns to an area where law, culture, politics, scientific research, medicine, and the thoughts and needs of contraceptive users intersect: the area of information. The chapter closes with a scan of those aspects of the environment that are most critical in generating the controversy that so often attends the development and use of modern contraceptive technologies.

The emphasis in this chapter is primarily on the United States. Even though we know that regulatory structures and legal frameworks differ significantly in many other countries in ways that could be illuminating, resources limited what the committee could deal with adequately. It may also be, at least at present, that breakthroughs in contraceptive research and development are not likely to occur without full-fledged U.S. participation. Finally, regulatory, legal, and political and legal decisions that are made in the United States continue to produce repercussions for other countries, particularly developing countries; examples include the controversy around Depo-Provera[1] and the persistent controversy in the United States around the abortion issue.

This is not to say that no other nation is present on the international contraceptive research and development stage. As perhaps the most prominent examples, Organon of The Netherlands and Schering AG of Germany are leading industrial players; until recently, French scientists at INSERM (*Institute National de la Santé et de Recherche Médicale*) were actively involved in the development of antiprogestins; India and China both have major research endeavors, and China is also a major producer of contraceptives; and The Wellcome Trust of the United Kingdom has recently committed £50 million to priorities in population and contraceptive research and development.

There are also informative similarities between the United States and other countries. Many European countries and the United Kingdom have experienced some of the same controversy around contraceptives for postcoital use that has been experienced in the United States in connection with RU 486 (Hughes 1995). Still, no nation is as litigious as the United States, although this may be changing (Steyer 1995), and few have a health system as driven by the market (Hutton et al. 1994). Each of these characteristics affect contraceptive research and development and the availability of contraceptive services.

REGULATORY INFLUENCES ON CONTRACEPTIVE RESEARCH AND DEVELOPMENT

Regulatory Developments Specifically Pertaining to Contraceptives

Changes in Requirements for Safety Data

Contraceptive products are subject to the same basic statutory and regulatory approval requirements as are other medical products in the corresponding regulatory category (i.e., drugs, biologics, or devices). Historically, however, the FDA has imposed special requirements on contraceptive products, particularly in the area of safety data, requirements which have had the practical result of delaying or obstructing the approval of such products. Among the most onerous was the long-standing requirement that new contraceptive drugs undergo long-term toxicology testing in several animal species, including seven-year studies in dogs and up to 10 years of study in monkeys. FDA's rationale for this unusually extensive testing was that contraceptives are intended for regular long-term use by millions of healthy women, most of whom have alternative contraceptive options, so that greater than usual rigor in ensuring long-term safety was necessary (NRC/IOM 1990).

This approach—though not lacking in logic—was, in its original form, somewhat exaggerated. Pregnancy, after all, poses its own set of health risks for many women, including serious complications for some women if the pregnancy is carried to term; these risks are likely to be far more sizable in developing countries where women's poor health, low economic status, and uneven access to good-quality care may be major factors. Thus, the risk-benefit calculus of approving a new contraceptive may not be quite as heavily weighted toward the reduction of product-associated risks as FDA's original model had it. At the same time, the calculation of risk in relation to both contraception and pregnancy is terribly complex; much debated; and highly various by age, culture, and socioeconomic environment. For instance, a young woman in the United States, even in a difficult socioeconomic environment, is unlikely to factor the possibility of maternal mortality into her "personal calculus of choice" about using contraceptives or getting pregnant (Zabin 1994), while a very young woman in a very remote village or urban slum in the developing world may do so as a matter of course. Similarly, older women in what is probably the majority of countries will construct their "burden-benefit" calculations with a keen awareness of the relationship between late childbearing and maternal mortality (Bulatao and Lee 1983; Scheper-Hughes 1995).

FDA's thinking on long-term toxicology studies has evolved over the years in the direction of greater flexibility. As noted in the 1990 NRC/IOM report, by 1987, the 10-year monkey study requirement had been eliminated and the seven-year dog (beagle) study requirement reduced to three years. The time and cost burden imposed by this latter test, however, was still substantial. In addition, the test was scientifically controversial because of the innately high risk of breast tumors in beagles, which, in turn, could increase the likelihood of "false positive" results.

The injectable contraceptive Depo-Provera (DMPA or depo-medroxypro-gesterone acetate) became something of a test case for the three-year beagle toxicology requirement. The Upjohn Company first sought FDA approval of this product in 1967. After a long and rather tortured regulatory history (NRC/IOM 1990), the FDA rejected the application, largely on the ground that the drug had produced a significant increase in benign and malignant mammary tumors in beagles. Subsequently, however, the results of large-scale epidemiologic studies of actual users of Depo-Provera in developing countries, conducted by the World Health Organization and others, became available and showed that DMPA had at most a weak association with an increased risk of breast cancer, and that such risk, if any, was of the same order of magnitude as that posed by oral contraceptives (Jordan 1992).

As a consequence, the FDA concluded that not only did "women using Depo-Provera run no greater risk for breast cancer (or any other type of cancer) than women taking other approved steroidal contraceptives," but that "at least in the case of [Depo-Provera], the results in the beagle did not accurately predict the effects in humans."[2] The agency accordingly eliminated the beagle test from the required toxicology testing for steroidal contraceptives (Jordan 1992) and approved Depo-Provera, on the ground that the "major safety issue of the possible relation between breast cancer and the use of this drug for contraception has been adequately addressed" (Corfman 1992).

With the elimination of the beagle testing requirement, the preclinical requirements for steroidal contraceptives have now been brought generally into line with those that apply to other categories of drugs, although their specifics still differ in certain respects (Jordan 1992). This represents a substantial step forward in reducing regulatory barriers to the development of contraceptive products.

Requirements for Contraceptive Methods Protecting Against Sexually Transmitted Diseases (STDs)

In other areas, however, the FDA continues to exhibit a restrictive approach to contraceptives that tends to delay product availability, sometimes in perplexing ways. On the one hand, the agency has responded to the AIDS emergency with greater flexibility and speed (Fox 1995; Washington Post 1995) and appeared to be disposed to extend that flexibility to those contraceptive methods that also offered protection against STDs. Nevertheless, the female condom, Reality, took 6.5 years to be approved. The producer, Wisconsin Pharmacal, attempted to gather clinical data justifying dual claims of protection against pregnancy and STDs, but was frustrated in that endeavor by the FDA and the product was ultimately approved only for contraception (J Trussell, personal communication, 1995). The matter of approval of vaginal contraceptives, discussed below, is another puzzling case in point.

Prevention of sexually transmitted infections is an unquestionably critical public health objective, and barrier contraception is on a very short list of ways that objective can be accomplished. As a public health agency, FDA clearly has the right, and the responsibility, to pay attention to this problem, including efforts to foster development of safe and effective barrier contraceptives that can also block STD infection (FDA 1990). But the other, and original, intended use of female barrier devices—to prevent pregnancy—is also an important public health concern. In this respect, FDA's approach to the basic issues of safety and efficacy for contraceptive products at times seems at odds with practical realities. Contraceptives are used by a wide variety of people, in a wide variety of settings, with a wide variety of motivations. Many of those users, particularly women at risk of an unwanted pregnancy, would be happy to have an inexpensive, safe, and convenient contraceptive product available when needed, even were the efficacy of such a product to be less than perfect, provided they are well informed about failure rates.

Again, the female condom serves as an example. In addition to the apparent confusion about STD prevention, the FDA also seemed to apply unrealistically high standards of efficacy to the product in terms of pregnancy prevention. Although the contraceptive efficacy of the female condom was shown to be the same as that for the sponge, cervical cap, and diaphragm (Trussell et al. 1994), the FDA insisted on comparing it with the male condom, despite the fact that a clinical trial of the male condom that conforms to modern standards of research design, execution, and analysis does not exist. Thus, while Reality's effectiveness in this regard was perhaps not as high as that of some alternative contraceptive products, it clearly offered much better protection than nothing. For a woman not using an alternative method, and whose partner was himself unwilling to use a condom, the female condom could well mean the difference between less-than-perfect (but still significant) protection and no protection at all. The question was raised: Why did not FDA simply require disclosure in the labeling of relative rates of efficacy and let women decide for themselves?

Other Issues Around Vaginal Contraceptives

Interestingly, FDA itself expressed an approach somewhat along these lines 15 years ago, in its comments on the report of the Advisory Panel on Over-the-Counter Vaginal Contraceptive Products. There the agency said: "FDA is . . . aware that there is a strong consumer interest in knowing the actual percentage effectiveness of each OTC vaginal contraceptive product. . . . FDA concurs with the Panel that the most valuable labeling is that which expresses effectiveness in terms of the percent of women for whom the product is effective under described conditions of use" (FDA 1980). This statement reflects what might be called a consumer-oriented approach to contraceptive products. The premise is: Give the consumer clear and reliable information about how contraceptive products actually perform (assuming, of course, a reproducible minimum level of safety and efficacy), and let her make her own decision about which product to use under which circumstances, the hypothesis being that greater variety of method choice will increase the likelihood that women will have authentic access to contraception when and as they need it.

However, unlike the changes in long-term toxicology testing, some of FDA's recent actions in the area of contraceptives seem to have been moving in the direction of less flexibility. Of particular note is the issuance by the agency in February 1995 of a notice of proposed rulemaking on vaginal contraceptive products that would require manufacturers of over-the-counter (OTC) vaginal contraceptive products to conduct expensive and time-consuming clinical trials and obtain approved new drug applications (NDAs) in order to continue to market their products (FDA 1995b). This proposal was based on the premise that the effectiveness of this category of products is dependent upon their final formulation. Therefore, FDA's argument goes, the typical OTC review approach of categorizing particular active ingredients as generally recognized as safe and effective, and allowing manufacturers to market those active ingredients in formulations of their choice as long as the inactive ingredients used are safe and suitable, would not work for OTC vaginal contraceptives.

The agency has attempted to mitigate the impact of the regulation by streamlining the data requirements for NDAs for currently marketed products (e.g., waiving the requirement for preclinical data for such applications) and by assuring manufacturers that they would have sufficient time to complete studies and submit data to FDA before the proposal took final effect. However, many OTC products are manufactured or marketed by smaller companies that will not have the resources or expertise to conduct full-scale clinical studies and put together an NDA. As the National Women's Health Network and the Boston Women's Health Book Collective observed in their written comments in mid-1995: "We believe that the proposed rule, which requires every manufacturer of spermicides designed to be used alone to conduct controlled contraceptive effectiveness trials, is over-burdensome, may lead to the withdrawal of some products, and will ultimately leave women with fewer methods of contraception available over-the-counter. . . . Our organizations do not object to the requirement that manufacturers conduct clinical studies of vaginal irritation" (National Women's Health Network 1995). The comments add that the contraceptive effectiveness of vaginal spermicides is known well enough to permit women to make reasonably well-informed choices. Were they, on the contrary, new products, both organizations would support both controlled trials of contraceptive effectiveness and vaginal irritation and studies of STD prevention.

While there is disagreement about whether enough is, in fact, known about the contraceptive efficacy of spermicides to allow reasonably well-informed choices, enthusiasm about lengthy and costly controlled effectiveness trials is hard to find. One possible approach might be development of less time-consuming research designs that would build on existing survey, clinical data, and/or current trials with microbicides or, perhaps, a comparative controlled contraceptive trial coordinated by a third party, with each manufacturer contributing a share of the cost (National Women's Health Network 1995). Another approach would take on the issue at a different level and require that the quality and quantity of clinical data on a particular product be reflected more explicitly in the product's labeling.

General Regulatory Developments

The drug development process, as a product of both science and society, evolves over time. In the early 1990s, several factors influenced that evolution: changing attitudes toward risks and benefits, the Prescription Drug User Fee Act of 1992, cooperation among international regulatory authorities, integration of computers into the drug review process, and a shift from the "honor system" to the "trust but verify" system of regulatory surveillance and enforcement (Mathieu 1994).

Changes in Regulation of Combination Products

Thus, recent years have brought a number of broader changes in how FDA reviews products generally; current internal and external pressures for further regulatory reform may produce even greater alterations (Lasagna 1995a). Several of the changes that have already occurred have significant implications for the agency's regulation of contraceptive products. Establishment in 1991 of a specific policy on FDA review of those products that combine elements of two or more of the three major product categories (drugs, biologics, and devices) has cleared away much of the procedural confusion that previously hampered the review of such products. Required by the Safe Medical Devices Act of 1990, FDA's rules on the regulation of these combination products assign jurisdiction within the agency on the basis of a product's "primary mode of action," and establish procedures for determining which component of the agency will handle the review of combination products (FDA 1991a). As part of this initiative, intercenter agreements were concluded between the drugs, biologics, and device centers specifying in more detail how particular products would be handled.

For contraceptive products that combine, for example, a device component with a drug component, the combination product policy reduces the chances of review delays caused by jurisdictional confusion within FDA. The intercenter agreement between the drug center and the devices center lists, for instance, a "condom, diaphragm, or cervical cap with contraceptive or antimicrobial agent" as an example of a combination product that is to be regulated by the device center under the statutory provisions pertaining to devices, on the grounds that such products have the "primary intended purpose of fulfilling a device function," although they also "have a drug component that is present to augment the safety and/or efficacy of the device" (FDA 1991a).

Further, the advent in 1992 of user fees and corresponding deadlines for FDA review of new drugs and biologics subject to user fee requirements, combined with FDA's overall efforts to manage the review process more efficiently, offer the prospect of faster review times generally for new contraceptive drugs and biologics. Average review times for new drugs seem to have dropped substantially since user fee requirements came into play, according to analysis carried out under the aegis of the White House task force on reinventing government (RIGO), although the time prior to acceptance of a new filing has increased (Clinton and Gore 1995). Another, more recent analysis, prepared by the U.S. General Accounting Office in response to a bipartisan congressional request, also found that there had been a considerable reduction in approval times for new drugs during 1987–1992 (Barnett 1995) and that the FDA is actually faster in approving drugs than its European counterparts (Schwartz 1995). The FDA's recently issued Annual Report to Congress showed that, in FY1994, the agency approved 93 percent of all drugs within a year of the companies' applications, surpassing the 55 percent benchmark mandated by the Prescription Drug User Fee Act (Associated Press 1995). The numbers may be debated by congressional and industry critics, yet there appears to be no industrial enthusiasm for diluting the advantages that the FDA approval stamp currently gives to products that have it, including some degree of legal protection and consumer confidence in their safety (Washington Post 1995).

Prospective Regulatory Changes

A number of changes being contemplated or implemented as part of current FDA reform initiatives could be of specific benefit to the development of contraceptive products. For instance, the reduction or elimination of requirements for FDA review of postapproval changes in manufacturing facilities or processes for drugs and biologics (BIO 1995; Clinton and Gore 1995), a concept that has already been implemented to some degree for biologics (FDA 1995b), is intended to reduce the regulatory burden on manufacturers of other products affected by those requirements, a category which includes contraceptives. The same is true for the proposed elimination of the costly and often irrelevant requirement for inclusion of an environmental assessment in most new drug applications (NDAs).[3] The biotechnology industry will also benefit from the recent issuance of proposed new rules that effectively allows FDA to treat well-characterized biotechnology products (e.g., monoclonal antibodies) like other drugs. The expectation is that this particular piece of reform will save biotechnology companies hundreds of millions of dollars and hasten passage of new biotechnology products through regulatory approval processes (Schwartz 1995).

Inclusion of Women in Clinical Trials

In July 1993, the FDA released a new Guideline for the Study and Evaluation of Gender Differences in the Clinical Evaluation of Drugs, which modifies and revises the section of its 1977 guidelines that recommended exclusion of women from Phase I and early Phase II of drug development. The new guidelines provide for the inclusion of women in those phases and state that the broad principles for that inclusion will also be applied to FDA approval processes for biological products and medical devices (IOM 1994a).

The exclusion of women from trials of contraceptives, products developed explicitly for women, is patently not an issue. What is an issue is the potential for interactions of new contraceptives with other drugs for which data on adverse effects and contraindications in women are lacking because women were excluded from the original trials. The importance of the pharmacokinetics of drugs is addressed in the 1988 FDA Guidelines for the Format and Content of the Clinical and Statistical Sections of New Drug Applications, which requires that consideration during drug development be given to effects on pharmacokinetics of estrogen replacement therapy and systemic contraceptives (IOM 1994a).

As women of reproductive age come to be increasingly included in the early phases of drug trials as a consequence of these new guidelines, there will be another issue, that is, the possibility of their becoming pregnant while they are participants in trials. This means that informed consent protocols must include information about contraception and the alternatives of voluntarily withdrawing from the study and terminating a pregnancy should conception take place (IOM 1994b). If the participant opts for contraception, this raises the issue of pharmacokinetics referred to above. Snow and Hall (1994) point to an apparent regional variability in pharmacologic response to contraceptives, specifically steroids. They also point to the limited and highly speculative state of the science in this regard, a situation that derives from study designs in the early phases of human trials. The WHO-recommended approach is that pharmacokinetic studies of contraceptive steroids be conducted separately from studies of the efficacy and side effects of those same steroids, in order to control for confounding with the research design. This precludes investigation of the relationships between pharmacokinetic variability among women and their experience of contraceptive side effects (Snow and Hall 1994).

LEGAL INFLUENCES ON CONTRACEPTIVE
RESEARCH AND DEVELOPMENT

Manufacturers' Concerns

Beyond the extensive regulatory requirements a potential contraceptive developer must contemplate when making product development decisions, there is the legal environment to consider. A pharmaceutical company generally expects to have some liability expenditure after marketing almost any product and will factor that anticipated expenditure into development calculations; in fact, companies may set aside a "kitty" for that purpose (IOM 1995a). As extensive as the regulatory process may be and as exhaustive in its consideration of possible unwanted effects on different categories of users, no clinical trial, no matter how well designed, can anticipate every single contingency when a product is marketed to what may be millions of consumers. Human physiology and individual medical and personal histories are simply too diverse and unpredictable, as are other contextual variables that cannot be incorporated into clinical trials. The law requires manufacturers to warn not only about *known* risks but about *foreseeable* risks that should have been known had the manufacturer applied "reasonable, developed human skills and foresight." While risks designated as "*unexpected and unknown*" will not trigger strict liability, sellers still are deemed to be experts and are imputed to have all "knowledge of the product's risks based on reliable and obtainable information" (Flannery and Greenberg 1994). Thus, development decision-making incorporates the assumption that a product *could* cause harm to some of its future users, some estimation of the magnitude of those problems, and prediction of the likelihood that a liability suit will result. Woven into these imponderables are concerns about the following:

- causing injury, whether from known or unknown side effects;
- loss of public confidence because of adverse publicity from lawsuits, whether lost or won;
- the costs ensuing from any legal action, even when the plaintiff's case is weak and liability is uncertain, including such indirect costs as work disruption, and the direct costs of litigation and settlement;
- delayed liability exposure from side effects that may not manifest for 5, 10, or 20 years;
- the potential for mass litigation, that is, class action lawsuits, particularly those that ensue from active recruitment of plaintiffs, some injured by the product, many not, and all of whom are "classed" together;
- government investigations by the FDA or by U.S. or state's attorneys after a lawsuit (Flannery 1995).

There are other issues. First, with most pharmaceuticals, a U.S. firm is likely to be marketing its product on a national scale, so that unpredictability almost inevitably derives from the variability among the individual product liability rules of as many as all 50 states, the District of Columbia, and two territories (Foote 1988; IOM 1990).

Second, there is the uncertainty introduced by having highly technical and complex scientific issues evaluated by a judge and jury untrained in the sciences (IOM 1994b).[4] This relative unfamiliarity may amplify the weight of personal feelings and opinions in final rulings. An ancillary consideration is that there seems to be a tendency for juries to be more sympathetic to injured plaintiffs than to large corporations.

Third, there is the manufacturer's inability to rely on FDA approval as protection against liability. As rigorous as FDA approval processes may be, most courts have held that obtaining FDA approval of a drug[5] does not provide a manufacturer with an absolute shield from state tort liability, although evidence of compliance with FDA warning regulations may be introduced as evidence of the adequacy of such warnings (Flannery and Greenberg 1994). This is addressed later in this chapter in the context of a government standards defense.

Fourth is the cost and unavailability of comprehensive general liability insurance, which includes product liability. This grew to be a big issue for contraceptive manufacturers and entities engaged in research in the 1980s. The reasons were both general—the size and number of liability awards soared in those years—and specific to contraceptives because they are used by so many women over long periods of time and because their risks may be latent for years and include risks to offspring (NRC/IOM 1990). Bigger corporations can self-insure or find other ways to secure the necessary insurance, but smaller companies and independent and nonprofit organizations do not have comparable avenues; for them, insurance is a more sizable impediment.

Finally there is the political climate. All aspects of liability pertain in a climate that is, for contraceptives, especially volatile and ideologically fraught because they are tethered to profound beliefs about abortion, the mechanisms of contraceptives, and conservative perspectives about family planning as a general matter. All this, in turn, tends to inflate the liability issue in virtually every dimension.

Product Liability Rules

Tort law encompasses civil wrongs where one person's conduct causes injury to another in violation of a duty imposed by law (Foote 1988). In the context of product liability, tort law encompasses both negligence, which is based on fault, and strict liability, which is based on no-fault principles (Prosser and Keeton 1984).

The objectives of product liability rules are to compensate individuals injured by unreasonably dangerous products, to deter the marketing of dangerous

or defective products, and to resolve disputes between those injured and manufacturers (Smith 1987). Since tort law is the province of the states, these rules
generally are created through common law, not statutory law; that is, they are
rules made for the most part by judges, not laws enacted by Congress or state
legislatures. There is no uniform federal product liability law that would preempt
those state rules (IOM 1994a; NRC/IOM 1990).

Liability pertains at two major junctures in the project development trajectory from laboratory to market. The first is during research, that is, during
clinical studies[6] when a product is applied to or ingested by a living human being.
The second is the liability of a manufacturer (and possibly a provider) after the
finished pharmaceutical product is launched on the market and public consumption begins. While legal action in these areas is in some respects based on the
same theories, there are significant differences between them.

There are five legal theories under which a product liability case can fall: (1)
express warranty, (2) implied warranty (both generally superseded by commercial codes in each state), (3) fraudulent misrepresentation (not commonly applied), (4) negligence, and (5) strict liability (see Table 7-1). It is the last two
areas that are pertinent to both product liability and research liability.

An additional theory underlies research liability: the theory of battery, which
is defined as unlawful and intentional bodily contact directed at another person
without that person's consent. In research liability cases, battery has to do with
use of an individual as a research subject without his or her knowledge or consent
and there may be a punitive element in damage awards (IOM 1994a). Battery
does not apply in product liability cases.

Negligence

Negligence in Product Liability Negligence is deviation from acceptable standards of conduct or standards of care. It entails breach of a legal duty owed by
the defendant to the plaintiff and injury consequent to that breach. To recover
damages for negligence, causation must be proved. An area of dissensus in
negligence theory is whether a defendant is liable for injuries to offspring that
occur as a result of any injury to the woman before the child's conception. In
most negligence cases, only compensatory damages are awarded, except for cases
of gross negligence, wherein some states allow a punitive element. Third parties
may also recover money damages for injury to a research participant caused by
negligence (Reisman 1992).

In product liability, a manufacturer can breach the "duty of care" in three
ways: (1) by adopting a design for the product that causes it to be unreasonably
dangerous; (2) making mistakes or omissions in the manufacturing process that
result in a properly designed product becoming unreasonably dangerous; (3) or
by failing to provide adequate warnings about the product's hazards and instructions concerning its use. In most jurisdictions, the manufacturer must warn only

TABLE 7-1 Five Theories of Liability

Theory	Explanation	Usage
Express Warranty	A written or oral affirmation of fact or promise made by the seller of the product to the buyer about the condition, efficacy, or safety of the product.	(1) Whether the seller actually made a statement of fact to the buyer about the product—expressions of opinions are not supportive; (2) the meaning or interpretation of said statements; (3) whether the statement was true or false; and (4) whether the product caused the plaintiff harm.
Implied Warranty	Representation by the seller that is implied in a contract for the sale of the product that the product is "merchantable"—"fit for the ordinary purposes for which such goods are used."	The seller must be a "merchant" and, in most states, manufacturers have been held to be so. Because sales are contracts, this presents a broad avenue for recovery against sellers of defective goods, but recovery is generally governed by the relevant provisions of the *Uniform Commercial Code* as adopted by each state.
Fraudulent Misrepresentation	Similar to warranty theory but the plaintiff must also prove fraud and deceit.	Plaintiffs must prove (1) that the defendant made a false representation about the product, (2) that the defendant knew the representation was false, (3) that the defendant intended to induce the plaintiff to act or refrain from acting on the basis of the misrepresentation, (4) that the plaintiff justifiably relied on the representation, and (5) that the plaintiff was injured thereby. [Product liability cases are not usually based on this theory owing to the common requirement of "clear and convincing" evidence.]

TABLE 7-1 Continued

Theory	Explanation	Usage
Negligence	Plaintiffs must show that: the defendant-manufacturer owed the plaintiff a "duty of care"; the defendant breached this duty of care; the plaintiff was injured; and the defendant's lack of care was the proximate cause of the injury. A manufacturer owes a duty of care to avoid an unreasonable risk of harm to the user of a product.	A manufacturer can be said to have breached this duty of care in three broad respects: (1) by adopting a design for the product that causes it to be unreasonably dangerous; (2) by making mistakes or omissions in the manufacturing process that result in a properly designed product becoming unreasonably dangerous; (3) or by failing to provide adequate warnings about the product's hazards and instructions concerning its use. As a general matter, only the medical provider—the "learned intermediary"—not the patient, must be directly warned.
Strict Liability	Relatively recent; plaintiff may recover without demonstrating negligence.	Plaintiff must demonstrate (1) design defect, including defective testing; (2) manufacturing defect; or (3) failure to warn.

SOURCE: National Research Council and Institute of Medicine. Developing New Contraceptives: Obstacles and Opportunities. L Mastroianni, PJ Donaldson, TT Kane, eds. Washington, DC: National Academy Press. 1990.

the medical profession, not the patient—the "learned intermediary" rule—and the adequacy of the warning is frequently in contention (Harper et al. 1986).

Negligence in the Context of Research. In research liability, legal actions for injury based on a negligence theory often involve the doctrine of "informed consent." There is a difference between the nature of consent needed to avoid a legal action for battery, which is a form of assent to a bodily intervention that is sometimes termed "simple consent," and what is needed to avoid an action for negligence, which requires "informed consent." The latter is defined as consent based on the disclosure of all facts, including the risks and benefits of the proposed intervention, as well as alternatives and their risks and benefits, that are necessary to form the basis of willing, uncoerced, intelligent consent by the patient to the procedure (Jonsen et al. 1982; Reisman 1992; Wadlington 1984). Legal action will be based on whether the information given to the participant before securing consent sufficiently warned of potential risks and whether the degree of disclosure was reasonable given the circumstances. Decisions in this area depend heavily on definitions of "adequacy" (Wadlington 1984). The statute of limitations that limits the number of years during which a legal action can be initiated is usually longer for a negligence action (IOM 1994a).

Strict Liability

Strict liability is fairly new in tort law, but this less-than-definitive theory leaves much room for interpretation. While a plaintiff must demonstrate more than simply some injury consequent to use, under this theory, use by a manufacturer of all possible care in design and manufacture does not absolve it from liability. Under strict liability, then, a person injured by a product can recover damages without having to show that the manufacturer was negligent.

The *Restatement of Torts (Second)*, a compendium of the views of leading legal scholars, recommends that the principle of strict liability not apply to products that present generic risks, termed "unavoidably unsafe" products, and cites vaccines and drugs as examples (Foote 1988). A manufacturer may be exempted from this general rule under the comment k exemption of the *Restatement*, Section 402A, which states that a drug is not "unreasonably dangerous" and the manufacturer is not subject to strict liability, as long as the drug is "properly prepared and marketed and a proper warning is given" (American Law Institute 1977). Comment k specifically refers to experimental drugs, "as to which, because of lack of time and opportunity for sufficient medical experience, there can be no assurance of safety" (Flannery and Greenberg 1994). However, though a manufacturer may keep a product from being considered "unreasonably dangerous" by giving appropriate warnings, the adequacy of these warnings is very often the legal issue brought into contention. Furthermore, while some state courts have consistently upheld this exception to strict liability, others have not (Foote 1988).

Manufacturers can generally satisfy their duty to warn for prescription and investigational drugs by informing physicians and investigators of any risks of harm. It then becomes the responsibility of the physician—the "learned intermediary"—to prescribe drugs only for appropriate indications and for monitoring their use (IOM 1994a). For prescription contraceptives, however, courts have reached differing conclusions as to whether manufacturers have a duty to warn consumers directly (Flannery and Greenberg 1994).

Liability for Injuries to Offspring

The greatest concern about liability is the possibility of injury to offspring when women of childbearing potential are included in clinical drug trials. Both researchers and manufacturers must not only be concerned with the health and well-being of the woman (or man) using its product—in our context a contraceptive product—but also with the future health of a child who might be born to that contraceptive user. These concerns reflect the experience with diethylstilbestrol (DES) and thalidomide and the ensuing realization that, as complex as proof of causation might be, the harm that might be alleged to result from *in utero* exposure to a drug is great. Other considerations are the greater length of the statute of limitations for cases of injury to children and the fact that a parent cannot waive a child's rights to sue (IOM 1994a). In fact, claims on behalf of a child of a contraceptive user can be filed against a manufacturer as many as 20 years after the child's birth, even when the birth itself may have occurred several years after the initial purchase of the product; this is because children's claims are typically tolled, which means that the statute of limitations does not begin to run during their minority (Clayton 1994). A highly specific "anticipatory release" signed by the parent *may* relieve the manufacturer of liability but, since this could generate future conflict between parent and child, it is typically disallowed (Clayton 1994).

Potential plaintiffs in a legal action for injuries to offspring include the living child and the parents. The most important questions are whether the child was born alive and what the parents would have done had they known about the risks: Would they have avoided the drug or put off procreation (Clayton 1994)? In the case of research, when the plaintiff is the child, the success of a legal action depends in part on the ability of the parents to show that they would not have participated in the research had they known about the risks (IOM 1994a). A child may bring an action for *wrongful life* when the parents claim that they would not have had the child if they had been informed of the risks; such actions have rarely been recognized by the courts. Parents who have a live but injured child might bring a *wrongful birth* action if they show that they would have avoided childbearing had they known of the risks (Clayton 1994). If the child is stillborn as a result of a research injury, some states allow the parents to bring an action for *wrongful death*. In some of those states, a wrongful death action for a stillborn child is allowed only if the child was deemed to have been a viable fetus at the time the injury occurred; in other states, a wrongful death action is allowed regardless of the fetus's initial viability.

Current Proposals for Tort Reform

If a manufacturer loses a suit, there are three kinds of damages that can be awarded to a claimant:

• Compensatory damages, which encompass economic damages for whatever economic injury may have occurred, for example, medical expenses, loss of income, or estimates of future judicial expenses; as well as

- Noneconomic damages, awarded to compensate for emotional distress, pain, and suffering; and
- Punitive damages[7] intended to punish and deter wrongdoing.

A punitive dimension in liability awards, once relatively rare, has become increasingly present in many tort judgments for damages (Flannery 1995; Peterson 1987). In response to that fact and to the growing numbers of cases and individuals entering into product liability litigation—and, of compelling interest, explosion in the dollar magnitudes involved—pressure for tort reform has mounted. Recognition of the need for a set of standards governing product liability on a federal level is, nevertheless, not new. Since at least the 101st Congress, members of both houses have made attempts to address the issue and some state legislatures have, for the first time, enacted legislation that, in some circumstances, limits damages awards against defendant manufacturers.[8]

The National Vaccine Injury Compensation Program (NVICP)

Beyond efforts at the state level, very specific federal reform legislation (H.R. 5184, 99th Cong. 2d sess., 1986) established the National Vaccine Injury Compensation Program (NVICP), essentially no-fault insurance against possible injuries from the seven pediatric vaccines children were mandated to receive in order to attend school in the United States. Beginning in the mid-1970s, a steady increase in numbers of vaccine-related lawsuits against manufacturers, as well as in the sizes of awards to plaintiffs, led to withdrawal of many companies from vaccine manufacturing and marketing (IOM 1985 and 1993). The NVICP was an attempt to compensate families of children adversely affected by government-mandated vaccines and to shore up the vaccine industry by eliminating liability risk through imposition of a vaccine excise tax. The trust fund into which the taxes were paid had a balance of about $620 million at the beginning of 1993, when the tax was lifted. In 1993, an IOM committee concluded that impact of the program was not yet clear (IOM 1993). Despite an apparent decrease in vaccine-related lawsuits and an increase in vaccine-related R&D, no company that had dropped out of vaccine manufacturing in the United States in the 1970s and 1980s had returned as of mid-1993. Nonetheless, foreign companies, many of which had traditionally shied away from the U.S. vaccine market, were readying themselves to enter it, either by applying for FDA licenses for their products or by entering into alliances with other companies and entities holding U.S. product licenses (IOM 1993). A very recent analysis of the effect of the NVICP indicates that industry now, 10 years later, views the program as "working" (Day 1996).

The program is regarded by some analysts as an inappropriate model for replication in other areas of health because of its loose handling of causation, among other matters (Wadlington, personal communication, 1995). However, it is not the only model: Analysis in the mid-1980s found that Denmark, Germany,

France, Japan, Switzerland, and the United Kingdom all had compensation programs for injuries whose reasonable cause was a vaccine mandated or recommended by law (IOM 1985). Replication in the area of contraception would encounter at least one contextual obstacle, that is, the difference in public perceptions of vaccines and contraceptives (Djerassi 1989). Vaccines are generally perceived as a public good that is also protective of the individual; the pediatric vaccines are seen as particularly protective of children who are in themselves generally perceived as a good thing. There is little or no perception of contraceptives as addressing a present or putative public health problem; thus, unlike vaccines, contraceptives are not seen as a public good.

Current Legislation

One outcome of this mounting concern is that two pieces of legislation, H.R.956 and S.565, passed the House and the Senate of the U.S. Congress in March and May 1995, respectively, and await reconciliation in conference. A third bill (H.R.10), included in the Republican Party's "Contract with America," contains many of the same legislative elements. The three bills are compared in Table 7-2.

It is perilous to take up the topic of legislation that is still in the making, since much of its content may change and, of course, there may be none.[9] After all, product liability legislation has been vigorously debated since it was first proposed in the early 1980s. Nonetheless, there are generic components whose inclusion in any final legislation could contribute significantly to enhancing the environment for improving existing contraceptives and developing new ones, in ways that will better respond to current national and international public health needs and demands. The most pertinent are the following:

A Government Standards Defense. This aspect of reform would standardize what some states have already adopted, that is, exclusion of the punitive element in awards for damages, assuming that there had been FDA review and approvals at appropriate junctures. The defense would not be available if the manufacturer withheld relevant information from the FDA (NRC/IOM 1990), nor would it prevent plaintiffs from receiving compensatory damages.

Punitive Limits. Another aspect of reform would be the imposition of limits on the size of punitive elements in awards and/or how those are awarded.

Limits on the Liability of Biomaterials Suppliers. Another element in tort reform would be limits on the liability of biomaterials suppliers.

Others. Other reform elements include caps on compensatory damages; modifications of statutes of repose and statutes of limitations; and issues related to pleadings found to be frivolous, including "loser-pays" provisions.

TABLE 7-2 Comparison of Pending Tort Reform Legislation, November 1995, United States

Area of Reform	H.R.956	S.565	H.R.10
Punitive Damages	Impose a $250,000 cap on punitive damages, or limit them to three times any economic losses. The bill would apply to any civil litigation, not just product disputes.	Cap at $250,000 or three times economic losses, which can include lost wages or medical expenses, whichever is greater. The bill would apply only to product liability cases.	Same cap would apply only to product liability actions and would require a specific showing of intentional malice for such awards.
Regulatory Approval Defense (Government Standards Defense)	Bar punitive damages in cases in which a medical device or drug had won approval from the FDA before the product was sold.	Provide no special exemptions from punitive damages against manufacturers of products that had won approval from the FDA.	Same as H.R.956.
Time Limits	Retain current law	Allow a plaintiff to bring a lawsuit up to two years after discovering both the cause of an injury and the injury itself. Under existing statutes of limitations, the clock begins to run as soon as a product causes an injury, even if the victim cannot detect it or cannot discern its source.	Same as H.R.956.

Frivolous Lawsuits	Expose plaintiffs found to have filed a frivolous lawsuit to the potential burden of having to pay the other side's legal fees and other sanctions.	Retain current law.	Same as H.R.956.
Statute of Repose	Limit the time for filing product liability cases for most products to 15 years after delivery.	Limit the time for filing a product liability suit to 20 years after a product is delivered. This limit would apply to durable goods such as machinery used in the work place, but not to toxic materials, nor to commercial trains or airplanes. States would be allowed to keep in place any law providing a shorter limit. The measure would retain the right of plaintiffs to file suits when the manufacturer issued a specific warranty guaranteeing the product beyond the 20-year term limit.	No time limit provision.

SOURCE: HJ Hyde. Products Liability Fairness Act of 1995; Biomaterials Access Assurance Act of 1995 (H.R. 956) [Common Sense Products Liability and Legal Reform Act of 1995.] Legi-Slate Report for the 104th Congress, Quick Bill, 7 August 1995.

Government Standards Defense

The 1990 NRC/IOM report on contraceptive development recommended that the U.S. Congress enact a federal product liability statute that would give contraceptive manufacturers credit for approval of contraceptive drugs and devices (and their labeling) by the FDA. The gist of such an "FDA Defense"— sometimes termed "Government Standards Defense" or "Regulatory Defense"— is as follows: If it is established that an injury-causing aspect of a contraceptive drug or device was in compliance with all applicable requirements of U.S. federal food and drug law at the time that drug or device was made or sold, then a manufacturer or seller of a contraceptive drug or device would not be liable under any of the relevant legal theories (misrepresentation, warranty, negligence, or strict liability) for any injury related to design, nor liable for failure to provide adequate warning or instruction regarding any danger associated with its use, nor liable if the FDA had *not* asserted that the contraceptive drug or device was *not* in compliance.

However, the defense would *not* be available if a claimant were able to establish that the manufacturer should have made design modifications or given different or additional warnings or instructions; if the manufacturer or seller knew or should have known of studies showing increased risk of harm from the contraceptive drug or device that indicated increased likelihood of serious injury; or if the claimant established that the FDA was not informed of dangers regarding the contraceptive drug or device that were known to the manufacturer or seller, and that the injury to the claimant or persons sharing the claimant's medical characteristics was attributable to such dangers (NRC/IOM 1990). The arguments for the FDA defense are that punitive elements of damage awards are meant to punish egregious behavior, not to punish companies that have complied with the strict rules of the regulatory system and could not have predicted the side effects alleged to have caused the injury.

Counterarguments are that the proposed legislation would protect irresponsible corporations at the expense of people victimized by faulty products (Mayer 1995; Schrage 1995). In general, manufacturers of all types of products have sought to limit their liability exposure and consumer groups have generally opposed these efforts. The pivotal issue appears to be that proposals for some kind of government standards defense have generally overlooked the widely held public belief that people are entitled to compensation for harm, particularly harm caused by negligence (Foote 1988). Other countries (e.g., New Zealand, Canada) have addressed comparable concerns through comprehensive accident compensation plans, of which the National Vaccine Injuries Compensation Program (NVICP) in the United States is an example. An indicator of the tensions over the concept of a government standards defense is the fact that, although such a provision appears in the bill passed by the House of Representatives, it is not included in the Senate-passed bill owing to fears that opposition to the provision would kill the possibility of passage. Nonetheless, it is very important to note that the argument for some kind of government standards defense does not do away with liability. FDA compliance is, indeed, a shield, but noncompliance makes that shield useless.

Arguments raised against a government standards defense often mention the histories of diethylstilbestrol (DES)[10] and the Dalkon Shield as illustrative of the risks to consumers inherent in such a defense. In these cases, however, the primary lesson may have less to do with the fact of corporate irresponsibility than it does with the perils of nonregulation. In the case of DES, it was not until 1962, with the amendments to the 1938 Food, Drug, and Cosmetic Act, that the FDA's jurisdiction was expanded and its character shifted from being a premarket notification system to being a premarket approval system (Merrill 1994). The Dalkon Shield came on the market in the late 1960s, when FDA approval was not yet required for devices. The device proved to carry large risks to the user and approval would not be likely today.

The Case of the Dalkon Shield The costs of the Dalkon Shield were high in several respects. After paying $250 million to settle approximately 4,400 suits, and after juries in 11 cases had awarded $24.8 million in punitive damages against it, the manufacturer, AH Robins, declared bankruptcy and was ordered to set up a trust fund to compensate those injured by its product (NRC/IOM 1990). As of October 1995, the Dalkon Shield trust had paid $1.42 billion to 185,000 women in the United States and 110 other countries, with another $800 million to be distributed by the end of the year and $654 million and 6,000 claimants remaining (Steyer 1995).

Another cost was that other manufacturers, notably G.D. Searle, a Monsanto Company subsidiary, whose Copper-7 and Tatum-T IUDs had been tested before receiving FDA approval and were never found defective, pulled those products off the market in 1986. Nonetheless, the company got some of the backwash from the general legal turbulence and has had to defend against 2,063 suits. At the end of 1995, over 20 years after Searle first started selling its intrauterine devices, 40 suits and 346 foreign complaints remained. Information from the company indicates that, unlike Robins, the costs of litigation did not have significant impact on the company or its parent. Of the total suits filed, 24 went to trial, of which Searle won 19 and lost five. Of the five losses, four cost a total of $689,300. The fifth, *Kociemba v. Searle*, considered somewhat aberrant, was an award of $8.75 million by a jury critical of Searle's testing and marketing of the IUD; of that total, $1 million was for emotional distress, $750,000 for pain and disability, and $7 million for punitive damages, the only award in any of the Searle trials that had a punitive element (Steyer 1995).

Searle was not alone in bearing costs from the Dalkon Shield experience. The costs to women were also high, surely to those who were injured and, to an unknowable degree, to those women who lost contraceptive options they would have had if the safe IUDs had not disappeared from the market.

Limits on Punitive Elements in Awards of Damages

Another area of proposed reform targets the excesses of punitive elements in damage awards. There appears to be no disposition toward total forgiveness of punitive damages; the objective is to standardize a national cap on punitive amounts. In general, it is proposed that there be an absolute cap of around $250,000 or some multiple or sum of compensatory damages. The argument is that this reform would allow manufacturers to estimate the potential costs of suits resulting from a new product and remove the uncertainty created by the disparate tort rules among the states. Some of the proposed reforms also include an "escape hatch," which provides the judge hearing the case the discretion to disallow the limits if the defendant's behavior is found to have been flagrantly negligent, in which instance the potential size of the punitive award will once again become essentially limitless. Punitive elements in awards would be predicated on clear and convincing proof of conscious, flagrant indifference to safety; compensatory damages would not be affected. Another option is the filing of criminal proceedings against those individuals responsible for the corporate behavior resulting in injury; this would punish the guilty rather than those who have no direct control over management decisions, that is, shareholders, employees, or the public. Yet another possible variation would be articulation of a set of explicit standards for behavior warranting punitive damage awards that would provide clearer guidance for judges and juries; those who propose this variation note that punitive damages thereby become more predictable in some respects and more precisely targeted on the kinds of behavior that most merit strong deterrence (Garber 1993).

The fundamental argument in favor of limits is that the states' patchwork of laws and unpredictable, arbitrary, and excessive punitive damage awards raise corporate costs; discourage research, development, and innovation; hurt the competitive position of U.S. companies in an increasingly international marketplace; and expose companies to risks that are disproportionate (Mayer 1995; Spayd 1995). One specific consumer perspective in support of limits is that threats of liability may motivate companies to take off the market drugs that are of identified toxicity but still needed by some subpopulation(s) willing to trade off the risks, because the costs of not having the medication available are so high (Mayer 1995).

Arguments against limits are that, first of all, they would encourage the marketing of unsafe products that could be more profitable, since predictability would permit industry to price them with greater assurance. Secondly, limits would dilute the primary deterrent value of punitive elements, that is, the unpredictability and arbitrariness that industry finds so unsettling. A more generic argument is that, as a general matter, egregious corporate conduct should be harshly punished without limits.

Limited Liability of Biomaterials Suppliers

Currently, suppliers of raw materials are held liable for damage awards even though they have no direct role in the use of their material as a biomaterial. In March 1993, as a result of many and costly claims related to its silicone breast implants,[11] Dow Corning stopped supplying silicone for permanent medical implants and reproductive, contraceptive, obstetric, and cosmetic applications. When DuPont was caught up in suits against Vitek, which made temporomandibular jaw (TMJ) implants using DuPont's Teflon as a component, the company discontinued supply of materials including Teflon, Dacron, and Delrin to the medical implant industry, and it appears that the supply of polyethylene, used for the bearing surface of all total joint replacements, will be exhausted by the end of the year as well (Greenberger 1995). Though the precipitating factors, as well as the corporate responsibility, are different in each case, the net effect is the same: the departure of these and other companies from this industrial area and a loss of materials badly needed for medical purposes. Particularly affected are small producers of finished implants who cannot guarantee the stringent indemnity insurance and other requirements for testing and consumer education that raw materials suppliers are now demanding (Baker 1995). Manufacturers of contraceptive devices that use silicone-based or analogous biomaterials, for example cervical caps and implants, will soon need to find other sources or re-engineer their products. It may be that offshore producers may be a source but, so far, non-U.S. producers seem reluctant to enter the U.S. market because of liability and insurance concerns.

The critical distinguishing factors in determining bulk supplier liability are whether the component was defective when it left the seller's control, whether the seller adequately warned of known or knowable risks associated with the buyer's intended use of the component, and whether the component was transformed into an entirely new and different product (Baker 1995). The Biomaterials Access Assurance Act of 1995 being considered in the U.S. Congress would expressly preempt all tort claims brought against biomaterials suppliers in state or federal courts. As currently written, the Act specifies that a biomaterials supplier is liable for harm to the consumer of the finished product only if the product supplied did not meet contract specifications; it also specifies that the supplier may not also be the device manufacturer. The buyer must also be producing implants approved by, and registered with, the FDA, pursuant to the Federal Food, Drug, and Cosmetic Act, an oblique reflection of the relevance of government standards to defense against liability. Whether this sort of statutory protection will entice bulk suppliers back into the medical device market cannot be predicted. The inevitable restructuring of this market will be driven by two forces: Large multinational corporations, with their deep pockets, will leave the field to smaller producers of biomaterials; at the same time, the probability that indemnification agreements will become standard in all supply contracts to the medical implant industry may drive out the smaller producers of medical implants who cannot afford to honor those agreements, some of whom would then be absorbed by larger companies (Baker 1995; Hyde 1995).

Liability Protection During Research

Another proposal, under internal consideration at the National Institutes of Health, contemplates a statutory product liability exemption for institutions, investigators, and manufacturers from claims for non-negligent injury occurring in PHS-funded research involving (1) human subjects and (2) use of an Investigational New Drug or Device (IND or IDE) approved by the FDA for testing (NIH 1995).

At present, with a few exceptions for small subpopulations, the only recourse for a human subject injured in a clinical trial is through the courts. Correspondingly, research institutions, investigators, and manufacturers who are not federal employees but are involved in PHS-funded research can be sued for any injury that may befall a subject of the research. This is so even though the drug or device and its use in the research has been made as safe as the current state of scientific knowledge is able to make it. In other words, it has been cleared by the FDA for human testing, the research protocol has passed scientific peer review and human subjects protection review by an Institutional Review Board (IRB); and the subject has given informed consent acknowledging the possibility of unknown risks at this stage of investigation. To protect themselves, manufacturers and institutions must purchase product liability insurance, often prohibitively expensive or simply unavailable. This constrains research and the marketing of new drugs and devices and has already affected development of new means of fertility regulation and the testing of new vaccines against infectious diseases. The constraint is especially severe for small businesses who, for the same reason, have been unable to proceed with clinical testing of devices developed in the Small Business Innovation Research (SBIR) program (NIH 1995).

The NIH is concerned, nonetheless, that a statutory exemption from product liability suits would be prejudicial for the rare injured subject who would, then, have no recourse whatsoever. This would be contrary to Guideline 13 of the International Ethical Guidelines for Biomedical Research Involving Human Subjects, which states that:

> Research subjects who suffer physical injury as a result of their participation are entitled to such financial or other assistance as would compensate them equitably for any temporary or permanent impairment or disability. In the case of death, their dependents are entitled to material compensation. The rights to

compensation may not be waived (Council for International Organizations of Medical Sciences [CIOMS] 1993).

Thus NIH recommends a companion legislative provision that would broaden the definition of "federal employee" for purposes of eligibility for benefits and compensation distributed under the Federal Employees' Compensation Act (FECA), an action for which there is precedent (NIH 1995). A similar proposal was offered in the form of a recommendation by the IOM committee that reviewed the Fialuridine (FIAU) Clinical Trials (IOM 1995a). The recommendation was that there be a system of no-fault compensation for research injury by government, sponsors, or some combination of both. In effect, this is another application of the Government Standards Defense, but during the research period rather than the postmarketing period. The NIH proposition would not require a waiver of rights to compensation, but rather would simply remove the risk of potentially excessive punitive awards from manufacturers or researcher(s) involved in clinical trials funded by the NIH.

Legal Cases Related to Contraceptive Development

The 1990 NRC/IOM contraceptive technology report, in its summary of trends in litigation involving contraceptives, noted that, while every single contraceptive method then available had been the subject of product liability litigation, the history of each was diversely patterned. Litigation around the intrauterine devices has been characterized by extremes—massive liability for one product, but only limited recovery by claimants in cases involving other IUDs. In the case of oral contraceptives, litigation has been characterized by its longrunning nature, an almost exclusive focus on warnings given by manufacturers about side effects, and only uneven success with defense premised on the learned intermediary rule. Most relevant to consideration of a government standards defense is that most courts hearing cases concerning oral contraceptives have held that compliance with FDA regulations does not, of itself, necessarily constitute adequate warning; FDA compliance is only considered along with all other evidence of whether, in the circumstances, the warning was adequate (*MacDonald v. Ortho Pharmaceutical; McEwen v. Ortho Pharmaceutical*). Finally, three other cases involving a diaphragm, a spermicide, and a condom were so variable in adherence to the rules of evidence that they must be considered anecdotal, if not aberrant (NRC/IOM 1990).

The Case of Norplant

The most substantial contemporary case of litigation involving a contraceptive is the current experience of Wyeth-Ayerst, the distributor of the silicone-coated levonorgestrel-containing implant, Norplant. With 2.3 million users elsewhere in the world, a cumulative five-year failure rate of only 3.7 percent,[12] virtually no reports of major problems, and 27,000 physicians trained by Wyeth-Ayerst in insertion techniques, Norplant looked like a safe, effective, long-term yet easily reversible approach to family planning (White 1995). Indeed, when it was introduced into the United States in February 1991, sales moved briskly and soon 1 million U.S. women had adopted the method. Norplant's sales in its first full year—its best—amounted to $141 million and ran at about 800 units a day (Kolata 1995).

However, American Home Products Corporation or Wyeth-Ayerst have now been served with over 500 lawsuits alleging injury as a result of the insertion, use, or removal of the Norplant System, with approximately 12,800 plaintiffs named in those suits. From 85–90 percent of the plaintiffs are located in Texas, where one lawyer alone accounts for over 5,300 plaintiffs. One-third of the suits are in state courts, principally in Texas, Illinois, and Indiana. Two-thirds of the suits were pending in federal courts and were consolidated for pretrial purposes in Beaumont, Texas, as master class action complaint MDL-1038,[13] on counts of negligence; product liability; various permutations of fraud, misrepresentation, and breaches of warranties; and allegations of scarring and side effects (U.S. District Court, Beaumont, Texas 1995). As of late 1995, court actions in Beaumont, Chicago, and San Francisco, were occupied with matters of class certification. The first state case likely to come to trial is *Ulrich v. Wyeth-Ayerst*, set for Superior Court in San Francisco in early 1996. The original allegation was infection at the implant site, but plaintiffs' counsel have recently recast the case as one involving an unspecified autoimmune disorder caused by Norplant's Silastic tubing.

In contemplating the ramifications of litigation, it is important to note that many other parties have been sued along with American Home Products and Wyeth-Ayerst. These include: physicians or health care providers (including Planned Parenthood), who were involved in either the insertion or removal of the implant, or treatment of plaintiffs; Leiras Oy, the manufacturer of Norplant or its parent company, Huhtamaki Oy;[13] Dow Corning, which supplied the Silastic tubing, or other Dow entities; Schering AG, the German company which supplies the bulk levonorgestrel; and the Population Council, which developed Norplant.

The impetus for the Norplant litigation appears to have come from attorneys for a group of breast implant plaintiffs who filed "cookie-cutter" complaints that were then picked up by other plaintiffs' lawyers. The allegations of injury fall roughly into three categories:

1. Removal difficulty claims, including those related to capsule displacement, lengthy removals, or improper insertion;

2. Levonorgestrel-related claims, including acne, headaches, depression, fatigue, mood swings, weight gain, weight loss, excessive bleeding, ovarian cysts,

increased intracranial hypertension, premature birth, birth defects, and other allegedly hormonal-related injuries; and

3. Silastic-related claims, including autoimmune problems, fear of silicone, and other injuries allegedly related to the hardened silicone elastomer tubing which contains the levonorgestrel.

The rates of removal difficulties are within the expected rates stated in the Norplant labeling, as are the reported adverse events attributed to the levonorgestrel component, which do not differ substantially from those alleged against oral contraceptives over the last 20 years. As for silicone issues, there is no reputable scientific opinion linking the Silastic tubing used in Norplant with any autoimmune or related problems in women; the silicone elastomer used as the delivery system for Norplant has been used for over 30 years in a wide variety of medical products, including catheters, shunts, pacemaker leads, joint replacements, and tubal litigation bands.

In late summer 1995, the FDA publicly reaffirmed its support for Norplant in written testimony before the Subcommittee on Human Resources and Intergovernmental Relations of the U.S. House of Representatives Committee on Government Reform and Oversight:

> One specific area where biological effects [of silicone] have been assessed is with the contraceptive implant, Norplant. This product is a piece of closed tubing of silicone elastomer filled with crystals of drug that delivers the drug over a five-year period. The biological safety of the tubing has been studied in laboratory and animal toxicity tests. The silicone materials caused the expected local reactions, but tests to detect immunologic reactions were negative. In addition, reported cases of autoimmune or potentially immune-related disorders among women using Norplant are consistent with the expected rate in this population (Kessler 1995).

In a subsequent *Talk Paper*, the agency announced that it had recently approved a new patient acknowledgement form that has been incorporated into the product's labeling, which allows patients to acknowledge receipt of information and the opportunity for thorough discussion regarding Norplant prior to insertion. The FDA was also developing information to help assure that patients are appropriately informed of the product's risks and benefits before implantation. It also wrote that its ongoing analysis of adverse reaction reports and postmarketing surveillance studies had found no basis for questioning the safety and effectiveness of Norplant when the product is used as directed in the labeling. FDA's review had already assessed the safety and effectiveness of the hormone levonorgestrel for long-term contraception and the safety of Norplant's silicone-based delivery system. The organized medical community also continues to support Norplant. Wyeth-Ayerst insists that it will stay with the product and will soon file a new drug application for Norplant II, a two-rod, three-year formulation (White 1995).

Nonetheless, the experience is seen as chilling (Economist 1995; Kolata 1995; White 1995). In addition, the method has also become a lightning rod for other sorts of controversy. Because it was perceived in some quarters as a way to control fertility in certain populations, Norplant has been used at times inappropriately, coercively, and even punitively, and a number of minority women's groups have charged that such pressures have been inequitably placed on women of color. This, of course, is not the fault of the manufacturers but it does add to the general weightiness of the atmosphere. Furthermore, the method has also been inaccurately determined to be an abortifacient, such that the State of Pennsylvania, which for the first time in recent history appropriated state funds for contraceptives, explicitly excluded Norplant, as well as Depo-Provera and IUDs from inclusion. Finally, there have been tensions over the cost of the method (U.S. Congress 1994), although those may be resolved soon in negotiations for a public-sector price. Nevertheless, the fact that women worldwide continue to use the method and find it appropriate to their needs provides testimony to the value of other perspectives.

Alternative Models

Any evaluation of tort, product liability, and regulatory systems must identify the criteria against which those systems are to be evaluated. As this report goes to press, the fate of product liability reform in the United States is uncertain and regulatory reform is still in process. Yet, even if there are changes, in the United States or elsewhere, those changes and any subsequent proposals for reform need to be evaluated in terms of the way they meet broader social and economic goals since they quite naturally serve a variety of goals and interests. For example, analysts who stress the goal of deterrence as a criterion for evaluating tort law assess the pressures that can be exerted so that product manufacturers and marketers will act to minimize the possibilities of accidental risks and maximize information to potential users about known risks and their prevention or minimization (Schwartz 1994). Analysts concerned with individualized justice will stress goals of access to compensation, while those more concerned with collective or distributive justice will focus on the just allocation of risks and of resources for compensation among populations of consumers. Finally, analysts concerned with market-incentive and consumer-choice goals will balance market accommodation of improved products and consumer choice against consumer protection and the innovator's just responsibility for avoidable and unavoidable defects in their products and services (Dewees and Trebilcock 1992). Since different models of legal and regulatory reform serve different objectives, priorities, and economic or ideologic interests, and since a model that advances one goal may obstruct or frustrate another, selection of the "right" model has to wait until those goals and interests have been determined and priorities ordered. Table 7-3 summarizes four alternative models of liability by way of reference.

TABLE 7-3 Alternative Models for the Reform of Tort Law

Fault-Based Liability Model

Conventional tort law bases liability on fault, meaning failure to maintain the standard of care and performance the law expects of those whose actions can harm others. Most actions bear minimal risks of harm to others that no amount of care can reduce, and victims bear these losses alone, subject to any insurance coverage they may arrange for themselves. Fault attracts liability through individual access to a system of remedy, particularly the court system. Historic distinctions between civil compensation of individuals proportionate to the injury they have suffered and criminal punishment of wrongdoers for their wrong against the community at large are blurred when civil courts award punitive damages for egregious wrongs proven by civil plaintiffs. Punitive damages are justified by proven egregious fault, but reward the individual victim who sues first with a windfall profit disproportionate to the compensable loss actually suffered, and may deplete the resources from which others equally harmed may recover just compensation. This model serves the goal of individualized remedy, but may defeat the goal of distributive justice.

Strict Liability Model

This model permits recovery of compensation without a plaintiff demonstrating a defendant's negligence or other fault. Responsive to the goals of consumer protection, it fixes product manufacturers and perhaps intermediaries with liability for even the irreducible minimum of defects that products cause. The justification is that manufacturers and others seek profits from the distribution of products known to result in injury to a broadly defined population, although not necessarily to any individual user. Manufacturers and others are made insurers for injuries associated with promotion of products, and the model claims to balance individuals' interests in compensation with manufacturers', distributors', and others' interest in profit from trade. This model accepts that potential manufacturers, etc., economically unable or unwilling to trade on this basis, will be deterred from entering or remaining in a market. Conviction that a product should be on the market in the public interest will disfavor this model over that of no-fault liability.

No-Fault Insurance Model

This model, of which the U.S. National Vaccine Injury Act of 1986 is an example, balances the social need of a product being available to the public with the need to ensure that those injured through its use receive convenient and effective compensation. Built into the system of public supply will be a means to accumulate funds, from which those proven to have suffered injury related to use of the product will recover just compensation for their financial losses and their pain and suffering. Means to develop compensation funds include special taxes collected by government; add-on user fees that distributors return to manufacturers from which to meet claims; and, for instance, government provision of funds from general revenues.

This model serves the goal of protecting individual users, innovators who serve a public interest in product development, and public service. The model serves distributive justice regarding products whose availability serves the public interest, but it denies the goal of individualized justice in that it excludes an individual victim of injury from entering the "forensic lottery" that offers the prospect of windfall riches in the form of punitive damages. An alternative is to afford victims the choice between, on the one hand, certain and prompt compensation for losses and for pain and suffering, and on the other hand, the delayed, uncertain outcome of no recovery or high reward through litigation.

TABLE 7-3 Continued

Reproductive Health Model

This model is less a discrete model of legal reform than it is a framework or context within which choice may be made among the models outlined above. This framework might favor fault-based liability over strict liability, or the no-fault insurance model over fault-based liability, on grounds of social justice and the importance of reproductive health to the well-being of individuals and countries. The framework would provide a range of public sector incentives to encourage the private sector to respond to reproductive health needs as and when they arise. This report has identified the need for combined barrier methods, male methods, postcoital and once-a-month methods, and novel non-barrier female methods with fewer systemic effects, and has pointed to the potential of immunocontraception for providing leads to innovation in some of these priority areas. The overall principle of this model would be the development and distribution of these and other means conducive to the protection and promotion of reproductive health. Public sector incentives might include financial, tax, and other such incentives as extension of a patent period for contraceptive and STD products to public and private organizations, or incentives to develop and publicize new means to improve reproductive health.

THE ROLE OF INFORMATION

Informed Consent, Informed Choice, and Consumer Education

This leads to a necessary but difficult intersection where we feel compelled to raise the following questions. First, are there other ways of making the liability climate more "temperate" without sacrificing the rights and recourse of consumers—in this case, the consumers of contraceptives—that principles of justice require? Second, does any of this intersect with other areas of rights, importantly the right to know? Third, without reference to law or penalty, what circumstances will produce the kind of information that is needed for individuals and families to freely and fairly determine the number and timing of the progeny they bring into the world?

Issues of Definition

Informed Consent in Tort Law "Informed consent" is the general principle of civil law describing the duty to disclose to a patient or user of some health technology the risks and benefits of a proposed intervention, as well as the optional or alternative technologies or courses of treatment that are available, so that the patient may exercise his or her judgment by balancing probable risks against probable benefits. It is this knowledge that constitutes the basis of willing, uncoerced, and intelligent consent by the patient or user to a proposed intervention (IOM 1989; Jonsen et al. 1982; Reisman 1992; Wadlington 1984).

Informed consent is a pivotal doctrine under the theory of strict liability. Under this theory, liability derives from negligence in failing to adequately disclose alternative choices and the risks of serious potential consequences, or "failure to warn." Legal action will be based on whether the information given to the participant before securing consent adequately warned of potential risks and whether the degree of disclosure was reasonable given the circumstances. Patients are seen as needing special information, since their mere compliance with what health professionals propose to do to them may not be considered in law to amount to true consent, so that liability may then arise for negligence. The doctrine is seen as protecting patient autonomy and reflects the view that, first, mature individuals have the legal right to make decisions that affect them, a concept developed by courts, originally in the United States (Cook and Dickens 1989) and, second, that physicians may not remain silent because divulgence might prompt the patient to forego needed therapy (Faden and Beauchamp 1986). While the legal individualism that leads to the doctrine of autonomy may not be favored in other cultures, even countries whose laws do not require informed consent recognize that the health professional—client relationship imposes on the professional special duties of assessment and disclosure before treatment is undertaken (Cook and Dickens 1989). Thus, decisions in this area depend heavily on definitions of adequacy (IOM 1994a; Wadlington 1984), as well on concepts of validity, understanding, and voluntariness (Gray and Osterweis 1986; IOM 1994a).

Informed Consent in Research While the term "informed consent" is used both in connection with tort law and in connection with research, it has somewhat different meanings in each context, differences that stem from the differing bases for liability in terms of which party is the defendant. A pharmaceutical company, for example, might be sued on the basis of the theory of strict liability; a researcher ordinarily would be sued only on the basis of negligence, including battery in certain cases (IOM 1994a). "Informed consent" also has a somewhat different meaning in the context of the processes of IRBs that are required for all research supported by the U.S. Public Health Service. IRBs are charged with the review of risk-benefit ratios, confidentiality protections, and procedures for selection of subjects. An IRB is also responsible for ensuring that investigators obtain the consent of participants and reviewing the protocols prepared for doing so, although they only rarely observe the process of obtaining consent itself (Robertson 1982). As women are increasingly included in clinical trials, there may be more coincidence between the universe of research and the tort system in connection with research-related injury (IOM 1994a). This possibility could also expand in the context of introductory trials, since those straddle the research and marketing phases squarely; this signals an area where work needs to be done on improved approaches to and standards for informed consent in international settings, as well as ensuring consistent and effective use of the procedure (WHO/HRP 1991).

Informed Choice The argument has been made that, as a legalistic term deriving in most respects from the practice of law, informed consent is limited as a principle of social policy. In law, informed consent has as its primary goal the legal protection of manufacturers and/or health providers; thus, another conceptual framework is needed whose primary orientation is the protection of the patient or client (Carpenter 1989).

As with informed consent, the principle of patient autonomy is pivotal in informed choice, as is the question of adequacy of information. However, the emphasis is on information for the protection of the patient or client, a desirable objective even if there were no threat of liability (Dukes and Swartz 1988). That protection is achieved by avoiding injury; injury, in turn, is avoided by fully informing potential users about all aspects of a product they are considering and encouraging them *not* to use that product if they find any of those aspects unacceptable. A key element is the informing process. The assumption here is that provision of correct information is insufficient in itself; presentation, intelligibility, and confirmation that the information has been understood are necessary components of insuring that individual choices are truly informed (Carpenter 1989).

The Notion of Informed Choice

The term "informed choice" has been accumulating currency in the family planning community and among women's advocacy groups (WHO/HRP 1991). Table 7-4 disaggregates the concepts of informed consent and informed choice in terms of their relevance to the stages of contraceptive research and development and adds a third term, "consumer education," as a member of the same conceptual family. All concepts clearly overlap.

Elsewhere in this report we observe that there is no "universal woman" to whom the information in the report or its recommendations are meant to apply in some inevitable, culture-blind fashion. Nonetheless, there are two principles in the women's agenda that are arguably universal: (1) the goal of enhancing women's control over their own bodies, including control over the occurrence and timing of pregnancy; and (2) equity in women's physical safety and well-being.

Other commonalities among women are objective circumstances that can make the legal premises of informed consent, as well as the practical premises of informed choice, virtually empty. True freedom to participate in a research trial or to use a given contraceptive depends on the client's access to alternative methods. Poor, illiterate women, especially, may often have little or no choice among either clinical services or methods (IOM 1995a). Many women worldwide lack access to the full and accurate information, sympathetic and respectful provider-client interaction, continuity of care, and availability of other basic reproductive health services that are the *sine qua non* for both informed consent,

TABLE 7-4 The Relative Roles of Informed Consent, Informed Choice, and Consumer Education

	Informed Consent	Informed Choice	Consumer Education
Research			
Clinical trials phases I–III	X		
Introductory trials	X	X	
Research *cum* Marketing			
Clinical provision of contraceptives/ contraceptive services	X[a]	X	X
Over-the-counter provision of contraceptives		X	X
Postmarketing research		X	X

[a]At present, informed consent sign-off sheets are used in connection with the provision of the Progestasert and Paragard IUDs and, imminently, Norplant.

where that operates in law, or for exerting informed choice (Bruce and Jain 1995; Carpenter 1989; WHO/HRP 1991). Women who are particularly needy are also likely to be particularly vulnerable to incentives in cash or kind for participating in trials. Furthermore, culture, language, and educational level condition understanding to such a degree that the users of contraception—female or male—are often neither informed, consenting, nor freely choosing research participants or consumers (IOM 1994a, WHO/HRP 1991).

Each of these potentiating situations enhances the likelihood that something will go wrong, if only because no contraceptive method is appropriate for all users and the range of their preferences, and none is free of side effects, although some are more severe for certain users than for others. Another potentiating circumstance resides in the nature of technology itself, independent of the possibility that information about some method side effects was not uncovered in premarketing clinical trials (Forrest 1994b). As the histories of oral contraceptives and intrauterine devices make clear, the first drug in a new therapeutic class is unlikely to be the optimal version. Incremental improvements after initial adoption play an important role in pharmaceutical and biological development and take place not only in industrial R&D laboratories but in clinical practice as well. Thus, new technologies retain some degree of uncertainty long after their initial adoption (Gelijns and Rosenberg 1994).

Another key element in making informed choices is having the knowledge on which to assess relative risks. For example, as maternal mortality rates associated with pregnancy and childbirth fall in most places in the world, and as those declines are perceived as real, the risk equation shifts and women will want different kinds of information on which to base their contraceptive decisions; they will also be less inclined to accept really bothersome contraceptive side effects (Germain and Dixon-Mueller 1993). Women who must confront unsafe abortion as the only alternative to contraception will want to understand their contraceptive options on the basis of efficacy. Other women may need information that will permit them to make tradeoffs between risks of an infection that could be lethal for them or their children, vis-à-vis anti-infective and/or contraceptive side effects. The point is that the parameters for decision-making around contraceptive and anti-infective use are more complex than ever, so that the knowledge for exercising informed choice is ever more critical.

Consumer Education

Chapter 6 discusses the restructuring of health services and the biomedical commodities industry as a component of health care reform efforts worldwide. Among the most relevant of these dynamics is the proliferation of health care delivery models which fall under the rubric of "managed care." These include a shift from hospital-based health care to any model that is cost-effective, including preventive interventions, particularly those that are cost-effective in the shorter as opposed to the longer term. Concurrent with these shifts is a consumer movement which incorporates notions of the "educated patient," patient autonomy, health promotion, client-centered care, and the significance of client-provider information exchange. In the context of contraceptive use and family planning, these have become standard themes. The point is often made that at least some of the failure rates associated with contraceptive methods (e.g., barrier methods) are a function of inadequate information and support (WHO 1991) or, as in the case of emergency contraception, an almost total lack of communication from provider to client. Furthermore, there is ample evidence that women everywhere, to a varying extent, are inadequately prepared by providers for the possibility of contraceptive side effects, their implications, and appropriate response.

One implication of all this is that accuracy of information, its level of completeness, intelligibility, and overall effectiveness, always important, are becoming critical to health care in general and to reproductive health in particular. Though by far from the only element in consumer education, the packaging and labeling of contraceptives play—or could play—a much more useful role in the educational process of clinicians and consumers than they now do (Guest et al.

1993). At present, the labels and inserts in contraceptive packaging are daunting visually and technically, a fact often attributed to exigencies imposed by the FDA and to concerns about liability. At the same time, the FDA only has jurisdiction to approve package inserts as accurate statements of the safety and efficacy of their contents; they are not in the business of approving new, perhaps more effective ways of informing consumers and clinicians.

Labeling and package inserts can be dismissed as a small matter, or at least smaller than other forces that impinge on the availability and use of contraceptives, such as the roles of the media and advocacy groups, and the ideas, information and, sometimes, misinformation that flow through them. Still, a single categorical location where intelligible, accurate information about the technical aspects of individual contraceptive technologies—their risks, side effects, contraindications, benefits, and proper use—is consistently available could serve to anchor the information base. It is also the case that the media pay attention to package labels; in the case of the Reality female condom, an apparent misreading of the label published in a major trade journal, sent the manufacturer's stock plummeting (AIDS Alert 1994).

Nor is labeling a small matter in its technical complexity, regulatory considerations, and legal implications; even "cosmetically" it will take considerable thought and work. And, even assuming that the method in question is physiologically and socially appropriate for use by a given population, there will always be some part of that population for whom newly accessible information will make no direct difference, either because it does not fit into the ways they calculate risk, or because they receive the information inadequately transmitted through an intermediary. Nor is there any easy way to calculate the costs and benefits of better labeling. Revising labeling in some generic way would inevitably impose costs, but these would seem unlikely to be crippling for large companies (IOM 1994c).[15] In a clinic setting, helping individuals make informed choices takes time and effort, both at a premium for busy health care providers who may also have patient load quotas. A well-informed consumer may decide not to use a product after all, and a possible sale does not occur, yet another cost. Still, these costs must be arrayed against others: the putative harm to a user or a user's progeny, the costs of compensating that harm, the costs to the reputation of the firm, and the costs to other appropriate consumers of losing an option when a contraceptive method is withdrawn from the market.

THE ENVIRONMENT

Whatever may come to pass in regulation, law, and improvements in information about contraception, after all is said and done, each of these is nested in individual and societal systems of belief and behavior. To an extent that is highly variable, chronologically and by local and national setting, contraception has evoked a sometimes stunning range of controversy. This situation persists, again with great variety, despite the fact that contraception has become an accepted fact of life for millions of individuals worldwide and despite major changes in attitudes concerning women's rights to equity and choice.

At the heart of controversy reside two fundamental clusters of issues: beliefs about human sexuality, especially female sexuality, and beliefs pertaining to abortion. In many parts of the world, sometimes as a correlate of economic reversals, controversy may be expressed in a resurgence of conservative ideologies regarding women, their sexuality, and their rights, a resurgence that may originate in religious fundamentalism, ethnic nationalism, or social conservatism in reaction to concerns about excessive sexual and personal freedom (IWHC/ UWI 1994).

Sexuality

The United States is no exception. One scholar quoted in the recent IOM study of unintended pregnancy (IOM 1995b) notes that "Few if any societies exhibit a more perverse combination of permissiveness and prudishness in their treatment of sexual issues" and adds that the U.S. popular media are "filled with sexual material, while, on the other hand, there is a noted absence of equal attention to contraception, responsible personal behavior, and values in sexual expression."

Other analysts point to the deep strains of ambivalence about contraceptives among some groups in the United States. In some cases, the ambivalence is rooted in economic inequality, racial discrimination, and a history sometimes marked with coercive or punitive uses of contraception (Samuels and Smith 1992; Segal et al. 1994). In others, it derives from the asynchrony between a tradition of high demand for technologic solutions, particularly in health, and the broad strain of technologic minimalism born in the 1960s. Another dimension of this line of thought includes worries about the "hypermedicalization" of women's health and the high priority that is placed by some women's advocacy groups on the need for women to have total control over their own fertility. A more specific ambivalence springs from disappointments as limitations and, in some cases, real deficiencies of new contraceptives are revealed in use in large populations (Forrest 1994b). Finally, there is an underlay of cynicism about the profit motives of the private sector, currently fueled by attention to issues of pharmaceutical pricing and the privatization of health care.

All these areas of dissonance necessarily affect the exchange of accurate information about sexual behavior, contraception, and the avoidance of unintended pregnancy (Chen 1995). At the same time, the disjoints foster dissatisfaction with current contraceptive methods and, somewhat ironically, strong support for continued research and development of new ones (Forrest 1994b).

Abortion

The other major element of this conceptual environment has to do with beliefs about childbearing and the relative rights of parents and offspring, with definitions of the beginning of viable life *ex utero*, and with the ways abortion and contraception are seen to overlap. This overlap, real or not, matters greatly, whether or not abortion is defined as in itself a contraceptive method; whether it is defined as a last recourse in case of contraceptive failure; whether a specific method is defined as having abortifacient effect, even though science may provide evidence that no such effect is in play; or whether artificial contraception is seen, in itself, to be morally wrong. The resurgence of abortion as a central theme in the current U.S. political campaign, attempts to reverse *Roe v. Wade*, and efforts to eliminate the national family planning program are ample indication of the durable, penetrating character of these matters. For example, the State of Pennsylvania just, for the first time, appropriated state funds for contraceptives but excluded Norplant, Depo-Provera, and IUDs from being provided because they are considered abortifacients, a definition that is scientifically incorrect.

There appears to be more clarity about current methods of emergency contraception, which are well accepted by medical and legal authorities in the United States and Europe as not being abortifacients, but as methods that either prevent fertilization altogether or stop the fertilized egg from implanting in the uterine wall. In other words, methods that prevent implantation from occurring, or perhaps even completing, are appropriately regarded as contraceptives, not abortifacients (Holt 1995).[16] The same clarity of perception may be less likely in connection with the antiprogestins, since these offer potential for a number of interventions across the whole menstrual cycle, before and after implantation, a matter that will require special consideration.

Revisiting the Analogy with Vaccines

Issues of regulation and liability were also central in the years of discourse around vaccines (IOM 1985 and 1993). Vaccines and contraceptives are alike in that neither is a curative drug for people who are already ill; rather, both are administered to healthy individuals to prevent a condition they may never get. As a result, adverse reactions are much more noticeable and less tolerated by the vaccinee (IOM 1993), so that both product categories have been especially susceptible to "superlitigation" (Djerassi 1989). However, as discussed earlier in this chapter and in Chapter 3, the vulnerability of the pediatric vaccines to litigation has been much attenuated by the National Vaccine Injury Compensation Program (NVICP) in the United States and was already less of an issue in the European countries, many of which had instituted some kind of vaccine injury compensation program (IOM 1985).

The vaccines market, after decades of modest, birth-driven growth, entered a phase of dramatic expansion beginning in the mid-1980s. As of 1995, global vaccines sales reached approximately $2.5 billion, a market size close to that of the global market for contraceptives (FIND/SVP 1996).[17] Part of the expansion is attributed to industry's gradual appreciation of the potential of the NVICP (Day 1996) and part to a confluence of other policy decisions, importantly the establishment of pediatric vaccination as part of the health care regimen for all newborns in most developed countries and intensification of vaccination campaigns in developing countries under the guidance of the World Health Organization (FIND/SVP 1996). WHO efforts were pivotal in raising immunization coverage of the developing world's children from about 10 percent in the late 1970s to 80 percent in many countries by the late 1980s. These efforts received further impetus from the 1990 World Summit for Children, where most of the world's nations committed themselves to achieving 90 percent national coverage by the year 2000 (UNICEF 1992). Consequent to the Summit, WHO, in conjunction with other United Nations' agencies, the World Bank, and the U.S. Agency for International Development, established an International Children's Vaccine Initiative (CVI) that is working toward development of a multivalent pediatric "supervaccine" that would require just one or two doses administered orally and would be heat stable, affordable, and have a low rate of side effects (IOM 1993).

The vaccines market was further driven by development of new, genetically engineered vaccines (HiB-related meningitis, hepatitis A, and hepatitis B), as well as efforts to develop vaccines for such key needs as prevention of AIDS (FIND/SVP 1996). Analysts also attribute vaccine market growth to recognition of the emergence and resurgence of diseases, appreciation of infectious etiologies for some chronic diseases, and mounting drug resistance (IOM 1992). Greater awareness of the cost-effectiveness of vaccines is also considered a factor (FIND/SVP 1996) and by subsidized bulk procurement for vaccine provision to developing countries that has been able to evoke positive commercial response (Mercer Management Consulting 1994). The bottom line is that there are over a dozen new pediatric vaccines in development,[18] in addition to almost two dozen diseases targeted for preventive vaccines for adults.[19] To these must be added efforts at developing therapeutic vaccines, obviously including AIDS, cancer, and herpes, and work in novel delivery systems, including liposomes, microspheres, and nanoparticles.

However, vaccines are not about human sexuality nor have they confronted anywhere near the diversity of public opinion that swirls around contraception. Furthermore, vaccines are not generically blurred as technologies *qua* technologies, nor are issues around their delivery as culturally fraught. Vaccines are what they are: They prevent disease and their modes of action are not confused by the public with any other purpose or effect. In addition, it is understood that vaccines are to be delivered by a provider in a formal health system and, while they may be required by law, they are not perceived as coercive except by small minorities who resist vaccination for their children largely on religious grounds. In contrast, the provider role in contraception is frequently brought into question (Forrest 1994b; Richter 1994).

CONCLUDING COMMENT

Despite the imperfection of the analogy between vaccines and contraceptives, the vaccine experience does inform us that the issues around particularly controversial medical products, whatever the sources of controversy, tend to be incremental and systemic in their resolution. The vaccine experience took time—two decades of working groups charged with solving "the vaccine problem," a decade of legislative attempts to construct a passable bill, and close to a decade for industry to perceive that the legislative remedy was effective. Change came from several sources—from a surge of discovery in the science; from legislative action that modified public policy; and, in lesser measure, from the decision of a major international procurer of commodities to seek professional assistance in assessing its processes and their impact. This does not mean that the same amount of time will be needed for improvement in the contraceptive landscape, nor will the solutions be the same. The central implication is that there is not likely to be any "silver bullet" solution to the dilemmas faced by the field of contraceptive research and development, but that each piece of the dilemma will need to be considered and addressed as part of a coherent strategy.

REFERENCES

AH Robins Company. 1988 Annual Report and Form 10-K. Richmond, VA: AH Robins Company. 1988.

AIDS Alert. Barriers to better condom "killing people"; regulatory, political hurdles stifle development. Atlanta, GA: American Health Consultants. 1994.

American Law Institute (ALI). Restatement (Second) of Torts §402A. 1977.

Associated Press. FDA Defends Its Drug Program. Washington, DC: 12 December 1995.

Baker FD. Effects of products liability on bulk suppliers of biomaterials. Food and Drug Law Journal 50:455–460, 1995.

Bankowski Z, J Barzelatto, AM Capron, eds. Ethics and Human Values in Family Planning: 22nd CIOMS Conference, Bangkok, Thailand, 19–24 June 1988. Geneva: WHO Special Programme of Research, Development and Research Training in Human Reproduction and Council for International Organizations of Medical Sciences. 1989.

Barnett AA. FDA criticized by Republicans despite success. Lancet 346:1617, 1995.

Biotechnology Industry Organization (BIO). FDA Regulatory Reform: A Proposal by the Biotechnology Industry Organization. Washington, DC: BIO. 27 February 1995.

Bruce J, A Jain. A new family planning ethos. The Progress of Nations. New York: UNICEF. 1995.

Bulatao RA, RD Lee. An overview of fertility determinants in developing countries. IN Determinants of Fertility in Developing Countries, Vol. 2. RA Bulatao, RD Lee, eds. New York: Academic Press. 1983.

Carpenter PF. Informed choice as a way to reduce risks and prevent injury. IN No Fault Compensation in Medicine: Proceedings of a Joint Meeting of the Royal Society of Medicine and the

British Medical Association, 12–13 January 1989. RD Mann, J Havard, eds. London: Royal Society of Medicine. 1989.

Carpenter PF. Perspectives of industry, the physician, and government: Responsibility, risk, and informed consent. IN New Medical Devices: Invention, Development, and Use. KB Ekelman, ed. Washington, DC: National Academy Press. 1988.

Cates W Jr., KM Stone. Family planning: The responsibility to prevent both pregnancy and reproductive tract infections. IN Reproductive Tract Infections: Global Impact and Priorities for Women's Reproductive Health. A Germain, KK Holmes, P Piot, JN Wasserheit, eds. New York: Plenum Press. 1992.

Chen V. A new social norm . . . all pregnancies intended. Carnegie Quarterly Fall–Winter:10–11, 1995.

Clayton EW. Liability exposure when offspring are injured because of their parents' participation in clinical trials. IN Women and Health Research: Ethical and Legal Issues of Including Women in Clinical Studies, Vol. 2, Workshop and Commissioned Papers, AC Mastroianni, R Faden, D Federman, eds. Washington, DC: National Academy Press. 1994.

Clinton W, A Gore. Reinventing Drug and Medical Device Regulations, 3. Washington, DC: Office of the President, Task Force on Reinventing Government. 1995.

Cook RJ. Antiprogestin drugs: Medical and legal issues. Family Planning Perspectives 21(6):267–272, 1989.

Cook RJ, BM Dickens. Ethics and human values in family planning: Legal and legislative aspects. IN Ethics and Human Values in Family Planning: 22nd CIOMS Conference, Bangkok, Thailand, 19–24 June 1988. Z Bankowski, J Barzelatto, AM Capron, eds. Geneva: WHO Special Programme of Research, Development and Research Training in Human Reproduction and Council for International Organizations of Medical Sciences. 1989.

Corfman P. Memorandum to the Record re Action on NDA 20-246, 27 October 1992. Rockville, MD: Food and Drug Administration. 1992.

Council for International Organizations of Medical Sciences (CIOMS). Guidelines for Biomedical Research Involving Human Subjects. Geneva: CIOMS. 1993.

Cunningham G, et al. Williams Obstetrics. 19th Edition, pp. 1335–1336. 1993.

Day K. Vaccine maker gets a shot in the arm. Washington Post, Business section, pp. 18–19, 11 March 1996.

Dewees D, M Trebilcock. The efficacy of the tort system and its alternatives: A review of the empirical evidence. Osgoode Hall Law Journal 30:58–138, 1992.

Dixon-Mueller R. Abortion *is* a method of family planning. IN Four Essays on Birth Control Needs and Risks. R Dixon-Mueller, A Germain, eds. New York: International Women's Health Coalition. 1993.

Djerassi C. The bitter pill. Science 245:345–361, 1989.

Dukes MNG, B Swartz. Responsibility for Drug-induced Injury. Amsterdam: Elsevier. 1988.

[The] Economist. On the needless hounding of a safe contraceptive method. pp. 113–114, 2 September 1995.

Faden RR, TL Beauchamp. A History and Theory of Informed Consent. New York: Oxford University Press. 1986.

FIND/SVP. Pharmaceutical Market Reports: Summary of Research Report on the World Market for Vaccines. New York: FIND/SVP. 1996.

Flannery EJ. Products Liability Issues and Tort Reform Update. Presentation to the Institute of Medicine Workshop on Private-Sector Participation in Contraceptive Research and Development: Opportunities, Challenges, Strategies, 11 May 1995. Washington, DC: Covington and Burling. 1995.

Flannery EJ, SB Greenberg. Liability exposure for exclusion and inclusion of women as subjects in clinical studies. IN Women and Health Research: Ethical and Legal Issues of Including Women in Clinical Studies, Vol. 2, Workshop and Commissioned Papers, AC Mastroianni, R Faden, D Federman, eds. Washington, DC: National Academy Press. 1994.

Food and Drug Administration (FDA). Talk Paper, 17 August 1995a.

FDA. Vaginal Contraceptive Drug Products for Over-the-Counter Human Use. Federal Register, 60:6892, 1995b.

FDA. Assignment of Agency Component for Review of Premarket Applications. Federal Register 56:58,754, 1991a.

FDA. Intercenter Agreement Between the Center for Drug Evaluation (CDER) and Research and the Center for Devices and Radiological Health (CDRH), section VII.A.2, 31 October 1991b.

FDA. Premarket Testing Guidelines for Female Barrier Contraceptive Devices Also Intended to Prevent Sexually Transmitted Diseases. 4 April 1990.

FDA. Vaginal Contraceptive Drug Products for Over-the-Counter Human Use: Establishment of a Monograph; Proposed Rulemaking. Federal Register 45:82,014, 1980.

Food Labeling and Nutrition News, Sample Issue, 4 January 1996.

Foote SB. Product liability and medical device regulation: Proposal for reform. IN New Medical Devices: Invention, Development, and Use. KB Ekelman, ed. Washington, DC: National Academy Press. 1988.

Foreman J. FDA allows Depo Provera as injectable contraceptive. Boston Globe p. 1, 30 October 1992.

Forrest JD. Contraceptive use in the United States: Past, present and future. Advances in Population, Vol. 2. London: Jessica Kingsley Publishers Ltd. 1994a.

Forrest JD. Acceptability of Contraceptives in the United States. Paper prepared for the *Ad Hoc* Group on Population of the International Council of Scientific Unions (ICSU). New York: The Alan Guttmacher Institute. 1994b.

Fox JL. For AIDS, the FDA may be reforming itself. Biotechnology 13:314–315, 1995.

Garber S. Products Liability and the Economics of Pharmaceuticals and Medical Devices. Santa Monica, CA: RAND Institute for Civil Justice. 1993.

Gelijns A, N Rosenberg. The dynamics of technological change in medicine. Health Affairs13(3):28–46, 1994.

Germain A, R Dixon-Mueller. Whose life is it, anyway? Assessing the relative risks of contraception and pregnancy. Women's health advocates and scientists talk about contraceptive technology. IN Four Essays on Birth Control Needs and Risks. R Dixon-Mueller, A Germain, eds. New York: International Women's Health Coalition. 1993.

Gray BH, M Osterweis. Ethical issues in a social context. IN Application of Social Science to Clinical Medicine and Health Policy. L Aiken, D Mechanic, eds. New Brunswick, NJ: Rutgers University Press. 1986.

Greenberger P. Memorandum: Press Conference on Biomaterials Availability Legislation, and Statement on Biomaterials Access Assurance Act. Washington, DC: Society for the Advancement of Women's Health Research. 1 February 1995.

Guest F, F Stewart, J Trussell, C Ellertson. Enhancing Safe and Effective Use of Oral Contraceptives. Paper prepared for meeting of FDA Fertility and Maternal Health Drugs Advisory Committee, 29 October 1993. Rockville, MD: Food and Drug Administration. 1993.

Harper F, F James, O Gray. Torts, 2nd ed., Vols. 3 and 5. Boston: Little, Brown and Company. 1986.

Holt R. Emergency Contraception: Working Paper on Pharmaceutical Company Involvement. Los Angeles, CA: Pacific Institute for Women's Health, Western Consortium for Public Health. 1995.

Hughes S. Emergency contraception—A hard pill to swallow? Scrip Magazine, September 1995:48–52.

Hunt AR, A Murray. Courting success: The Republican Contract with America sets its sights on the legal system. SmartMoney, March 69–70, 1995.

Hutton J, M Borowitz, I Oleksy, BR Luce. The pharmaceutical industry and health reform: Lessons from Europe. Health Affairs 13(3):98–111, 1994.

Hyde HJ. Products Liability Fairness Act of 1995; Biomaterials Access Assurance Act of 1995 (H.R. 956) [Common Sense Products Liability and Legal Reform Act of 1995]. Legi-Slate Report for the 104th Congress, Quick Bill, 7 August 1995.

Institute of Medicine (IOM). Review of the Fialuridine (FIAU) Clinical Trials. FJ Manning, M Swartz, eds. Washington, DC: National Academy Press. 1995a.

IOM. The Best Intentions: Unintended Pregnancy and the Well-Being of Children and Families. S Brown, L Eisenberg, eds. Washington, DC: National Academy Press. 1995b.

IOM. Women and Health Research: Ethical and Legal Issues of Including Women in Clinical Studies, Vol. 1. AC Mastroianni, R Faden, D Federman, eds. Washington, DC: National Academy Press. 1994a.

IOM. Women and Health Research: Ethical and Legal Issues of Including Women in Clinical Studies, Vol. 2, Workshop and Commissioned Papers. AC Mastroianni, R Faden, D Federman, eds. Washington, DC: National Academy Press. 1994b.

IOM. Nutrition Labeling: Issues and Directions for the 1990s. D Porter, RO Earl, eds. Washington, DC: National Academy Press. 1994c.

IOM. The Children's Vaccine Initiative: Achieving the Vision. VS Mitchell, NM Philipose, JP Sanford, eds. Washington, DC: National Academy Press. 1993.

IOM. Emerging Infections: Microbial Threats to Health in the United States. J Lederberg, RE Shope, SC Oaks Jr., eds. Washington, DC: National Academy Press. 1992.

IOM. Medical Professional Liability and the Delivery of Obstetrical Care, Vol. I. Washington, DC: National Academy Press. 1989.

IOM. Vaccine Supply and Innovation. Washington, DC: National Academy Press. 1985.

International Women's Health Coalition, and Women and Development Unit, University of the West Indies Challenging the Culture of Silence: Building Alliances to End Reproductive Tract Infections. [Report of a Conference on Reproductive Tract Infections among Women in the Third World, Barbados, March 1992]. P Antrobus, A Germain, S Nowrojee, rapporteurs. New York: International Women's Health Coalition. 1994.

Jones EF, JD Forrest, SK Henshaw, J Silverman, A Torres. Pregnancy, Contraception, and Family Planning Services in Industrialized Countries. New Haven: Yale University Press. 1989.

Jonsen AR, M Siegler, WJ Winslade. Clinical Ethics: A Practical Approach to Ethical Decisions in Clinical Medicine. New York: Macmillan. 1982.

Jordan A. FDA requirements for nonclinical testing of contraceptive steroids. Contraception 46:499–509, 1992.

Kessler DA. Testimony Before the Subcommittee on Human Resources and Intergovernmental Relations of the House Committee on Government Reform and Oversight. Washington, DC, 1 August 1995

Kolata G. Will the lawyers kill off Norplant? New York Times, Section 3, p. 1, 28 May 1995.

Lasagna L. Impact of Funding and Policy Changes on the Food and Drug Administration. Manuscript submitted for publication. Boston: Tufts Center for the Study of Drug Development. July 1995a.

Lasagna L. What's Wrong with the FDA? Unpublished manuscript. Boston: Tufts Center for the Study of Drug Development. July 1995b.

Levine C. Women and HIV/AIDS research: The barriers to equity. Evaluation Review 14(5):447–463, 1990.

Lewin T. Fears, suits and regulations stall contraceptive advances. New York Times, Business section, pp. 1, 12, 27 December 1995.

Macklin R. Ethics and human values in family planning: Perspectives of different cultural and religious settings. IN Ethics and Human Values in Family Planning: 22nd CIOMS Conference, Bangkok, Thailand, 19–24 June 1988. Z Bankowski, J Barzelatto, AM Capron, eds. Geneva: WHO Special Programme of Research, Development and Research Training in Human Reproduction and Council for International Organizations of Medical Sciences. 1989.

Mathieu M. New Drug Development: A Regulatory Overview, 3rd ed. Waltham, MA: Parexel International Corporation. 1994.

Mayer CE. Getting personal on product liability: Two lawmakers' opposing views stem from their own painful experiences. The Washington Post, pp. D1–4, 7 March 1995.

Mercer Management Consulting. Summary of UNICEF Study: A Commercial Perspective on Vaccine Supply. New York: Mercer Management Consulting. 1994.

Merrill RA. Regulation of drugs and devices: An evolution. Health Affairs 13(3):47–69, 1994.

National Institutes of Health. Fiscal Year 1997 Legislative Proposal: Products Liability Exemption for PHS IND and IDE Research. Bethesda, MD: National Institutes of Health. 1995.

National Institutes of Health (NIH). Long-term Effects of Exposure to Diethylstilbestrol (DES), NIH Workshop, Falls Church, VA, 22–24 April 1992.

National Research Council and Institute of Medicine. Developing New Contraceptives: Obstacles and Opportunities. L Mastroianni Jr, PJ Donaldson, TT Kane, eds. Washington, DC: National Academy Press. 1990.

National Women's Health Network. Memorandum to Dockets Management Branch, Food and Drug Administration: Vaginal Contraceptive Drug Products for Over-the-Counter Human Use (Docket No. 80N-0280). Washington, DC: National Women's Health Network. 2 June 1995.

Newbille CI. The "injectable contraceptive"—Depo Provera: Cause for alarm, not celebration. Health and Fitness 1:6, 1993.

Peterson MA. Civil Juries in the 1980s. Santa Monica, CA: Rand Institute for Civil Justice. 1987.

Prichard JRS. Canadian Feral/Provincial/Territorial Review on Liability and Compensation Issues in Health Care. Toronto: University of Toronto Press. 1990.

Prosser W, P Keeton. Prosser and Keeton on Torts, 5th ed. St. Paul, MN: West Publishing. 1984.

Reisman EK. Products liability: What is the current situation and will it change (and how) when more women are included in studies? Paper presented at the Women in Clinical Trials of FDA-Regulated Products Workshop, Washington, DC, Food and Drug Law Institute, 5 October 1992.

Richter J. Beyond control: About antifertility vaccines, pregnancy epidemics and abuse. IN Power and Decision: The Social Control of Reproduction. G Sen, R Snow, eds. Cambridge, MA: Harvard University Press. 1994.

Robertson JA. The law of institutional review boards. UCLA Law Review 25:484–549, 1982.

Samuels SE, MD Smith, eds. Norplant and Poor Women. Menlo Park, CA: The Henry J. Kaiser Family Foundation. 1992.

Sathyamala C. Depot-medroxyprogesterone acetate and breast cancer: A critique of the WHO's multinational case control study. Medico Friend Circle Bulletin 220:1-5, 1995.

Scheper-Hughes N. Death Without Weeping: The Violence of Everyday Life in Brazil. Berkeley: University of California Press. 1995.

Schrage M. Shielding companies from suits is just industrial policy in disguise. The Washington Post, p. B3, 10 March 1995.

Schwartz GT. Reality in the economic analysis of tort law: Does tort law really deter? University of California at Los Angeles Law Review 42:377–444, 1994.

Schwartz J. FDA revises biotechnology rules: Changes are designed to consolidate and speed approval process. Washington Post, Federal Page, p. A19, 13 November 1995.

Segal SJ, GP Talwar, RG Edwards. The Agenda for Contraceptive Research. Paper prepared for the Ad Hoc Group on Population of the International Council of Scientific Unions (ICSU). New York. 1994.

Sivin I. International experience with NORPLANT® and NORPLANT®-2 contraceptives. Studies in Family Planning 19(2):81094, 1988.

Smith SD. The critics and the "crisis": A reassessment of current conceptions of tort law. Cornell Law Review 72:765–798, 1987.

Snow R, P Hall. Steroid Contraceptives and Women's Response: Regional Variability in Side-Effects and Pharmacokinetics. New York: Plenum Press. 1994.

Spayd L. America, the plaintiff: In seeking perfect equity, we've made a legal lottery. The Washington Post, Outlook section, 5 March 1995.

Squires S. DES daughters and their children. The Washington Post, February 19:14. 1991.

Steyer R. Searle nearing end of lawsuits over Copper 7 contraceptive. St. Louis Post-Dispatch, p. 1-E, 15 October 1995.

Swenson S. Depo-Provera: Loopholes and double standards. Hastings Center Report 17:3, 1987.

Trussell J, K Sturgen, J Strickler, R Dominik. Comparative contraceptive efficacy of the female condom and other barrier methods. Family Planning Perspectives 26(2):66–72, 1994.

United Nations Children's Fund (UNICEF). The State of the World's Children 1992. New York: Oxford University Press. 1992.

United States Congress, House of Representatives. Impact of the high cost of long-term contraceptive products on federally sponsored family planning clinics, welfare reform efforts, and women's health initiatives. Hearing before the Subcommittee on Regulation, Business Opportunities, and Technology of the Committee on Small Business, 103rd Congress, 2nd session. Washington, DC, 18 March 1994.

United States District Court for the Eastern District of Texas, Beaumont Division. Memorandum Opinion and Order Granting Plaintiffs' Motion to Remand (Case No. 1:94CV5006). Beaumont, TX, 17 March 1995.

Wadington W. Breaking the silence of doctor and patient (review of J. Katz's The Silent World of Doctor and Patient). The Yale Law Journal 93(8):1640–1651, 1984.

Washington Post. Editorial: Drug Regulation and Reform. 5 December 1995.

White K. Contraceptive makers chilled by court challenges. Journal of Women's Health 4(3):223–224, 1995.

World Health Organization. Creating Common Ground: Women's Perspectives on the Selection and Introduction of Fertility Regulation Technologies—Report of a Meeting Between Women's Health Advocates and Scientists, 20–22 February 1991. Geneva: WHO/Special Programme of Research, Development and Research Training in Human Reproduction and the International Women's Health Coalition. 1991.

World Health Organization Collaborative Study of Neoplasia and Steroid Contraceptives. Depo-medroxyprogesterone Acetate (DMPA) and Cancer: Memorandum from a WHO Meeting. Bulletin of the WHO 64(3):375–382, 1986.

Zabin LS. Addressing adolescent sexual behavior and childbearing: Self esteem or social change. Women's Health Issues 4:93–97, 1994.

NOTES

1. Although Depo-Provera was manufactured and marketed by a U.S. company (Upjohn), the U.S. Food and Drug Administration (FDA) did not approve it for routine contraceptive use until 1993 because, among other reasons, the FDA concluded that other contraceptives were equally or more convenient, safe, and effective. This decision made the drug unavailable to countries with a "country of origin approval rule" even though, unlike the United States, some of those countries had no alternatively available or appropriate contraceptives (Cook and Dickens 1989). At the same time, there was much debate around the fact that the drug was eventually licensed for contraceptive use in over 90 countries while the FDA continued to withhold approval, a circumstance considered by some analysts as constituting an "ethical double standard" (Swenson 1987). At the same time, other

groups—for example, the National Black Women's Health Project and Women of All Red Nations (WARN) in the United States, and several women's advocacy groups in India—expressed concern about Depo-Provera (Foreman 1992; Newbille 1993; Sathyamala 1995, Swenson 1987). Concerns have tended to fall into two categories: issues of side effects and the method's potential for coercive applications.

2. Beagle dogs were found to respond differently to steroid hormones, at the receptor site and systemically, than do humans. As a result, regulatory bodies in other countries and the WHO toxicology review committee all agreed that beagle dogs were inappropriate as testing models for steroid use in humans.

3. The NDA is the vehicle through which drug sponsors obtain FDA authorization to market a new pharmaceutical in interstate commerce. In the NDA, the sponsor proposes that a compound be approved, and uses clinical data, nonclinical data, and other information to show that the drug is safe and effective for the proposed indication (Mathieu 1994).

4. The Supreme Court recently rejected the long-standing *Frye* rule, which required that any proposed scientific testimony must have received general acceptance of its reliability by the relevant scientific community before the court would admit it into evidence. In *Daubert v. Merrell Dow Pharmaceuticals*, the Court explained that *Frye*'s general acceptance standard was superseded by the adoption of the Federal Rules of Evidence. Under the Federal Rules, the trial judge makes a flexible determination of whether the evidence rests on a reliable foundation and is relevant to the task at hand. The effect this change will have on the liability climate is unknown (IOM 1994a).

5. The rule for devices is different. Courts have concluded that state tort claims relating to medical devices are preempted under a provision of the Federal Food, Drug, and Cosmetic Act, 21 U.S.C. Section 360K(a) (E. Flannery, personal communication, 1996).

6. The term "clinical studies" encompasses a wide range of activities. In pharmaceutical testing, it usually refers to randomized clinical trials, using either a placebo or an established therapeutic as the control. Clinical studies also include the early-phase safety studies in health volunteers, postmarketing studies to expand indications for use or investigate safety and effectiveness in special populations, and investigations of the outcome of health interventions (Flannery and Greenberg 1994).

7. "Punitive damages" is really a term of art. The more accurate statement is that there is an element of punishment in many tort judgments for damages (W Wadlington, personal communication, 1995). We use the term, however, because it is less cumbersome.

8. E.g., Arizona, Colorado, New Jersey, Ohio, Oregon, and Utah have passed legislation that allows the manufacturer of an FDA-approved product to assert a government standards defense in response to claims for punitive damages (Ariz. Rev. Stat. Ann. §12-701[A][1992]; Colo. Rev. Stat. Ann. §13-21-403[1] [West 1989]; N.J. Stat. Ann. §58C-5[c] [West 1987]; Ohio Rev. Code Ann. §2307.80C [Anderson 1996]; Oreg. Rev. Stat. Ann. §30.927 [1995]; Utah Code Ann. §78-18-2[1] [1995]). In addition, two states, Illinois and North Dakota, have adopted a defense to punitive or exemplary damages for products that have been approved by a state or federal regulatory agency with authority to approve the product in question (Ill. Rev. Stat. §5/2-2107 [1996] [state or federal]; N.D. Cent. Code §32-03.2-11 [1995] [federal]. (NRC/IOM 1990; M Powell, personal communication, July 1996).

9. The House and Senate accepted the conference report, referred to as H.R. 956, but the President vetoed the bill and the veto override attempt failed. This was reported in the press (cf. *Wall Street Journal*, 3 May 1996, p. A12), too late to permit incorporation of that information into the body of this document. This outcome means that the issue remains an issue..

10. DES was a synthetic estrogen widely prescribed in the 1940s and 1950s to prevent miscarriage by enthusiastic physicians who overlooked large, controlled clinical trials indicating that DES was ineffective and focused instead on smaller studies in which the drug appeared to show promise (Levine 1993). In the late 1960s and early 1970s, the drug was found to be clearly causative of grave injury to the offspring of pregnant women who had taken it, primarily their female offspring (NIH

1992). The ensuing legal actions were numerous and costly, with over a thousand pending nationwide as of February 1991 (Squires 1991). Of high relevance for the area of research liability were the awards for battery made to women involved in clinical trials of DES who had not been informed that they were part of a study (IOM 1994a). The experience encouraged exclusion of pregnant and potentially pregnant women from clinical research and the writing of FDA guidelines to reinforce that practice (IOM 1994a).

11 . Dow Corning was to be the largest contributor ($2 billion) to the $4.2 billion class action settlement reached in 1994 among breast implant manufacturers (including Bristol-Myers Squibb, Minnesota Mining and Manufacturing, and Baxter International) and the approximately 400,000 women signed up to participate in the settlement. However, Dow filed for bankruptcy in May 1995 and withdrew. The settlement remains the largest liability settlement in U.S. history and, since an additional 7,000 women are filing individual suits (Kolata 1995), the costs can only rise.

12. This failure rate is based on clinical trials with two types of Norplant capsules: the original hard capsules and newer soft capsules. Cumulative failure rates through the end of five years were 4.9 percent for the hard capsules and only 1.6 percent for the capsules made of soft tubing (Sivin 1988). Leiras Oy, Norplant's manufacturer, now only uses soft tubing.

13. MDL = Multidistrict litigation.

14. In February 1996, Huhtamaki Oy announced that negotiations were under way on the sale of its pharmaceutical division, Leiras, to an international pharmaceutical company. ". . . The operating environment for Leiras has changed, hence our decision to concentrate on the foods division." This may have a major impact on the availability and/or price of Norplant implants for public-sector purchasers of the product. It is not clear at the time of this writing whether the decision is in any way related to the company's experience with Norplant and what that might imply.

15. The FDA estimates that implementation of nutrition labeling required under the recently enacted Dietary Supplement Health and Education Act will cost that industry from $52 to $85 million to implement (Food Labeling and Nutrition News 1996).

16. According to medical textbooks, pregnancy begins when the process of implantation of the ovum in the uterine wall is complete. Implantation is not generally regarded as complete until 28 to 31 days from the first day of a woman's last menstrual period, assuming regular cycles (Cunningham 1993; Holt 1995). This prevailing medical opinion has been followed by policy makers and courts in Europe and the United States (*e.g., Brownfield v. Daniel Freeman Marina Hosp., 256 Cal. Rptr. 240, 245 [Ct. App. 1989]; Margaret S. v. Edwards, 488 F. Suppl. 181, 191 [E.O. La. 1980]*).

17. The pediatric vaccines accounted for over 60 percent of that market, U.S. sales for slightly under half. The market is expected to enter a period of more modest growth through the 1995–1999 forecast period, followed by a second surge after the year 2000, fueled by the introduction of vaccine products to treat diseases for which there is now no preventive vaccine, the growth of mega- or multivalent vaccines, and the WHO "supervaccine" (FIND/SVP 1996).

18. Acute infantile gastroenteritis; DTaP-HIB; DTaP-IPV-HIB; group A and group B streptococcus; hemophilus influenzae type B; malaria; meningococcus A,B, and C; pertussis; pneumoccocal disease; polio; pseudomonas infections; and respiratory syncytial virus.

19. Cholera; dengue fever; gonorrhea; group B streptococcus; helicobacter pylori; hepatitis A, B, C, D, E, and X; herpes virus; human B19 parvovirus vaccine; influenza; Lyme disease; rheumatoid arthritis; staphylococcus aureus infections; traveler's diarrhea; and a range of new adjuvants.

8

Recommendations

This study began with three questions.

The first was: Is there really a need for new contraceptives and, if so, why?

The second was: If, as has been said, the field of contraceptive research and development has somehow lost the energy that characterized it at the time of what is called the "first contraceptive revolution," are there new prospects in the science that could reenergize it?

The third was: Given such prospects, would they be sufficient to accomplish that revitalization; if not, why not; and what sort of climate and resources would be required for that to happen? Thus, the Institute of Medicine and this study committee were challenged not only with investigating what the new science had to offer, but with examining the climate for collaboration between the public and private sectors in translating those offerings so as to meet the need and demand for new contraceptive options.

Throughout its work, the committee sought to frame its exploration and possible response to these issues around contraceptive research and development in a way that might offer a fresh outlook on the subject. Four concepts seemed to merit integration into such a framework: the idea of a "woman-centered agenda," the challenge of unintended pregnancy, consideration of contraceptives from both the perspective of need and market demand, and new possibilities for collaboration between the sectors.

The committee concluded that there *is* indeed a need for new contraceptives, as well as evidence of a real market for them. While the existing array of contraceptive options represents a major contribution of science and industry to human well-being, nonetheless it fails to meet needs in significant populations;

furthermore, the costs of that failure are high, for societies, for families, and for individuals. The committee also found that an agenda for contraceptive research and development that is "woman-centered" to be reasonable, just, and also market-worthy. The challenge is to find creative ways to elicit the best response from the scientific and industrial communities in a conducive climate that protects the integrity of inquiry and the safety of consumers.

The issue of climate is central. The aspects of context that press on every effort to provide safe and effective contraceptive technologies are complex and reflective of deeply rooted differences and deeply held beliefs. In addition, there is the current atmosphere of fiscal austerity in so much of the world, an atmosphere that cannot be ignored. At the same time, what is to be done about real, urgent, and unmet needs that affect public health and well-being everywhere? The committee opted for a set of recommendations that are neither glamorous nor sweeping. They are, instead, unified by their practicality, located in the middle ground of policy, and intended to respond to what seem to be the needs of a significant majority.

Finally, the committee chose to use this closing chapter to simply list its recommendations, without elaboration and divided into two main sections: first, the criteria for and the prospects of the science and, second, the elements of context that will need to be affected if the science is to advance significantly and the needs and demands of individuals and families are to be met. The reader is referred to the summary at the very outset of this report which frames each recommendation in the larger setting to which it corresponds. Each presentation serves a slightly different policy objective for different audiences, while the report as a whole is meant as a review of the various key dimensions of this very complicated but very essential topic.

THE PROSPECTS OF THE SCIENCE

Recommendation 1. The committee recommends that priorities for new research be assessed against the preference criteria presented in a new "woman-centered agenda" and that existing public-sector contraceptive research and development portfolios be reassessed similarly. Such an approach highlights the need for improvements and new advances in contraceptives for women, and in areas where there are few or inadequate options, namely:

• Methods that act as chemical or physical barriers to conception and to transmission of sexually transmitted diseases, including the human immunodeficiency virus (HIV);
• Menses-inducers and once-a-month methods targeted at different points in the menstrual cycle;
• Methods for males that would expand their contraceptive choices and responsibility.

Recommendation 2. Modern scientific methods now exist that can identify genes whose products are involved solely in reproduction and are therefore prime targets for inhibition of conception. Fundamental research on the cells, tissues, and organs that contribute to conception can now be carried out with a new and incisive precision using tools of modern biology. The committee recommends, therefore, that priority be accorded to work with genes whose products are truly specific and urges attention to the fact that investment in basic research in contraception will be essential if work with these elements is to proceed with reasonable dispatch. Absent such investment, it is hard to see where innovative new approaches to contraception will come from.

Recommendation 3. Toward development of new contraceptive methods for females and for males, the areas of specific research that have come to light during this study and that this committee believes deserve the greatest attention in the shorter and longer terms are presented in Boxes 8-1 and 8-2.

Recommendation 4. The committee believes that the field of immunocontraception holds promise: for contraception, for innovative approaches to barriers to infection, and for areas of science with broader applications. The committee recommends the emphases presented in Box 8-3.

Recommendation 5. The committee urges that the research and development of anti-implantation and postimplantation methods be pursued as a response to a major public health need and to evidence of demand. Nonetheless, because the area of postimplantation is so controversial and thus unlikely to attract investment by large pharmaceutical companies, partnerships between smaller firms and nonprofit organizations may represent the most appropriate avenues for research, in the United States and elsewhere. The committee recommends this area of research and development as a priority for funders for whom this controversy is not constraining. Research on monthly methods up to and including implantation should also have high priority.

ADVANCING THE SCIENCE AND TRANSLATING UNMET NEED INTO MARKET DEMAND

Recommendation 6. The committee recommends that, to make a full range of contraceptive products accessible to consumers and to increase demand for contraceptive products to something closer to the level of unmet need, there should be continued and sufficient government support of contraceptive services—for males as well as females—particularly for low-income individuals and particularly in developing countries. The committee also recommends that third-party payers, who bear the costs and may reap the benefits of the health status of their covered populations, include contraception as a covered service. Ideally, family

---

Box 8-1
Approaches to New Contraceptive Methods for Females

Vaginal Methods (Barriers)

Short-to-medium term:

- identifying agents that are spermiostatic rather than spermicidal
- developing antifertility agents that inhibit virus and/or other pathogenic organisms in the vagina
- modifying mucous secretions from cervical epithelial cells to prevent sperm passage

Monthly Methods and Menses-inducers

Short term:

- evaluating combinations of antiprogestins, antiestrogens, and inhibitors of enzymes involved in steroid synthesis to induce menses

Long term:

- understanding factors involved in blastocyst implantation
- developing specific luteolytic agents

Inhibition of Ovulation

Long term:

- inhibiting ovulation using nonpeptide GnRH antagonist/hormone combinations
- understanding the mechanism controlling follicular rupture as a way to prevent ovulation while permitting development of the corpus luteum

Inhibition of Fertilization

- inhibiting sperm-egg fusion, acrosome reaction induction, and sperm transport
- understanding the molecular basis of follicular atresia and luteinization, to provide leads for specific induction of atresia in the dominant follicle

---

planning services and the management of sexual health would be integrated as components of comprehensive reproductive health services.

Recommendation 7. The committee recommends that consideration be given to a multilateral approach that would enlist the participation of public agencies and private philanthropic organizations toward support for an extension of the Global

---

Box 8-2
Approaches to New Contraceptive Methods for Males

Short term:

• inhibiting LH and FSH secretion by combinations of progestin/androgen as long-acting injectables or implants

Long term:

• targeting spermatogenesis using inhibition of FSH secretion, or FSH action using receptor blockers
• inhibiting meiosis
• affecting epididymal function to disrupt sperm maturation
• inducing premature acrosomal activation
• identifying genetic loci that affect gamete development or behavior, and developing inhibitors of these functions

---

Box 8-3
Approaches to Immunologic Contraception for Females and Males

• pursuit of multideterminant sperm immunogens and early conceptus antigens
• increased research on antibodies to reproductive hormones and their receptors
• increased research on the local immune response of the female reproductive tract
• emphasis on immunologic methods protective against HIV (human immunodeficiency virus), HSV (herpes simplex virus), and HPV (human papilloma virus)

Contraceptive Commodity Programme that would create incentives for the development of *new* contraceptives. Since contraceptive procurement is already tiered and since both purchasers and vendors appear to accept that as a fact of life, an additional tier might be constructed for volume commitments for procurement of *new* contraceptives at prices that would constitute an incremental attraction to industry and still be feasible for countries able and willing to expand the range of contraceptives available to their populations.

Recommendation 8. The committee strongly endorses continued public sector support of, first, basic research in innovative areas of reproductive biology as a source of new leads for contraceptive research and development and, second, in the applied research that will bring the most promising leads to fruition. The committee believes that the greatest value added will accrue to strategies focused on attracting investment in those smaller domestic and foreign firms able and willing to do upstream research in contraceptives or in a fundamental reproductive mechanism of particular promise. In this connection, the committee calls attention to the new Consortium for Industrial Collaboration in Contraceptive Research, whose purpose is to catalyze funding for feasibility studies and matching industry investment in early-stage contraceptive research and development in priority areas of the woman-centered agenda. The committee believes this initiative to be a creative and potentially high-payoff mechanism for sponsor investment.

Recommendation 9. The committee recommends that approval guidelines be developed as quickly as possible for the high-priority area of vaginal microbicides and spermicides, as a first step toward clarifying requirements for clinical trials and monitoring of novel contraceptives in general. A consensus conference on this topic is recommended, perhaps convened by the World Health Organization. Of special concern in this specific context are guidelines for what would constitute clinically significant levels of anti-infective efficacy, as well as risk of possible fetal exposure.

Recommendation 10. The committee reiterates the 1990 NRC/IOM committee recommendation that the U.S. Congress enact a federal product liability statute that gives contraceptive manufacturers credit for FDA approval of contraceptive drugs and devices. When the FDA has considered the relevant health and safety data on a contraceptive product, has approved the product, and has required warning and instructions to accompany it, it is sound national policy to make this approval available to manufacturers as a limited defense and not to penalize them for something they could not have known at an earlier point. Because the statute would interact with postmarketing surveillance efforts, this recommendation would be more compelling were formal postmarketing surveillance studies to be generally required. This said, the committee adds emphatically that it endorses a government standards defense only in the context of existing levels of rigor and scrutiny in approval processes and presentation of all relevant data by manufacturers.

Recommendation 11. The committee believes that users of contraceptives have a right to information about them that is balanced, accurate, and intelligible. Significant sources of such information are the labels and inserts that are integral to pharmaceutical packaging. The legal, regulatory, educational, sociocultural, scientific, and even artistic aspects of these packaging elements are large and complex, so that modifying them significantly will require cross-disciplinary and cross-sectoral effort. The committee urges that this topic be addressed soon, for two reasons. First, balanced, accurate, and intelligible contraceptive packaging is of potential benefit to contraceptive users, health providers, manufacturers, and entities concerned with public health and welfare, since it could contribute to the more appropriate and wiser use of contraceptive technologies. Second, the activity in itself offers the opportunity for much-needed dialogue within and across sectors, genders, classes, and systems of belief.

CLOSING COMMENT

Despite the undeniable richness of the science that could be marshaled to give the women and men of the world a broader, safer, more effective array of options for implementing decisions about contraception, childbearing, and prevention of sexually transmitted disease, dilemmas remain. These dilemmas have to do with laws and regulations, politics and ideology, economics and individual behavior, all interacting in a very complex synergy that could lead to the conclusion that nothing can be done to resolve the dilemmas because everything needs to be done.

This committee examined the development of vaccines for the world's children as an experience with many analogies to contraceptive research and development. That experience informs us that the dilemmas around controversial medical products, whatever the sources of controversy, tend to be incremental and systemic in their resolution. Modification of the terrain for vaccine research and development took time—two decades of working groups charged with solving "the vaccine problem," a decade of legislative attempts to construct a passable bill, and close to a decade for industry to perceive that the legislative remedy was effective. Change came from several sources—from a surge of discovery in the science, from legislative action that modified public policy, from leadership at national and international policy levels, and from the decision of a major international donor to seek outside guidance in assessing its processes and their impact.

This does not mean that the same amount of time will be needed for improvement in the contraceptive landscape, nor will the solutions be the same. The central implication is that there is not likely to be a "silver bullet" solution to the dilemmas faced by the field of contraceptive research and development. Each piece of the dilemma will have to be tackled in cumulative fashion as part of a coherent strategy, each resolution improving matters somewhat and eventually amassing enough weight to tip the balance in a more positive direction. What this study committee has tried to do is identify a relatively small set of emphases and changes that, altogether, could turn the field around, but that, even partially implemented, could open up the field to freer, more equitable access to those who require its fruits.

Appendixes

A

Female Methods

Horacio Croxatto, M.D.
Instituto Chileno de Medicina Reproductiva, Santiago

Michael Harper, Ph.D., Sc.D.
Center for Reproductive Medicine, Baylor College of Medicine

Donald McDonnell, Ph.D.
Department of Pharmacology, Duke University Medical Center

Wylie Vale, Ph.D.
*The Clayton Foundation Laboratories for Peptide Biology,
The Salk Institute, La Jolla, Calif.*

INTRODUCTION

The advent of modern molecular and cell biology has permitted a detailed look at the regulation of ovarian secretory function, follicular and oocyte maturation, and ovulation. This, in turn, has disclosed targets within the ovary which, at the current time, appear to have the greatest potential for leading to the development of a deliverable contraceptive within the next 10 to 15 years.

INTERFERENCE WITH PREFERTILIZATION EVENTS

General

Oocyte maturation and ovulation are coordinated by a series of cascading signals involving the brain, pituitary, and gonads. Fertility in mammals is modulated by multiple factors including length of day, availability of food, exposure to stressors, illness, presence or evidence of potential mates and competitors, and breast feeding. The final common pathway for the effects of this external and internal sensory information on fertility is the collection of GnRH (gonadotropin-releasing hormone)-producing neurons in the hypothalamus that provide this neuropeptide to the anterior pituitary gland via a local vascular connection. The

351

pituitary gonadotropes respond to GnRH by secreting the gonadotropins, LH (luteinizing hormone) and FSH (follicle-stimulating hormone); these act in concert with each other and with many other local ovarian factors to control steroidogenesis and release of mature oocytes. Each regulatory component is a potential target for interfering with oocyte maturation and ovulation and hence fertility. Among possible contraceptive targets are receptors and transcriptional regulators for GnRH, activin, inhibin, gonadotropins, and intragonadal paracrine/autocrine factors; however, much basic and applied work is still needed to generate specific pharmacologic tools for controlling these molecules.

Brain

Contraception can be achieved by preventing production of GnRH, a strategy that would only require steroid replacement at a physiologic level with potential health benefits. The maintenance of GnRH expression may be dependent upon tissue-specific transcription factors which, if sufficiently restricted, could be blocked pharmacologically. GnRH action can be prevented by synthetic analogues or specific antibodies. The GnRH-producing cells in the hypothalamus secrete this peptide in a rhythmic fashion that is critical for normal gonadotropin secretion and work is under way to determine the cellular and molecular basis of the "GnRH pulse generator." Pharmacologic disruption of pulse parameters can have differential effects on the secretion of the two pituitary hormones, FSH and LH; thus, it may be possible to selectively disorganize gametogenesis. Superimposed upon the GnRH pulse generator are numerous neural and hormonal inputs mediated by monoamines, neuropeptides, prostaglandins, nitric oxide, sex and adrenal steroids, thyroid hormones, cytokines, and peptide growth factors that stimulate or inhibit GnRH production. Some of these could be targets for contraception, provided that cell-type-specific drugs could be developed.

Hypothalamus and Pituitary

The production of both LH and FSH is dependent upon receipt of periodic pulses of GnRH from the hypothalamus. GnRH binds to the GnRH receptor, a serpentine, G protein-coupled receptor, and induces its second messengers. The exposure of the pituitary to persistently high levels of GnRH or to potent long-acting agonist analogues (superagonists) results in an initial stimulation that is followed by desensitization secondary to receptor down-regulation and attenuation of receptor signal transduction.

Prolonged superagonist administration suppresses both LH and FSH secretion leading to hypogonadism. Superagonists are now on the market for several indications—including precocious puberty and the treatment of hormone-dependent neoplasias and dysplasias. These agents inhibit fertility in females and males, reduce steroid production, and induce postmenopausal symptoms. Thus, any continuous use of superagonists as contraceptives will necessitate steroid replacement therapy.

An alternative approach, involving agents that bind to the GnRH receptor, is to inhibit gonadotrope functions with GnRH receptor antagonists. These compounds have the advantage of producing an immediate suppression of gonadotropin secretion, thereby avoiding transient stimulation of the gonadotropes, gonads, and steroid-dependent tissues. However, much higher doses of the presently available antagonists must be delivered than in the case of the agonists. The development of potent, orally active antagonists would provide a means of reversibly suppressing gonadal functions. Screening of chemical and microbiological libraries with high throughput GnRH receptor assays may provide leads for further optimization. These antagonists, given with steroid replacement, should be very effective contraceptives in both women and men. Furthermore, because GnRH antagonists do not transiently stimulate sex hormone production, they would be more appropriate than agonists for the treatment of steroid-dependent neoplasia and dysplasia. The recent development of tissue-specific steroids raises the possibility that new steroids might be found that are specific for GnRH cells of the hypothalamus or pituitary gonadotropes.

The selective regulation of pituitary FSH is achieved physiologically by the interplay of GnRH, gonadal steroids, and peptide hormones/growth factors. There are reports in the literature of the existence of a small peptide, FSH-releasing factor (FRF), that acts at the pituitary level to stimulate FSH but not LH. If such a putative factor were identified and found to be physiologically necessary for normal FSH production, then blockers of this peptide would suppress fertility. Activin, a dimeric peptide growth factor produced locally within the pituitary, is probably the key trophic factor maintaining expression of FSH. Activin has little effect on LH production in most systems. Two inhibitors of activin have been identified, inhibin and follistatin. Inhibin, a heterodimeric protein structurally related to activin (they share a common subunit) blocks the responses of some (but not all) cells to activin; follistatin binds to activin and bioneutralizes it. Both proteins reduce the production of FSH in animals and suppress follicular development. Inhibin is secreted by the ovary under FSH stimulation and provides a negative feedback signal that shuts off further secretion of that pituitary hormone; follistatin is produced locally and serves to limit all effects of activin. The binding and signaling receptors for activin have been cloned and it may be possible to develop small molecules that would interfere with these functions. The way inhibin blocks activin is currently unknown, but studies of this process may provide insight for developing inhibin-mimetics. Because inhibin only suppresses a subset of activin effects, such drugs may be relatively specific to suppression of reproduction (DePaolo et al. 1991; Vale et al. 1994, 1990).

The finding that activin and inhibin can uncouple the transcription of FSHß from that of LHß provides evidence for the existence of distinct intracellular regulatory pathways for the two proteins that may be exploitable.

Follicular Development

A unique organ, the ovary is made up of hundreds of thousands of primary follicles that die during the lifetime of a female. Of the 400,000 follicles found in the human female at puberty, only about 400 will ever make it to ovulation.

From before birth, and throughout the reproductive years, small cohorts of follicles start growing continuously, one after the other, out of the pool of primary follicles. The vast majority undergo atresia after reaching different stages of growth. Beginning with puberty, growing follicles are periodically subjected to a process of recruitment and selection, from which a dominant follicle emerges in each menstrual cycle. This follicle proceeds to grow to maturity, a condition that makes it responsive to the ovulatory stimulus. The fact that a single follicle is selected to complete the process of maturation in each menstrual cycle is remarkable. This dominant follicle survives the other partners of its cohort, which enter atresia, and it proceeds to ovulation. It has been suggested that this process is regulated in part both by hormonal gradients within the ovary and by the ability of the developing follicle to respond to these signals by virtue of its physical location. However, the fidelity of the system and the usual outcome, that is, the production of one ovum, suggests that follicle selection is a tightly controlled process, the molecular basis for which has yet to be determined.

It has been established that most ovarian cell turnover occurs as a consequence of programmed cell death or apoptosis, an important cellular process by which superfluous or unwanted cells are deleted from an organism during tissue remodeling and differentiation. Although not identical in all cells, it has received much attention recently as a consequence of the identification of several transcription factors involved in regulating the process and the definition of the external stimuli that modulate the function of these proteins. Within the ovary, several substances have been shown to modulate the rate of cellular apoptosis by acting as follicular survival factors or mediators of cell death. From among the factors identified thus far, gonadotropins, steroid hormones, cytokines such as IGF-1, and interleukins seem likely to be important (Artini et al. 1994; Erickson and Danforth 1995).

Modulation of Ovarian Follicle Apoptosis as a Potential Contraceptive Approach

Follicular atresia is a well-regulated apoptotic event and not the result of cell necrosis. The ovary is a unique tissue with massive cell death throughout reproductive life. As suggested above, more than 99 percent of ovarian follicles endowed at early life are destined to undergo apoptosis. Based on extensive literature dealing with follicle selection and ovulation, as well as recent analysis of follicle apoptosis and follicle recruitment, one can propose a multistep model for the life cycle of ovarian follicles (Figure A-1).

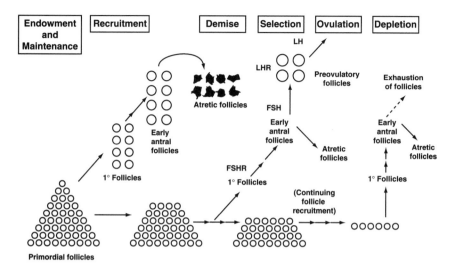

FIGURE A-1 Life cycle of ovarian follicles. FSH = follicle-stimulating hormone; FSHR = follicle-stimulating hormone receptor; LH = luteinizing hormone; and LHR = luteinizing hormone receptor. SOURCE: Prepared for this report by Aaron Hsueh.

At early stages of ovarian development, a fixed number of primordial follicles are endowed in the ovary. Later on, no mitosis of germ cells can be detected in the ovary, and gradual depletion of the follicle pool begins as subpopulations of follicles initiate growth. As they reach the early antral stage, all follicles undergo degeneration through apoptosis. However, after the activation of the hypothalamic-pituitary axis at puberty, circulating gonadotropins (mainly FSH) act as survival factors to prevent the demise of a small subgroup of early antral follicles (Hsueh et al. 1994). From these, a dominant follicle is selected for final maturation and ovulation.

Throughout reproductive life, the cyclic process of follicle recruitment, atresia selection, and ovulation continues until the follicle pool is exhausted around the time of reproductive senescence (or menopause in women). Ovarian cell apoptosis in early antral follicles, before their final selection into preovulatory ones, represents a unique stage for contraceptive intervention. Recent studies have demonstrated that gonadotropins, estrogens, growth hormone, growth factors (IGF-I, EGF/TGFβ, basic FGF), a cytokine (interleukin-1), and nitric oxide act in concert to ensure the survival of preovulatory follicles. In contrast, androgens, interleukin-6, and gonadal GnRH-like peptide are apoptotic factors. The selection of these follicles and their continuing maturation can be blocked by treatment with antagonists for the follicle survival factors or by increasing the levels of apoptotic factors. Promising candidates include the FSH blockers, such as deglycosylated FSH antagonists, and the extracellular fragments of FSH receptors that may serve as a neutralizing binding protein. These agents would act in an ovary-specific manner. It should be realized, however, that this approach must be complemented with physiologic replacement therapy, since preventing the emergence of the dominant follicle would probably lead to hypoestrogenism. The fact that all but one follicle within a selected cohort degenerates indicates that selective regulation of atresia within the ovary actually occurs. Understanding the molecular events that control follicle selection could have a major impact on contraceptive research.

Disruption of the Ovulatory Process

The ovulatory process comprises several coordinated changes that occur in mature follicles, triggered by the ovulatory stimulus (the gonadotropin surge). They include resumption of meiosis, cumulus expansion with detachment from the mural granulosa, onset of luteinization expressed as a new steroidogenic pattern, and the collagenolitic cascade that leads to rupture of the follicle wall and release of follicle contents. Although all these events are triggered by the same stimulus, they can be dissociated by specific pharmacologic interventions. It is therefore possible to prevent follicular rupture without interfering with luteinization and steroidogenesis. In other words, although the oocyte is prevented from leaving the follicle to be fertilized, at the same time the normal hormonal oscillations of the menstrual cycle are preserved. Recent data indicate that LH uses at least three signal transduction pathways to produce follicular rupture: CAMP-dependent protein kinase, the protein kinase C, and the calcium/calmodulin-dependent protein kinase II pathway (Kugu et al. 1995). In addition, the LH surge induces the expression of the prostaglandin synthase 2 gene (PGS-2), which codes for an enzyme whose activity is essential for follicular rupture. This enzyme could be selectively inhibited, eliminating ovulation without blocking luteinization and the synthesis of steroid hormones (Morris and Richards 1993, 1995). Luteinizing hormone induces prostaglandin endoperoxide synthase-2 and luteinization *in vitro* by A-kinase and C-kinase pathways (Sirois 1995).

It should also be possible to intervene with the onset of meiosis, advancing it to such a point that, by the time the oocyte is released, it is no longer fertilizable. Meiotic cell division is a process, unique to the gonads, which is designed to permit the exchange of genetic material between maternal and paternal DNA. While this process of what is essentially the creation of genetic diversity is tightly regulated, because of its unique mode and site of action it has potential as a realistic target for contraceptive intervention. Based on work in mammalian cells, as well as in species as diverse as *Drosophila* and *Xenopus*, it has become clear that meiotic and mitotic cell division and the way they are regulated are sufficiently distinct to assume that process-specific regulatable targets can be identified. One point of intervention might be the regulation of progression of primary oocytes from prophase I to metaphase II (Grigorescu et al. 1994). The oocyte contained in each follicle rests in an animated state, arrested in the prophase I of the first meiotic division, until the follicle matures and receives the ovulatory stimulus. The ovulatory stimulus has the peculiar property of stimulating resumption of meiosis only of the oocyte contained in the mature follicle. The processes that maintain the oocyte in a quiescent stage for between 12 and 50 years remain largely unknown. Fully grown oocytes resume meiosis when they are separated from granulosa cells or when isolated cumulus-oocyte complexes are stimulated with FSH. This has led to the concept that the cell layer surrounding the oocyte produces a substance—oocyte maturation inhibitor (OMI)—which is inhibitory, and that the ovulatory stimulus releases this inhibition and adds a stimulatory factor for germinal vesicle breakdown (GVB), a prerequisite for completion of meiosis. Purines produced by follicular cells and transmitted to the oocyte via gap junctions are known to be involved in preventing resumption of meiosis (Downs 1993).

Unusual sterols present in human follicular fluid and bovine testis have been shown recently to activate mouse oocyte meiosis *in vitro* and are believed to play a crucial role in the resumption of meiosis in mammals (Byskov et al. 1995). It is likely that synthetic analogues may be efficient both as agonists and as antagonists for pharmacologic manipulation of the onset of meiosis. An intracellular factor that regulates the transition from first meiotic prophase to metaphase II— maturation promoting factor (MPF)—has been identified and determined to be a heterodimer comprised of the regulatory subunit cyclin B and the catalytic subunit, the cyclin-dependent protein kinase p34cdc2 (Dorce 1990).

These concepts introduce two specific areas that must be investigated further, one to define the precise chemical messenger(s) responsible for keeping the oocyte in the dormant state, the second to define the events responsible for the termination of dormancy and the resumption of meiosis. There are, of course, specific concerns about intervention in the process of meiosis. Most of these deal with the possibility of consequences from interfering with the process of genetic exchange and any effects on an ovum or resulting fetus were an oocyte to escape regulation by a pharmaceutical agent. Although these are valid considerations, they are premature until such time as the events that regulate the meiotic process are defined.

Granulosa Cell-specific Targets

The granulosa cell layer is the innermost lining of the follicle wall and surrounds the oocyte. Under the influence of FSH, granulosa cells proliferate and produce estradiol. It is likely that targeting the FSH receptor (different ways to achieve this are discussed in Appendix B) would be useful in interrupting the process of follicular development. However, the ensuing decrease in circulating estrogens on a long-term basis would be contraindicated, owing to the important role of estrogen in regulating the processes responsible for maintenance of bone mass and cardiovascular tone, and in regulating vasomotor function (Barzel 1988), so that FSH receptor blockers would have to be given in conjunction with steroid replacement therapy. The new generation of tissue-selective steroid receptor agonists, for example, raloxifene, may be available for use in contraception.

It is not clear that blocking FSH actions in the granulosa cell has to result only from a pharmacological action at the receptor. It is possible that an understanding of the intermediate steps from the cell surface to the nucleus, and of the genes within the ovary that respond to this hormonal stimulus, may permit the development of specific agents that uncouple the synthesis of estrogen from other gene products required for follicular development.

Ovary-specific Gene Transcription

One of the most exciting areas of reproductive research has to do with whatever is involved in determining the expression and role of novel hormone-dependent transcription factors within the ovary, including follicular and corpus luteum cells and the oocyte. In the last 10 years, the cloning and characterization of the steroid hormone receptors has been accomplished and has assisted in our understanding of the mechanism of action of the reproductive hormones estrogen and progesterone (Evans 1988). The specific impact of these observations will be discussed below. Emanating from this research was the unexpected finding that the family of proteins to which the steroid hormone belongs comprises up to 50 members that are related structurally but, for many of which, no ligands have been identified (O'Malley 1991).

These "orphan receptors" are so structurally related to those of the steroid receptors that it is considered likely that some, if not all, will be found to have an endogenous ligand. This contention has received some support from the discovery in 1992 of a ligand for the orphan nuclear receptor RXR (Heyman et al. 1992). This ligand is 9-cis retinoic acid, a metabolite of retinoic acid. Since then, progress has been slow in defining specific ligands for other such receptors, although agents that regulate their biological activity indirectly have been identified. In this category, the identification of a nuclear receptor that responds to the addition of farnesyl pyrophosphate (FAR) (Forman et al. 1995) and a family of related receptors (peroxisome proliferator-activated receptors [PPAR]) that are transcriptionally regulated by fatty acid derivatives, are intriguing examples of an emerging new endocrinology (Kliewer et al. 1992). Of particular relevance to reproduction is the recent discovery that the transcriptional effects of melatonin, a hormone intimately involved in reproduction, are manifested through the orphan receptor RZR (Becker-Andre et al. 1994). A combination of melatonin and a synthetic progestin is being studied as a novel type of oral contraceptive preparation.

It is possible that the slow pace of the discovery of ligands for additional orphan receptor members of this subfamily may indicate that they do not, in fact, have ligands but are regulated in other ways. This contention is supported by a series of independent findings that indicate that some orphan receptors can be activated by membrane depolarization, as well as by agents such as dopamine and nerve growth factor that act at the cell surface (Power et al. 1991; Lydon et al. 1992). Nevertheless, the recent discovery that the orphan receptor PPARγ is the target for the biological efficacy of the thiazolidinediones, a class of drugs used for the treatment of non-insulin-dependent diabetes, indicates that these receptors are realistic pharmaceutical targets (Lehmann et al. 1995). The discovery of this compound, which binds to PPARγ with high affinity and permits it to activate target gene transcription, is an important result from a pharmaceutical perspective. It demonstrates that, without knowing whether or not an orphan receptor has an endogenous ligand, it can be regulated by a synthetic pharmaceutical in a manner that impacts on a relevant biological process. This paradigm is likely to be reiterated with other orphan receptors, some of which may be relevant to oocyte maturation.

More research into the role of nuclear hormone receptors in the regulation of the transcriptional program within the oocyte and in the ovary is needed. The recent finding that the nuclear receptor germ cell nuclear factor (GCNF) is restricted in expression to developing gametes and is detectable in all stages of oocyte development justifies this contention (Chen et al. 1994). Although a direct link between its expression and function has not yet been established, GCNF's unique pattern of expression would imply a critical function. Efforts to identify the target genes that are responsive to GCNF, as well as identification of an endogenous ligand or a synthetic molecule that could regulate its transcriptional activity, will be required at a minimum to evaluate its potential role as a target for contraception. In addition to GCNF, the nuclear receptor SF-1 (steroidogenic factor-1) may also play a key regulatory role in gametogenesis (Ikeda et al. 1994; Lala et al. 1992; Luo et al. 1994). This receptor, identified initially as a positive transcriptional regulator of steroidogenic enzymes, has now been determined to have a much more central effect on gonadal development.

Although a ligand has not yet been identified, there have been significant advances in our understanding of the biology of SF-1. In recent published experiments in which the SF-1 protein has been genetically disrupted in mice, it was determined that the ensuing progeny failed to develop gonads and their pituitary lacked gonadotropes. The mechanism by which SF-1 may exert its regulatory activities is just beginning to become clearer. The gene-encoding Mullerian inhibiting substance (MIS), a cytokine required for male reproductive tract development, is positively regulated by SF-1 (Shen et al. 1994). All these examples illustrate the impact of basic nuclear factor research on our understanding of the molecular events underlying the development of reproductive capacity.

Steroid Hormone Receptors

In addition to more attention to new targets in the ovary, much progress will be made by taking a fresh look at targets that are already established. In particular, the actions of steroid hormones at the gonadal/pituitary/hypothalamic axis, a well-defined series of targets acted upon by existing oral contraceptives, could advance to a new level by developments in our understanding of the steroid hormone receptor signal transduction pathways. The cloning of the estrogen and progesterone receptors and the ability to use these tools to dissect the progester-one- and estrogen-mediated signal transduction pathways indicate that, in addition to the receptor, its environment impacts on the biological efficacy of the hormone.

A recent and unexpected finding is that different ligands induce distinct alterations in receptor structure, the consequence of which is that these ligands can then promote unique sets of protein-protein interactions and subsequently regulate gene transcription in a differential manner (Allan et al. 1992). One of the most striking examples of this process is the observation that estradiol and tamoxifen, ligands for the estrogen receptor, induce distinct conformational changes within the receptor, with distinct biological consequences *in vivo* (McDonnell et al. 1995; Tzukerman et al. 1994). In this instance it has been shown that tamoxifen functions as an antagonist of the estrogen receptor in the breast and as an agonist in bone and in the cardiovascular system. The splitting by tamoxifen of the desirable and undesirable effects of estrogen receptor activation reinforces the notion that tissue- or process-specific steroid receptor modulators can be developed. Exploitation of these observations should lead to the generation of novel compounds with improved therapeutic efficacy.

Support is needed for basic studies of the hormones and growth factors, their receptors, and intracellular signaling mechanisms mediating the neuroendocrine and gonadal regulation of reproduction. Strategies for interfering with this regulation can target critical molecules for blockade or inappropriate expression through development of orally-active or very long-acting small molecules. In the long term, gene therapy approaches may permit the utilization of biosynthetic molecules, including larger proteins produced by biosynthetic organoids with extended but finite life spans.

Recommendations

Based on our current understanding of the state of research in the regulation of ovarian function and oocyte development, we make the following recommendations:

1. The mechanisms underlying the pulsatile release of GnRH and the differential regulation of FSH and LH synthesis and secretion should be elucidated.

2. Specific molecular events associated with maintenance of oocytes in prophase I, and release of this block by the ovulatory stimulus only in mature follicles, should be defined. This should be accompanied by a determination of the suitability of these targets for pharmacological intervention.

3. The horizons of apoptosis research should be expanded to include the developing follicle as a target. Apoptosis research in diverse areas, including this one, could "cross-fertilize" these complementary fields of research and perhaps produce benefit to each other. One very important research objective is to understand the mechanism by which the dominant follicle progresses while other developing follicles undergo atresia.

4. Examination of molecular and cellular aspects of follicular development, definition of key "players" and their specific targets, and identification of endogenous and synthetic ligands should be major research objectives.

5. Studies should be undertaken to elucidate the factors that control follicular rupture, since inhibition of this process would be an ideal way to prevent fertilization through simulation of a normal nonconception cycle with unaltered steroid patterns, steroid levels, and cycle length.

6. Established targets, for instance, the steroid hormone receptors, should be reexamined, the rationale being the recent observation that tissue-selective compounds can be developed to control specific subsets of genes that are regulated by the natural hormone.

INTERFERENCE WITH POSTFERTILIZATION EVENTS

After ovulation, the oocyte enters the oviduct (fallopian tube) and progresses into the ampullary segment, where it may be fertilized if it is met by capacitated spermatozoa that retain their fertilizing potential. Fertilization could be prevented by interventions that hinder the sperm from reaching the ampullary segment, by causing the sperm to undergo a premature acrosome reaction, by blocking sperm binding to the zona pellucida, by changing the consistency of the zona to prevent sperm penetration, or by premature aging of the oocyte. Once fertilization has occurred, the fertilized egg is retained in the ampullary segment of the oviduct for the next 72 hours. During this period, it undergoes several mitotic cycles so that, after traversing the isthmic segment, which takes only hours, it reaches the uterus at the 8- to 12-cell stage. It then lies free in the uterus for another three to four days while undergoing continued mitotic cycles, reaching first the morular stage and then undergoing cavitation to form a blastocyst (Croxatto 1995). Even before attachment to the endometrial epithelium, the blastocyst commences to cause changes in the endometrium, for example, increased blood flow at the future site of attachment. After attachment, the trophoblastic cells of the blastocyst start to invade through the endometrial epithelial lining into the stromal compartment, where the stromal cells begin a process of differentiation known as decidualization. Implantation is considered the process that starts with attachment and ends with decidualization. Concomitant with implantation in primates, the trophoblastic cells of the embryo start to secrete chorionic gonadotropin (CG), which is necessary for maintenance of the corpus luteum and continued progesterone production. Progesterone is an essential requirement for the establishment and maintenance of early pregnancy.

Oviductal and/or Myometrial Function

Based on the fact that agents that accelerate oviductal transport of eggs in polyovular animals with cornuate uteri also decrease the number of embryos that implant successfully, it has been felt for many years that, if the developing embryos could be expelled from the oviduct prematurely, then pregnancy would not take place. While this effect has been demonstrated in animals, at the moment there is no good proof that this is the case in humans. On the contrary, placement of human *in-vitro*-fertilized embryos in the uterus at a very early developmental stage (equivalent to what would happen if the embryo were expelled prematurely from the oviduct) has produced viable human offspring. It has been established that the main reason why embryos arriving prematurely in the uterus do not implant in some animals is because they are rapidly expelled from the uterus (Adams 1980; Ortiz et al. 1991). Close to the time when embryos normally enter the uterus, the activity of the myometrium changes so that, instead of being expelled, the embryos are retained. The human may differ in that the shift from expulsion to retention may occur much earlier than in it does in rodents; it is also possible that the different shape of the uterus makes the expulsive mechanism less efficient. In any event, it would appear that, for effective contraception, a drug that would accelerate tubal transport should also cause expulsion of the embryo from the uterus by itself or, in combination with an oxytocic agent, stimulate uterine contractility. On the other hand, an agent that stimulated only enough uterine contractility to cause embryonic expulsion, even when the embryo entered the uterus at the normal time, would also provide effective contraception. In the human female there is a three-day window from the moment the egg enters the uterus until blastocyst adhesion to the endometrium begins. By accelerating tubal transport, this window could be widened to six days, during which time expulsion of the egg could be achieved.

Recent data indicate that the time at which the early-stage embryos pass from the oviduct to the uterus is dictated in some species predominantly by ovarian sex steroids; in others, this is due to substances secreted by the embryo during its journey through the oviduct. Two of the substances involved appear to be prostaglandin E_2 (PGE_2) (Weber et al. 1991 [mare]) and platelet-activating factor (PAF) (Velásquez et al. 1995 [hamster]). Since the human oviduct does not respond with accelerated transport to acute increases in estrogen or progesterone levels (Croxatto 1995), it is likely to belong to that class of mammals in which the embryo itself, rather than ovarian steroids, control its passage to the uterus. Until this is confirmed and the substance involved is identified, it will be difficult to assess the feasibility of using this natural mechanism to put this process out of phase.

Hormonal treatments that cause retention of embryos in the oviducts of animals also reduce their fertility, but this approach does not appear applicable to human females because of the likelihood that it would cause an intratubal (ectopic) pregnancy. This complication, which does not occur in nonprimates, can be life-threatening in human females. New understanding of the regulation of embryo transport may result in new approaches to contraception that would act at the tubal and/or myometrial level.

Postcoital Contraception

Estrogens, Progestins, and Estrogen/progestin Combinations

As indicated earlier, administration of estrogens soon after coitus to nonprimates causes a notable decrease or suppression of fertility; it was for this reason that estrogens were first tried as a method of emergency contraception in women. Large-scale trials of various estrogens showed that, in human females, estrogens were moderately effective in preventing pregnancy when taken within 72 hours after a single mid-cycle act of intercourse (Blye 1973; Haspels 1994). The exact mode of action of this treatment is unknown. For the reasons given above, it is not likely that embryo transport through the oviduct is accelerated; what may be involved is either expulsion of the embryo from the uterus, disruption of the synchronous development of the endometrium with that of the embryo that is necessary for implantation, or ovulation blockade.

One drawback of this treatment is the extent of side effects, especially nausea and vomiting. To alleviate these consequences, the therapy has been modified to a combined estrogen/progestin regimen. This reduces side effects, although it does not eliminate them, at the same time that the window of efficacy remains unaltered (Yuzpe et al. 1982; Yuzpe and Lancee 1977). Another emergency contraceptive approach is vaginal administration of steroids, the objective of which is to increase efficacy and reduce gastrointestinal side effects. One piece of research that should be implemented is formulation of pills for postcoital contraception for vaginal administration, with performance to be comparable to that of orally administered pills. Progestins alone ("minipills") have also been used and seem to be effective (Farkas et al. 1981; Ho and Kwan 1993).

A major advantage of combination therapy is that, although in the United States no postcoital contraceptive preparation is marketed as such, administration of four marketed oral contraceptive pills taken two and two, 12 hours apart, provides effective postcoital contraception. This is not widely known among either providers or users who might need such treatment. However, because of the probable disruption of the menstrual cycle produced by such therapy, it is not suitable for use cycle after cycle or where there are multiple acts of unprotected intercourse in any single cycle.

Antiprogestins

Current antiprogestins are synthetic steroids that bind to the progesterone receptor and prevent the transcription activation that is normally initiated by the ligand-receptor complex. Since the antiprogestin mifepristone has been shown to terminate pregnancy when given after a missed menses, it has also been tried as a postcoital contraceptive. In two trials in which mifepristone was given at the dose of 600 mg orally within 72 hours after unprotected intercourse to a total of 597 women, there was not a single pregnancy; there were nine pregnancies among 589 women similarly treated with estrogen/progestin or progestin-only formulations (Glasier et al. 1992; Webb et al. 1992). This low failure rate indicates that this particular antiprogestin is an effective postcoital contraceptive. In both studies, the incidence of nausea and vomiting was significantly lower than has been the case with other presently available compounds. Nevertheless, menstrual delay was more common in the group receiving mifepristone.

Postcoital emergency use of mifepristone is being studied further by the Special Programme of Research, Development, and Research Training in Human Reproduction of the World Health Organization (WHO/HRP 1995). An ongoing clinical trial comparing single doses of 10, 50, and 600 mg taken within five days of unprotected intercourse is expected to be completed in 1996.

Mifepristone can delay ovulation due to temporary arrest of the growth of the dominant follicle, can offset the positive feedback of estrogen on the discharge of gonadotropin from the pituitary gland, and can disrupt the required secretory changes of the endometrium. These features make an antiprogestin effective for preventing either fertilization or implantation, depending on the stage of the menstrual cycle at which it is taken. Conceivably, a combination of estrogen and an antiprogestin could be more effective than either compound alone and would permit reduction in the amount of each ingredient, with a concomitant reduction in side effects.

Anti-implantation Agents

Targeting Hormones

Antiestrogens given in small single doses during the 24 hours prior to implantation can specifically inhibit implantation in species such as the rat and the mouse, which require a surge of endogenous estrogen to initiate the implantation process. However, these compounds have not been shown to be effective in species such as the rabbit and the hamster, which require only progesterone and need no maternal estrogen to initiate implantation (Harper 1972).

The situation in primates is more complex. Since there is a rise in plasma estrogen levels in primates around the time of implantation, it was thought for some time that they, too, would require estrogen for implantation. However, a series of experiments in which monkeys were ovariectomized after ovulation and mating and given only progesterone replacement indicated that pregnancy could occur normally. Furthermore, recent studies in women with premature ovarian failure who used *in vitro* fertilization and embryo transfer to overcome their infertility showed that a combination of estrogen and progesterone during the first half of the artificial cycle, followed by progesterone alone starting several days before the transfer and continuing through the implantation period, was perfectly adequate to ensure pregnancy (see Harper 1992 for discussion). Similar results have been demonstrated in monkeys (Ghosh et al. 1994). Thus, it is clear that maternal estrogen is not required at the time of implantation to initiate that process in primates. However, there have been several studies in primates where antiestrogens were given after ovulation and before implantation and produced an antifertility effect (Harper 1992).

In any event, a lack of progesterone action on the uterus always leads to pregnancy failure. There are three ways to prevent progesterone from acting on its target organs and each has its limitations. One way is to prevent synthesis of progesterone by enzyme inhibitors, for example, azastene or epostane (Crooij 1988; Schane et al. 1978; Snyder and Schane 1985). Epostane (200 mg orally every 6 hours for 7 days) terminated pregnancy in about 80 percent of women up to the eighth week of pregnancy, but nausea was a common side effect (Bigerson and Odlind 1987; Crooij et al. 1988). The main problem with this approach is that it may affect synthesis of adrenal steroids.

A second approach is to intercept progesterone in the circulation by specific antibodies. This could be achieved on a long-term basis by active immunization (Hillier et al. 1975; Nieschlag and Wickings 1978; Rider et al. 1985). A possible drawback would be exposure of the endometrium to the action of unopposed estrogen. However, administration of a synthetic progestin, not crossreactive with the antiprogesterone antibody, during the last quarter of the cycle would produce withdrawal bleeding regardless of other events in the cycle. This is a potentially interesting target.

The third approach is to block progesterone action at the receptor level using antiprogestins. Mifepristone has been administered to primates and to human females within the time frame between ovulation and implantation to assess effects on the endometrium and on fertility. A single dose of 10 mg administered 5 to 8 days after the LH surge produced marked asynchrony between glandular and stromal elements of the endometrium (Greene et al. 1992), an effect which presumably would be incompatible with implantation. Single doses of 2 or 10 mg/kg given 2 days after ovulation to rhesus monkeys were highly effective for preventing pregnancy (Ghosh and Sengupta 1993). Similarly, administration of 200 mg on the second day after the LH surge caused retarded endometrial development in human females (Swahn et al. 1990), as well as reduced fertility (Gemzell-Danielsson et al. 1993).

It is also plausible that combinations of progesterone synthesis inhibitors with progesterone receptor blockers might be more effective than either alone (Birgerson and Odlind 1987; Birgerson et al. 1987; Crooij et al. 1988; Selinger et al. 1987). Since most of these hormonal manipulations result in making endometrial development out of synchrony with or hostile to the embryo, a combination of an anti-estrogen and an antiprogestin might also be effective. Until recently, except for the WHO/HRP research team, no one has been able to conduct the required human trials, even though there has been extensive clinical experience with such candidate compounds for other indications. India and the People's Republic of China have recently supported work in this neglected field.

Cell-adhesion Molecules

One of the first events in the implantation process is the attachment of the blastocyst to the uterine epithelial surface, an effect possibly accomplished by cell-adhesion molecules. Under appropriate conditions, functional and structural changes occur at the apical surfaces of epithelial cells lining the endometrial cavity which permit blastocyst attachment. Carbohydrates appear to be intimately involved in cell–cell adhesion. Synthesis of the histo-blood group H-type-1 antigen is hormonally regulated and is expressed in the endometrial epithelium at the peri-implantation period in several species, including the human. It is thought that endometrial carbohydrates carrying the H-type-1 antigen may be involved in the initial blastocyst adhesion (Kimber 1994; Kimber et al. 1995).

The integrins are a family of cell-adhesion molecules. The distribution of several α and β integrin subunits has been studied in the human endometrium during the menstrual cycle. It was noted that the collagen/laminin receptors (α_2, α_3, and α_6) were expressed mainly on the epithelial cells, whereas the fibronectin receptor (α_5) was found mainly in the stroma. The two subunits of the vitronectin receptor ($\alpha_v\beta_3$) and integrin $\alpha_4\beta_1$ varied throughout the cycle, with α_v increasing throughout the cycle and β_3 only appearing abruptly on day 20, and α_4 decreasing about day 24. Changes in the expression of these integrins may define the putative period of uterine receptivity for blastocyst attachment (Ilesanmi et al. 1993; Lessey 1994; Lessey et al. 1992, 1994; Schultz and Armant 1995). Blockade or disruption of this expression of integrins might also provide a specific means of preventing implantation.

Another cell surface glycoprotein with potential importance in blastocyst adhesion is a high molecular weight glycoprotein identified by mouse ascites golgi antibodies. This glycoprotein involves N-acetyl-galactosamine and other determinants, is secreted from the endometrial glands in the human during the period of uterine sensitivity for implantation (Kliman et al. 1995), and is thought to be involved in the initial adhesion phase of implantation.

Mucins are *O*-linked glycoproteins present on the apical surface of epithelial cells (Strous and Dekker 1992). Mucin domains can extend for 200–500 nm from the cell surface (Jentoft 1990). A high density of such glycoproteins on apical cell surfaces could block access to the cell membrane. Muc-1 (also known as episalin) is a member of this family of mucin glycoproteins. Muc-1 expression (protein and message) is found only in the endometrial epithelial cells of mouse uterus. It is high at proestrus and estrus and is barely detectable on day 4 of pregnancy (just prior to implantation). Using steroid-treated ovariectomized mice, it was shown that Muc-1 was stimulated by estrogen and down-regulated by progesterone and antiestrogens owing to inhibition of estrogen action (Braga and Gendler 1993; Surveyor et al. 1995). It seems reasonable, therefore, to argue that loss of Muc-1 is necessary, though not sufficient, to generate the receptive state for implantation. Muc-1 is also found in granulated metrial cells of the mouse decidua by day 8 of pregnancy. This is unusual since Muc-1 is considered to be an epithelial differentiation marker (Braga and Gendler 1993). If manipulation of Muc-1 expression is to serve as a basis for a contraceptive approach, ways of decreasing it prematurely or delaying its down-regulation would have to be found. It may prove difficult to obtain a sufficient degree of asynchrony between the development of uterine receptivity and the embryo to constitute a reliable method of contraception.

Heparin-binding epidermal growth factor (HB-EGF) binds to the EGF receptor and is a mitogen for keratinocytes and fibroblasts. Its binding to the EGF receptor and its biological activity are potentiated by heparin sulfate proteoglycans, which are present in high amount in the basal lamina of the luminal epithelium. At least in the rat, HB-EGF is regulated by progesterone with expression in the uterine stromal cells and suppression in epithelial cells. It appears that it is involved in the development and maintenance of the decidual cells that are required for subsequent stages of implantation after attachment. The decidualizing stimulus first causes differentiation in the stromal cells underlying the epithelium and then is propagated to other stromal cells. Thus, HB-EGF may be important for establishing uterine receptivity for implantation and causing stromal cell proliferation (Zhang et al. 1994a). Its appearance can be blocked by antiprogestins and thus may be a good contraceptive target (Zhang et al. 1994b).

Two new adhesion molecules have recently been described, trophinin and tastin. Trophinin is an intrinsic membrane protein which mediates self-binding, while tastin is a cytoplasmic protein whose role is to permit trophinin to act as a cell-adhesion molecule. These molecules are associated with the cytoskeleton and have been found on monkey blastocyst trophectoderm and human endometrial luminal epithelium at the beginning of the appearance of the period of receptivity (Fukuda et al. 1995). The functional significance of these factors in implantation remains to be determined, but they may also be useful new leads for a contraceptive acting to prevent blastocyst attachment.

Clearly, prevention of attachment of the blastocyst to the endometrial lining could be an attractive possibility for developing a novel method of contraception. Much basic work still remains to be done to establish which of the cell-adhesion molecules are crucial for this process. Unless agents that act in this manner have a long biological half-life, there will also be practical difficulties in determining the optimal time during the cycle for administration.

Cytokines/Growth Factors

Within the last 10 years there has been a veritable explosion of research and interest in a variety of endogenous glycoproteins that are known as growth factors and/or cytokines. The importance of many of these agents, especially members of the interleukin family, for regulation of the immune system is now well established. However, the study of mutant mouse strains or production of transgenic mice with the gene for a particular cytokine disabled (the so-called "knockout" mouse) has recently revealed that some of these cytokines also regulate endometrial functions (Harvey et al. 1995). Several candidates have been proposed for an essential role in implantation.

Interleukin-1 is used to designate two structurally related proteins, IL-1α and IL-1β, with a molecular mass of about 17,000 daltons. Both proteins bind to the same receptor (IL-1R) and mediate similar actions. The receptor is also in two forms, IL-1 type I and type II, of which the type I receptor binds both IL-1α and β and the function of the type II receptor is unknown. IL-1α is present in mouse (message and protein) uterus during the preimplantation period and appears to be hormonally regulated since it peaks just before implantation (De et al. 1993; Tackacs et al. 1988). IL-1β mRNA has been found in human endometrium, as has the IL-1R which peaks in the luteal phase (Simón et al. 1993a, 1993b; Tabizzadeh et al. 1990). Furthermore, IL-1β, which is increased during endometrial decidualization, also acts as a modulator of the degree of decidualization (Frank et al. 1995). The action of IL-1 on its receptor can be inhibited by an endogenous inhibitor, the IL-1α receptor antagonist. Treatment of mice with the IL-1R antagonist during the preimplantation period prevented pregnancy (Simón et al. 1994). Experiments to repeat these results have been only partially successful and the critical importance of IL-1 in implantation *per se* remains to be established.

In a mutant inbred mouse strain that has undetectable levels of colony-stimulating factor-1 (CSF-1), breeding of homozygous males and females results in a failure of implantation. This effect is not specific to the maternal reproductive tract, because breeding the homozygous females with heterozygous males results in a certain degree of rescue of the pregnancy, which may indicate an embryonic function in this rescue (Pollard et al. 1991). This may mean that CSF-1 might also be a critical factor for implantation. It regulates gene expression and induces synthesis of another cytokine, tumor necrosis factor-α (TNF-α). In these homozygous mutant mice, TNF-α expression in the reproductive tract was not different from that in mice with normal CSF-1 levels (Hunt et al. 1993). When defective early development of mouse embryos is induced by exogenous CSF-1, preimplantation development can be restored to normal by TNF-α or granulocyte macrophage colony-stimulating factor but not by transforming growth factor ß1 (Tartakovsky and Ben-Yair 1991). Interestingly, TNF-α inhibits decidualization of human endometrial stromal cells *in vitro* (Inoue et al. 1994), so that the balance between CSF-1 and TNF-α may be critical for normal progression of the implantation process. In human endometrial stromal cells in culture, secretion of macrophage CSF is progesterone dependent and should therefore be increased during the luteal phase of the cycle (Hatayama et al. 1994; Kariya et al. 1994). Short-term blockade of CSF-1 action to prevent implantation may be free of the side effects such as osteopetrosis that are seen in the mutant animals.

Leukemia inhibitory factor (LIF) is a 38- to 67-kDA glycoprotein, which can be secreted or remain cell-associated. LIF exerts actions on a variety of different cell types. The results of experiments in mice with the gene for LIF mutated are very promising. Homozygous mice deficient in LIF appeared normal except for being approximately 25 percent smaller than wild-type animals. Homozygous males were fertile and produced offspring from both normal and heterozygous females. In contrast, homozygous females mated to wild-type heterozygous or homozygous males did not become pregnant. These females were not sterile because normal blastocysts were found in the uterus on both day 4 (the day of implantation) and day 7, which indicates that implantation was delayed. Such blastocysts when transplanted to wild-type females implanted normally but when wild-type blastocysts were transplanted to the homozygous females, implantation did not occur. Replacement therapy with recombinant LIF (without the glycosylation) induced implantation of some blastocysts in the homozygous mice. Expression of LIF mRNA in the uteri of pseudopregnant mice was similar to that seen in pregnant mice, suggesting that the embryo was not involved in this expression (Bhatt et al. 1991; Stewart et al. 1992).

These results clearly indicate that, in the mouse, LIF production by and action on the uterus is a critical factor for initiation of implantation. In the mouse both LIF message and protein is regulated by estrogen (Bhatt et al. 1991; Yang et al. 1996), and the mouse is a species requiring estrogen for blastocyst implantation. The importance of LIF in the implantation process in other species, especially those not requiring estrogen, has not been established; this is of crucial importance for relevance to the human.

At the same time, there is some supporting evidence from other species. LIF protein, LIF receptor, and gp130 have been shown to peak in the uteri of both pregnant and pseudopregnant rabbits before implantation, in a similar fashion to mice (Yang et al. 1994, 1995a, 1995b). Since the rabbit does not require estrogen for induction of implantation, it would seem likely that LIF in this species is regulated differently from the mouse. Indeed, this has proved to be the case. LIF protein uterine levels are increased by progesterone and unaltered by estrogen. In endometrial specimens from women during nonconception cycles, both LIF message and protein are low or absent during the proliferative phase and high during the secretory phase, remaining high to the end of the cycle (Charnock-Jones et al. 1994; Kojima et al. 1994). LIF secretion from human endometrial cell cultures, however, shows a peak at the mid-luteal phase (around the time of implantation in a conception cycle) (Chen et al. 1995). LIF and IL-6 are both found in pig uterine secretions just prior to embryo attachment (Anegon et al. 1994). The reason for the discrepancy between message and protein levels and secretion in the human may be due to changes between cell-associated and secretory forms or between conception and nonconception cycles. In mice and rabbits, no examination was done for LIF expression in pseudopregnant animals after the equivalent time of implantation in pregnant animals. In sum, the data in hand suggest that LIF may be an important lead in the development of specific anti-implantation agents.

There are, nonetheless, some possible problems. There are significant similarities in primary amino acid sequences and predicted secondary structures of LIF with other cytokines, e.g., oncostatin M (OSM), IL-6, ciliary neurotrophic factor (CNTF), and granulocyte colony-stimulating factor (G-CSF) (Horseman and Yu-Lee 1994; Rose and Bruce 1991). These structurally related cytokines modulate differentiation in a variety of cells so that there is a possibility that, in some cells at least, they could substitute for each other, although the present understanding is that LIF and related cytokines are not functionally equivalent (Piquet-Pellorce et al. 1994) despite similarities in receptor structure (see below). The importance of LIF is underscored by the high degree of conservation in the coding regions and high degree of similarity of the protein across species (Willson et al. 1992).

Actions of these cytokines on cells are mediated through membrane-bound receptors. Binding of these cytokines to their receptor complexes activates a signal transduction pathway, resulting in rapid tyrosine phosphorylations, followed by activation of a protein kinase cascade and early gene responses. These appear to be nonreceptor tyrosine kinases. Specificity of response may be ensured by intracellular structure of the cytokine receptor dictating which signaling molecules are activated and expression levels of signaling molecules in the different cell types (Taniguchi 1995). Similarities between the receptor signal transducing units of CNTF, G-CSF, IL-6, IL-11, and LIF have been reported (Horseman and Yu-Lee 1994). There are two LIF receptor types, a high- and a low-affinity type (Hilton et al. 1988; Yamamoto-Yamaguchi et al. 1986). The cloned LIF receptor (LIFR) only binds LIF with low affinity, but after the binding of a common receptor component gp130 (the signal transduction unit for IL-6R), LIFR is converted to the high-affinity type (Gearing et al. 1991, 1992). The receptors for all the above cytokines involve gp130 binding, acting as a signal transduction unit. The IL-6R comprises a homodimer of gp130, but OSMR,

LIFR, and CNTFR involve only one gp130 subunit plus the LIFR β subunit, all complexed with a third element, a specific α subunit, which may be membrane-bound or act as a soluble factor, and regulate the binding of factors to the β subunits (Davis et al. 1993; Hirano et al. 1994; Ip et al. 1992; Murakami et al. 1993). Receptor activation results from binding of gp130 which converts the α:β complexes to the high-affinity form. These receptor components constitutively associate with Jak-Tyk kinases, which are activated by receptor dimerization (Lütticken et al. 1994; Murakami et al. 1993; Stahl et al. 1994). A family of proteins known as STATs (signal transduction and activation of transcription) are involved in the actions of many polypeptide ligands on cells. STAT3 is activated through phosphorylation on tyrosine as a DNA binding protein by the LIF-IL-6-CNTF family of ligands (Zhong et al. 1994). Selection of the particular substrate STAT3 is specified not by the particular Jak activated but by the tyrosine-based motifs in the receptor components gp130 and LIFR (Stahl et al. 1995). Blockade of the tyrosine kinases prevents phosphorylation of the receptor subunits and gene induction.

Since gp130 is involved in signal transduction for all members of this receptor family, inactivation of the gp130 signaling function may not provide a good contraceptive target owing to lack of specificity. Nevertheless, inhibition of tyrosine kinase activity itself has been suggested as a potential drug target (Levitzki and Gazit 1995), although whether sufficient specificity can be ensured is again an unresolved question. However, specific blockade of the formation of the LIFR α:β complex, given the essential need of LIF for implantation, appears a much more appealing target, if it can be established that LIF plays the same role in other species that it does in the mouse. Such inhibition targeted at the essential LIFR α subunit should provide the specificity needed to avoid interference with function of OSM, CNTF, and IL-6. Although LIF has actions at sites other than the uterus, the fact that the mutant mice deficient in LIF were apparently normal gives hope that short-term inhibition of LIF action in the uterus will be without other adverse consequences.

Studies in nonhuman primates have identified a variety of other growth factors whose secretion by the endometrium is hormonally regulated. There are cell-specific changes in gene expression of the receptors for insulin-like growth factor I (IGF-I) and epidermal growth factor (EGF), and for the secreted proteins IGF-binding protein 1 and retinol-binding protein (Fazleabas et al. 1994). In human endometrial cell cultures, IGF-I, its receptor, and the IGF-binding proteins 1–4 are all localized to the epithelial cells and highest at the early- to mid-secretory phase of the cycle (Tang et al. 1994). It is postulated that these changes are modulated by the embryo and are essential for implantation. However, at present the data are purely correlative. Fibroblast growth factors (FGFs) are involved in angiogenesis, cell growth, and cell differentiation, and disruption of the gene for FGF-4 in mice causes severe inhibition of the growth of the blasto-cyst inner cell mass (the cells that form the embryo) and failure of pregnancy just after implantation (Feldman et al. 1995). FGFs have a dual receptor system; one component is the FGF receptor with an extracellular ligand-binding domain and an intracellular tyrosine kinase domain, and the other is a series of heparin or heparin sulfate proteoglycans required for FGF binding. There are several binding sites for these proteoglycans on FGF, and thus design of compounds able to modulate FGF action should be possible (Ornitz et al. 1995).

In summary, there are several new and promising approaches that could form the basis for a once-a-month contraceptive pill. Yet, all this research must still be brought to proof of concept stage and, even when an LIFR blocker that blocks implantation is developed, many questions will remain. There will be a need to determine specific dosages and frequencies, all of which will depend on the half-life of the compound being used. Will it be necessary to deliver the agent locally, or will an oral preparation suffice? If the agent is given too late, will the effect be simply a normal pregnancy and is there a risk of a teratogenic effect? Is there likely to be a shortening of the cycle that causes difficulties in determining the time for optimal dosing in the next cycle? Obviously, there are difficulties; still, those may be fewer than those produced through hormonal manipulation, making the approach worthy of further investigation.

Inhibition of hCG Production

As discussed above, peptide agonists and antagonists of GnRH have been developed and their actions in blocking the central hypothalamic-pituitary axis have been extensively investigated as a method of contraception in both men and women, as discussed above. Investigations are under way to develop nonpeptide antagonists since they are likely to be simpler and cheaper. Whether such agents could block the action of trophoblast GnRH in stimulating the hCG secretion necessary for luteal support and pregnancy maintenance is unknown. It may also be that other factors are involved in regulation of early hCG production that might be amenable to attack. Inhibition of the early hCG production necessary for luteal maintenance would cause early pregnancy failure without disrupting menstrual cyclicity.

Induction of Luteolysis

In nonprimates, it has been relatively easy to develop agents that cause luteolysis, that is, premature demise of the corpus luteum with interference in progesterone secretion and consequent failure of pregnancy. In primates, in whom the mechanisms of luteal support appear to differ significantly from those of nonprimates, this has proven difficult. At this time, induction of luteolysis does not appear to be a promising avenue, but basic research on regulation of the corpus luteum may provide new leads. One alternative means to achieve the same effect is by blockade of progesterone synthesis in the corpus luteum. Such a functional luteolysis has been demonstrated following administration of either azastene or epostane during the luteal phase of the cycle to rhesus monkeys (Schane et al. 1978; Snyder and Schane 1985); in pregnant monkeys, pregnancy was terminated (Schane et al. 1978). Even with a luteolytic agent in hand, it might prove to be effective only during the period before the trophoblast provides luteal support, although this was not the case with the progesterone synthesis inhibitors (Asch et al. 1982; Snyder and Schane 1985). In such cases, the agent would not be luteolytic at the end of the cycle but only until the peri-implantation period, after which cycle disruption might ensue.

Expected Menses Induction

Another possible once-a-month contraceptive modality aims at insuring the occurrence of endometrial sloughing at the time of expected menses, regardless of whether or not an embryo has implanted. Since progesterone is essential to maintain the integrity of the endometrium, it is theoretically possible that a single high dose of an antiprogestin given at, or shortly before, the time of expected menses might achieve this purpose. Mifepristone has been given as a single dose of 600 or 400 mg, or 100 mg for four consecutive days in the late luteal phase to women who had detectable levels of the β subunit of hCG; actual failure rates, expressed as percentages of subjects continuing to be pregnant, were from 17 to 19 percent. This level of efficacy is similar to that observed after use of mifepristone to interrupt pregnancy when given up to 11 days after a missed menses. In order to improve effectiveness, WHO/HRP is conducting a two-center study in which mifepristone is followed by administration of misoprostol, an orally active prostaglandin that has been shown to increase significantly the rate of pregnancy termination when both are combined after missed menses. Data from this study may be available during 1996.

Recommendations

Available evidence suggests that there are several promising targets that can be pursued now and we therefore make the following recommendations:

1. There should be expeditious examination of combinations of antiprogestins and other hormonal or antihormonal drugs, given orally or vaginally, as a method of emergency or once-a-month contraception. A more effective combination could be developed in a relatively short time frame.
2. Studies in nonhuman primates should be conducted to develop the concept and test the safety of immunization against progesterone as a simple and easily reversible contraceptive method.
3. The most promising of the adhesion molecules should be studied to deter-

mine how essential they are for initial blastocyst attachment to the endometrial epithelium.

4. Experiments using active or passive immunization should be conducted to determine whether, for example, LIF is essential for implantation in species other than the mouse. If such experiments prove positive, then means to disrupt uterine LIF function for a short period should be sought; the most specific approach would appear to be through interference with binding of the specific LIFRα subunit. Examination of the obligatory requirement for other growth factors/cytokines should be carried out.

5. Nonpeptide GnRH antagonists, which would be useful for applications both before and after fertilization, should be developed.

REFERENCES

Adams CE. Retention and development of eggs transferred to the uterus at various times after ovulation in the rabbit. Journal of Reproduction and Fertility 60:309–315, 1980.

Allan GF, X Leng, ST Tsai, et al. Hormone and antihormone induce distinct conformational changes which are central to steroid receptor activation. Journal of Biological Chemistry 267:19513–19520, 1992.

Anegon I, MC Cuturi, A Godard, et al. Presence of leukemia inhibitory factor and interleukin 6 in porcine uterine secretions prior to conceptus attachment. Cytokine 6:493–499, 1994.

Artini PG, C Battaglia, G D'Ambrogio, et al. Relationship between human oocyte maturity, fertilization and follicular fluid growth factors. Human Reproduction 9:902–906, 1994.

Asch RH, CG Smith, et al. Luteolytic effect of azastene in the nonhuman primate. Obstetrics and Gynecology 59:303–308. 1982.

Barzel US. Estrogens in the prevention and treatment of postmenopausal osteoporosis. American Journal of Medicine 85:847–850, 1988.

Baumann H, GG Wong. Hepatocyte-stimulating factor. III. Shared structural and functional identity with leukemia inhibitory factor. Journal of Immunology 143:1163–1167, 1989.

Becker-Andre M, I Wisenberg, N Schaeren-Wiemers, et al. Pineal gland hormone melatonin binds and activates an orphan of the nuclear receptor superfamily. Journal of Biological Chemistry 269:28531–28534, 1994.

Bhatt H, LJ Brunet, CA Stewart. Uterine expression of leukemia inhibitory factor coincides with the onset of blastocyst implantation. Proceedings of the National Academy of Sciences, USA 88:11408–11412, 1991.

Birgerson L, A Lund, V Odlind, et al. Termination of early human pregnancy with epostane. Contraception 35:111–120, 1987.

Birgerson L, V Odlind. Early pregnancy termination with antiprogestins: A comparative clinical study of RU 486 given in two dose regimens and epostane. Fertility and Sterility 48:565–570. 1987.

Blye RP. The use of estrogens as postcoital contraceptive agents. American Journal of Obstetrics and Gynecology 116:1044–1050, 1973.

Braga VMM, SJ Gendler. Modulation of Muc-1 mucin expression in the mouse uterus during the estrus cycle, early pregnancy and placentation. Journal of Cell Science 105:397–405, 1993.

Byskov AG, CY Andersen, L Nordholm, et al. Chemical structure of sterols that activate oocyte meiosis. Nature 374:559–562, 1995.

Charnock-Jones DS, AM Sharkey, et al. Leukemia inhibitory factor mRNA concentration peaks in human endometrium at the time of implantation and the blastocyst contains mRNA for the receptor at this time. Journal of Reproduction and Fertility 101:421–426, 1994.

Chen D-B, R Hilsenrath, Z-M Yang, et al. Leukaemia inhibitory factor in human endometrium during the menstrual cycle: Cellular origin and action on production of glandular epithelial cell prostaglandin *in vitro*. Human Reproduction 10:911–918, 1995.

Chen F, AJ Cooney, Y Wang, et al. Cloning of a novel orphan receptor (GCNF) expressed during germ cell development. Molecular Endocrinology 8:1434–1444, 1994.

Crooij MS. Antiprogestins. European Journal of Obstetrics and Gynecology and Reproductive Biology 28:129–132, 1988.

Crooij MJ, CC deNooyer, BR Rao, et al. Termination of early pregnancy by the 3β-hydroxysteroid dehydrogenase inhibitor epostane. New England Journal of Medicine 319:813–817, 1988.

Croxatto HB. Gamete transport. IN Reproductive Endocrinology, Surgery and Technology. E Adashi, JA Rock, Z Rosenwaks, eds. Philadelphia: Lippincott-Raven. 1995.

Davis S, TH Aldrich, N Stahl, et al. LIFRß and gp130 as heterodimerizing signal transducers of the tripartite CNTF receptor. Science 260:1805–1808, 1993.

De M, TR Sandford, GW Wood. Expression of interleukin 1, interleukin 6 and tumor necrosis factor a in mouse uterus during the peri-implantation period of pregnancy. Journal of Reproduction and Fertility 97:83–89, 1993.

DePaolo LV, M Shimonaka, RH Schwall, et al. *In vivo* comparison of the follicle-stimulating hormone-suppressing activity of follistatin and inhibin in ovariectomized rats. Endocrinology 128:668–674, 1991.

Dorce M. Control of M-Phase by maturation-promoting factor. Current Opinions in Cell Biology 2:269–273. 1990.

Downs SM. Factors affecting the resumption of meiotic maturation in mammalian oocytes. Theriogenology 39:65–79, 1993.

Erickson GF, DR Danforth. Ovarian control of follicle development. American Journal of Obstetrics and Gynecology 172:736–747, 1995.

Evans RM. The steroid and thyroid hormone receptor superfamily. Science 240:889–895, 1988.

Farkas M, G Apró, M Sas. Clinico-pharmacological examination of Postinor (0.75 mg d-norgestrel). Therapeutica Hungarica 29:22–30, 1981.

Fazleabas AT, S Hild-Petito, HG Verhage. Secretory proteins and growth factors of the baboon (*Papio anubis*) uterus: Potential roles in pregnancy. Cellular Biology International 18:1145–1153, 1994.

Feldman B, W Poueymirou, VE Papaioannou, et al. Requirement of FGF-4 for postimplantation mouse development. Science 267:246–249, 1995.

Forman BM, E Goode, J Chen et al. Identification of a nuclear receptor that is activated by farnesol metabolites. Cell 81:687–693, 1995.

Frank GR, AK Brar, H Jikihara, et al. Interleukin-1ß and the endometrium: An inhibitor of stromal cell differentiation and possible autoregulator of decidualization in humans. Biology of Reproduction 52:184–191, 1995.

Fukuda MN, T Sato, J Nakayama, et al. Trophinin and tastin, a novel cell adhesion molecule complex with potential involvement in embryo implantation. Genes and Development 9:1199–1210, 1995.

Gearing DP, MR Comeau, DJ Friend, et al. The IL-6 signal transducer, gp130: An oncostatin M receptor and affinity converter for the LIF receptor. Science 255:1434–1437, 1992.

Gearing DP, CJ Thut, T VandenBos, et al. Leukemia inhibitory factor is structurally related to the IL-6 signal transducer gp130. EMBO Journal 10:239–248, 1991.

Gemzell-Danielsson K, M-L Swahn, et al. Early luteal phase treatment with mifepristone (RU 486) for fertility regulation. Human Reproduction 8:870–873, 1993.

Ghosh D, P De, J Sengupta. Luteal phase oestrogen is not essential for implantation and maintenance of pregnancy from surrogate embryo transfer in the rhesus monkey. Human Reproduction 9:629–637, 1994.

Ghosh D, J Sengupta. Anti-nidatory effect of a single, early post-ovulatory administration of mifepristone (RU 486) in the rhesus monkey. Human Reproduction 8:552–558, 1993.

Glasier A, KJ Thong, M Dewar, et al. Mifepristone (RU 486) compared with high dose estrogen and progestogen for emergency postcoital contraception. New England Journal of Medicine 327:1041–1044, 1992.

Greene KE, LM Kettel, SS Yen. Interruption of endometrial maturation without hormonal changes by an antiprogesterone during the first half of luteal phase of the menstrual cycle: A contraceptive potential. Fertility and Sterility 58:338–343, 1992.

Grigorescu F, MT Baccara, et al. Insulin and IGF-1 signaling in oocyte maturation. Hormone Research 42:55–61, 1994.

Harper MJK. The implantation window. Baillière's Clinical Obstetrics and Gynecology 6:351–371, 1992.

Harper MJK. Agents with antifertility effects during preimplantation stages of pregnancy. IN Biology of Mammalian Fertilization and Implantation. KS Moghissi, ESE Hafez, eds. Springfield, IL: C.C. Thomas. 1972.

Harvey MB, KJ Leco, MY Arcellana-Panlilio, et al. Roles of growth factors during peri-implantation development. Molecular Human Reproduction 10:712–718, 1995.

Haspels AA. Emergency contraception: A review. Contraception 50:101–108, 1994.

Hatayama H, H Kanzaki, M Iwai, et al. Progesterone enhances macrophage colony-stimulating factor production in human endometrial stromal cells in vitro. Endocrinology 135:1921–1927, 1994.

Heyman RA, DJ Mangelsdorf, JA Dyck, et al. 9-cis retinoic acid is a high affinity ligand for the retinoid X receptor. Cell 68:397–406, 1992.

Hild-Petito S, HG Verhage. Secretory proteins and growth factors of the baboon (*Papio anubis*) uterus: Potential roles in pregnancy. Cell Biolology International 18:1145–1153, 1994.

Hillier SG, GV Groom, et al. Effects of active immunization against steroids upon circulating hormone concentrations. Journal of Steroid Biochemistry 6:529–535, 1975.

Hilton DJ, NA Nicola, D Metcalf. Specific binding of murine leukemia inhibitory factor to normal and leukemic monocytic cells. Proceedings of the National Academy of Sciences USA 85:5971–5975, 1988.

Hirano T, T Matsuda, K Nakajima. Signal transduction through gp130 that is shared among the receptors for the interleukin 6 related cytokine subfamily. Stem Cells 12:262–277, 1994.

Ho PC, MSW Kwan. A prospective randomized comparison of levonorgestrel with the Yuzpe regimen in post-coital contraception. Human Reproduction 8:389–392, 1993.

Horseman ND, L-Y Yu-Lee. Transcriptional regulation by the helix bundle peptide hormones: Growth hormone, prolactin, and hematopoietic cytokines. Endocrine Review 15:627–649, 1994.

Hsueh AJ, H Billig, A Tsafriri. Ovarian follicle atresia: Hormonally controlled apoptotic process. Endocrine Review 15:707–724, 1994.

Hunt JS, H-L Chen, et al. Normal distribution of tumor necrosis factor-α messenger ribonucleic acid and protein in the uteri, placentas, and embryos of osteopetrotic (*op/op*) mice lacking colony-stimulating factor-1. Biology of Reproduction 49:441–452, 1993.

Ikeda Y, WH Shen, et al. Developmental expression of mouse steroidogenic factor-1, an essential regulator of the steroid hydroxylases. Molecular Endocrinology 8:654–662, 1994.

Ilesanmi AO, DA Hawkins, BA Lessey. Immunohistochemical markers of uterine receptivity in the human endometrium. Microscopic Research Technique 25:208–222, 1993.

Inoue T, H Kanzaki, M Iwai, et al. Tumor necrosis factor α inhibits *in vitro* decidualization of human endometrial stromal cells. Human Reproduction 9:2411–2417, 1994.

Ip NP, SH Nye, TG Boulton, et al. CNTF and LIF act on neuronal cells via shared signaling pathways that involve the IL-6 signal transducing receptor component gp130. Cell 69:1121–1132, 1992.

Jentoft N. Why are proteins O-glycosylated? Trends in Biochemical Science 15:291–294, 1990.

Kariya M, H Kanzaki, T Hanamura, et al. Progesterone-dependent secretion of macrophage colony-stimulating factor by human endometrial stromal cells of nonpregnant uterus in culture. Journal of Clinical Endocrinology and Metabolism 79:86–90, 1994.

Kimber SJ. Carbohydrates as low affinity binding agents involved in initial attachment of the mammalian embryo at implantation. IN Early Fetal Growth and Development. RHT Ward, SK Smith, D Donnai, eds. London: Royal College of Obstetricians and Gynecologists Press. 1994.

Kimber SJ, IM Illingworth, SR Glasser. Expression of carbohydrate antigens in the rat uterus during early pregnancy and after ovariectomy and steroid replacement. Journal of Reproduction and Fertility 103:75–87, 1995.

Kliewer SA, K Umesono, DJ Noonan, et al. Convergence of 9-cis retinoic acid and peroxisome proliferator signaling pathways through heterodimer formation of their receptors. Nature 358:771–774, 1992.

Kliman HJ, RF Feinberg, LB Schwartz, et al. A mucin-like glycoprotein identified by MAG (mouse ascites golgi) antibodies: Menstrual cycle-dependent localization in human endometrium. American Journal of Pathology 146:166–181, 1995.

Kojima K, H Kanzaki, M Iwai, et al. Expression of leukemia inhibitory factor in human endometrium and placenta. Biology of Reproduction 50:882–887, 1994.

Kugu K, AM Dharmarajan, S Preutthipan, et al. Role of calcium/calmodulin-dependent protein kinase II in gonadotropin-induced ovulation in *in vitro* perfused rabbit ovaries. Journal of Reproduction and Fertility 103:273–278, 1995.

Lala DS, DR Rice, KL Parker. Steroidogenic factor 1, a key regulator of steroidogenic enzyme expression, is the mouse homolog of fushi tarazu-factor 1. Molecular Endocrinology 6:1248–1258, 1992.

Lehmann J, L Moore, TA Smith-Oliver, et al. An antidiabetic Thiazolidinedione is a high affinity ligand for peroxisome proliferator-activated receptor PPARg. Journal of Biological Chemistry 270:12953–12956, 1995.

Lessey BA. The use of integrins for the assessment of uterine receptivity. Fertility and Sterility 61:812–814, 1994.

Lessey BA, AJ Castelbaum, CA Buck, et al. Further characterization of endometrial integrins during the menstrual cycle and in pregnancy. Fertility and Sterility 62:497–506, 1994.

Lessey BA, L Damjanovich, C Coutifaris, et al. Integrin adhesion molecules in the human endometrium: Correlation with the normal and abnormal menstrual cycle. Journal of Clinical Investigation 90:188–195, 1992.

Levitski A, A Gazit. Tyrosine kinase inhibition: An approach to drug development. Science 267:1782–1788, 1995.

Luo X, Y Ikeda, KL Parker. A cell-specific nuclear receptor is essential for adrenal and gonadal development and sexual differentiation. Cell 77:481–490, 1994.

Lütticken C, UM Wegenka, J Yuan, et al. Association of transcription factor APRF and protein kinase Jak1 with the interleukin-6 signal transducer gp130. Science 263:89–92, 1994.

Lydon JP, RF Power, OM Conneely. Differential modes of activation define orphan subclasses within the steroid/thyroid receptor superfamily. Gene Expression 2:273–283, 1992.

McDonnell DP, DL Clemm, T Herman, et al. Analysis of estrogen receptor function *in vitro* reveals three distinct classes of antiestrogens. Molecular Endocrinology 9:659–669, 1995.

Morris JK, JS Richards. Luteinizing hormone induces prostaglandin endoperoxide synthase-2 and luteinization *in vitro* by A-kinase and C-kinase pathways. Endocrinology 136:1549–1558, 1995.

Morris JK, JS Richards. Hormone induction of luteinization and prostaglandin endoperoxide synthase-2 involves multiple cellular signaling pathways. Endocrinology 133:770–779, 1993.

Murakami M, M Hibi, N Nakagawa, et al. IL-6-induced homodimerization of gp130 and associated activation of a tyrosine kinase. Science 260:1808–1810, 1993.

Nieschlag E, EJ Wickings. Biological effects of antibodies to gonadal steroids. Vitamins and Hormones 36:165–202, 1978.

O'Malley BW. Steroid hormone receptors as transactivators of gene expression. Breast Cancer Research and Treatment 18:67–71, 1991.

Ornitz DM, AB Herr, M Nilsson, et al. FGF binding and FGF receptor activation by synthetic heparin-derived di- and trisaccharides. Science 268:432–436, 1995.

Ortiz ME, G Bastias, O Darrigrande, HB Croxatto. Importance of uterine expulsion of embryos in the interceptive mechanism of postcoital oestradiol in rats. Reproduction, Fertility, and Development 3:333–337, 1991.

Piquet-Pellorce C, L Grey L, A Mereau, et al. Are LIF and related cytokines functionally equivalent? Experimental Cell Research 213:340–347, 1994.

Pollard JW, JS Hunt, W Wiktor-Jedrzejczak, et al. A pregnancy defect in the osteopetrotic (*op/op*) mouse demonstrates the requirement for CSF-1 in female fertility. Developmental Biology 148:273–283, 1991.

Power RF, JP Lydon, OM Conneely, et al. Dopamine activation of an orphan of the steroid receptor superfamily. Science 252:1546–1548, 1991.

Rider V, A McRae, RB Heap, et al. Passive immunization against progesterone inhibits endometrial sensitization in pseudopregnant mice and has antifertility effects in pregnant mice which are reversible by steroid treatment. Journal of Endocrinology 104:153–158, 1985.

Rose TM, AG Bruce. Oncostatin M is a member of a cytokine family that includes leukemia-inhibitory factor, granulocyte colony-stimulating factor, and interleukin 6. Proceedings of the National Academy of Sciences of the USA 88:8641–8645, 1991.

Schane HP, JE Creange, AJ Anzalone, et al. Interceptive activity of azastene in rhesus monkeys. Fertility and Sterility 30:343–347, 1978.

Schultz JF, DR Armant. ß₁- and ß₃-class integrins mediate fibronectin binding activity at the surface of developing mouse peri-implantation blastocysts. Journal of Biological Chemistry 270:11522–11531, 1995.

Selinger M, IZ Mackenzie, MD Gillmer, et al. Progesterone inhibition in mid-trimester termination of pregnancy: Physiological and clinical effects. British Journal of Obstetrics and Gynaecology 94:1218–1222, 1987.

Shen WH, CC Moore, Y Ikeda, et al. Nuclear receptor steroidogenic factor 1 regulates the Mullerian inhibiting substance gene: A link to the sex determination cascade. Cell 77:651–661, 1994.

Simón C, A Frances, GN Piquette, et al. Embryonic implantation in mice is blocked by interleukin-1 receptor antagonist. Endocrinology 134:521–528, 1994.

Simón C, GN Piquette, A Frances, et al. Interleukin-1 type I receptor messenger ribonucleic acid (mRNA) expression in human endometrium throughout the menstrual cycle. Fertility and Sterility 59:791–796, 1993a.

Simón C, GN Piquette, A Frances, et al. Localization of interleukin-1 type I receptor and interleukin-1ß in human endometrium throughout the menstrual cycle. Journal of Clinical Endocrinology and Metabolism 77:549–555, 1993b.

Sirois J. Induction of prostaglandin endoperoxide synthase-2 by human chorionic gonadotropin in bovine preovulatory follicles *in vivo*. Endocrinology 135:841–848, 1995.

Snyder BW, HP Schane. Inhibition of luteal phase progesterone levels in the rhesus monkey by epostane. Contraception 31:479–486, 1985.

Stahl N, TG Boulton, T Faruggella, et al. Association and activation of Jak-Tyk kinases by CNTF-LIF-OSM-IL-6ß receptor components. Science 263:8833–8841, 1994.

Stahl N, TJ Faruggella, TG Boulton, et al. Choice of STATs and other substrates specified by modular tyrosine-based motifs in cytokine receptors. Science 267:1349–1353, 1995.

Stewart CC, P Kaspar, LJ Brunet, et al. Blastocyst implantation depends on maternal expression of leukemia inhibitory factor. Nature 359:76–79, 1992.

Strous GJ, J Dekker. Mucin-type glycoproteins. Critical Reviews in Biochemistry and Molecular Biology 27:57–92, 1992.

Surveyor GA, SJ Gendler, L Pemberton, et al. Expression and steroid hormonal control of Muc-1 in the mouse uterus. Endocrinology 136:3639–3647, 1995.

Swahn ML, M Bygdeman, S Cekan, et al. The effect of RU 486 administered during the early luteal phase on bleeding pattern, hormonal parameters and endometrium. Human Reproduction 5:402–408, 1990.

Tabibzadeh S, KL Kaffka, PG Satyaswaroop, et al. Interleukin-1 (IL-1) regulation of human endometrial function: Presence of IL-1 receptor correlates with IL-1-stimulated prostaglandin E_2 production. Journal of Clinical Endocrinology and Metabolism 70:1000–1006, 1990.

Tackacs L, EJ Kavacs, MR Smith, et al. Detection of IL-1α and IL-1ß gene expression by *in situ* hybridization: Tissue localization of IL-1 mRNA in the normal C57BL/6 mouse. Journal of Immunology 141:3081–3094, 1988.

Tang X-M, MJ Rossi, BJ Masterson, et al. Insulin-like growth factor I (IGF-I), IGF-I receptors, and IGF binding proteins 1–4 in human uterine tissue: Tissue localization and IGF-I action in endometrial stromal and myometrial smooth muscle cells *in vitro*. Biology of Reproduction 50:1113–1125, 1994.

Taniguchi T. Cytokine signaling through nonreceptor protein tyrosine kinases. Science 268:251–255, 1995.

Tartakovsky B, E Ben-Yair. Cytokines modulate preimplantation development and pregnancy. Developmental Biology 146:345–352, 1991.

Tzukerman MT, A Esty, D Santioso-Mere, et al. Human estrogen receptor transcriptional capacity is determined by both cellular and promoter context and mediated by two functionally distinct intramolecular regions. Molecular Endocrinology 8:21–30, 1994.

Vale W, L Bilezikjian, C Rivier. Reproductive and other roles of inhibins and activins. IN The Physiology of Reproduction. E Knobil, JD Neill, eds. New York: Raven Press. 1994.

Vale W, A Hsueh, C Rivier. The inhibin/activin family of hormones and growth factors. IN Handbook of Experimental Pharmacology, Vol. 95/11: Peptide Growth Factors and Their Receptors II. New York: Springer Verlag. 1990.

Velásquez LA, JG Aguilera, HB Croxatto. Possible role of platelet-activating factor in embryonic signaling during oviductal transport in the hamster. Biology of Reproduction 52:1302–1306, 1995.

Webb AMC, J Russell, M Elstein. Comparison of Yuzpe regimen, danazol and mifepristone (RU 486) in oral postcoital contraception. British Medical Journal 305:927–931, 1992.

Weber JA, DA Freeman, DK Vanderwall, et al. Prostaglandin E_2 hastens oviductal transport of equine embryos. Biology of Reproduction 45:544–546, 1991.

Willson TA, D Metcalf, NM Gough. Cross-species comparison of the sequence of the leukaemia inhibitory factor gene and its protein. European Journal of Biochemistry 204:21–30, 1992.

WHO, Special Programme of Research, Development, and Research Training in Human Reproduction (WHO/HRP), Task Force on Postovulatory Methods of Fertility Regulation. Menstrual regulation by mifepristone plus prostaglandin: Results from a multicentre trial. Human Reproduction 10:308–314, 1995.

Yamamoto-Yamaguchi Y, M Tomida, M Hozumi. Specific binding of a factor inducing differentiation to mouse myeloid leukemic M1 cells. Experimental Cell Research 164:97–102, 1986.

Yang Z-M, D-B Chen, S-P Le, MJK Harper. Differential hormonal regulation of leukemia inhibitory factor (LIF) in rabbit and mouse uterus. Molecular Reproduction and Development 43:470–476, 1996.

Yang Z-M, S-P Le, D-B Chen, MJK Harper. Temporal and spatial expression of leukemia inhibitory factor in rabbit uterus during early pregnancy. Molecular Reproduction and Development 38:148–152, 1994.

Yang Z-M, S-P Le, D-B Chen, et al. Expression patterns of leukemia inhibitory factor receptor (LIFR) and the gp130 receptor component in rabbit uterus during early pregnancy. Journal of Reproduction and Fertility 103:249–255, 1995a.

Yang Z-M, S-P Le, D-B Chen, et al. Leukemia inhibitory factor (LIF), LIF receptor and gp130 in the mouse uterus during early pregnancy. Molecular Reproduction and Development 42:407–414, 1995b.

Yuzpe AA, WJ Lancee. Ethinylestradiol and dl-norgestrel as a postcoital contraceptive. Fertility and Sterility 28:932–936, 1977.

Yuzpe AA, RP Smith, AW Rademaker. A multicenter clinical investigation employing ethinyl estradiol combined with dl-norgestrel as a postcoital contraceptive. Fertility and Sterility 37:508–514, 1982.

Zhang Z, C Funk, D Roy, et al. Heparin-binding epidermal growth factor-like growth factor is differentially regulated by progesterone and estradiol in rat uterine epithelial and stromal cells. Endocrinology 134:1089–1094, 1994a.

Zhang Z, C Funk, SR Glasser, et al. Progesterone regulation of heparin-binding epidermal growth factor-like factor gene expression during sensitization and decidualization in the rat uterus: Effects of the antiprogestin ZK 98.299. Endocrinology 135:1256–1263, 1994b.

Zhong Z, Z Wen, JE Darnell Jr. STAT3: A STAT family member activated by tyrosine phosphorylation in response to epidermal growth factor and interleukin-6. Science 264:95–98, 1994.

B

Male Methods

David W. Hamilton, Ph.D.
*Department of Cell Biology and Neuroanatomy,
University of Minnesota Medical School*

Patricia M. Saling, Ph.D.
*Department of Obstetrics and Gynecology and
Department of Cell Biology,
Duke University Medical Center*

INTRODUCTION

The ideal male contraceptive should be safe, effective and reversible and should not have an effect on libido. In addition, it should be self-administered with little training and require neither elaborate surgical procedures nor prolonged periods of either abstinence or alternative contraceptive techniques to be effective. The biology of the male reproductive tract puts certain limitations on the development of novel contraceptive strategies yet, because of the unique features of cells in the male reproductive tract, new possibilities are presenting themselves that need to be carefully addressed.

Current Options

Contraceptive options for men are extremely limited. By far the most common contraceptive method in use today is the condom and, barring unforeseen complications such as puncture, this method can be highly effective both in contraception and in protection against sexually transmitted diseases for both men and women. A major advantage of the condom is that its effect is immediate and it does not require periods of abstinence or, indeed, use of other contraceptive approaches to be effective. Reversal is also immediate.

Vasectomy, on the other hand, which is the other most common and effective form of contraception used by men today (e.g., Wang et al. 1994), requires alternative contraceptive techniques for varying periods after the operation until there are no longer sperm in the ejaculate (azoospermia). Vasectomy also has the disadvantage of requiring a surgical procedure, although the degree of invasion is minimal (especially with nonscalpel vasectomy [NSV] with chemical or other methods of vas occlusion); however, reversal requires a more elaborate surgical procedure, with return of fertility dependent upon numerous unknown factors. Furthermore, vasectomy provides no protection against transmission of sexually transmitted infections.

Variations on the theme of vasectomy have been suggested over the years, for example, valves that regulate vasal fluid flow (Kuckuck et al. 1975), and interruption of control of the vas musculature (Amobi and Smith 1995). A promising approach has been developed in China where percutaneous intravasal injection into the vas lumen of a quick-curing polymer results in a plug that effectively blocks seminal flow (Zhao et al. 1992). Still, this approach also requires a period of alternative contraceptive use until azoospermia is achieved (as much as 12 months [Chen et al. 1992]), although reversal is a simple and apparently effective procedure of merely removing the plug and does not require elaborate microsurgery.

These mechanical methods rely on restricting movement of sperm into the female reproductive tract. An equally effective strategy could be to render sperm inactive prior to ejaculation or to produce azoospermia with drugs. In the following sections we provide an overview of research in male contraception and suggest strategies that might be employed to develop effective contraceptives for men. In order to provide some rationale for different strategies, we begin with a brief excursion into the structure and regulation of function in the male reproductive tract.

Overview of the Male Reproductive Tract

In developing contraceptives for men, it is obviously essential to take into account the dynamics of the male reproductive system, particularly spermatogenesis. Spermatogenesis is a precisely timed process whose regulation is a poorly understood, complex set of interactions among many cell types. Post-testicular sperm maturation is also highly complex, regulated as it is by circulating factors from the testis and from other organs, as well as by factors derived from intraluminal secretions of the testis itself. The intricacy of these processes is well recognized, but most of its details are unknown. The contraceptive strategy employed, therefore, will depend upon where in the male reproductive tract intervention occurs.

Gross Structure

Sperm are produced in the seminiferous tubule of the testis; are then released into the lumen of the tubule as immature cells, unable to fertilize eggs; and are carried by bulk flow through the rete testis and efferent ductule into the single, coiled tubule that comprises the epididymis. Movement of sperm into the epididymis from the testis is rapid, but as sperm traverse the efferent ductules, >90 percent of the water in the fluid that surrounds them is removed (Crabo 1965). This, in turn, produces a viscous, sperm-containing epididymal fluid that, over a time span of a week or more, is moved slowly through the epididymis by contractions of the smooth muscle surrounding the duct. During this transit, sperm acquire the ability to fertilize eggs through metabolic and other biochemical changes, and also develop the ability to move progressively; these modifications are collectively termed "sperm maturation." The matured sperm are stored in the tail of the epididymis until ejaculation, at which time they move through the vas deferens and its ampulla; mix with secretions of the prostate, seminal vesicle, and bulbourethral glands; and exit through the penile urethra. From the time spermatogonia begin to differentiate into sperm until the time of ejaculation, the cellular and fluid environment, which is progressively modified, contributes to germ cell maturation, eventually assuring their ability to fertilize eggs. Contraceptive strategies can be developed that target events throughout this journey, that is, during the processes of sperm maturation.

The Testis   The seminiferous tubule is comprised of a structurally complex epithelium surrounded by muscle-like myoid cells, interstitial cells, and fluid. It is in this tubule that spermatogonia form into highly specialized sperm. The epithelium essentially comprises two cell types: Sertoli cells and germ cells. Three additional cell types—myoid cells, Leydig cells, and "immune cells"—surround the epithelium. Sertoli cells are tall, columnar somatic cells that extend from the base of the epithelium to the lumen of the duct. They surround and nurture the differentiating germ cells and, by means of structural specializations termed Sertoli–Sertoli junctions, segregate the germ cells undergoing meiosis (spermatocytes) and spermiogenesis (spermatids) from macromolecules in the blood and lymph vascular systems. Owing to this process of segregation—the so-called blood–testis barrier—the only germ cells accessible to macromolecules borne by blood or lymph are spermatogonia and early spermatocytes, although we do not know how or whether blood-borne factors affect spermatogonia.

Germ cells undergo well-defined maturational events that comprise spermatogenesis, a process that begins at puberty with mitotic divisions of the primitive, Type A spermatogonia. This is followed by subsequent cell divisions—the number varies by species—of most of the daughter cells. Some daughter cells do not differentiate further; rather, these "resting" spermatogonia provide stem cells for future spermatogenetic events. The Type A spermatogonia that continue to divide eventually differentiate into Type B spermatogonia that are committed to enter meiosis. Once germ cells enter meiosis they are termed spermatocytes. The first meiotic division, carried out by primary spermatocytes, has a long prophase (see Dym 1983, or other histology texts for more detailed descriptions) and so these cells are frequently seen in histological sections of the seminiferous epithelium. The second meiotic division, carried out by secondary spermatocytes, has a short duration; as a consequence, these cells are more rare in histological sections than primary spermatocytes. Upon completion of meiosis, the cells enter spermiogenesis and begin the long process of differentiation from essentially round cells to highly polarized, highly differentiated sperm. In the human, the total process of spermatogenesis takes ~64 days. In animals, the process takes less time but, interestingly, experimental studies to date have not been able to alter the timing of spermatogenesis.

Germ cells comprise a histologically complex group of cells; the complexity derives in part from the fact that spermatogenesis, in humans, occurs in patches along the length of the seminiferous tubule and the patches are not all in synchrony. Within patches, however, there is synchronous differentiation. If one were able to sample one patch over the 64 days of spermatogenesis different cell associations, or stages (seven have been defined in the human), would be seen because of the timing of each phase (that is, mitosis, meiosis, and spermiogenesis). This lack of synchrony throughout the testis poses a major problem for the design of strategies for interrupting spermatogenesis, since it essentially determines *a priori* that any interruption of spermatogenesis would require at least a two-month delay before there was any noticeable decrease in sperm in the ejaculate.

The myoid cells that surround the seminiferous epithelium have contractile properties. They release a glycoprotein, termed PmodS (Skinner and Fritz 1985) that affects Sertoli cells by activating the IP_3 signaling pathway, although the function of PmodS is not known. Leydig cells produce testosterone, which supports spermatogenesis and also acts in the negative long-loop feedback system that regulates release of luteinizing hormone (LH) and follicle stimulating hormone (FSH) (see below). There is considerable evidence that the "immune" cells (e.g., macrophages) affect Leydig cell functions (Hutson 1994).

Interactions among these various major cell types in the testis have been amply documented. For instance, Sertoli cell products interact with germ cells to regulate their differentiation (see Sharpe 1993) and, recently, it has been shown that germ cells produce factors that affect Sertoli cell function (Onoda and Djakiew 1990, 1993). In addition, as described above, interstitial cells produce factors that affect Sertoli cells and possibly germ cells. In the aggregate, the observations on cell–cell interactions at the level of the testis ("short-loop feedback mechanisms") are extensive and could be targeted for contraceptive intervention.

The Excurrent Ducts and Accessory Organs of Reproduction   When sperm leave the testis and enter the first part of the epididymis, they are not capable of fertilizing eggs; it is the progression through the epididymis that results in their ability to fertilize. The maturation experienced by sperm in the epididymis involves both metabolic changes and interactions with the secretions of the epididymis and accessory organs of reproduction that lead to molecular modifications of the sperm surface (see below).

Regulation of Function in the Male Reproductive Tract

In addition to the regulation of function at the level of the seminiferous tubule through short-loop mechanisms mentioned above, there are endocrine feedback loops that support sperm development in the seminiferous tubule. These "long-loop interactions" (recently reviewed by McLachlan et al. 1995) are mediated by hormones produced in the brain and the gonads, the so-called hypothalamic-pituitary-gonadal axis. Secretion of the hypothalamic decapeptide GnRH (gonadotropin-releasing hormone) by hypothalamic neurons in the pituitary leads to release of the gonadotropins LH (luteinizing hormone) and FSH (follicle-stimulating hormone) from gonadotroph cells in the anterior pituitary. LH and FSH are carried to the testis in blood, where LH stimulates production of testosterone by Leydig cells and FSH interacts with Sertoli cells to affect synthesis of proteins that are secreted both into the luminal compartment of the tubule and the blood vascular system (e.g., inhibin). Testosterone, carried by the blood and lymph, interacts with both the hypothalamus and pituitary to inhibit LH release, while inhibin inhibits FSH release.

Regulation of function of the excurrent ducts occurs both by blood-borne factors, such as testosterone, and by factors not yet fully characterized that are secreted by the testis and carried through the tubule lumen where they can effect expression of proteins and glycoproteins secreted by the epididymis. Increasing evidence indicates that sperm, as well as innervation of the excurrent ducts, can directly affect epithelial cell function (Douglass et al. 1991).

The long-loop feedback system has, in fact, already been targeted in a number of studies on male contraception (see Wang et al. 1994) by using such compounds as steroids and GnRH agonists and antagonists that have been previously used in studies on humans and for which toxicological information is available. Studies attempting interruption of the long-loop feedback mechanisms have involved injections of androgens to inhibit hypothalamic and pituitary functions related to gonadotropin release (e.g., Handelsman et al. 1992). Azoospermia was accomplished after variable periods of administration and, at the end of treatment, sperm returned to the ejaculate and the individuals were fertile. Similar strategies have been attempted using GnRH agonists and antagonists, but required ancillary injections of androgens to obviate loss of libido (Bagatell et al. 1993). (See Chapter 4 herein for further discussion of these approaches.)

Potential Targets for Male Contraceptive Development

In addition to the endocrine feedback loops referred to immediately above, there are many cellular and molecular events in the male reproductive tract that are unique to that tract. We would like to address potential areas of future research in two areas: the testis and the excurrent ducts.

Inhibition of FSH Secretion and/or FSH Action

Follicle-stimulating hormone (FSH) is a hormone produced by the anterior pituitary that regulates testicular function by binding to high-affinity receptors located in males exclusively on Sertoli cells. In mammals, the absolute requirement for FSH in the maintenance of adult spermatogenesis is controversial; however, it does appear to be generally agreed that in humans, as in nonhuman primates, qualitatively normal spermatogenesis requires FSH as well as testosterone (Zirkin et al. 1994). Therefore, contraceptive attack directed against either FSH or its receptor, if unique determinants are present, may offer a method to disrupt spermatogenesis without affecting steroid hormones.

FSH is a heterodimeric 30 kD glycoprotein that contains about 30 percent carbohydrate. The hormone is composed of noncovalently associated subunits, an α chain 92 residues in length and a β chain 111 residues in length. The FSH α subunit has a close structural relationship with the α subunits of LH, hCG and TSH (thyroid-stimulating hormone), whereas the β subunit is unique and is considered to be responsible for the receptor specificity of FSH. The FSH receptor is an integral membrane protein containing the usual seven-pass transmembrane structure conserved for interaction with G-proteins at the cytoplasmic face of the plasma membrane. The extracellular domain of the FSH receptor is, however, unusually large for this class of receptor. The receptor exists in the membrane of the Sertoli cell as a homotetramer, and ligand-blot studies indicate that FSH binds only to the tetrameric form of the FSH receptor.

Molecular details of the interaction of FSH with its receptor have been studied through the use of synthetic peptides corresponding to regions of the primary sequence of either FSH or its receptor, as well as by site-directed mutagenesis. These analyses reveal that the interaction between hormone and receptor is quite complicated. FSH appears to utilize different sites to effect receptor binding and signal transduction (Valove et al. 1994): FSH-βArg[35] is critical for efficient receptor binding but not for signal transduction whereas, in contrast, a specific oligosaccharide attached at FSH-αAsn[52] has been reported to be critical for signal transduction but not receptor binding. Reciprocal studies dealing with the FSH receptor have mapped the linear nonhomologous sequence Arg[265]–Ser[296] as important for FSH binding. These characteristics of the FSH/FSH receptor system suggest several possible and quite specific contraceptive tactics.

Alteration of FSH Secretion   Since the action of FSH is limited to the Sertoli cell alone, absence of FSH in the adult male would not be expected to lead to adverse side effects; indeed, trials that have been conducted thus far support this contention (see above). These studies utilized GnRH analogues or androgens to affect the long feedback pathway and produce infertility. The major stumbling block in this regard appears to be the metabolic clearance rate of either the androgens or the GnRH analogues. Some attention has been given to development of long-acting esters of testosterone (see Wang et al., 1994) but, to date, treatment still requires unacceptably frequent injections.

Targeting of Unique Sequences of FSH for Immunologic Destruction Since FSH-β is considered to be responsible for the receptor specificity of FSH, linear sequences—particularly those involved in binding to the receptor—could be targeted by specific neutralizing antibodies. Thus, after defining the optimally immunogenic epitopes, individuals could be immunized with synthetic peptides corresponding to those epitopes. The desired consequence would be the elicitation of specific antibodies that would bind to FSH in the circulation and prevent the hormone's interaction with its receptor. Compared to the foregoing approach, this strategy has the advantage of greater selectivity; however, it has potentially adverse side effects relative to the anterior pituitary, which is not protected from immunological attack and could possibly be destroyed by cell-mediated immunity since it is the site of FSH synthesis. This would be analogous to the ovarian failure encountered in mammalian experiments with immunization with ZP3. One strategy that might be employed to circumvent this difficulty would be the identification of exclusive B-cell epitopes, if present, in the linear sequence of FSH-β used as immunogen. Such exclusive B-cell epitopes would be predicted to elicit only specific antibodies without the cytotoxic arm of the immune response. Nevertheless, it may turn out that exclusive B-cell epitopes are not, in fact, present in the targeted sequence, or that the epitope is not sufficiently immunogenic on its own to generate blocking antibodies.

Interference with FSH Binding to the FSH Receptor Because the biological effects of FSH are exerted through activation of its receptor on Sertoli cells, methods that prevent FSH receptor activation are predicted to disturb spermatogenesis. At least two different strategies can be considered as ways to produce this effect: (1) direct interference with hormone-receptor interaction by generation of specific anti-FSH receptor antibodies or mimetopes, or (2) indirect interference by preventing proper assembly of the functional tetrameric receptor.

Direct Interference with Hormone-Receptor Interaction Current evidence suggests that the extracellular domain of the FSH receptor contains unique sequences that could be selectively targeted by antibodies or mimetopes so as to prevent FSH binding. This target is located at an accessible site since, although the sperm-producing portion of the testis is protected by the blood–testis barrier, the basal surface of Sertoli cells bears the FSH receptors and is available to the circulation. A potential disadvantage of this strategy is that the agent—antibody or mimetope—that binds to the FSH receptor may itself activate the receptor; this would obviate any contraceptive effect. Studies of receptor activation in a variety of other systems have revealed that both activating and nonactivating antibodies may be directed against epitopes in the extracellular domains of various receptors; in the case of the FSH receptor, exploration of this possibility would be required, using both *in vitro* and animal model assays.

Indirect Interference with Hormone-Receptor Interaction   As indicated above, FSH binding studies indicate that the hormone binds only to tetrameric FSH receptors. This means that any strategies that would prevent proper assembly of receptor subunits would effectively block receptor action. For most oligomeric receptors, assembly occurs intracellularly; improperly assembled receptors are retained within the cell and not inserted into the plasma membrane. Assuming that specific targets within the FSH receptor sequence can be identified—a reasonable assumption—the novel task is to determine how to prevent proper assembly. As far as we know, the information needed to achieve this objective is not available, but understanding of protein trafficking within cells is advancing at a remarkable rate and it can be anticipated that some strategies will be available in the future.

Control of Meiosis

Meiosis is the process by which the number of chromosomes in a diploid nucleus (2N) is reduced to the haploid state (1N) by cell division. There are two cell division cycles in meiosis; meiosis I and meiosis II. The former involves DNA synthesis and results in two daughter cells each of which are diploid. In the latter, there is no DNA synthesis, so that the four daughter cells that result from this division are haploid. Meiosis occurs only in germ cells and in no other cells in the body in both males and females and the basic mechanism underlying meiosis is the same in both sexes. However, there are dramatic differences between the two sexes in the way the process takes place. In males, meiosis is a continuous event, that is, once they have been initiated, the two cell divisions in meiosis are carried to completion. In the female, on the other hand, meiosis is arrested at the end of prophase in the first meiotic division and at metaphase in the second division. The first arrest can be years in duration and is relieved only when the oocyte is stimulated to grow in preparation for ovulation. The second arrest is relieved at fertilization.

The basic question that arises, therefore, is: Why are there no meiotic arrests in the male similar to those in the female? The next question is: Can the mechanisms of arrest in the female be utilized in developing an approach to meiotic arrest in males that would be an effective contraceptive? The first meiotic arrest in females appears to be heavily dependent upon cAMP-dependent protein kinase A. In view of the general importance of this system in other cells in the body—in other words, it is very far from being specific—it does not seem likely that altering activity of this system would be a rewarding strategy.

On the other hand, arrest of meiosis II appears to involve at least one unique germ cell protein, Mos, although there probably are other factors involved as well but it is not clear exactly when transcription occurs and studies to date are contradictory. In one study, c-mos was found to be transcribed in the male during meiosis, but the message was not translated until spermiogenesis began (Chapman and Wolgemuth 1994); in another study, c-mos was found expressed before meiosis (Van der Hoorn et al. 1991). This means that the protein is expressed either too late or too early to have an effect on meiosis in the male. One can speculate that if the protein was expressed *during* meiosis, then meiotic arrest would occur and would block further development of sperm. Targeting cells in the adluminal compartment of the blood/testis barrier is discussed below, but this is potentially such a powerful approach to fertility regulation that renewed investigation of the barrier is warranted.

Genetic Manipulation of Sperm

An ideal male contraceptive would interfere with the production or maturation of sperm without affecting testis function in any other way, including any reduction of hormone secretion or libido. An attack on developing germ cells within the testis would be a very direct approach to the disruption of sperm production. As spermatogonia differentiate into spermatocytes, they begin to advance toward the lumen of the seminiferous tubule. As noted above, primary spermatocytes engage in the first meiotic division to generate secondary spermatocytes; the latter cells undergo the second meiotic division to give rise to haploid spermatids. No further divisions occur: Spermatids differentiate into sperm (during spermiogenesis) and are liberated into the lumen of the seminiferous tubule. The progenitor spermatogonia are located at the base of the seminiferous tubule, are unprotected by the blood–testis barrier, and are therefore available to perturbation by agents distributed through the circulation. In contrast, the population of germ cells that initiates meiosis (primary spermatocytes) become protected by the blood/testis barrier during the first meiotic division. At that point, the germ cells are no longer directly accessible to the circulation. As an alternative to targeting spermatogonia, it may be possible to use Sertoli cells as a route of delivery to postmeiotic germ cells. This would be fairly complex since a two-stage delivery system would be necessary (targeting first to Sertoli cell, and then to germ cell), but it would make use of the extensive communicating junctions that exist between Sertoli and germ cells.

Utilization of techniques developed for gene therapy should allow the targeting of accessible germ cells. In standard gene therapy, a stem cell population is targeted and new genes are inserted into these cells to overcome the effects of damaged genetic material. In a contraceptive context, these same techniques, for example, targeting surface components specific to spermatogonia, could be used but, instead of correcting a malfunction, a defect would be introduced. Sertoli cells could also (perhaps more easily?) be targeted in this way, and genes introduced that would disable normal function. In essence, this would be a "Sertoli cell knockout." Since the number of Sertoli cells limits the number of germ cells undergoing differentiation, the efficiency of this approach might not have to be near 100 percent to achieve a large impact on sperm numbers. The important task of identifying germ cell processes that are amenable to this strategy remains; several possible sites of contraceptive attack are described below. The creation of "conditional knockouts" in mice has been described wherein a specified gene was inactivated selectively in a particular cell type. These findings, which remain to be exploited for contraceptive development, pave the way for the selective inactivation of specific genes. In the context of the epididymis, for instance, one could envisage "knocking out" genes that encode epididymal secretory proteins that are important in maturing the sperm surface either by binding directly to the surface or by modifying it enzymatically. In this way, critical determinants of the sperm surface would not appear properly, leading to compromised function during fertilization.

Disturbance of Normally Functioning Transcription Factors   An important approach to disrupting sperm production would be to interfere with differentiation itself. Spermatogenesis is under elaborate, yet strict, control both spatially and temporally. This control is exerted in part by transcription factors, proteins that bind to DNA with the effect of switching genes on or off. Although this field is relatively unexplored in terms of germ cells, it can be imagined that the schedule of transcription factor expression is extremely important. Inappropriate expression of a transcription factor, either absence of expression when needed or overexpression, is likely to have profound effects on differentiation. Transcription factors specific to germ cells have already been identified (Chen et al. 1994), making this topic a very attractive one to pursue. Since spermatogonia are not protected by the blood–testis barrier, events that occur in this population should be emphasized with this approach until it can be established that the delivered agent can operate postmeiotically.

As a specific example, an attractive process to target with this approach would be the replacement of nuclear histones with protamines. This replacement process is exclusive to developing sperm cells and occurs in spermatids. Spermatocytes, however, synthesize protamines, highly charged basic proteins that, when complexed with DNA, are thought to facilitate the dense chromatin packing found in the sperm head. Failure to package the chromatin in this way could have important implications for chromatin structure or stability.

Among other processes that might be targeted productively are any that are unique to sperm development, for instance, acrosome formation (see below). Like histone/protamine replacement, acrosome formation normally occurs in postmeiotic germ cells. Nevertheless, several of the acrosomal contents are synthesized much earlier, some as early as in late spermatogonia/early spermatocytes. Thus, thorough understanding of these fundamental processes of spermatogenesis will assist in identifying possible targets.

Mapping of Genes Responsible for Fertility and/or Infertility Classic genetic techniques offer an alternative approach to trying to identify unique transcription factors or processes involved in sperm production. Many of the processes of meiosis and gamete production are highly conserved across all animal phyla, and important information can be gained from the study of well-established model systems, with the aim of then relating that information back to the human situation. For instance, the genetics of *Drosophila* have been studied extensively. Of the ~4,000 genes in the total genome, mutation of ~400 of them causes sterility in females; of these, ~150 are without any obvious effects elsewhere in the organism (see Chapter 5). Parallel studies for male fertility might identify a similar subset of mutations. While all of these mutations are unlikely to have human correlates, some of them may serve as a previously unrecognized site for contraceptive focus.

Inhibition of Acrosome and Tail Formation

Two important events in sperm development are, first, formation of the acrosome and, second, the establishment of the longitudinal polarity of the cell by attachment of centrioles to the nucleus leading to formation of the sperm tail. These events occur in no other cells in the male and are therefore potentially susceptible to unique intervention for contraception. As far as we know, these processes are not regulated by hormones.

Interference with Acrosome Formation The acrosome is bound tightly to the outer surface of the nuclear envelope, just deep to the plasma membrane overlying the sperm head. It is a product of the Golgi apparatus (Thoren-Tjomsland et al. 1988) and first appears morphologically in spermatids; however, it has been shown that the mRNA for acrosomal contents can be synthesized as early in pachytene spermatocytes. During spermiogenesis, selected vesicles in the trans-Golgi network begin to accumulate a granular content and fuse into a large acrosomic body that moves from the Golgi to attach to the nucleus. The remaining Golgi is partially lost in residual bodies and phagocytosed by Sertoli cells, although portions of Golgi membranes remain in the cytoplasmic droplet found on the sperm tail. The trans-Golgi network in most somatic secretory cells faces away from the nucleus toward the apical surface of the cells. In somatic cells, secretory vesicles move from the Golgi toward the apical plasma membrane to eventually fuse with it and release their contents. In contrast, the trans-Golgi network in spermatids faces toward the nucleus so that the forming acrosomic body is ideally placed to move to the nucleus. In essence, the acrosome is a secretory vesicle that stores its products during the later phases of spermiogenesis and post-testicular maturation until a signal is given by the binding of sperm to the zona pellucida to release the contents (see below). Since formation of the acrosome is absolutely essential for fertility, it seems reasonable that interfering with the process could result in sperm that could not fertilize an egg.

There are several questions that arise about formation of the acrosome that may provide a strategy for interrupting either its formation or its function:

- What mechanisms are involved in orientation of the Golgi apparatus that are different from those found in most somatic cells?
- What signals target acrosomic contents to only a subset of vesicles in the trans-Golgi network?
- What structural features participate in coalescence of the acrosomic vesicles?
- What are the mechanisms for tight interactions between the membrane of the acrosomic body and the nuclear membrane?

Interference with Centriole Attachment and Sperm Tail Formation   Like the acrosome, the sperm tail is essential for fertility. The tail derives from centrioles but, in sperm, the flagellum that forms is highly modified compared to those in other cells. Centrioles and the Golgi apparatus in most somatic cells are structurally closely related to form the cytocentrum. In all cells, centrioles have the potential to germinate cilia or flagella, but only in spermatids do the centrioles migrate around the periphery of the cell to bind tightly to the nuclear envelope 180 degrees away from the attachment of the acrosome. The first indication of tail formation is movement of the centrioles to lie just deep to the plasma membrane. They then appear to migrate around the cell and, at a certain point, move toward the nucleus, pulling with them the plasma membrane in the region. The centrioles bind to the outer nuclear membrane, becoming highly modified themselves; the longitudinal centriole germinates the axoneme that comprises the sperm tail. All of these modifications, as well as the formation of the mitochondrial sheath, fibrous sheath, the annulus, and outer dense fibers, are unique events that occur only in spermatids. Presumably these unique events require unique processes to bring them about, which can be targeted for contraceptive intervention.

Alteration of Sperm Surface Proteins During Spermatogenesis and Post-Testicular Development

During spermatogenesis, sperm acquire a highly polarized morphology, with a quadripartite structure consisting of a head, which contains the haploid genome, a midpiece, a principal piece, and an end piece. The extreme state of compartmentalization observed in this cell at maturity extends as well to the organization of the sperm plasma membrane, where both lipids and proteins are organized into highly regionalized domains. Many questions about the formation and maintenance of the membrane domains remain, but at least some domains are thought to be important functionally. During spermiogenesis, when the haploid cell is remodeled, many of these domains make their first appearance, although several are refashioned during post-testicular maturation in the epididymis.

Several sperm proteins thought to be important in fertilization have been identified and their appearance in the membrane of the developing sperm is being charted (Bartles 1995). Although few studies dealing with the development of membrane domains have been conducted directly with human sperm, human homologues for some of the nonhuman tracked proteins have been identified and are presumed to behave similarly. Many of these fertilization-related proteins are inserted into the plasma membrane during spermatogenesis and display a restricted distribution from the start, whereas others are more uniformly distributed in testicular sperm but are directed into domains during epididymal passage. Both fertilin and PH-20 represent sperm proteins important for fertilization that fall into the latter category (Myles and Primakoff 1991). In testicular sperm, while both these proteins are distributed over the entire sperm surface, they are restricted during epididymal transit to specialized regions of the sperm head. *In vitro* studies of guinea pig sperm indicate that this redistribution can be affected by trypsin treatment of immature sperm, giving rise to the notion that redistribution is proteolysis-dependent *in vivo*. This sort of alteration is presumably caused by secretory products of the epididymal epithelium; disruption of the elaboration of such components will be considered in the following section. In terms of intrinsic sperm structure and its relationship to fertilizing capacity, however, these concepts give rise to possible contraceptive strategies.

Disruption of Membrane Domains   A conserved feature of all mammalian sperm analyzed to date is the extreme regionalization of membrane components. While membrane domains are also a common feature of somatic cells, they are rarely built to such an extent. Although at present the specific function(s) of this polarized organization in any cell type is not clear, germ cells invest heavily in elaborating and maintaining this organization. As more becomes known about the cellular components involved in generating and maintaining membrane domains, it may be possible to target these pathways so that domain formation is disrupted. The absence of a high local concentration of a particular sperm protein in a defined region, or the inability of specific components to couple to appropriate intracellular constituents, are likely to lead to dysfunctional sperm.

Disruption of Delivery of Fertilization-related Proteins to the Membrane   As mentioned earlier, fertilin is delivered to the membrane of the developing sperm cell during spermatogenesis; in fact, initial delivery to the surface occurs in spermatids. Eddy and O'Brien (1994) have hypothesized that the temporal regulation of surface expression may be responsible for directing proteins to the correct surface domain. If this concept is accurate, then alteration of the timing of protein expression could subtly disorder the intricate organization of the sperm membrane, with infertile sperm as the result. Of course, fertilin need not be the sole sperm protein that could be targeted with this strategy: Any fertilization-related protein that displays a restricted surface distribution in the mature sperm would be an equally attractive candidate. Indeed, it may be that emphasis on fertilization-related proteins is unnecessary, since the inappropriate timing of any surface protein may so disrupt the positioning of other functional components that detrimental effects would ensue.

Interruption of Epididymal Function

In addition to serving as a sperm reservoir, the epididymis provides an environment for morphological and biochemical alterations in the sperm that are necessary for fertility, that is, the "sperm maturation" that takes place during the one- to two-week period that sperm require for passage through the single convoluted tubule that comprises this organ. Whereas the morphologic changes that occur with maturation are fairly subtle, the functional changes effected are essential for the sperm's fertilizing ability. These include the capacity for (1) vigorous motility; (2) productive interaction, both binding and acrosomal exocytosis, with the egg's extracellular matrix, the zona pellucida; and (3) productive interaction with the egg's plasma membrane. These functions of the epididymis, and indeed the maintenance of the organ itself, are androgen-dependent; in the absence of androgen, the epididymis decreases dramatically in size and sperm maturation does not occur.

Thus, transit through this post-testicular site confers on sperm the ability to fertilize an egg; as such, it constitutes what may be among the best locations for contraceptive attack for several reasons. First, the epididymis is an end-organ for hormone action but apparently is not itself involved in hormone synthesis *in vivo*. Second, the only known functions of the epididymis, that is, transit, maturation, and storage, involve sperm exclusively. Third, sperm are fully formed genetically in the testis and are fairly inert biosynthetically upon arrival in the epididymis. Consequently, compared to manipulations of the testis, contraceptive strategies directed toward the epididymis are considerably less likely to produce adverse hormonal or genetic side effects.

Much of the sperm surface appears to be remodeled during maturation and modifications have been detected in all types of plasma membrane components, including lipids, proteins, and carbohydrates. Several theories have been advanced with regard to the mechanisms involved in these changes, including (1) modification (glycosylation, phosphorylation, and so forth) or unmasking (hydrolysis, either limited or complete) of preexisting components; (2) redistribution of preexisting components; or (3) binding of new components to preorganized domains at the sperm surface following synthesis and secretion by the epididymal epithelium. Sperm surface changes are mediated by products of the epididymal epithelium secreted into the lumen of this tubule. Although the specific components of the epididymal fluid that are responsible for maturing sperm have not been fully identified, it is clear that the composition of the fluid is complex and changes dramatically along the length of the tubule, suggesting that different components of the sperm surface may be modified at different locations along the length of the epididymis.

Although the molecular details of sperm maturation are not well known, it is clear nevertheless that this is an ideal organ to target for contraception. Several possible approaches are outlined below but they are just a beginning. Further research into the molecular mechanisms underlying sperm maturation are very likely to be richly rewarding in their potential to produce novel strategies of a sort that we may not even have imagined.

Modification of Expression of Epididymal Proteins Important in Sperm Maturation   Several proteins that are secreted into epididymal fluid and subsequently adsorbed onto the sperm surface have been identified in humans and in other mammalian species. We do not yet know whether any of these proteins are essential for sperm maturation, since it is only recently that techniques have become available that suggest the feasibility of this kind of approach (Gu et al. 1994). If further research supports feasibility, then the modified expression of such critical proteins would constitute an excellent strategic avenue for male contraceptives.

Application of Epididymis-specific Antiandrogens   As indicated earlier, the functioning of the epididymis depends upon androgen. Impaired delivery of androgen to this site markedly disrupts a large number of parameters, including the secretion of glycosidases known to modify the sperm surface. Recent progress in the administration of organ-specific antiestrogens makes it possible to consider a parallel route for the delivery of antiandrogens to the epididymis. If such an agent were to become available, it might be one of the best ideas for reversible contraception in the male.

Immunoneutralization of Epididymal-specific Proteins   If epididymis-specific proteins that are important in human epididymal and/or sperm function were to be identified, a highly likely possibility, then it should be possible to target these for neutralization by specific antibodies using an immunocontraceptive approach. Just as might be the case for females, males would be immunized with a peptide corresponding to an epididymal-specific portion of the protein of interest. The probability is that the antibodies generated would have considerably better access to epididymal cells than they would to testicular cells, since the blood–testis barrier is not present in the epidiymis.

Regulation of the Inhibition of Immune Reactions by Sperm

A little recognized aspect of sperm development is the fact that, in many species, proteins secreted by the seminal vesicle are immunosuppressive and attach covalently to the sperm surface by a transglutaminase-catalyzed reaction. This phase of sperm maturation may be as important to the viability of sperm in the female tract as any of the events that occur in the epididymis, since the sperm would be essentially immunologically silent and would evade the female immune system (see review by Hamilton 1994). Whether similar events occur in human males and females are unknown.

Induction of Premature Acrosome Reaction

During the gamete interactions that lead to fertilization, one of the regulators of success is the appropriate occurrence of exocytosis in the sperm cell. Normally, this event occurs after the sperm has bound to the egg's protective coat, the zona pellucida, and the enzymes released from the sperm's acrosome permit penetration through this egg coat. Inappropriate release of the acrosomal enzymes when the sperm is some distance from the egg results in infertility.

Recently, progress has been made in defining some of the sperm proteins important in triggering exocytotic release of the acrosome. One of these is termed ZRK (zona receptor kinase), a ZP3 receptor that has the structure of a receptor tyrosine kinase (Burks et al. 1995). It is thought that sperm binding to ZP3 in the zona promotes the oligomerization of ZRK and thereby activates the receptor by autophosphorylation, by analogy with the mechanism of activation for other well-characterized receptor tyrosine kinases. Thus, strategies of the type described just below that would influence the premature occurrence of any of these events—either directly or indirectly—is likely to have profound consequences for fertility.

Delivery of a ZP3-mimic to Sperm in the Male   Theoretically, a reagent that binds ZRK and is multivalent or minimally bivalent could aggregate these ZP3 receptors and activate them. Activation would lead to exocytosis and premature release of the acrosomal enzymes. Either peptide or nonpeptide reagents could be considered as ZP3 mimics; it should be possible to identify these with relative straightforwardness since the primary structure of ZRK is known and there is at least some initial information about ligand binding sites. Delivery of such a mimic could occur in the epididymis and thus potentially be present on sperm for a relatively long period of time. Alternatively, the ZP3 mimic could be targeted to any of the accessory organs of the male reproductive tract—seminal vesicles, prostate, Cowper's glands, or bulbourethral glands—with the choice made on the basis of targeting potential, stability of mimic, etc., and therefore be applied to the sperm surface at ejaculation.

There are, at the outset, at least two possible problems with this approach. One is that sperm binding to the natural ligand ZP3 normally occurs after sperm capacitation, which is a poorly defined final maturational phase accomplished within the female reproductive tract during which both the intrinsic (e.g., increased membrane fluidity) and the extrinsic (e.g., glycosylation) structure of the sperm membrane are modified. Therefore, the binding of a multivalent ZP3 mimic to sperm prior to capacitation, as proposed here, may not be sufficient to stimulate exocytosis. The other is that sperm are present at high concentration in the epididymis, particularly the cauda epididymidis; the accessibility of such a reagent to sperm in the male reproductive tract would have to be extremely high for this approach to be effective.

Identification of the Acrosome Reaction-Eliciting Substance Produced by t-Bearing Sperm Although the strategy outlined above is attended by caveats, it turns out that there is actually a natural method of producing precisely this effect. It has been known for several decades that mouse sperm heterozygous for a mutation in the T-locus will make equivalent amounts of t-bearing and wild-type sperm. However, when mated, there is a transmission distortion for the t-bearing sperm such that 95 percent of the offspring are also heterozygous for the T-locus mutation. This phenomenon has been studied extensively and found to depend on the ability of the t-bearing sperm to provoke premature acrosome reactions in the wild-type population (Brown et al. 1989). The mechanism(s) underlying this effect are completely unknown, and further study of this system could reveal the component(s) that evoke this effect.

Inhibition of Gamete (Sperm–Egg) Interaction

Sperm–egg interaction can be broken down into at least the following six steps (Saling 1995):

1. Cumulus layer penetration
2. Primary binding to the zona (ZP3-mediated)
3. Triggering of acrosomal exocytosis
4. Secondary binding to the zona (probably ZP2-mediated)
5. Penetration through the zona pellucida
6. Fusion between the sperm and egg plasma membranes.

Since each of these events is necessary for fertilization under normal circumstances, potential blockade of any step would impair, if not prevent, fertility. Sperm proteins associated with individual steps of gamete interaction have also been identified recently, which permits selective focus on particular steps and/or proteins. To develop a male-directed contraceptive aimed at eventually blocking these events requires detailed knowledge about the proteins that will be attacked, both in terms of their mechanisms of action as well as potential modification during epididymal transit. An appropriate location for attack appears to be the epididymis, principally for the reasons outlined above; as such, we have already dealt with general strategies that might be employed for this purposes earlier in this paper. There are also in this category strategies using specific sperm proteins.

• **PH-20:** It may turn out that the role of PH-20 in secondary binding depends upon glycosylation. Delivery of antiandrogens to the epididymis might alter expression of the glycosidase required for this effect and therefore result in a PH-20 protein on the sperm surface that is 90 percent less effective in secondary binding to the zona.

• **Fertilin:** We have already referred to the fact that proteolytic processing of fertilin in the epididymis is required for redistribution of the protein to the appropriate subcellular domain in mature sperm. Were the protease responsible for this effect to be identified, it might be possible to design a "conditional knockout" of the gene encoding this enzyme in the epididymis, thereby preventing fertilin redistribution and functioning.

• **ZRK:** This ZP3 receptor appears to be sperm-specific, which may make it attractive for an immunocontraceptive strategy. If antibodies directed against the extracellular domain of ZRK were able to gain access to the epididymal lumen and bind to ZRK on sperm, either or both of two events might occur: (1) steric blockade of sperm–ZP3 interaction or (2) premature release of the acrosome. Both of these events are predicted to lead to infertility. Because of the extremely large number of cells that would require neutralization, optimized delivery of any reagent would be essential.

Concluding Remarks

This paper has followed the general discussion at the symposium on New Frontiers in Contraceptive Technology held at the Institute of Medicine in December 1994[1] and expands on some of the more general concepts that emerged during that meeting. The fundamental message is that there are many plausible targets for development of contraceptives for males. The largest obstacle to targeting the male reproductive tract is its biology. Approaches to inhibition of spermatogenesis (for example, work with the long-loop feedback system) and vasectomy show that infertility is not produced immediately and that lag times can be long. Behavior in men does not conform well to such delays or, in fact, to regimen in general. Still, this does not mean that all approaches will entail comparable problems. Further developments in this field can come only through cooperative interactions among scientists in academia and in industry, and by prioritizing allocation of resources sufficient to achieve the goals.

REFERENCES

Amobi NI, IC Smith. Differential inhibition in the human vas deferens by phenoxybenzamine: A possible mechanism for its contraceptive action. Journal of Reproduction and Fertility 103:215–221, 1995.

Bagatell CJ, AM Matsumoto, RB Christensen, et al. Comparison of a gonadotropin releasing-hormone antagonist plus testosterone (T) versus T alone as potential male contraceptive regimens. Journal of Clinical Endocrinology and Metabolism 77(2):427–432, 1993.

Bartles JR. The spermatid plasma membrane comes of age. Trends in Cell Biology 5:400–404, 1995.

Brown J, JA Cebra-Thomas, JD Bleil, et al. A premature acrosome reaction is programmed by mouse t haplotypes during sperm differentiation and could play a role in transmission ratio distortion. Development 106:769–773, 1989.

Burks DJ, R Carballada, HDM Moore, et al. Interaction of a tyrosine kinase from human sperm with the zona pellucida at fertilization. Science 269:83–86, 1995.

Chapman DL, D Wolgemuth. Regulation of M-phase promoting factor activity during development of mouse male germ cells. Developmental Biology 165(2):500–506, 1994.

Chen ZW, YQ Gu, XW Liang, et al. Safety and efficacy of percutaneous injection of polyurethane elastomer (MPU) plugs for vas occlusion in man. International Journal of Andrology 15(6):468–472, 1992.

Chen F, AJ Cooney, Y Wang, et al. Cloning of a novel orphan receptor (GCNF) expressed during germ cell development. Molecular Endocrinology 8:1434–1444, 1994.

Crabo BG. Studies on the composition of epididymal content in bulls and boars. Acta Veterinaria Scandinavica 6 (Suppl.5):1–94, 1965.

Douglass J, SH Garrett, JE Garrett. Differential patterns of regulated gene expression in the adult rat epididymis. Annals of the New York Academy of Sciences 637:384–398, 1991.

Dym M. The male reproductive system. IN Histology. L Weiss, ed. New York: Elsevier Biomedical. 1983.

Eddy EM, DA O'Brien. The Spermatozoon. IN The Physiology of Reproduction. E Knobil, JD Neill, eds. New York: Raven Press. 1994.

Gu H, JD Marth, PC Orban, et al. Deletion of a DNA polymerase beta gene segment in T cells using cell type-specific gene targeting. Science 265:103–106, 1994.

Hamilton DW. Local immunity and sperm processing in the male reproductive tract. IN Local Immunity in Reproductive Tract Tissues. PD Griffin, PM Johnson, eds. New York: Oxford University Press. 1994.

Handelsman DJ, AJ Conway, LM Boylan. Suppression of human spermatogenesis by testosterone implants. Journal of Clinical Endocrinology and Metabolism 75(5):1326–1332, 1992.

Hutson JC. Testicular macrophages. International Review of Cytology 149:99–143, 1994.

Kuckuck L, GS Chhina, SK Manchanda. Development and initial evaluation of a vas deferens valve. Indian Journal of Physiology and Pharmacology 19(1):20–27, 1975.

McLachlan RI, NG Wreford, DM Robertson, et al. Hormonal control of spermatogenesis. Trends in Endocrinology and Metabolism 6:95–101, 1995.

Myles DG, P Primakoff. Sperm proteins that serve as receptors for the zona pellucida and their post-testicular modification. Annals of the New York Academy of Sciences 637:486–493, 1991.

Onoda M, D Djakiew. Modulation of Sertoli cell secretory function by rat round spermatid protein(s). Molecular and Cellular Endocrinology 73:35–44, 1990.

Onoda M, D Djakiew. A 29,000 Mr protein derived from round spermatids regulates Sertoli cell secretion. Molecular and Cellular Endocrinology 93:53–61, 1993.

Saling PM. Gamete interactions leading to fertilization in mammals: Principles, paradigms, and paradoxes. IN Reproductive Endocrinology, Surgery, and Technology. EY Adashi, JA Rock, Z Rosenwaks, eds. New York: Raven Press. 1995.

Sharpe R. Experimental evidence for Sertoli-germ cell and Sertoli-Leydig cell interactions. IN The Sertoli Cell. L Russell, M Griswold, eds. Clearwater, FL: Cache River Press. 1993.

Skinner MK, IB Fritz. Testicular cells secrete a protein under androgen control that modulates Sertoli cell function. Proceedings of the National Academy of Sciences, USA 82:114–118, 1985.

Thoren-Tjomsland G, Y Clermont, L Hermo. Contribution of the Golgi apparatus components to the formation of the acrosomic system and chromatoid body in rat spermatids. Anatomical Record 221:591–598, 1988.

Valove FM, C Finch, JN Anasti, et al. Receptor binding and signal transduction are dissociable functions requiring different sites on follicle-stimulating hormone. Endocrinology 135:2657–2661, 1994.

Van der Hoorn FA, JE Spiegel, MF Maylie-Pfenninger, et al. A 43 kD c-mos protein is only expressed before meiosis during rat spermatogenesis. Oncogene 6(6):929–932, 1991.

Wang C, R Swerdloff, GMH Waites. Male contraception: 1993 and beyond. IN Contraceptive Research and Development 1984 to 1994: The Road from Mexico City to Cairo and Beyond. PFA Van Look, G Pérez-Palacios, eds. Delhi: Oxford University Press. 1994.

Zhao SC, SP Zhang, RC Yu. Intravasal injection of formed-in-place silicone rubber as a method of vas occlusion. International Journal of Andrology 15(6):460–464, 1992.

Zirkin BR, C Awoniyi, MD Griswold, et al. Is FSH required for adult spermatogenesis? Journal of Andrology 15:273–276, 1994.

NOTE

1. The proceedings from this meeting, including a participants list, are included in this report as Appendix E.

C

Immunocontraceptive Approaches

John Christian Herr, Ph.D.
Department of Cell Biology and The Center for Recombinant Gamete Contraceptive Vaccinogens, University of Virginia

INTRODUCTION

The concept of an immunocontraceptive might be stated as follows: A formulation of certain molecules is injected or taken orally by a man or woman, resulting in the production by his or her own body of circulating antibodies or immune effector cells that interrupt reproductive processes and sustain a period of infertility, without side effects. As of the summer of 1995, no immunocontraceptive had been marketed in any country, either for human or veterinary application.

This review discusses some general concepts regarding contraceptive immunization, reviews several promising immunogen candidates, identifies hurdles on the path to developing an immunocontraceptive, and cites new approaches that may offer opportunities for significant scientific advances.

Differences Between Traditional Vaccines and Immunocontraceptives

The vaccine paradigm was established nearly two centuries ago when, in 1796, Edward Jenner inoculated an 8-year-old boy with cowpox and effectively prevented smallpox. Since then, many vaccines have been developed, their purpose being to provide protection against debilitating or life-threatening micro-organisms. The purpose of an antifertility immunogen is to prevent fertility or early pregnancy. Traditional immunization against micro-organisms may often be the only means available for controlling a given disease; in the case of contraception, alternative methods are already available.

Another major difference is that traditional vaccines are also based on, and directed against, foreign antigens contained in the disease-causing micro-organism; in contrast, antifertility immunization is directed against isologous antigens from the egg, sperm, or certain reproductive hormones. Since isologous antigens may not be as immunogenic as foreign antigens, development of sustained immune responses to them may be difficult, owing in part to mechanisms of immunologic tolerance.

Finally, the ideal traditional vaccine confers long-term protective immunity, usually aided by boosting throughout the lifetime of the individual as a result of exposure to the natural antigen. Because it will be generally desirable for an immunocontraceptive to be reversible, the immunity induced should be of relatively short duration, that is, measured in months or a few years, and should not be boosted naturally by exposure to the target antigen; in other words, insemination should not boost a sperm-based immunocontraceptive.

THE PATHWAY TO DEVELOPMENT OF AN IMMUNOCONTRACEPTIVE

The pathway for development of an immunocontraceptive follows a series of steps not unlike those followed in traditional vaccine development. These include: (1) fundamental discovery and characterization of appropriate immunogens derived from reproductive hormones and/or from the sperm, egg, egg investments, conceptus, or accessory reproductive organs; (2) development of methods for producing the immunogens to high standards of purity through (a) genetic engineering of genes encoding specific immunogens, (b) peptide syntheses, or (c) isolation of the antigen from natural sources; (3) production and purification of immunogens under good laboratory practices (GLP); (4) formulation of immunogen doses; (5) small animal and primate testing of immunogen formulations for immunogenicity, safety, and efficacy; (6) evaluation of mechanisms of immunogen action; (7) human trials for immunogenicity, safety, and efficacy, using formulations produced under good manufacturing practices (GMP); and (8) development of diagnostics to monitor infertility status in recipients of effective immunogens.

The first step—discovery and characterization of immunocontraceptive components—is perhaps the most complicated; it is also the stage at which many research projects currently stand. This step is subdivided into several milestones: (1) definition of events or processes in reproduction accessible to immune intervention; (2) identification of molecules (immunogens) whose elimination or neutralization will have an antifertility effect; (3) biochemical characterization of the structure of the immunogen(s); and (4) determination of whether the immunogen is unique to the reproductive event or tissue targeted and is absent in all other tissues.

In considering which molecules might be best for a contraceptive immunization, consideration should be given to events in the process of reproduction that are accessible to immune intervention. For purposes of simplification, mammalian reproduction may be divided into several key stages, each of which may offer an opportunity for intervention: (1) gamete production (spermatogenesis and oogenesis); (2) gamete shedding and transport (copulation; sperm transport in the cervix, uterus, and oviduct; ovulation and oviductal transport of the cumulus mass); (3) gamete interaction (capacitation, the acrosome reaction, penetration of the egg investments, fusion with the oolemma); (4) blastocyst transport and hatching; and (5) implantation. All of these events can theoretically be inhibited by eliciting an immune response directed against functionally and structurally important molecules that are accessible to immune effectors (antibody or cell mediated).

Many cells and cellular products are involved in the stages of mammalian reproduction enumerated above, including hypothalamic, pituitary, and gonadal hormones; gamete surface components, including proteins, glycoproteins, and glycolipids; and secretions of reproductive organs including cervical, uterine, oviductal, prostatic, and seminal vesicular secretory products. Thus, the field of potential targets would seem to be extensive. However, there are criteria that should be applied to this universe of possible candidates, in order to identify those suitable for development of immunocontraceptives for clinical use (Griffin 1990). These criteria are discussed immediately below; their specifications narrow the range of targets considerably.

Criteria for Candidate Prioritization

Relevance. An antifertility immunogen should be based on a molecule involved in and essential for the process of reproduction, so that immunological neutralization, blockage, or removal of the antigen will cause infertility.

Specificity. In order to avoid complications, it is particularly important that the molecules selected for immunocontraceptive development exhibit tissue specificity, that is, that they are secreted or expressed only in the intended target tissue. This issue should be addressed at the immunogen discovery phase rather than later during toxicological and teratological safety studies, so as to avoid unnecessary effort and expense studying unsuitable immunogens. The potential complications of immunization with contraceptive vaccines include: (1) immediate hypersensitivity and anaphylactic responses; (2) delayed hypersensitivity responses; and (3) autoimmune response and autoimmune disease owing to immune reaction with endogenous antigens of the immunized subjects (Tung 1986). Many of these concerns may be obviated by selection of non-crossreactive immunogens specific to the reproductive target tissues.

Existence of a Homologous Animal Model. The target antigen should, ideally, have an identical or closely related form and function in an animal model in which immunogenicity, safety, and efficacy studies can be carried out.

Accessibility. The target antigen must be accessible to antibody or sensitized lymphocytes in the circulation and/or lumen of the genital tract of the recipient. The target antigen must therefore be secreted by the target cells and/or appear displayed on the surface membrane or glycocalyx of the target cells. In the case of sperm, which undergo remodeling of the sperm surface after the acrosome reaction, this criterion includes the inner-acrosomal membrane, which is the limiting membrane on the anterior portion of the sperm head after the completion of the acrosome reaction. "Coating antigens" derived from the male sex accessory glands might also be included.

Amplitude. The concentration of neutralizing antibodies induced by immunization is important. Not only must sufficient antibody be induced, but it must be induced in the right place and at the right time. The amount of antibody must be sufficient to neutralize the target antigen to achieve contraceptive efficacy as well as safety. Thus knowledge of the concentration of the target molecule is important, as is information on fluctuations in its concentration. The neutralizing concentrations of antibody must be available at the appropriate location in the circulation or lumen of the reproductive tract at the time when the antigen is accessible. Negative effects of too high an antibody response must also be avoided. Insoluble immune complex formation in the circulation in vascular sites may provoke immunopathology (immune complex diseases). Immediate and delayed hypersensitivity reactions may occur in the reproductive organs. Thus, a balance must be struck between reaching an amplitude of antibody or immune effector cells necessary to achieve contraceptive efficacy while, at the same time, avoiding inflammatory complications.

The immunogens chosen for incorporation into an immunocontraceptive must include epitopes recognized by most, if not all, recipients. In an outbred population such as the human race, variability in host responsiveness to any single epitope is likely to be large. A given immunogen may be effective in one group but ineffective in another. This implies that a formulation that includes a variety of immunogens to which all groups respond has the best likelihood of achieving high contraceptive efficacy.

Transience. Reproductive antigens that are present only transiently or in low concentrations have some advantages: (1) The risk of chronic formation of immune complexes is minimized; (2) The immune response will be called into effect only when the antigen is present; (3) Excess antigen is not likely to overwhelm available antibody.

Synthetic Capability. Capacity to synthesize the immunogens in large quantities under good laboratory and good manufacturing practices is an important practical requirement for selecting molecules for clinical testing. Use of the natural tissues as starting materials for immunocontraceptive production is possible; however, isolation processes from natural sources are much more difficult to control from the standpoint of safety than are standard synthetic or genetic engineering procedures. For example, isolating a sperm antigen from human semen would require safety assurances that viruses such as HIV and hepatitis B were absent from the starting semen preparation. Thus, recombinant proteins and synthetic peptides offer important advantages.

The Timing of Intervention

Pre- and Postfertilization Immunocontraception

Based on assumptions regarding their hypothesized mechanism of action, immunocontraceptives based on antigens associated with the sperm, egg, or early conceptus are frequently referred to as pre- or postfertilization immunocontraceptives, although such designations are largely speculative since the mechanism of action of any immunocontraceptive is only partially understood. The basic hypotheses are, first, that an antibody to a sperm membrane component would act in the oviduct to prevent fertilization or to agglutinate or lyse sperm during passage through the female tract; in other words, immunocontraception would take place prior to fertilization, that is, a *pre*fertilization method. In contrast, an immunocontraceptive based on antibody to chorionic gonadotrophin, which is a product of the early embryo's syncytiotrophoblast, would act within the uterus to induce early abortion and would therefore be a *post*fertilization intervention.

Gender Focus

The emphasis in research to date has been on methods of immunizing women, either to prevent fertilization or early pregnancy. This focus has been a function of historical developments in reproductive biology in which detailed knowledge about female reproductive biology has preceded understandings about the male reproductive system. This is partly because women are most immediately concerned with conception and its implications and partly for a range of cultural reasons.

Biologic considerations also come into play. For example, both men and women would seem to be equal candidates for immunocontraceptive approaches using formulations based on sperm antigens, since natural models of infertility due to antisperm antibodies occur in both males and females. In males, antisperm antibodies arise following vasectomy in all animal models studied and in human males (Linnet 1983). Indeed, the lowered incidence in male fertility observed following vasectomy reversal (vasovasostomy or reasnatomosis) may be due to immunologic mechanisms. Women also exhibit antisperm antibodies and, in some women with unexplained infertility, levels of these antisperm antibodies may be quite high (Mathur et al. 1981). Yet, despite the capability of both men and women to develop antisperm antibodies, development of amounts of such antibody sufficient to reduce fertility in the female reproductive tract appears much more feasible, simply by virtue of numbers. The numbers of sperm in the oviduct at the time of fertilization may only be in the tens, possibly hundreds; the number of sperm requiring immunologic interdiction in the male tract is on the order of 10^8 to 10^9. Thus, generating contraceptive titers of antisperm antibody in the oviduct is a less challenging prospect than producing a comparable effect in the male reproductive tract.

ANTIGENS WITH CONTRACEPTIVE POTENTIAL

The molecules that have been considered as contraceptive immunogens fall into the following groups:

1. Reproductive hormones. This group consists of two basic, somewhat overlapping subsets:

 • A group which includes the hypothalamic gonadotropin-releasing hormone, GnRH; the pituitary gonadotrophins, luteinizing hormone (LH) and follicle-stimulating hormone (FSH); and the gonadal steroids; and
 • A group which includes hormones produced by the conceptus such as human chorionic gonadotrophin (hCG), a glycoprotein hormone produced by the placental syncytiotrophoblast.

2. Other antigens of the trophoblast and early embryo.
3. Egg-surface antigens. This category encompasses the protein constituents of the oolemma, the zona pellucida, and possibly the corona radiata.
4. Sperm-surface antigens. This category subsumes proteins associated with the sperm plasma membrane and the acrosomal membranes. Proteins associated with the inner-acrosomal membrane are of interest, since this membrane becomes the limiting membrane of the anterior sperm head following the acrosome reaction, an event occurring prior to fertilization. Antigens secreted by the accessory organs of the male reproductive tract (epididymis, seminal vesicles, and prostate) that bind to and coat the sperm surface are also possible immunogens in this group.

Reproductive Hormones as Antigens

GnRH-based Immunogens for Both Males and Females

The decapeptide gonadotrophin-releasing hormone (GnRH) is synthesized in the hypothalamus. It regulates the synthesis of the pituitary gonadotrophins, LH and FSH, that are the key regulators of spermatogenesis and oogenesis. LH acts on Leydig cells and luteal cells to regulate steroid synthesis. FSH acts on the seminiferous epithelium to stimulate spermatogenesis at puberty in males, and on the theca and granulosa cells to stimulate follicular maturation in females. The role of FSH during the later stages of sexual life in the male is less well understood, but it appears to be important for spermatogonial proliferation.

A GnRH formulation offers a particularly promising approach to a reversible male contraceptive. The mechanism of action of such a formulation posits the following cascade of events: a rise in circulating anti-GnRH antibodies would reduce levels of GnRH, LH, and FSH; levels would then fall, steroid production would subsequently decline, and spermatogenesis would cease (Bremner et al. 1986). Secondary effects, including decrease in testicular size, possible decline in libido, and alterations in secondary sexual characteristics, are practical drawbacks to the commercial acceptance of this formulation. Current GnRH formulations have coupled this decapeptide to various carriers, including tetanus toxoid, and have found that, in rats inoculated with GnRH-TT immunogen on five occasions over a 15-week period, there was atrophy of the testes and accessory sex organs (prostate and seminal vesicles), decreased testosterone as antibodies to GnRH increase, suppressed spermatogenesis, and a decline in libido (Ladd et al. 1989). At the same time, because the formulation shrinks male sex accessory glands, it has been viewed as a possible treatment for prostatic carcinoma or benign prostatic hyperplasia and is being tested in men with prostate cancer under Population Council sponsorship at The University of Texas at San Antonio; similar studies are being conducted through the National Institute of Immunology in Delhi, India.

Thus, to become marketable as a contraceptive for males, a GnRH formulation would require supplementation with testosterone to maintain libido and avoid alterations in secondary sexual characteristics (Ladd et al. 1988). Key to possible acceptance will be the ability to deliver correct doses of supplementary androgen to achieve those objectives. In addition, because administration of exogenous androgen is well known for decreasing LH and FSH through the pituitary feedback loop, it could also reinforce contraceptive action by depressing LH and FSH and inhibiting spermatogenesis. Development of slow-release formulations of androgen, possibly coupled to transdermal delivery, may constitute an important parallel technology that is necessary for success in developing a GnRH immunocontraceptive for men. Reversibility will also be pivotal and appears to be possible. Immunized rats supplemented with testosterone display normal sexual behavior yet still show 100 percent infertility; after cessation of immunization, antibody titers have gradually fallen, testosterone production returned, and testis and accessory gland weights have increased (Bremner et al. 1986; Ladd et al. 1989).

The GnRH approach has also been tested on female primates, whose menstrual cyclicity has been impaired in response to administration of a GnRH formulation. However, because of an accompanying decline in estrogen synthesis which could be associated with eventual osteoporosis, application of this formulation would be inappropriate for some percentage of women (Talwar et al. 1993). Use of a GnRH formulation has also been contemplated for use during the postpartum period, the objective being to prolong the anovulatory period that occurs during the period of postpartum amenorrhea that is induced by lactation. Researchers have concluded that concerns about possible effects on infants of anti-GnRH antibodies being passively transferred through breast milk have largely been laid to rest, since there appears to be no active uptake of these antibodies by the infant gut. A phase I human immunogenicity trial of a GnRH-DT (diphtheria toxoid) immunogen is currently under way in postpartum women at two centers in India.

FSH Immunogen for Males

Immunization of male monkeys with sheep FSH has led to a high degree of contraceptive efficacy (Moudgal et al. 1988b). The immunogen in this case was isolated from natural sources (sheep pituitaries) and formulated with aluminum hydroxide gel as an adjuvant. Doses of 1.0, 0.3, 0.1, and 0.1 mg were given at days 1, 20, 40, and 70, followed by a booster 100 days thereafter (Moudgal and Aravindan 1993). A 70 percent reduction in sperm count (oligospermia) was observed three months after the start of injection. Flow cytometry of testicular cells harvested on day 80 indicated that the primary spermatocyte population had been reduced by >90 percent, the spermatogonial population by 32 percent, and the round spermatid population by 53 percent; testis weight decreased by only 10 percent (Moudgal et al. 1988a, 1988b, 1992). Fertility testing in monkeys was started as early as 90 days after immunization and ten immunized males, fertile prior to immunization, were cohabitated with at least five females each on days 9 to 14 of the menstrual cycle. The efficacy of the FSH formulation was excellent: None of 52 mated females became pregnant (Moudgal et al. 1992). Furthermore, toxicity studies in rats and monkeys have shown no complications, even in monkeys immunized for over five years, and the formulation's contraceptive effect is reversible; following cessation of boosting and fall in antibody titers, sperm counts gradually returned to normal and 9 out of 10 monkeys regained fertility (Moudgal and Aravindan 1993).

Among the possible hormone-based male immunocontraceptives that have undergone trial, the FSH formulation is the only one that does not require supplementation with exogenous androgens. Although the formulation has no effect on androgen-dependent libido and should therefore be at least theoretically acceptable to the human male, and although it does not produce azoospermia (total absence of sperm), the formulation does cause acute oligospermia (reduced sperm numbers), a state that is compatible with infertility, and the sperm that are produced in immunized animals are not only reduced in numbers but are immature and of poor quality.

As indicated, the FSH formulation is currently made with hormone obtained from sheep pituitaries. Future work on this contraceptive immunogen is likely to move toward a formula based on recombinant proteins or synthetic peptides corresponding to epitopes of human or primate FSH. As an avenue for a commercially acceptable, effective, reversible male contraceptive, the FSH formulation is one of the more promising possibilities.

Immunogens of the Early Conceptus

The human chorionic gonadotrophin (hCG) formulations are the most extensively studied, are furthest along the development pathway, and serve as a model for a postfertilization immunocontraceptive. The hCG hormone is a glycoprotein produced by the placental trophoblast. It has a molecular weight of approximately 38 kd and a carbohydrate content of 30 percent. The hCG molecule is comprised of two dissimilar, noncovalently linked subunits designated α and β (Alexander 1992). Because the hormones FSH, LH, thyroid-stimulating hormone (TSH), and hCG have a similar α subunit, antibodies to the whole hCG molecule crossreact with these hormones (Kharat et al. 1990). As a consequence, formulations based on whole hCG are open to possible immunopathologic complications resulting from impairment of FSH, LH, or TSH functions or immune complex formation. Because the β subunit is distinctive in this regard, a formulation based upon this subunit offers a possibility of greater specificity.

The hCG hormone responds to several criteria for a suitable contraceptive target. It is made in appreciable amounts in a physiologically active form only in pregnancy (specificity) and in trophoblastic or nontrophoblastic cancers. Its synthesis starts at the preimplantation stage of blastocyst development, being detectable on day 21 of the menstrual cycle, and increases rapidly after implantation as the mass of the trophoblast expands (accessibility) (Talwar et al. 1993).

The precise mechanism(s) by which an hCG formulation might exert antifertility effects are unknown, but there are several possibilities. First, because the hCG hormone is the stimulus for continued maintenance of the corpus luteum and progesterone production which, in turn, sustains the endometrium in a receptive state for receiving the embryo, it may play a direct role in implantation. In other words, not only does hCG act early but it is vital for pregnancy to occur. Antibodies to hCG that would be induced by an hCG formulation might inactivate the hormone's biologic activity and thereby interrupt the βhCG-dependent events of corpus luteum maintenance and endometrial receptivity, in so doing interrupting implantation.

Another possible mechanism of action is by direct immune attack on the hCG-producing cells of the peri-implantation blastocyst (Stevens 1988). Unlike steroid contraception, which blocks ovulation and replaces natural steroids with synthetic compounds, ovulation and sex steroid synthesis should continue when hCG formulations are used.

The hCG Formulation from Natural Sources Pregnancy urine is the source of the hCG that has been used in a formulation being tested at the National Institute of Immunology in India (Talwar et al. 1981, 1990, 1994). Since women are generally tolerant to the β subunit of hCG, in this formulation the β subunit has been chemically linked to a foreign carrier molecule, tetanus toxoid, to mobilize T helper cell function. Women immunized with this βhCG-TT conjugate develop antibodies to both hCG and tetanus toxoid, so that the formulation confers protection against tetanus. When the immunogen is administered four times at two-week intervals, menstrual regularity is maintained, ovulation is undisturbed, uterine biopsies appear to remain normal, and titers are sustained for a year, after which the response declines to near zero levels between 300 and 500 days following immunization. Immune complexes formed as a result of the presence of antibody appear to be appropriately handled by the body's scavenging system. Studies in hyperimmune monkeys showed that no immune deposits were detected in the pituitaries, choroid plexus, or kidneys after repeated challenge with hCG.

At the same time, because the antibody titers achieved with this vaccine were highly variable, several modifications to the formula have been made. The first injection now contains an adjuvant, SPLPS (sodium phthalyl derivative of lipopolysaccharide), which boosts antibody response. Attempts were also made to enhance the formulation's immunogenicity by (1) making a mixture of the β subunit of *ovine* LH conjugated to diphtheria toxin (βLH-DT) and the hCG-TT, or (2) by forming a heterospecies dimer (HSD) consisting of the β subunit of *ovine* LH and the β subunit of hCG.

The HSD formulation proved to be the most immunogenic in humans, and phase II trials have been conducted with this formulation at a dose of 300 μg per injection (Talwar et al. 1992; Talwar et al. 1994). The formulation was highly effective in those women who had reached sustained serum concentrations of anti-hCG antibody of at least 50 ng/ml (Talwar et al. 1994). However, these protective levels are only reached in 80 percent of the women inoculated. Thus, 20 percent of women did not achieve contraceptive protection with the current formulation. Another drawback is the lag that occurs after a woman is first immunized but before titers reach protective levels. Women receive three injections at six-week intervals; a three-month period is required for protection to be conferred, so that there is a window at the outset of the therapy during which a woman is unprotected.

The current hCG formulation that is derived from natural materials appears safe, with no major complications observed and with ovulation continuing to occur in inoculated women. With improvements in delivering this immunogen, either through use of slow-release biodegradable microspheres or administration of live recombinant antigen through vaccinia viruses (Talwar et al. 1992, 1993), it is possible the formulation might achieve levels of protection that could make it a commercially viable product. The results from human trial of this hCG formulation (Talwar et al. 1994) are of general importance to the field of immunocontraceptives since they demonstrate for the first time "proof of principle": that is, if sufficient levels of antibody are generated to a defined reproductive antigen, a sustained period of contraception occurs and, as the antibody titers decline to preimmunization levels, fertility is restored.

A Synthetic hCG Peptide Formulation   This formulation is being developed under sponsorship of the World Health Organization (Jones et al. 1988). It has already been tested in women for immunogenicity (phase I) (Jones 1990), and phase II efficacy trials in humans were under way as of 1995.

Because the C-terminal region of β hCG is unique to this subunit and because antibodies directed to it do not crossreact with LH, considerable effort has been directed toward development of a peptide formulation based on the C terminus. A series of peptides have been synthesized representing sequences from 6 to 47 amino acids of the C terminus. Since peptides of fewer than 20 amino acids showed relatively lower immunogenicity and induced antibodies incapable of neutralizing hCG (Stevens 1988) and peptides of 35 amino acids or more in length consistently produced antibodies capable of neutralizing hCG, only peptides of this length or longer have been utilized in subsequent development. These peptides require coupling to a carrier to elicit the optimum antibody response and bovine gamma globulin, tetanus toxoid, and diphtheria toxin have all been tested as potential vehicles.

Data on actively immunized marmosets (Hearn et al. 1988) and baboons (Stevens 1976) showed an hCG peptide formulation to be capable of blocking fertility at an early stage of pregnancy, with no discernible alterations of menstrual cycling. In baboons (n = 15) receiving a control injection of diphtheria toxin alone, 14 of 20 ovulatory menstrual cycles resulted in pregnancy, for a 70 percent fertility rate. In baboons inoculated with the hCG peptide coupled to diphtheria toxin, 2 of 44 menstrual cycles resulted in pregnancy, a 4.6 percent fertility rate. Thus, this hCG formulation was 95 percent efficacious. These studies were conducted over three menstrual cycles following completion of the immunization regimen (Stevens 1979).

The hCG peptide formulation that has now progressed to a phase I human clinical trial for immunogenicity is composed of a synthetic oligopeptide corresponding to the amino acid sequence 109–145 of the C terminus of βhCG (Jones et al. 1988). The peptide is conjugated to diphtheria toxoid to form a hapten-carrier complex and a water-soluble adjuvant, muramyl dipeptide (MDP), is incorporated into the aqueous phase of the formula. Prior to injection, a saline-oil emulsion is created, with an oil phase consisting of 4 parts squalene to 1 part mannide monooleate as an emulsifying agent (Stevens et al. 1981, 1990).

To date, 30 premenopausal human female subjects, already surgically sterilized prior to the study, were inoculated with this formulation (Jones et al. 1988). Subjects were assigned to five dosage groups of six subjects each, with each subject receiving a variable dose intramuscularly, injected twice six weeks apart, with the highest dose being 1 mg peptide in 0.5 ml of vehicle. The study revealed that significant levels of antibodies to hCG were attained in the female subjects (Jones 1990). Animal teratology studies are under way with this formulation, and a phase II efficacy study in humans was begun in Sweden. However, because of problems with both vehicle and adjuvant, as of this writing, trials were suspended. Still, this synthetic peptide immunocontraceptive bears close watching.

Egg-surface Antigens

At least three glycoproteins, ZP1, ZP2, and ZP3, have been identified in the zona pellucida of pig, human, mouse, and rabbit eggs, homologies among the zona proteins in these species having been identified (Hedrick 1993). Pig zona pellucida has been injected into mice (Millar et al. 1989), dogs (Mahi-Brown et al. 1988), rabbits (Skinner et al. 1984), and monkeys (Sacco et al. 1990), and in each species significant inhibitory effects on fertility have been observed.

For example, immunization of 50 female squirrel monkeys with 200 μg each of ZP3 (isolated from pig zona), in conjunction with Freund's adjuvant, induced significant antibody titers. The monkeys were followed for four breeding seasons. For the first two years, the group immunized with ZP3 had no pregnancies, while the controls had a 16 percent fertility rate. In the third and fourth breeding seasons, 6 percent of the immunized group became pregnant versus a 21 percent pregnancy rate in controls. The monkeys showed initial disturbances in ovarian function as measured by estradiol and progesterone assays. However, by 10–15 months postimmunization, normal hormonal function had returned as assessed by both hormone determinations and histological observation of normal folliculogenesis (Sacco et al. 1990). There have been similar contraceptive effects in marmosets immunized with porcine ZP3; however, induction of high-titer antibodies to the zona were invariably associated with the appearance of ovarian pathology and depletion of the primordial follicle pool (Paterson et al. 1992).

Severe ovarian disease (Taguchi et al. 1980a,b; Tung et al. 1987), termed autoimmune oophoritis, has been induced by injecting zona proteins in other models, particularly rabbit (Skinner et al. 1984) and mouse (Rhim et al. 1992). In rabbits, injection of pig zona pellucida caused loss of growing follicles, a failure to ovulate in response to hCG, and increased levels of FSH and LH in serum compared to control animals (Skinner et al. 1984). In mice, a synthetic peptide corresponding to amino acids 328→342 of ZP3 has been shown to induce autoimmune oophoritis (Rhim et al. 1992).

These findings suggest that a zona-based formulation might induce immunologic attack on many of the eggs in the ovary and, in effect, induce a type of premature ovarian failure, in other words, induced menopause, a finding that has somewhat diminished enthusiasm for zona-based immunocontraceptives. Still, in theory, zona antibodies could exert their potential contraceptive effects through two mechanisms: (1) inhibition of sperm–zona interaction, as demonstrated by *in vitro* and passive immunization experiments (East et al. 1984); and (2) induction of autoimmune oophoritis. If antibodies could be developed that would act only to block fertilization without causing oophoritis, the path to an immunocontraceptive based on the zona pellucida would clear.

It is in this area that the research challenges lie. One possible approach is to define epitopes that induce antibodies without inducing T cell responses. Studies with peptides derived from the zona proteins may offer some experimental insights into those B cell epitopes that may be incorporated into an immunocontraceptive but not cause ovarian disease.

Sperm-surface Antigens

Background

Immunizing women with sperm to render them infertile is not a new concept. It was proposed many years ago (Baskin 1932; Rosenfeld 1926) and a U.S. patent (2,103,240) was awarded to Baskin for a nonspecific spermatoxic vaccine and for the process involved in its production (Katsh 1959). Despite 12 claims made in the patent, there is no record in the literature as to whether the patented product achieved the objectives stated. Immunization with human seminal plasma proteins or diluted semen resulted in anaphylactic responses in several women, usually after the seventh to tenth injection; inoculation with sperm antigen did not (Otani et al. 1971). Similar hypersensitivity reactions to seminal plasma antigens have been recorded elsewhere (Bernstein et al. 1981).

In animal models, injection of female rabbits with sperm membrane extracts has been shown to significantly reduce fertility (Menge et al. 1979). Rabbit sperm precoated with specific monoclonal antibodies prior to insemination also have shown reduced fertility (Naz et al. 1984). Kummerfeld and Foote achieved a 98 percent suppression of fertility in female rabbits injected with ejaculated, epididymal- or amylase-treated sperm (Kummerfeld and Foote 1976); similarly, virtually complete fertility suppression was obtained in female rabbits after immunization with homologous sperm (Muñoz and Menge 1978).

With crude complex sperm extracts demonstrating some contraceptive efficacy, the principal research effort has been directed subsequently toward identifying and characterizing individual sperm molecules that have similar antifertility effects. A number of antigens have been described that first appear during spermatogenesis and then persist on the mature sperm. As a class, these antigens are often referred to as "intrinsic differentiation antigens," as opposed to extrinsic or coating antigens of sperm. Such differentiation antigens often fulfill the important criterion of tissue specificity discussed above. Several promising sperm antigens are discussed below in connection with possible mechanisms of action induced by a sperm-based immunocontraceptive.

The overall purpose of studies of sperm-based molecules is to develop an immunocontraceptive that will induce antibodies in the female reproductive tract

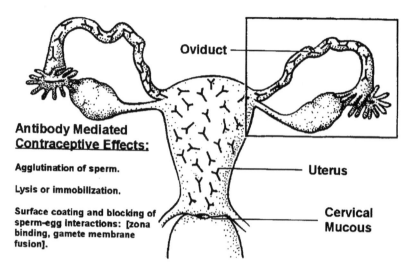

Antibody Mediated
Contraceptive Effects:

Agglutination of sperm.

Lysis or immobilization.

Surface coating and blocking of
sperm-egg interactions: [zona
binding, gamete membrane
fusion].

Oviduct

Uterus

Cervical
Mucous

FIGURE C-1   Diagram of the female reproductive tract indicating the levels at which antibodies to sperm, if present in cervical mucus or uterine or oviductal secretions, might act to agglutinate, lyse, or immobilize sperm. Insert shows region highlighted in Figures C-2 and C-3.

at sufficient levels to block fertilization. It is envisioned that antibodies developed by this formulation will act to agglutinate, immobilize, or coat the sperm in the oviduct, uterus, cervix, or vagina (see Figure C-1). Thus, the formulation will exert its effects before the fertilization event, as a "prefertilization contraceptive." This contraceptive strategy is deemed to have the highest likelihood of widespread acceptance by individuals of varied religious, ethical, and political persuasions.

Multideterminant Sperm Immunocontraceptives

An ideal sperm immunocontraceptive might contain sperm-specific immunogens that would induce antibodies to all the sperm-surface domains that are accessible to antibody, that is, the sperm head, midpiece, and tail plasmalemma, as well as the inner-acrosomal membrane that forms a major part of the anterior surface of the sperm head following the acrosome reaction. This concept guides the work in this field overall and suggests that there is an opportunity for various groups, each working on individual immunogens, to eventually combine their efforts to create the "ultimate immunocontraceptive."

As sperm progress through the female reproductive tract, immune effectors in female secretions may exert contraceptive effects that act in various regions (see Figure C-1). There are numerous possibilities. Antisperm antibodies present in cervical mucus might agglutinate or lyse sperm in the vagina prior to sperm passage through the cervix. Sperm, coated with surface antibody, might be prevented from swimming through and penetrating cervical mucus, a condition often referred to clinically as the "shaking phenomenon" that is well described in the literature on sperm-cervical mucus interaction. Another possibility is that sperm might either be trapped or lysed by antibodies present in uterine secretions so that they are prevented from reaching the oviduct or, perhaps, antibody coating of sperm might interfere with the critical process of capacitation. Antibodies present in oviductal fluid might likewise bind to sperm antigens and prevent the key steps in fertilization that occur in the oviduct. Finally, antibodies to sperm-surface domains, if present in oviductal fluids or embedded in the zona pellucida (which is permeable to immunoglobulins) might coat key sperm receptors at any of the key stages of sperm-egg interaction: penetration of the cumulus mass, zona binding, capacitation, induction of the acrosome reaction, shedding of the acrosomal ghost, penetration of the zona pellucida, binding to the oolemma, or internalization of the spermatozoon by the egg (see Figure C-2 and Figure C-3).

LDH-C$_4$ LDH-C$_4$ (also referred to as LDH-X in older literature) is an isoenzyme of lactate dehydrogenase, a glycolytic enzyme that is found only in male

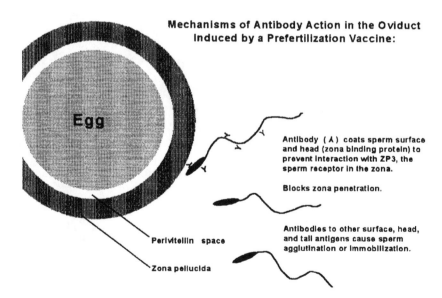

Mechanisms of Antibody Action in the Oviduct Induced by a Prefertilization Vaccine:

Egg

Antibody (A) coats sperm surface and head (zona binding protein) to prevent interaction with ZP3, the sperm receptor in the zona.

Blocks zona penetration.

Antibodies to other surface, head, and tail antigens cause sperm agglutination or immobilization.

Perivitellin space

Zona pellucida

FIGURE C-2   Possible mechanism of antibody action to a sperm-surface antigen where antibody coats the sperm head to prevent sperm binding to the zona pellucida and blocks zona penetration.

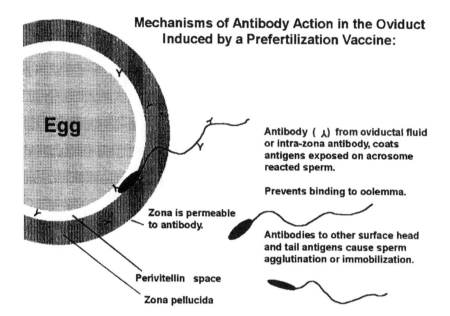

Mechanisms of Antibody Action in the Oviduct Induced by a Prefertilization Vaccine:

Egg

Antibody (λ) from oviductal fluid or intra-zona antibody, coats antigens exposed on acrosome reacted sperm.

Prevents binding to oolemma.

Zona is permeable to antibody.

Antibodies to other surface head and tail antigens cause sperm agglutination or immobilization.

Perivitellin space

Zona pellucida

FIGURE C-3 Possible mechanism of antibody action to a sperm antigen which is on the acrosomal membrane. Antibody in the zona pellucida and oviduct fluid coats the sperm antigen, preventing interaction of the sperm with the oolema.

germ cells, thus fulfilling the important criterion of tissue specificity (Goldberg 1977, 1975; Wheat and Goldberg 1983). The complete amino acid sequence for human LDH-C_4 has been deduced from cDNAs (Millan et al. 1987); in addition to being one of the best characterized human sperm proteins, it is the sperm antigen that has undergone the most extensive animal and primate testing (Lee et al. 1982; Hogrefe et al. 1987, 1989; Wheat and Goldberg 1985). LDH-C_4 first appears with the onset of puberty during prophase of the first meiotic division of the primary spermatocyte. The protein is found within the mature sperm in association with the midpiece, where it appears localized both to the mitochondrial sheath and, to a lesser extent, to plasma membrane overlying the midpiece and principal piece. As far as we know, LDH-C_4 is never expressed in female tissues and because of its stage-specific expression in primary spermatocytes, it is also sequestered from the immune system of the male by the blood–testis barrier.

In considering the mechanism of action of an LDH-C_4 antigen, the following considerations are germane. Although primarily an intracellular constituent, LDH-C_4 is presumably accessible to immune attack owing to its presence to some degree on the plasma membrane overlying the midpiece. Antibodies to LDH-C_4 partially suppress fertility in female mice and rabbits, the antibodies cause some agglutination, and in some cases complement mediated lysis. Both auto- and isoimmunogenic responses to LDH-C$_4$ have been noted in mice and rabbits (Goldberg 1973; Lerum and Goldberg 1974). Oviductal fluids are a transudate of serum. Although the contraceptive mechanism is not entirely known, what seems to happen is that high titers of circulating antibody to LDH-C$_4$ result in quantities of antibody in the oviduct that are sufficient to agglutinate or lyse oviductal sperm, thus preventing fertilization. Ovulatory cycles in these animal models were not affected by immunization, nor were other deleterious side effects noted.

A formulation consisting of purified mouse LDH-C$_4$ was injected into female baboons, which subsequently underwent fertility testing. In the experimental group, 8 of 30 matings resulted in pregnancy for a 27 percent fertility rate; 21 of 29 matings in the control group resulted in pregnancy, a 72 percent fertility rate. A second formulation based on mouse LDH-C$_4$, consisting of a synthetic peptide (amino acids 5–16, coupled to diphtheria toxoid), has also been shown to reduce fertility in female baboons. Ten of 14 baboons in the control group became pregnant (71 percent fertility), compared to 3 of 14 baboons in the experimental group, a 21 percent fertility rate (Goldberg 1990).

More recently, a formulation based on another human LDH-C$_4$ sequence (amino acids 9–20) was fertility-tested in female baboons. In the control group 8 of 15 animals became pregnant (53 percent), compared to 2 out of 14 animals in the experimental group (15 percent). If the pregnancy rate is scored as the number of pregnancies occurring per number of cycles of mating, the controls had 8 pregnancies in 34 cycles of mating (23 percent), whereas the experimental group had 2 pregnancies out of 45 mated cycles (4 percent). The contraceptive effect was reversed within one year after the last immunization (O'Hern et al. 1995), nor have there been detectable side effects with LDH-C$_4$ immunization in baboons in any of the studies to date (O'Hern et al. 1995). The thinking is that, since serum antibody levels were not directly correlated with infertility in these studies, cell-mediated immunity rather than humoral immunity might be the critical effector mechanism.

It is clear that an immunocontraceptive based upon the sperm-derived LDH-C$_4$ immunogen has a contraceptive effect in primates, although not currently of a magnitude sufficient to suggest a product that is competitive with oral contraceptives. Nevertheless, this antigen is a likely candidate for inclusion in a mixture of immunogens to form a multideterminant immunocontraceptive. Because LDH-C$_4$ has undergone primate tests and has repeatedly shown that a sperm antigen can reduce fertility, it is serving as the model for other sperm antigen development programs. A new formulation of the hC9-20 peptide from LDH-C$_4$ has been prepared by coupling to a promiscuous T cell epitope from tetanus toxoid; in 1995, fertility studies were under way in animals (monkeys).

RSA-1 The RSA-1 differentiation antigen appears on the surface of rabbit pachytene spermatocytes and on the surface of rabbit sperm. This molecule is a potent autoantigen, and polyclonal as well as monoclonal reagents to this molecule inhibit fertilization. RSA-1 fulfills several criteria for a zona pellucida binding protein (O'Rand et al. 1984, 1988, 1993a).

A family of RSA peptides in the 14–18 kDa range has been observed and the human homologue (Hspa18) of the rabbit sperm autoantigen RSA has been cloned (Lea et al. 1993). The cloned molecule, termed hSp17 to distinguish it from the native molecule, is 151 amino acids in length, with a predicted mass of 17,534 daltons. The human Sp17 sequence is 76.7 percent identical to a rabbit 17-kd sperm autoantigen, termed RSA. The amino terminus hSp17 has 43 percent identity with a known protein from human testis, the cAMP-dependent, protein kinase, type II α regulatory subunit.

Human Sp17 has been studied by Northern analysis and all data indicate that it is testis specific. A recombinant hSp17 has been generated and an antisera made to the recombinant protein (rec-hSp17). This anti-rec hSP17 recognizes a doublet of 29 kDa on Western blots of human sperm extracts. The antigen has been localized by immunofluorescence on both the human sperm head and tail. Human Sp17 binds fucoidan and human zona with saturation kinetics. Further, hSp17 is recognized by sera from vasectomized men who have antisperm antibody titers, indicating that hSpa18 is a human sperm autoantigen (Lea et al. 1993).

The mouse homologue of hSp17 has also been cloned, sequenced, and expressed. Mouse Sp17 is 74 percent identical to rabbit and 72 percent identical to human. When female mice are immunized with mSp17, they make an antisera that reacts with a 24-kDa band on Western blots. Fertility testing in mice with a peptide (p10G) derived from the rabbit autoantigen RSA reduced fertility by 80 percent in those animals that developed high titers (O'Rand et al. 1993b). Both human and mouse recombinant Sp17 have been synthesized and tested in mice, and a significant decrease in fertility has been observed (Yamasaki et al. 1995).

Tcte-1   A recently cloned mouse gene within the T complex appears to encode a sperm-specific protein known as Tcte-1 (Sarvetnick et al. 1990). The Tcte-1 gene product is a 56-kD protein that possesses certain properties of an egg-binding protein including interaction with ZP3. Antibodies to Tcte-1 bind principally to the plasma membrane overlying the head of acrosome-intact mouse sperm and compete with mouse ZP3 for binding to the sperm head. In addition, antibodies to Tcte-1 inhibit the binding of mouse sperm to mouse eggs (L. Silver, personal communication, 1995). Since Tcte-1 is a candidate for an egg-binding protein on the sperm head, a Tcte-1 formulation could inhibit fertilization if sufficient antibodies were generated in the oviduct to block this protein or induce sperm lysis. Because the product of the Tcte-1 gene is the same molecular mass as sp56 (a protein previously identified as an egg-binding protein by photoaffinity labeling using purified mouse ZP3 and the Denny-Jaffee reagent [Bleil et al. 1988]), there is considerable interest in Tcte-1 and it is considered promising for immunocontraceptive development. Immunogenicity and fertility tests of recombinant forms of Tcte-1 in mice could take place in the not too distant future.

PH-20   PH-20 is an integral membrane protein of 64 kDa, present on both the plasma membrane and inner-acrosomal membrane of guinea pig sperm. The protein is anchored in the plasma membrane by phosphatidylinositol and undergoes proteolytic processing during the acrosome reaction (Phelps et al. 1988). Some monoclonal antibodies to PH-20 block sperm interaction with the zona pellucida, suggesting that PH-20 is a zona pellucida binding protein (Primakoff et al. 1985).

PH-20 has provided the field of sperm-based immunocontraceptives with a compelling model for continuing the quest for a human immunocontraceptive based on sperm components (Primakoff et al. 1988). Immunization of female guinea pigs with PH-20 purified from the natural source (sperm) has provided remarkable evidence that full but reversible contraception can be achieved. Two injections of PH-20 were given over a one-month period and the animals were mated two months after the first injection. Of 25 immunized females, none became pregnant, a 100 percent contraceptive effect; in contrast, out of 36 controls, 34 became pregnant (94 percent fertility) (Primakoff et al. 1988). No further immunizations were given to the female guinea pigs and they continued to be mated. By 6 months after the first injection, 17 percent of the animals conceived; by 9–11 months, 46 percent had regained fertility (Primakoff et al. 1988). PH-20 cDNAs have been cloned for both guinea pig and human, and primate testing of the PH-20 formulation to determine its immunogenicity is likely in 1996. Because of the 100 percent contraceptive efficacy shown in the guinea pig model, the outcome of primate trials of PH-20 are awaited with high expectations.

At the same time, in view of a finding of hyaluronidase activity associated with the molecule (Gmachl et al. 1993), some caution with regard to PH-20's tissue-specificity is appropriate, since this finding raises the question as to whether PH-20 or PH-20 domains are present in other tissues that express hyaluronidase. An extensive RT-PCR study of PH-20's tissue-specificity, including bone marrow and circulating blood elements, may be warranted to confirm—or not confirm—the molecule's testis-specificity.

SP-10   In 1985 and 1986, the World Health Organization sponsored workshops to identify sperm antigens that could function as potential immunogens (Anderson et al. 1987). The human sperm protein SP-10 was identified as a potential contraceptive immunogen, both on the basis of its apparent germ cell specificity, as well as on the basis of functional assays that indicated that a monoclonal antibody (MHS-10) specific to SP-10 was able to inhibit sperm penetration in a hamster egg penetration assay (Anderson et al. 1987).

Electron microscopic immunocytochemical studies using the MHS-10 monoclonal antibody have indicated that the human SP-10 protein is localized to the developing acrosome of round and elongating spermatids and remains associated with the acrosomal matrix and membranes of mature sperm (Herr et al. 1990a; Kurth et al. 1991). By immunofluorescence microscopy in intact human sperm, the SP-10 antigen is found to be distributed as a cap-shaped fluorescent pattern on the anterior sperm head. After induction of the acrosome reaction with ionophore, SP-10 remains associated with the inner-acrosomal membrane and the equatorial segment, where it displays immunofluorescent images of a faint acrosomal cap or a fluorescent equatorial bar on the acrosome-reacted sperm (Herr et al. 1990b). This finding is relevant to the hypothesized mechanism of action of an SP-10 antigen, since the equatorial segment and postacrosomal regions of the sperm are thought to be involved in the initial interaction of the sperm surface with the egg plasma membrane.

The Inner-acrosomal Membrane as a Target for Immunocontraception

While considerable attention has been given to sperm plasmalemma antigens as targets for immunocontraception, less consideration has been given to components associated with the acrosomal membranes. Human sperm must undergo the acrosome reaction in order to penetrate the zona pellucida (Singer et al. 1985) so as to fuse with the egg plasma membrane (Sathananthan and Chen 1986). After the acrosome reaction, the acrosomal contents are externalized and the inner-acrosomal membrane then becomes the limiting membrane of the anterior sperm head (Nagae et al. 1986; Yudin et al. 1988). Most sperm observed on the human zona after one minute of binding *in vitro* have intact acrosomes, but the numbers of acrosome-reacted sperm on the zona rapidly increase with time as the zona acts as a potent inducer of the reaction (Cross et al. 1986). The combined events of zonal binding and acrosome reaction have been referred to as "primary binding," an event presumably mediated in humans by interaction between zonal proteins and a human equivalent of the ZP3 receptor (Bleil et al. 1988). Penetration through the zona is mediated by components released from the acrosome and exposed on the inner-acrosomal membrane; the latter process is referred to as "secondary binding." After penetration of the zona, initial fusion between sperm and egg in humans, as in other eutherian animals, is thought to occur between the plasma membrane over the equatorial segment of the sperm and the egg plasma membrane (Bedford et al. 1979). The SP-10 molecule resides within the acrosomal compartment in association with the acrosomal membranes and is observed on the inner-acrosomal membrane and equatorial segment of acrosome-reacted sperm. Thus, the proposed mechanism of contraceptive action of a SP-10 based immunocontraceptive is induction of sufficient titers of anti-SP-10 within the oviductal fluids to bind (agglutinate/lyse) the relatively few acrosome-reacted sperm found there, thus inhibiting sperm/egg interaction. (Included in this concept is the notion that the zona pellucida is permeable to immunoglobulins, and that anti-SP-10 antibody of serum origin may infiltrate the zonal matrix during follicle maturation and remain embedded in the zona during oviductal passage.) SP-10 thus fulfills the criterion of transience noted at the beginning of this paper. The molecule is exposed during a key step of the fertilization process but remains within the acrosomal compartment until the acrosome reaction is initiated.

It is important to consider acrosomal antigens as two categories that have some significant differences in terms of the criteria listed at the beginning of this paper. The first group comprises antigens that have both a plasma membrane form and an intra-acrosomal form (e.g., PH-20 [hyaluronidase]); the second group comprises antigens that are restricted in the mature sperm to the acrosomal membranes and matrix (e.g., acrosin, SP-10). Proteins that have dual localizations both on the sperm plasma membrane and within the acrosome are accessible to antibody at many stages of sperm transport within the female tract. However, proteins that are restricted to the acrosomal membranes and matrix afford a much narrower window for immunologic interdiction and contraceptive action; such antigens within the acrosomal compartment become accessible to antibody as the acrosome reaction is initiated, fusion pores form, hybrid vesicles develop, and the acrosomal membranes and matrix are exposed to the surrounding medium.

Restricted localization of acrosomal proteins to the matrix and membranes of the acrosomal compartment has both advantages and disadvantages from the perspectives of contraceptive development. As an advantage, intra-acrosomal proteins (which remain sequestered until initiation of the acrosome reaction) may afford precise staging of immunizing action to events occurring after sperm-zona binding. In theory, this targeted timing of action should offer an attractive model for a prefertilization immunocontraceptive. On the other hand, it must be appreciated that, for inhibition of fertilization to occur *in vivo*, antibody to intra-acrosomal antigens must be generated at sufficient levels in the oviduct and/or zona pellucida to contact these antigens at the egg surface within the narrow window of time when these antigens "decloak" and are accessible. Antibody levels must be sufficient to block one or several stages in the cascade of events involving primary and secondary binding to the zona, induction of the acrosome reaction, shedding of the acrosomal ghost, penetration of the zona pellucida, and binding to the oolemma. Sperm plasma membrane antigens should undoubtedly receive the major focus of attention in research efforts; it is still too soon to tell whether intra-acrosomal antigens will have a place as one component of a multideterminant immunocontraceptive.

OTHER NEW APPROACHES

This review has touched on only a few of the potential immunogens that may eventually become the immunocontraceptive of the future. New methods and experimental approaches are emerging that offer unprecedented opportunities and challenges for new investigators in the immunocontraceptive arena.

New Delivery Systems

An important application of the human intra-acrosomal protein SP-10 model has been to insert the SP-10 gene into avirulent *Salmonella* for use in oral administration. The advent of recombinant DNA technology has enabled foreign genes to be expressed in *Salmonella*, thus converting this bacterium into an efficient delivery system for the induction of immune responses to the expressed antigens. *Salmonella typhimurium* strains with deletions of the adenylate cyclase (cya) and cyclic AMP receptor protein (crp) genes are avirulent and immunogenic, at the same time that they retain their ability to colonize gut-associated lymphoid tissue (GALT) and internal organs (Curtiss and Kelly 1987). Since *S. typhimurium* naturally invades and persists in GALT (Carter and Collins 1974), oral immunization with attenuated *Salmonella* expressing foreign antigens stimulates antigen-specific secretory, humoral, and cellular immune responses (for a review, see Curtiss et al. 1990). A cDNA sequence encoding human SP-10 was cloned on an asd+ vector and expressed to a high level in an avirulent Delta cya, Delta crp, and Delta asd strain of *S. typhimurium*. Oral immunization of female BALB/c mice with this recombinant *Salmonella* elicited high-titer anti-SP-10 IgG antibodies in serum and IgA antibodies in vaginal secretions. Anti-SP-10 antibody titers could be further elevated by secondary and tertiary oral administrations of the recombinant *Salmonella*.

These quite recent results are the first indication that a gene encoding a human sperm antigen can be delivered in an oral immunogen vector and induce a secretory immune response against sperm-specific antibodies in the reproductive tract. This discovery could lead to the development of a simple, safe, efficient, and easy to use immunocontraceptive and opens the way for development of additional vectors that induce secretory immunity in the female reproductive tract (Srinivasan et al. 1995).

Novel Antigens

Because the sperm, egg surface, early embryo, and embryonic membranes represent unique differentiated cell types, it is likely that quite a few candidate immunogens will eventually be discovered that will be both specific for the gametes and/or conceptus (specificity) and will also be presented on the cell surface (accessibility). In the case of the sperm, for example, use of lectins and monoclonal antibodies has revealed antigens that cover the entire sperm surface or show a mosaic of topographically restricted domains. Some domains overlie anatomically and functionally distinct regions of cytoplasm; some antigens arise during spermatogenesis; some are secreted by the epididymis and bind to the sperm during epididymal maturation; and some antigens coat the sperm surface at the time of ejaculation when sperm mix with the secretions of the accessory glands. There may well be similar differentiation markers on the trophectoderm, the hatched blastocyst, or the oolemma. Thus, a rich opportunity awaits new investigators who would seek to define and characterize novel surface antigens of the gametes and early conceptus, and to manipulate their encoding genes so as to produce recombinant immunogens.

Vectorial Labeling and 2-D Electrophoresis

One direction for research characterizing immunogen candidates is to create data bases from 2-D electrophoresis and to couple this method with vectorial labeling to define surface antigens on egg, sperm, or trophoblast (Naaby-Hansen et al. 1995). Presented with the problem of defining which antigens on the sperm might be appropriate for inclusion in an immunocontraceptive, knowledge of which proteins are exposed on the sperm surface would provide a key rationale for candidacy. A two-dimensional gel protein data base for the majority of human sperm proteins has been created (Naaby-Hansen et al. 1995) and both isoelectric focusing (IEF) and nonequilibrating gel electrophoresis (NEPHGE) have been employed to separate human sperm proteins, which were then stained with silver to obtain protein spots over a range of pH four to ten. Using vectorial labeling of the sperm surface with I^{125} as well as surface biotinylation this data base has provided definition of a repertoire of the major proteins exposed on the human sperm surface. The Western blotting method with antibodies to known proteins was employed in conjunction with autoradiography of surface-labeled proteins to co-identify individual protein spots and thus validate the surface labeling procedure and to orient known proteins on the 2-D map. The 2-D gels were stained, the gel images were digitized, and now data from more than 50 2-D gels representing sperm proteins from eight different people has been digitized. A consensus repertoire, termed the "sperm protein encyclopedia" which contains 1,293 silver-stained human sperm proteins that have been assigned coordinates, molecular weight, pI, and shape of spot. Vectorial labeling with biotin has shown 214 surface proteins. None of the controls for known intercellular proteins were labeled.

This approach to designing a sperm-surface-directed immunocontraceptive will require (1) microsequencing selected surface proteins after 2-D preparative SDS-PAGE; (2) developing oligonucleotide probes for cloning and sequencing these proteins; and (3) tissue-specificity studies.

Mixtures of Immunogens

The results noted for the hCG formulation, which currently shows an 80 percent efficacy, and the LDH-C4 formulation, which shows roughly 75 percent efficacy, highlight the fact that an immunocontraceptive product has yet to be achieved with efficacy equal to the 95 percent usually quoted for oral steroid pills. The FDA requirement that each component of a pharmaceutical consisting of several compounds must be tested in its own right for safety and efficacy has, to date, focused attention on the testing of single-component formulations. With several immunogens now being tested as single compounds, it is likely that a future test of a multideterminant formulations, possibly consisting of several sperm antigens or several sperm antigens in conjunction with hCG, will occur in the coming years.

Gene Therapy

As noted at the outset, the traditional paradigms for immunization began with Jenner's use of cowpox to induce immunity to smallpox, the first example of injection of a closely related, less virulent strain of a virus to attenuate or inactivate disease organisms. With the advent of subunit vaccines consisting of molecules from the organism that were particularly immunogenic or were capable of inducing neutralizing antibodies, the fundamental concept then moved beyond using whole organisms. With advances in protein chemistry came the possibility of using synthetic peptides based on important epitopes or immunodominant regions and, more recently, with recombinant DNA technology, there is now the capability for selectively attenuating organisms, engineering and expressing recombinant protein subunits, and developing immunogens consisting of recombinant proteins.

Another quantum leap in the field builds on the work by Wolff et al. (1990). The research showed that skeletal muscle fibers randomly distributed in the muscle belly expressed the plasmid DNA encoding several reporter proteins, apparently taking up the DNA without a need for special delivery systems such as calcium precipitation or gene guns. DNA expression continued for several months and the plasmids are not integrated into the genome but persist as episomes. Subsequent analysis by the Liu group (Ulner et al. 1993) confirmed the Wolff paradigm and showed that antigens expressed in skeletal muscle after direct naked DNA injection are presented to the immune system: Plasmid DNA-encoding influenza A nucleoprotein, driven by either Rous sarcoma virus or cytomegalovirus promotors and injected into mouse skeletal muscle, generated both specific antibody to nucleoprotein and nucleoprotein-specific cytotoxic lymphocytes. Furthermore, this immune response also protected mice upon subsequent challenge with a heterologous strain of live influenza A virus. It has also been reported that cDNA expression vectors encoding interleukin 2 or interleukin 4, when injected into mouse skeletal muscle, cause expression of these proteins and in vivo cytokine effects (Raz et al. 1993). Further gene inoculation of human immunodeficiency virus envelope protein (pM160) into mouse muscle also has been shown to generate antibodies to HIV (Wang et al. 1993).

Thus, it would seem that the principle of naked DNA innoculation is established. The possibility is now at hand to pursue development of DNA vaccination into muscle, using genes encoding immunogens—from the sperm, egg, or early conceptus—with potential contraceptive effects, an area potentially rich for discovery but with potential products at some distance in the future.

REFERENCES

Alexander NJ. Contraceptive vaccine development. IN Vaccine Research and Developments. W Koff, H Six, eds. New York: Marcel Dekker. 1992.

Anderson DJ, PM Johnson, WR Jones, et al. Monoclonal antibodies to human trophoblast and sperm antigens: Report of two WHO-sponsored workshops, 30 June 1986, Toronto, Canada. Journal of Reproductive Immunology 10:231–257, 1987.

Baskin MJ. Temporary sterilization by the injection of human spermatozoa: A preliminary report. American Journal of Obstetrics and Gynecology 24:892, 1932.

Bedford JM, HDM Moore, LE Franklin. Significance of the equatorial segment of the acrosome of the spermatozoa in eutherian mammals. Experimental Cell Research 119:119–126, 1979.

Bernstein L, B Englander, J Gallagher, et al. Localized and systemic hypersensitivity reactions to human seminal fluid. Annals of Internal Medicine 94:459, 1981.

Bleil JD, JM Greve, PM Wassarman. Identification of a secondary sperm receptor in the mouse egg zona pellucida: Role in maintenance of binding of acrosome-reacted sperm to egg. Developmental Biology 128:376–385, 1988.

Bremner WJ, AM Matsumotoa. Endocrine control of human spermatogenesis: Possible mechanism for contraception. IN Male Contraception: Advances and Future Prospects, GI Zatuchni, A Goldsmith, JM Spieler, JJ Sciarra, eds. Philadelphia: Harper and Row. 1986.

Carter PB, FM Collins. The route of enteric infection in normal mice. Journal of Experimental Medicine 139:1189–1203, 1974.

Cross NL, P Morales, JW Overstreet, et al. Two simple methods for detecting acrosome-reacted human sperm. Gamete Research 15:213–226, 1986.

Curtiss R III. Attenuated *Salmonella* strains as live vectors for the expression of foreign antigens. IN New Generation Vaccines, GC Woodrow, MM Levine, eds. New York: Marcel Dekker. 1990.

Curtiss R III, SM Kelly. *Salmonella tymphimurium* deletion mutants lacking adenylate cyclase and cyclic amp receptor protein are avirulent and immunogenic. Infectious Immunology 55:3035–3043, 1987.

Dunbar BS, AB Dudkiewicz, DS Bundman. Proteolysis of specific porcine zona pellucida glycoproteins by boar acrosin. Biology of Reproduction 32:619–630, 1985.

East IJ, DR Mattison, J Dean. Monoclonal antibodies to the major protein of the murine zona pellucida: Effects on fertilization and early development. Developmental Biology 104:49, 1984.

Freemerman AJ, RM Wright, JC Herr. Cloning and sequencing of baboon and cynomolgus monkey intra-acrosomal protein SP-10 and comparison with human SP-10 and mouse sperm antigen 63. Molecular Reproduction and Development 34:140–148, 1993.

Gmachl M, JS Sagan, S Ketter, et al. The human sperm protein PH-20 has hyaluronidase activity. FEBS 336, 545–548, 1993.

Goldberg E. LDH-C4 as an immunocontraceptive model. IN Gamete Interaction: Prospects for Immunocontraception, NJ Alexander, PD Griffin, JM Spieler, GMH Waites, eds. New York: Wiley-Liss. 1990.

Goldberg E. Isozymes in testes and spermatozoa. IN Isozymes: Current Topics in Biological and Medical Research, Vol. 1. MC Rattazzi, JG Scandalios, GS Whitt, eds. New York: Alan R. Liss. 1977.

Goldberg, E. Lactate dehydrogenase-X (crystalline) from mouse testes. IN Methods in Enzymology, Vol. XLI: Carbohydrate Metabolism, Part B. New York: Academic Press. 1975.

Goldberg E. Infertility in female rabbits immunized with lactate dehydrogenase X. Science 181:458, 1973.

Golden WL, C von Kap-Herr, BE Kurth, et al. Refinement of the localization of the gene for human intra-acrosomal protein SP-10 to band q24 of chromosome 11 by nonisotopic in situ hybridization. Genomics 18:446–449, 1993.

Griffin PD. Strategy of vaccine development. IN Gamete Interaction: Prospects for Immunocontraception. NJ Alexander, PD Griffin, JM Spieler, GMH Waites, eds. New York: Wiley-Liss. 1990.

Hearn JP, AA Gidley-Baird, JK Hodges, et al. Embryonic signals during the preimplantation period in primates. Journal of Reproduction and Fertility 36(Suppl.):49, 1988.

Hedrick JL. The pig zona pellucida: Sperm binding ligands, antigens and sequence homologies. IN Reproductive Immunology. PM Johnson, F Dondero F, eds. New York: Raven Press. 1993.

Herr JC, CJ Flickinger, M Homyk, et al. Biochemical and morphological characterization of the intra-acrosomal antigen SP-10 from human sperm. Biology of Reproduction 42:181–193, 1990a.

Herr JC, RM Wright, E John, et al. Identification of human acrosomal antigen SP-10 in primates and pigs. Biology of Reproduction 42:377–382, 1990b.

Herr JC, K Klotz, J Shannon, RM Wright, et al. Purification and microsequencing of the intra-acrosomal protein SP-10: Evidence that SP-10 heterogeneity results from endoproteolytic processes. Biology of Reproduction 47:11–20, 1992.

Herr JC, RM Wright, CJ Flickinger, et al. Assignment of the gene for human intra-acrosomal protein SP-10 to the p12->q13 region of chromosome 11. Journal of Andrology 12(5):281–287, 1991.

Hogrefe HH, JP Griffith, MG Rossmann, et al. Characterization of antigenic sites on the refined 3A structure of mouse testicular lactate dehydrogenase-C4. Journal of Biological Chemistry 262:13155–13162, 1987.

Hogrefe HH, PTP Kaumaya, E Goldberg. Immunogenicity of synthetic peptides corresponding to flexible and antibody-accessible segments of mouse lactate dehydrogenase (LDH)-C4. Journal of Biological Chemistry 264:10513–10519, 1989.

Jones WR. Lessons from an anti-hCG contraceptive vaccine trial. IN Gamete Interaction: Prospects for Immunocontraception. NJ Alexander, PD Griffin, JM Spieler, GMH Waites, eds. New York: Wiley-Liss. 1990.

Jones WR, J Bradley J, SJ Judd, et al. Phase I clinical trial of a World Health Organization birth control vaccine. Lancet 1:1295, 1988.

Katsh S. Immunology, fertility and infertility: A historical survey. American Journal of Obstetrics and Gynecology 77:946, 1959.

Kharat E, NS Nair, K Dhall, et al. Analysis of menstrual records of women immunized with anti-hCG vaccines inducing antibodies partially cross-reactive with hLH. Contraception 41:293–299, 1990.

Kummerfeld HL, RH Foote. Infertility and embryonic mortality in female rabbits immunized with different sperm preparations. Biology of Reproduction 14:300–305, 1976.

Kurth BE, K Klotz, CJ Flickinger, et al. Localization of sperm antigen SP-10 during the six stages of the cycle of the seminiferous epithelium in man. Biology of Reproduction 44:814–821, 1991.

Ladd A, G Prabhu, Y-Y Tsong, et al. Active immunization against gonadotrophin-releasing hormone combined with androgen supplementation is a promising antifertility vaccine for males. American Journal of Reproductive Immunology 17:121, 1988.

Ladd A, Y-Y Tsong, J Lok, et al. Active immunization against LHRH: I: Effects of conjugation site and dose. American Journal of Reproductive Immunology 22:56, 1990.

Ladd A, Y-Y Tsong, G Prabhu, et al. Effects of long-term immunization against gonadal function. Journal of Reproductive Immunology 15:85–101, 1989.

Lea I, RT Richardson, EE Widgren, et al. Cloning and sequencing of human Sp17, a sperm zona binding protein. Molecular Biology of the Cell 4:248a, 1993.

Lee CY, JH Huan, E Goldberg. Lactate dehydrogenase from the mouse. IN Carbohydrate Metabolism, Part D, Methods in Enzymology. WA Wood, ed. New York: Academic Press. 1982.

Lerum JE, E Goldberg. Immunological impairment of pregnancy in mice by lactate dehydrogenase X. Biology of Reproduction 11:108, 1974.

Linnet L. Clinical immunology of vasectomy and vasovasostomy. Urology 22:101, 1983.

Liu M-S, R Aebersold, C-H Fann, et al. Molecular and developmental studies of a sperm acrosome antigen recognized by HS-63 monoclonal antibody. Biology of Reproduction 46:937–948, 1992.

Madhwa Raj HG. Effects of active immunization with follicle stimulating hormone (FSH) on spermatogenesis in the adult crab-eating monkey: Evaluation for male contraception. IN Immunological Approaches to Contraception and Promotion of Fertility. G Talwar, ed. New York: Plenum Press. 1986.

Mahi-Brown CA, R Yanagimachi, ML Nelson, et al. Ovarian histopathology of bitches immunized with porcine zonae pellucidae. American Journal of Reproductive Immunology and Microbiology18:94, 1988.

Mathur S, ER Baker, HO Williamson, et al. Clinical significance of antisperm antibodies in infertile couples. Fertility and Sterility 36:486, 1981.

Menge AC, H Peegel, ML Riolo. Sperm fractions responsible for immunologic induction of pre- and postfertilization infertility in rabbits. Biology of Reproduction 20:931, 1979.

Millan JL, CE Driscoll, KM LeVan, et al. Epitopes of human testis-specific lactate dehydrogenase deduced from a cDNA sequence. Proceedings of the National Academy of Sciences, USA 84:5311–5315, 1987.

Millar SE, SM Chamow, AW Baur, et al. Vaccination with a synthetic zona pellucida peptide produces long-term contraception in female mice. Science 246:935, 1989.

Moudgal NR. A need for FSH in maintaining fertility of adult male subhuman primates. Archives of Andrology 7:117–125, 1981.

Moudgal NR, GR Aravindan. Induction of infertility in the male by blocking follicle-stimulating hormone action. IN Immunology of Reproduction. R Naz, ed. Boca Raton, FL: CRC Press. 1993.

Moudgal NR, GS Murthy, AL Rao, et al. Development of FSH as a vaccine for the male—A status report on the recent researches carried out using the bonnet monkey M. radiata. IN Proceedings of the International Symposium on Immunological Approaches to Contraception and Promotion of Fertility. GP Talwar, ed. New York: Plenum Press. 1986.

Moudgal NR, GS Murthy, N Ravindranath, et al. Contraception through regulation of endogenous FSH secretion: Prospects for the male. IN Human Reproduction and Contraception, S Takagi. GI Zatuchni, eds. Japan: Professional Postgraduate Services. 1988a.

Moudgal NR, GS Murthy, N Ravindranath, et al. Development of a contraceptive vaccine for use by the human male: Results of a feasibility study carried out in adult male bonnet monkeys (Macaca radiata). IN Contraceptive Research for Today and the Nineties. GP Talwar, ed. New York: Springer Verlag. 1988b.

Moudgal NR, N Ravindranath, GS Murthy, et al. Long-term contraceptive efficacy of vaccine of ovine follicle-stimulating hormone in male bonnet monkeys (Macaca radiata). Journal of Reproduction and Fertility 96(1):91–102, 1992.

Muñoz MG, AC Menge. Infertility in female rabbits isoimmunized with subcellular sperm fractions. Biology of Reproduction 18:669, 1978.

Naaby-Hansen S, JC Herr. A 2-D protein database for the human spermatozoa. Journal of Andrology 16 Jan.–Feb., Suppl.), 1995.

Nagae T, R Yanagimachi R, P Srivastava, et al. Acrosome reaction in human spermatozoa. Fertility and Sterility 45:701–707, 1986.

Naz RK, BB Rosenblum, AC Menge. Characterization of a membrane antigen from rabbit testes and sperm isolated by using monoclonal antibodies and effect of its antiserum on fertility. Proceedings of the National Academy of Sciences, USA 81:857, 1984.

O'Hern PA, Bambra CS, M Isahakia, et al. Reversible contraception in female baboons immunized with a synthetic epitope of sperm-specific lactate dehydrogenase. Biology of Reproduction 52:331–339, 1995.

O'Rand MG. Sperm–egg recognition and barriers to interspecies fertilization. Gamete Research 19:315–328, 1988.

O'Rand MG, J Beavers, EE Widgren, et al. Inhibition of fertility in female mice by immunization with a B-cell epitope, the synthetic sperm peptide, P10G. Journal of Reproductive Immunology 25:89–102, 1993a.

O'Rand MG, RT Richardson, N Yamasaki. Zona pellucida binding of mammalian spermatozoa. Journal of Reproductive Development 39(Suppl.):43–44, 1993b.

O'Rand MG, EE Widgren, SJ Fisher. Sperm antigens relevant to infertility. IN Perspectives in Immunoreproduction. S Mathur, CM Fredericks, eds. New York: Hemisphere Publishing. 1988.

O'Rand MG, EE Widgren, SJ Fisher. Characterization of the rabbit sperm membrane autoantigen, RSA, as a lectin-like zona binding protein. Developmental Biology 129:231, 1984.

Otani Y, I Hiroshi, S Inoue, et al. Immunization of human female with human sperm and semen. International Journal of Fertility 16:19, 1971.

Paterson M, T Koothan, K Morris, et al. Biology of Reproduction 46:523–534, 1992.

Phelps BM, P Primakoff, D Koppel, et al. Restricted lateral diffusion of PH-20, a pi-anchored sperm membrane protein. Science 240:1780, 1988.

Primakoff P, H Hyatt, D Myles. A role for the migrating sperm surface antigen Ph-20 in guinea pig sperm binding to the egg zona pellucida. Journal of Cell Biology 101:2239, 1985.

Primakoff P, W Lathrop, L Woodman, et al. Fully effective contraception in female guinea pigs immunized with the sperm protein PH-20. Nature 335:543–546, 1988.

Raz E, A Watanake, SM Baird, et al. Systemic immunologic effects of cytokine genes injected into skeletal muscle. Proceedings of the National Academy of Sciences, USA 90:4523, 1993.

Rhim SH, SE Millar, F Robey, et al. Autoimmune disease of the ovary induced by an 8 amino acid zona pellucida peptide. Journal of Clinical Investigation 89:28, 1992.

Rosenfeld SS. Semen injections with serologic studies. American Journal of Obstetrics and Gynecology 12:385, 1926.

Sacco AG, EC Yurewicz, MG Subramanian, et al. Analysis of the porcine zona pellucida Mr = 55,000 antigen for contraceptive use. IN Reproductive Immunology. L Mettler, D Billington, eds. Amsterdam: Elsevier. 1990.

Sarvetnick N, JY Tsai, H Fox, et al. A mouse chromosome 17 gene encodes a testes-specific transcript with unusual properties. Immunogenetics 31:283, 1990.

Sathananthan AH, C Chen. Sperm–oocyte fusion in the human during monospermic fertilization. Gamete Research 15:177–186, 1986.

Singer SL, H Lambert, JW Overstreet, et al. The kinetics of human sperm binding to the human zona pellucida and zona-free hamster oocyte *in vitro*. Gamete Research 12: 29–39, 1985.

Skinner SM, T Mills, HJ Kirchick, et al. Immunization with zona pellucida proteins results in abnormal ovarian follicular differentiation and inhibition of gonadotropin-induced steroid secretion. Endocrinology 115:2418, 1984.

Srinivasan J, S Tinge, R Wright, et al. Oral immunization with attenuated *Salmonella* expressing human sperm antigen induces antibodies in serum and the reproductive tract. Biology of Reproduction 53:462–471, 1995.

Stevens VC. Development of hCG antifertility vaccine. IN Perspectives in Immunoreproduction. S Mathur, CM Fredericks, eds. New York: Hemisphere Publishing. 1988.

Stevens VC. Human choronic gonadotropin: Properties and potential immunological manipulation for clinical application. IN Clinics of Obstetrics and Gynecology, Vol. 6. W. Jones, ed. London: W.B. Saunders. 1979.

Stevens VC. Perspective on development of a fertility control vaccine from hormonal antigens of trophoblast. IN Development of Vaccines for Fertility Regulation: A World Health Organization Symposium. Copenhagen: Scriptor. 1976.

Stevens VC, B Cinader, JE Powell, et al. Preparation and formulation of an hCG antifertility vaccine: Selection of an adjuvant and vehicle. American Journal of Reproductive Immunology 6:315–321, 1981.

Stevens VC, JE Powell, M Rickey, et al. Studies of various delivery systems for hCG vaccine. IN Gamete Interaction: Prospects for Immunocontraception. NJ Alexander, PD Griffin, JM Spieler, GMH Waites, eds. New York: Wiley-Liss. 1990.

Taguchi O, Y Nishizuka. Autoimmune oophoritis in thymectomized mice: T cell requirement in adoptive transfer. Clinical Experiments in Immunology 42:324, 1980a.

Taguchi O, Y Nishizuka, T Sakakura, et al. Autoimmune oophoritis in thymectomized mice: Detection of circulating antibodies against oocytes. Clinical Experiments in Immunology 40:540, 1980b.

Talwar GP, SK Gupta, AK Tandon. Immunologic interruption of pregnancy. IN Reproductive Immunology. N Gleicher, ed. New York: Alan R. Liss. 1981.

Talwar GP, O Singh, R Pal, et al. A vaccine that prevents pregnancy in women. Proceedings of the National Academy of Sciences USA 91:8532–8536, 1994.

Talwar GP, O Singh, R Pal, et al. Vaccines against LHRH and HCG. IN Immunology of Reproduction. R Naz, ed. Boca Raton, FL: CRC Press. 1993.

Talwar GP, O Singh, R Pal, et al. Anti-hCG vaccines are in clinical trials. Scandinavian Journal of Immunology 36(Suppl. 11):123, 1992.

Talwar GP, O Singh, R Pal, et al. Experiences of the anti-hCG vaccine of relevance to development of other birth control vaccines. IN Gamete Interaction: Prospects for Immunocontraception. NJ Alexander, PD Griffin, JM Spieler, GMH Waites, eds. New York: Wiley-Liss. 1990.

Tung KSK. Immunopathologic consideration of antifertility vaccines. IN Male Contraception: Advances and Future Prospects. Philadelphia: Harper and Row. 1986.

Tung KSK, S Smith, C Teuscher, et al. Murine autoimmune oophoritis, epididymoorchitis, and gastritis induced by day 3 thymectomy. Immunology. American Journal of Pathology 126:293–302, 1987.

Ulner JB, JJ Donnelly, SE Parker, et al. Heterologous protection against influenza by injection of DNA encoding a viral protein. Science 259:1745, 1993.

Wang B, KE Ugen, U Svikartan, et al. Proceedings of the National Academy of Sciences, USA 90:4156, 1993.

Wheat TE, E Goldberg. Antigenic domains of the sperm-specific lactate dehydrogenase C4 isozyme. Molecular Immunology 22:643–649, 1985.

Wheat TE, E Goldberg. Sperm-specific lactate dehydrogenase C4: Antigenic structure and immunosuppression of fertility. IN Isozymes: Current Topics in Biological and Medical Research, Vol. 7. MC Retezzi, JG Scandalios, GS Whitt, eds. New York: Alan R. Liss. 1983.

Wolff JA, RW Malone, P Williams, et al. Direct gene transfer into mouse muscle *in vivo*. Science 247:1465, 1990.

Wright RM, E John, K Klotz, et al. Cloning and sequencing of cDNAs coding for the human intra-acrosomal antigen SP-10. Biology of Reproduction 42:693-701, 1990.

Yamasaki N, RT Richardson, MG O'Rand. Expression of the rabbit sperm protein Sp17 in COS cells and interaction of recombinant Sp17 with the rabbit zona pellucida. Molecular Reproduction and Development 40(1):48–55, 1995.

Yudin AI, W Gottlieb, S Meizel. Ultrastructural studies of the early events of the human sperm acrosome reaction as initiated by human follicular fluid. Gamete Research 20:11–24, 1988.

D

Part 1: Barrier Methods

Lourens J.D. Zaneveld, Ph.D., D.V.M.
Department of Obstetrics and Gynecology, Rush University,
Rush-Presbyterian-St. Luke's Medical Center

Deborah J. Anderson, Ph.D.
Fearing Research Laboratory, Department of Obstetrics,
Gynecology, and Reproductive Biology,
Brigham and Women's Hospital and Harvard Medical School

Kevin J. Whaley, Ph.D.
Department of Biophysics, The Johns Hopkins University

INTRODUCTION

This chapter has two parts. The first describes approaches to development of novel vaginal agents and formulations with potential for preventing both conception and STD transmission. To facilitate understanding of these approaches, we present background information on the nature of chemical formulations, the functional activity of spermatozoa, and the infective mechanisms of sexually transmitted pathogens. The second part of the chapter presents some of the theoretical underpinnings of mucosal immunity, an area that offers hope of bridging the large and present gap between contraception and prevention of sexually transmitted disease.

The need to focus on sexually transmitted diseases in connection with contraception reflects a growing, if reluctant, recognition of several large sociomedical facts: that the prevalence of these diseases is mounting in much of the world; that their transmission is not limited to small or distant populations engaging in aberrant sexual behavior; that their immediate and more remote sequelae can be dire; and that, biologically and behaviorally, contraception and disease prevention will be necessary partners, at least sometimes, for significant numbers of people and for the foreseeable future.

While effective contraceptive technology for females has been available for several decades, very few contraceptive methods—the condom and some vaginal formulations and devices—also protect against sexually transmitted diseases (STDs) (Claypool 1994). Of these, only the condom offers protection against the whole spectrum of these diseases, including HIV, and only the female condom and vaginal formulations and devices can be controlled directly by women. Attempts to limit the spread of HIV and other STDs through behavioral modification, encouraging condom use and fewer sexual partners, for example, have proved insufficient to the large task of stemming transmission of these diseases (Stein 1993). Furthermore, understanding about alternative, nonpenetrative sexual practices ("outercourse") that are both protective and satisfying would appear to be limited, although recent empirical data in large population samples are lacking (Greenwood and Margolis 1981; Norman and Cornett 1995; Norsigian 1994). Women experience particular difficulties owing to underlying gender power inequalities that constrain their ability—sometimes severely—to protect themselves from HIV infection, given the absence of a protective technology they could use, if necessary, without a partner's consent (Stein 1990).

New emphasis on developing contraceptive agents that have the additional, critical characteristic of preventing STDs is also being driven by the realization that sexually transmitted diseases other than HIV elevate the risk of HIV transmission (Berkley 1991; Wasserheit 1992); by the increasing rates of heterosexual transmission of HIV infection; by realization of women's greater vulnerability to infection (Mann et al. 1992; Stein 1993); and by women's need to control their own protection against infection and/or conception.

Globally, most women are at greatest risk of acquiring HIV through heterosexual vaginal intercourse with an infected man (Mayer and Anderson 1995). To avoid infection via this route, a preventive method must establish an effective barrier between the infectious elements in genital secretions and those cells of the female reproductive tract that are susceptible to infection. Such a barrier may be physical (such as that provided by condoms), chemical (such as that provided by an intravaginal microbicide), some combination of a physical and a chemical barrier (such as a condom and an intravaginal microbicide), or immunologic (such as topically applied monoclonal antibodies or mucosal immunogens).

The ideal vaginal microbicide should be colorless, odorless, tasteless, stable at room temperature with a long shelf life, easy to use, fast-acting for an appropriate duration after insertion, effective pre- and postcoition, affordable, available without prescription, and safe for use at least once or twice daily. While it would be desirable to develop some microbicides that do not kill sperm, because women who only sometimes want to prevent pregnancy will always want to prevent STD infection, this paper focuses on chemical barriers that may be able to block *both* conception and STD transmission, that is, "prophylactic contraception" (Cone and Whaley 1994).

In so doing, however, there is no intention to disparage the present and future value of physical barrier methods. The diaphragm and cervical cap can provide some protection against disease transmission (Rosenberg et al. 1992) and are appropriate for use by some women, although much is unknown about their efficacy, utilization, and protective power (Stein 1993; Stratton and Alexander 1993).

Vaginal topical formulations had received very little research attention until recently. Advances have relied on serendipitous discovery or relatively minor changes in existing methods and, overall, have failed to solve the most critical problems associated with these formulations. Nevertheless, scientists have accumulated much new knowledge about sperm and genital tract physiology over the past three decades. Combined with recent progress in biochemistry, pharmaceutics, and engineering, such knowledge should make it possible now to compensate for previous lack of progress in this increasingly critical area.

MECHANISMS OF FERTILIZATION BY SPERMATOZOA

During ejaculation, spermatozoa are often placed near the cervix, trapped within the seminal coagulum. As the coagulum liquefies, the spermatozoa are released and enter cervical mucus, a process of penetration that can occur as rapidly as 1.5 to 3 minutes after ejaculation. The primary mechanism whereby spermatozoa pass through cervical mucus appears to be their motility, although other factors such as enzymatic digestion of the mucus may also play a role. The amount of time viable spermatozoa remain in the vagina is not well studied but appears to vary from two to six hours.

Successful sperm penetration into and through cervical mucus occurs primarily during the mid-cycle of the menstrual period, at which time the cervical mucus may contain micelles that guide spermatozoa toward the uterus. At other times in the cycle, particularly the luteal phase, cervical mucus is "hostile" to spermatozoa and does not allow penetration. Even at the optimal period, only about 0.1 to 1 percent of ejaculated spermatozoa pass through the cervix. Still, many spermatozoa become trapped in the cervical crypts and can be released at a later date, potentially providing a constant source of spermatozoa for about four days. Passage of spermatozoa through the uterus and fallopian tubes (oviducts) relies on sperm motility, contractions of the tract, and the motion of cilia on the endothelial surface. Because the uterotubal junction and the fallopian tube isthmus also present a barrier to sperm transport, only about 5,000 spermatozoa actually reach the site of fertilization.

At the time of fertilization, an oocyte is surrounded by three layers. These are, from the outside inwards, the cumulus oophorus, the corona radiata, and the zona pellucida. The fertilizing spermatozoon has to pass through all these layers to contact the oocyte itself. In addition, it must penetrate the vitelline (egg plasma) membrane and decondense inside the ooplasm. Penetration through the oocyte's protective layers requires the use of lytic enzymes, associated with the acrosome of the spermatozoon. Good evidence suggests that hyaluronidase helps sperm pass through the cumulus; acrosin, a serine proteinase, helps it penetrate the zona pellucida. Sperm motility, ligand-receptor interactions, and other factors are also required for sperm penetration.

Just before or just after it contacts the zona pellucida, the spermatozoon undergoes a morphologic change called the acrosome reaction. This extracellular or exocytotic event results in the disappearance of the sperm's outer acrosomal membrane and surrounding plasma membrane; dispersal of the acrosome proper; activation of proacrosin; and release of acrosomal contents, with acrosin being of particular importance. While sperm penetration through the cumulus oophorus can occur in the absence of the acrosome reaction—presumably because hyaluronidase is associated with the external membranes—sperm passage through the zona pellucida is not possible without this reaction. An early acrosome reaction, such as one that occurs in the vagina, will result in premature release of acrosomal contents and, most likely, in an inability of the spermatozoon to fertilize.

Proper timing of the acrosome reaction is controlled by capacitation in the female genital tract, an activation process resulting in removal of inhibitory substances from the sperm surface; by possible modification of the sperm's plasma membrane; and by changes in motility patterns. Ejaculated spermatozoa cannot undergo the acrosome reaction unless they are capacitated. Capacitation can occur in all parts of the female genital tract, with the possible exception of the vagina, and requires at least four hours. However, it probably occurs as a continuous process while the spermatozoa are being transported through the cervix, uterus, and fallopian tubes, so that a spermatozoon is fully or mostly capacitated by the time it reaches the oocyte. Final steps in the capacitation process may occur during sperm passage through the cumulus oophorus.

Recently, biochemical aspects of capacitation and the acrosome reaction have received significant attention as possible targets for intervention (Dunbar and O'Rand 1991; see also Appendixes B and C in this volume). The former appears to involve impeding maturation and the acrosome reaction by preventing changes in the sperm's plasma membrane or, in contrast, attempting to induce a premature acrosome reaction that would render sperm unable to meld with an egg. The acrosome reaction, like other exocytotic processes, requires certain physiological conditions such as ligand interaction with surface receptors, activation of second messenger systems, protein phosphorylation, ionic and osmotic changes, and, ultimately, membrane fusion, vesiculation, and disappearance.

MECHANISMS OF INFECTION BY SEXUALLY TRANSMITTED PATHOGENS

Sexually transmitted diseases are caused by a variety of organisms, including bacteria (aerobic and anaerobic), chlamydia, mycoplasmas, ureaplasmas, spirochetes, fungi, flagellates, amoebae, worms, and viruses. Each of these organisms has different biologic properties, conferring widely diverse mechanisms of infection and pathogenesis (see Chapter 2 and Chapter 5).

TABLE D-1 Susceptible Sites for Sexually Transmitted Disease Infection in the Lower Female Genital Tract

	Vulva	Vagina	Endocervix	WBCs of Vascular Origin
Treponema pallidum	X	X	X	
Haemophilus ducreyi	X	X		
Neisseria gonorrhoeae		X		
Candida albicans		X		
Trichomonas vaginalis		X		
Chlamydia trachomatis		X		
Cytomegalovirus				X
Epstein Barr virus				X
Herpes simplex virus	X	X	X	
Hepatitis B virus		X	X	
Human papillomavirus	X	X	X	
Human immunodeficiency virus, type 1	?	?	X	X

SOURCE: Derived from: P Stratton, NJ Alexander. Prevention of sexually transmitted infections. Infectious Disease Clinics of North America 7(4):841–859, December 1993; W Cates, KM Stone. HIV, other STDs, and barriers. IN Barrier Contraceptives: Current Status and Future Prospects, CK Mauck, M Cordero, HL Gabelnick, et al., eds. New York: Wiley-Liss. 1994.

The most common human STD pathogens and their primary sites of infection are listed in Table D-1. Effective vaginal microbicides must block infection by directly and efficiently killing these organisms or by blocking or inactivating molecular mechanisms underlying infection. Current detergent vaginal formulations have broad-spectrum cytolytic properties that may be effective against several STD pathogens but may also damage epithelial and other genital tract cells and disrupt normal vaginal flora. Ligand/receptor molecules located on the surface of STD pathogens and their host cells—which are responsible for pathogen attachment and entry—are obvious targets for microbicide action. While these molecular structures have not been fully characterized for most STD pathogens, researchers are intensively seeking them today, importantly including HIV-AIDS.

Human Immunodeficiency Virus (HIV) Type 1

The infectiousness of HIV is highly variable and there are still surprising gaps in understanding of its transmission, including the factors affecting amount and timing of virus shedding, the roles of vaginal and seminal antibodies, and the effects of exogenous or endogenous hormones (Mayer and Anderson 1995; Stratton and Alexander 1994). Partner studies have provided much of the information we do have. They indicate that the following factors affect rates of HIV transmission: (1) mean numbers of sexual contacts and/or types of sexual practices; (2) differences in infectivity of partners depending on disease stage, symptomatology, and therapeutic drug status; (3) potential differences in infectivity of various clades of HIV-1; and (4) intrinsic biological differences between infecting or susceptible partners. Specific risk factors specific to heterosexual transmission of HIV-1 include: (1) sex during menstruation; (2) anal intercourse; (3) traumatic sex; (4) advanced HIV disease stage of infected partner; (5) zidovudine therapy (negative association); (6) age of the female partner; (7) choice of contraceptive method; and (8) concomitant STD infections (bacterial vaginosis, candidiasis, chancroid, chlamydia, gonorrhea, herpes simplex, human papilloma virus, syphilis, and trichomoniasis have all been associated with HIV transmission) (Mayer and Anderson 1995; Stratton and Alexander 1993).

The cell biology and molecular mechanisms of HIV-1 sexual transmission are areas where much remains to be learned. It is known that HIV-1 is present in semen and cervicovaginal secretions, both in cell-free and cell-associated forms, and data from both *in vitro* and *in vivo* primate studies indicate that each of these forms may be capable of transmitting infection. Cell-free HIV-1 in genital-tract secretions may infect Langerhans cells, lymphocytes, and/or macrophages residing within the epithelial layer of mucosal surfaces in the vagina, foreskin, and penile urethra. Infection could occur via CD4, Fc, complement, or other receptors as yet unknown. If genital lesions or microabrasions are present, HIV-1-infected white blood cells (WBCs) in genital-tract secretions could infect by direct access to target cells in connective tissue (resident and extravasated WBCs). Furthermore, *in vitro* studies indicate that HIV-infected WBCs may have the capacity to adhere to mucosal epithelium and transmit HIV directly to these cells (Mayer and Anderson 1995).

Numerous biologic variables can affect HIV levels in semen and cervicovaginal secretions and may also influence HIV transmission rates. Leukocytospermia (inflammation of the genital tract) in men has been associated with higher HIV-1 titres in semen. This phenomenon may be due to recruitment of HIV-1-infected cells to the genital tract; induction of edema and capillary dilation, both of which increase the potential for erosion and escape of blood lymphocytes and monocytes into the intravascular space and lumen; and/or activation of lymphocytes that could make them more capable of producing HIV-1. In women, several variables can affect infectious HIV-1 titres in genital-tract secretions, including: (1) inflammation of the genital tract; (2) menstruation, which introduces infected peripheral blood cells into vaginal secretions; (3) factors elevating vaginal pH, which is normally acidic and confers protection against STDs, including HIV-1; (4) cervical ectopy; and (5) hormonal factors that influence the thickness of the epithelial layer and the production of protective mucus (Mayer and Anderson 1995).

An open—and highly significant—question is whether HIV is carried solely by somatic cells in semen or whether it is carried by the sperm themselves. If the former is the case, contraception is not necessary for prevention of sexually transmitted infection, so that a primary technologic need is for a virucide/microbicide; individuals can then decide whether they wish to contracept as well, but it is a separate decision. However, if the latter is the case, contraception becomes an essential concomitant of disease prevention (Stein 1993).

The healthy human vagina has several natural defense mechanisms against STD pathogens. The stratified squamous epithelium lining of the vagina and ectocervix is generally several cell layers thick, conferring physical protection against most invading organisms. Copious amounts of mucins produced during certain stages of the menstrual cycle also provide a physical barrier to pathogens. In addition, the vagina and cervix are both capable of mounting antibody and cell-mediated immune responses to genital tract infections, and cervicovaginal secretions contain a number of nonspecific antibacterial and antiviral defense agents, including lysozymes, polyamines, zinc, H_2O_2, lactoferrin, and B-defensins (Cohen et al. 1990). Finally but quite importantly, the predominant normal vaginal microflora—lactobacillus organisms—help to maintain low pH conditions that are hostile to most viral and bacterial pathogens (Voeller et al. 1992b).

Unfortunately, a number of situations perturb these natural protective mechanisms. Menopause and progestin-dominated hormonal therapies, for example, cause thinning of the squamous epithelial layer and reduction in cervical mucus production. Intercourse and vaginal infections, whose coincidence is not uncommon, can cause an elevation in vaginal pH, disarming this effective protective mechanism. And, although currently marketed vaginal topical contraceptives may, in fact, be buffered at acidic pH, the buffering capacity of semen itself elevates the vaginal pH substantially (Masters and Johnson 1980).

APPROACHES TO THE DEVELOPMENT OF NOVEL VAGINAL FORMULATIONS

Pivotal Issues

The Balance Between Protection and Perturbation

The functional activity of both spermatozoa and pathogenic microbes can be prevented by killing or inactivating them. The former strategy employs spermicides and microbicides. The latter relies on agents that inhibit the functional activity of spermatozoa and microbes so that they are unable to enter, respectively, the oocyte or the vaginal/cervical epithelium and target cells. Although these inactivating agents are more appropriately called spermistats and microbistats, the terms *spermicide* or *microbicide* are still frequently used for all antifertility and antimicrobial agents. Candidate classes of these compounds include detergents and surfactants, iodophores, carbohydrates, antibodies, antiviral drugs, defensins, and pyocins.

Many of the chemical formulations that are currently available for use as vaginal contraceptives, in addition to their contraceptive properties, can confer some protection against such STD infections as *Neisseria gonorrhea, Trichomonas vaginalis,* and *Chlamydia trachomatis* (Rosenberg et al. 1987, 1992). However, like microbicides, spermicides act as cytotoxins, often destroying vaginal and cervical cell membranes (Patton et al. 1992). As a consequence, the protective capacity of these formulations erodes under frequent and/or prolonged use, largely because their potential effects on normal vaginal flora and on the vaginal/cervical epithelium create perturbations that can actually promote the possibility of STD transmission (Kreiss et al. 1992; Niruthisard et al. 1991, 1992). This means that, if vaginal formulations are to be used more often for STD prevention, they will have to be nonirritating, nontoxic, and not upset the normal vaginal environment. In other words, such formulations must produce no lasting impact on the normal vaginal flora and their work in maintaining the vaginal milieu and its naturally acidic pH, nor should they compromise the vaginal or cervical epithelium. Each formulation will therefore need to be rigorously tested for any proinflammatory effects that could promote transmission of STD pathogens, notably HIV-1.

Efficacy

A topical formulation used for purposes of vaginal contraception consists of one or more active ingredients and a base (carrier) to deliver them. Both are important and each presents particular challenges to researchers and users. Typically, an active ingredient makes up only about 5–10 percent of an entire formulation; at least this is the case for those products that are on today's market, primarily surfactants or detergents such as nonoxynol-9, octoxynol-9, menfegol, and benzalkonium chloride (Haslett 1990; Hatcher and Warner 1992; Mauck et al. 1994). The activity of these products resides in their ability to dissolve lipid components in the cell membrane or viral envelope. Since these agents have approximately the same properties and potency, marketed formulations differ primarily in their base composition—either jellies, creams, foams, suppositories, tablets, films, or sponges. Because the active ingredients in these formulations all act by immobilizing or killing spermatozoa, they are usually referred to as "spermicides."

The contraceptive use-effectiveness of existing formulations varies greatly from study to study (Trussell 1994). Reported failure rates range from 2 percent to over 40 percent, with typical rates falling between 15 and 20 percent (Sobrero 1989), much higher than desirable. The limited efficacy of these formulations, their brief longevity after vaginal placement and effects on coital spontaneity, together with leakage and consequent "messiness," surely constrain consumer interest in available vaginal contraceptives.

Although the relatively poor efficacy of available vaginal contraceptive formulations can be partly blamed on improper use, some animal experiments have shown that the efficacy of many current products may be low even with more reliable use (Homm et al. 1976; Zaneveld et al. 1977). This implies that either their active ingredients and/or their distribution/delivery systems are in some way ineffective; because good comparative studies are rare, it has been difficult to discern where, exactly, the primary limitations reside.

Furthermore, because many pathogens—for instance, HIV, the herpes viruses, and chlamydial elementary bodies—are cell-associated, the margin between toxicity and efficacy is narrow. There is nothing unique about the membrane of an infected cell that permits a surfactant to distinguish it from the membrane of a healthy cell, though the cells of intact genital mucosa may be protected to some extent by a coating of mucus.

Finally, *in vitro* spermicidal efficacy does not necessarily translate into *in vivo* contraceptive efficacy (Quigg et al. 1988). Thus, without *in vivo* studies, it is not possible to state with certainty whether an agent with spermicidal properties is also contraceptive (Zaneveld 1994a, 1994b), nor are *in vitro* spermicidal comparisons adequate to the task of assessing the relative contraceptive activity of different formulations.

The Base

Because an active ingredient is only as effective as its delivery system allows, the formulation's base requires careful attention. Not only can the nature of a given base "make or break" the active ingredients, but can, in itself contribute to prevention of STD infections and conception, an attribute that should enhance the overall acceptability of vaginal topicals to women. The following characteristics of a good base are particularly important:

• A good base should spread rapidly and evenly over the vaginal and cervical surface, forming a slightly adhesive film.
• Optimally, this film should be impenetrable to microbes and, if possible, spermatozoa.
• The film should remain in place for prolonged periods of time, including during intercourse, providing long-acting protection.
• Leakage and consequent "messiness" should be minimal.
• Finally, the formulation should be somehow buffered at an acidic pH so as to retain a pH below 4.5 even in the presence of semen.

New Technologies

Many complicated biochemical processes are required for successful fertilization. Inhibition of any of these processes can lead to infertility, providing a large number of potential attack sites for new contraceptive agents, both chemical and immunologic. Yet, to date, only a few researchers have taken advantage of advances in knowledge to develop novel vaginal contraceptives.

New information can also be utilized to identify agents that can prevent both conception and STD infection. Tissue and/or cell invasion is required for both spermatozoa and pathogenic microbes to reach their target sites. Such invasion requires the activity of lytic enzymes, binding proteins, receptor-ligand interactions, fusion, endo- and exocytotic events, and a myriad of other processes. Each of these events is susceptible to inhibition, which would in turn prevent invasion. It is possible, if not likely, that spermatozoa and certain pathogenic microbes use some identical mechanisms of invasion. If so, the same agent could be used to prevent both occurrences (see Table D-2).

Detergents and Surfactants

Several detergents are already licensed in one country or another for intravaginal use as contraceptive agents. These include nonoxynol-9, the most commonly used, as well as menfegol, octoxynol, and benzalkonium chloride. Like the phospholipids that constitute cell membranes, detergents have hydrophobic and hydrophilic domains and exhibit activity that derives from their ability to dissolve lipid components in the cell membrane or viral envelope. Improvements on nonoxynol-9 may come from removing low molecular weight toxic components from the polydispersed N9 mixture (Klebanoff 1992; Walter et al. 1991a, 1991b), from improving dispersion/distribution, by providing for triggered release (Quigg 1991), or by lowering the detergent dose. In order to extend the spectrum of activity or longevity of action, low concentrations of nonoxynol-9 could be combined with other agents, for example, other detergents (Psychoyos 1994), beta-lactoglobulin (Neurath et al. 1996), antivirals (De Clercq 1993; Tsai et al. 1995), or zinc (Krieger and Rein 1992; Mardh et al. 1980; Williams 1980).

Milk Fatty Acids

Lipids found in human milk and epidermis display antibacterial and antiviral activity (Isaacs et al. 1990). Microbial killing by milk lipids is primarily due to the free fatty acids and monoglycerides that are released from milk triglycerides by lipases. At high concentrations, lipophilic molecules may be expected to have activity on sperm membranes that is similar to their activity on the membranes of other cells (Thormar et al. 1987).

Chlorhexidine

Chlorhexidine is a broad-spectrum antiseptic used in a prescription oral rinse. It is a positively charged molecule at physiological pH and binds to negative sites

TABLE D-2 Potential Targets and Mechanisms for Agents that Prevent Pregnancy and/or Sexually Transmitted Diseases

Target	Mechanism	Intended Effect
Sperm		
Nonoxynol-9	Surfactant	Spermicidal
C31G	Surfactant	Spermicidal
Chlorhexidine	Surfactant	Spermicidal
Peroxides	Membrane active	Spermicidal
Antibody (MAb)	Agglutination	Decreased forward motility
	Shaking phenomenon	Decreased forward motility
Magainin	Pore formation	Spermicidal
Decapacitation factor	Blocks capacitation	No acrosome reaction
Progesterone	Activates calcium channels	Premature acrosome reaction
AGB	Acrosin inhibitor	Fertilization blocked
Sulfonated polystyrene	Acrosin inhibitor	Fertilization blocked
	Agglutination	Decreased forward motility
ZP mimics	Blocks ZP binding	Fertilization blocked
Acidic buffer	Maintains low pH	Spermicidal
Zinc	Blocks capacitation	Blocked fertilization
Neem	Membrane-active	Spermicidal
Squalamine	Membrane-active	Microbicidal
Pathogen		
Nonoxynol-9	Disrupts membrane/envelope	Microbicidal
C31G	Disrupts membrane/envelope	Microbicidal
Chlorhexidine	Disrupts membrane/envelope	Microbicidal
Milk fatty acids	Disrupt membrane/envelope	Microbicidal
Peroxides	Membrane-active	Microbicidal
Antibody	Agglutination	Immune exclusion
Docosanol	Disrupts membrane/envelope	Microbicidal (enveloped viruses)
CAM mimic	Decoy	Adhesion blocked
Sulfated polymer	Coats cells	Adhesion blocked
	Coats virus	Fusion blocked
AGB	Protease inhibition	Adhesion blocked
Protegrins	Pore-formation	Microbicidal
Acidic buffer	Maintains low pH	Microbicidal
Zinc	Binds proteins	Microbicidal
Neem	Membrane-active	Microbicidal
Squalamine	Membrane-active	Microbicidal
PMPA	Reverse transcriptase inhibition	Anti-HIV
Cervicovaginal Environment		
1. Mucus		
Acidic buffer	Lowers or maintains pH	Microbicidal
Lactoferrin	Fe binding	Inhibits Fe-dependent pathogens
Lysozyme	Enzymatic bacteriolysis	Bactericidal
Zinc	Protein binding	Microbicidal
Sulfonated polystyrene	Increases viscosity	Decreased sperm migration
Chlorhexidine	Increases viscosity	Decreased sperm migration

TABLE D-2 Continued

Target	Mechanism	Intended Effect
Mucopolysaccharidase inhibitor	Increases viscosity	Decreased sperm migration
Lubricating gels	Increases lubricity	Trauma reduction
2. Epithelium		
Docosanol	Membrane-active	Microbicidal (enveloped viruses)
B-lactoglobulin	Blocks HIV receptors	Anti-HIV
Squalamine	Inhibits Na^+/H^+ exchange	Anti-HIV
C31G	Fibrin formation	Trauma repair
Lubricating gels	Prevents abrasions	Pathogen entry blocked
Zinc sulfate	Promotes wound healing	Pathogen entry blocked
3. Immune System		
Cytokines	Activate macrophages	Phagocytosis
Antibodies	Interaction with mucus	Immune exclusion
	Agglutination	Immune exclusion
	Blocks adhesion	Immune exclusion
4. Commensals		
Acidic buffers	Decreases acid-intolerant bacteria	Increased lactobacillus
Peroxides	Decreases peroxide-intolerant bacteria	Increased lactobacillus
Lactobacillus	Microbial competition	Decreased pathogens

SOURCE: Original table prepared for this paper by D Anderson and K Whaley, 1996.

on cell surfaces; this leads, in turn, to altered permeability, cellular leakage, and precipitation or coagulation of cytoplasmic proteins. Chlorhexidine has been shown to be spermicidal (Sharman et al. 1986), to inactivate HIV, and to cause changes in cervical mucus that prevent penetration by spermatozoa (Chantler et al. 1989).

C31G

C31G is an equimolar mixture of two synthetic, amphoteric surface-active compounds shown to have broad-spectrum antimicrobial properties (Corner et al. 1988). Its active agents are alkyl dimethyl glycine and alkyl dimethyl amine oxide, and the alkyl chain length (C-12 to C-16) is representative of the natural distribution of the fatty acids of coconut oil. The surfactant properties of C31G would suggest potential for activity against sperm and enveloped viruses; it also appears to promote wound healing (Michaels et al. 1983).

Docosanol

1-Docosanol, a 22-carbon-long saturated alcohol, has been shown to inhibit lipid-enveloped viruses (Katz et al. 1994), inhibiting viral replication by interfering with fusion or early intracellular events surrounding viral entry into target cells (Katz et al. 1991). Since such a large percentage of the molecule becomes associated with cell membranes, docosanol can be expected to have some activity on sperm function.

Neem

Neem oil extracted from the seeds of *Azadirachta indica* has been shown to have antiviral, antibacterial, and antifungal activity (National Research Council 1992). The antifertility activity of vaginally applied neem oil has been established in rabbits and monkeys (Talwar et al. 1994). Neem oil can also inhibit spermatogenesis, sperm–egg interaction, implantation, and can act as an abortifacient. Its precise mechanism of action is not clearly understood, but may be due to immunomodulatory activity such as enhanced phagocytic activity and induced production of gamma interferon.

Squalamine

Squalamine is an aminosterol antibiotic first isolated from the shark (Moore et al. 1993). A condensation of an anionic bile salt, it has just recently been chemically synthesized (Sadownik et al. 1995). Squalamine exhibits potent bactericidal activity against both gram-negative and gram-positive bacteria, is fungicidal, and also induces osmotic lysis of protozoa. One mechanism of action may be an inhibition of sodium-hydrogen exchangers on cell surfaces that produces changes in intracellular pH. Such a mechanism may prove to be spermicidal and might influence HIV's ability to infect target cells.

Serine Proteinases and Their Inhibitors

Different types of serine proteinase inhibitors are now known to be able to inhibit HIV replication without cytotoxicity (Bourinbaiar and Nagorny 1994; Hallenberger et al. 1992; Hattori et al. 1989). It is also known that spermatozoa utilize a trypsin-like serine proteinase (acrosin) for penetration through the zona pellucida and that certain acrosin inhibitors are potent contraceptives when placed vaginally in animal models. Aryl 4-guanidinobenzoates such as 4'-acetamidophenyl 4-guanidinobenzoate (AGB) have been found to be more contraceptive than nonoxynol-9 (Kaminski et al. 1985) and it was recently reported that AGB is also a potent anti-HIV agent (Bourinbaiar and Lee-Huang 1994b). N-α-tosyl-L-lysyl-chloromethylketone (TLCK) has also been found to inhibit both HIV infectivity (Bourinbaiar and Nagorny 1994) and fertilization when placed vaginally (Zaneveld et al. 1970).

Acidic Buffers

Since sperm are inactivated by acidity (Shedlovsky et al. 1942), it appears that in neutralizing the vagina, the alkalinity of semen enables more sperm to reach and enter the cervix (Masters and Johnson 1980). When this "window of neutrality" is, in effect, "opened" by semen, it stays open for at least two hours after intercourse. This unfortunately can facilitate the sexual exchange of STD pathogens that otherwise would be killed by the acid and gives those pathogens additional time to reach target cells in the new host. Exposing cell-free HIV to the acid pH ranges normally found in healthy vaginal secretions reduces both its infectivity and the survival of HIV-infected lymphocytes (Voeller and Anderson 1992a, 199b). Even mild acidity (pH 5) has been shown to inhibit other STD pathogens, e.g., *Neisseria gonorrhoeae* (Zheng et al. 1994).

Peptides

Magainin, a peptide isolated from frogs, is a cationic peptide that is antibacterial, antifungal, antiprotozoan, antiviral, and antispermatozoal (de Waal et al. 1991; Edelstein et al. 1991). These peptides are able to adopt an amphiphilic alpha-helix structure in a hydrophobic environment and can punch holes in the cell walls of infecting organisms.

Defensins are complexly folded and amphipathic peptides which, while rich in antiparallel beta-sheet, are devoid of alphahelical domains (Ganz and Lehrer 1994). Their unusually broad antibacterial spectrum encompasses gram-positive and gram-negative bacteria, many fungi, mycobacteria, spirochetes, and several enveloped viruses (Lehrer et al. 1993; Schonwetter et al. 1995). The antimicrobial properties of defensins result from their insertion into target cell membranes and the formation of voltage-sensitive channels.

There are many antibacterial peptides that are inhibited by seminal plasma, but magainin II and a synthetic peptide of a 37-Kd cationic antimicrobial protein have been shown to inhibit sperm motility (D'Cruz et al. 1995). Gramicidin, a peptide antibiotic used in the former Soviet Union as an active component of contraceptive gels and foams, also exhibits anti-HIV activity (Bourinbaiar and Lee-Huang 1994a).

Sulfated Polymers

We have known for over two decades that polyanionic substances, particularly sulfated polysaccharides, are able to interfere with the virus adsorption process, including HIV (DeClercq 1993). A sulfonated polystyrene polymer has been shown to be contraceptive in rabbits (Homm et al. 1985); the polymer is known to agglutinate spermatozoa, alter sperm-cervical mucus interaction and inhibit sperm acrosin (Foldesy et al. 1986).

H_2O_2 or Peroxidases

When combined with H_2O_2 and a halide, peroxidases form a powerful anti-microbial system that is effective against a variety of microorganisms, including viruses (Klebanoff and Coombs 1991). The proposal has been made to add hydrogen peroxide and/or peroxidases (derived from animals or produced by genetic engineering) to vaginal formulations. These products may work in conjunction with H_2O_2-generating lactobacilli in the vagina.

Monoclonal Antibodies (MAbs)

Antibodies in mucus play a major role in preventing mucosal transmission of disease. Monoclonal antibodies of human origin, expected to be potent, flexible, specific, sturdy, and inexpensive, can now be developed to serve as natural protective agents for mucosal surfaces (Cone and Whaley 1994; Ma et al. 1995). Both contraception and prevention of viral STDs with MAbs have been demonstrated in animals, and controlled release of antibodies for long-term topical passive immunoprotection permits this technology to be noncoitally related as well (Sherwood et al. 1996). Monoclonal antibodies are a technology almost two decades old yet, while used in many fields, including human health, they have been significantly underutilized in contraception. Nonetheless, MAbs offer a pathway to "prophylactic contraception," a concept within reproductive health that bridges the mechanisms of mucosal transmission of sperm as well as pathogens (see Table D-3).

TABLE D-3 Fertilization and STD Infections Prevented by Polyclonal and Monoclonal Antibodies

Antigen	Species
Polyclonal antibodies for prevention of fertilization	
Semen	Rabbits
Oocytes/ZP	Mice/rats
Sperm	Mice
LDHC4	Mice/baboons
Inhibin	Hamsters/marmosets
Monoclonal antibodies for prevention of fertilization	
Sperm	Rabbits
ZP2/ZP3	Mice
Sperm	Mice
Sperm	Rabbits
Sperm	Rabbits
Polyclonal antibodies	
Hepatitis B	Humans
Chlamydia	Mice
HSV-2 (herpes simplex virus-2)	Mice
Treponema pallidum	Hamsters
Treponema pallidum	Rabbits
Candida albicans	Mice
HIV/SIV (human immunodeficiency virus/ simian immunodeficiency virus)	Monkeys
Monoclonal antibodies	
HIV gp 120	Chimpanzees
HIV gp 120	hu-PBL-SCID mice
HSV-1/gD	Mice
HSV-1/gB	Mice
HSV-2/gD	Mice
HSV-2/gD	Mice

SOURCE: Adapted from: RA Cone, KJ Whaley. Monoclonal antibodies for reproductive health: Part I. Preventing sexual transmission of disease and pregnancy with topically applied antibodies. American Journal of Reproductive Immunology 32:114–131, 1994.

Part 2: Mucosal Immunologic Approaches

Deborah J. Anderson, Ph.D., and Alison J. Quayle, Ph.D.
Fearing Research Laboratory, Brigham and
Women's Hospital and Harvard Medical School,
Department of Obstetrics, Gynecology, and Reproductive Biology

INTRODUCTION

Development of effective immunocontraceptives awaits the identification and genetic engineering of appropriate molecular sequences and their expression in immunogenic form. It also depends on the ability to deliver immunogens to achieve the desired effect at the appropriate site within the male or female reproductive tract. Since both the lower female and the male genital tract mucosa are considered part of the common mucosal system, there is an implication that mucosa-targeted immunization would induce effective genital tract immune responses. In this paper, we review the basic principles of mucosal immunology of the male and female genital tracts and explore options that might become available for mucosal immunization, both for purposes of contraception and protection against infectious disease.

GENERAL MUCOSAL IMMUNOLOGY

Antibody-mediated (Secretory) Mucosal Immunity

The mucosal membranes of the body include the respiratory tract, conjunctiva, intestinal tract, mammary glands, and the urogenital tracts of the male and female. These mucosal surfaces cover a vast surface area, estimated at around 400 square meters, and are constantly exposed to environmental antigens. In contrast to the lymphoid organs, the majority of plasmacytes in mucosal-associated organs are of the immunoglobulin A (IgA) isotype (80 percent, compared to 30 percent in the lymphoid organs) and the predominant antibody in external secretions is usually secretory immunoglobulin A (SIgA). More SIgA is synthesized by the immune system than any other isotype (Ma et al. 1995; Mestecky and McGhee 1993). Approximately 70–80 percent of all Ig-producing plasma

Adapted from: Quayle AJ, DJ Anderson. Induction of mucosal immunity in the genital tract and prospects for oral vaccines. IN Birth Control Vaccines. R Raghugpathy, GP Talwar, eds. Austin, TX: R.G. Landes. 1995.

cells are located in the intestinal mucosa, making this organ the largest reservoir of immune cells in the entire body (Brandtzaeg et al. 1993).

Given the importance of the mucosal system and the fact that the human body actually synthesizes and secretes more antibodies into mucus than it does into blood, it is surprising that so little is known about how the secreted antibodies function in mucus to protect the human mucosal surfaces. Some known effector actions are: (1) agglutinating pathogens; (2) blocking pathogen interactions with target cells; (3) trapping pathogens in mucus; (4) helping to regulate protective commensals (e.g., vaginal flora); and (5) secreting or neutralizing pathogens that have penetrated the mucosal surface (Cone and Whaley 1994; Franek et al. 1984; Mazanec et al. 1993). A significant advantage of using polymeric secretory type antibodies for topical application would be the extraordinary potency created by their polyvalency, which increases their avidity and, because of their structure, their particular potency in processes of agglutination (Cone and Whaley 1994; Hornick and Karush 1972; Raff et al. 1991). In addition, sIgAs persist longer in mucosal secretions than IgG because of resistance to proteolysis. Furthermore, they cause less inflammation because of a low capacity to bind complement. These unique attributes of sIgA would seem to be appealing areas for expanded research.

Despite their apparent importance for mucosal protection, few investigators or companies seem to have attempted to develop IgA monoclonal antibodies. This has been particularly the case for sIgA, despite the fact that it is the first line of defense against infectious agents (Ma et al. 1995) and is the isotype least likely to cause the inflammatory responses that IgG can initiate (Cone and Whaley 1994; McGhee et al. 1992). The emphasis has been on IgG, at least partly because of the prominence of blood in concepts of vital functions (Cone and Whaley 1994), and those IgA MAbs that have been developed have been used by most companies for therapeutic purposes rather than for promoting sexual health. This picture may be modified by discoveries of the potential applicability of transgenic plants for large-scale production of recombinant sIgA for passive mucosal immunotherapy (Ma et al. 1995).

Historically, the study of mucosal immunity can be traced back over 200 years (Mestecky and McGhee 1989). Classical scientific studies began in the late eighteenth century, when Pasteur and his pupils demonstrated that oral immunization with the appropriate killed bacterium could protect animals from a number of enteric infections (Gay 1924; Mestecky and McGhee 1989). The concept of an independent local immune defense system was initially proposed by Besredka in 1919 after finding that rabbits orally immunized with killed *Shigella* were protected against dysentery, irrespective of serum antibody titre (Besredka 1919). The findings from this study were later tested in a clinical setting when thousands of humans were orally immunized against dysentery and typhoid fever (Besredka 1927).

Scientific endeavor in the 1960s and 1970s laid the foundations for contemporary understandings of the mucosal immune system. In 1963, Tomasi and Zigelbaum reported a predominance of IgA in human colostrum, saliva, and urine samples in comparison to serum (Tomasi and Ziegelbaum 1963) and immuno-histochemical studies suggested that this must be locally produced since IgA-secreting plasma cells were 20 times more abundant than IgG-secreting plasma cells in the human intestine (Crabbe et al. 1965). Later studies showed that the plasma cells in mucosa predominantly produced IgA dimers or polymers (Brandtzaeg 1973) associated with a 15kD glycopeptide "joining" (J) chain that is also a component of pentameric IgM (Halpern and Koshland 1970; Mestecky et al. 1971). This contrasts with the IgA-producing plasma cell populations in the bone marrow, spleen, and lymph nodes, which synthesize the predominantly monomeric IgA found in serum. Immunoglobulin A (Hanson 1961; Tomasi et al. 1965) and IgM (Brandtzaeg 1975) in secretions were found to be associated with secretory component, and both isotypes were shown to be translocated to external secretions by a transepithelial transport mechanism (Brandtzaeg et al. 1968 and 1970). In brief, polymeric IgA binds to secretory component that is expressed on the basolateral surface of epithelial cells. This complex is endocytosed and the resulting vesicle transcytosed, fusing with the apical membrane and finally re-leasing the secretory component-IgA complex into the lumen (see Brandtzaeg et al. 1993 for review).

Although immune cells are found throughout the mucosae, antigen uptake and induction of immune responses occur predominantly in specialized inductive sites. These are the gut-associated lymphoreticular tissues (GALT) which in-clude the Peyer's patches (PP), the appendix in some animals, solitary lymph nodes and small follicles, and the bronchus-associated lymphoreticular tissue (BALT) (Mestecky and McGhee 1993). The Peyer's patches are distinct nod-ules, visible to the naked eye and predominantly located in the small intestine; in young adult humans, they number approximately 200 (Cornes 1965). Each PP has a B-cell zone consisting of a number of follicles with germinal centers, a parafollicular or T-cell-dependent area, and a dome region with a lymphocyte- and macrophage-rich corona overlain by a specialized epithelium. This epithe-lium is cuboidal (in contrast to the columnar epithelium lining the remainder of the gut [Bockman and Cooper 1973]), with no goblet cells and little mucus, and has special antigen-sampling cells called microfold (M) cells (Owen and Jones 1974). The M cells pinocytose and phagocytose antigen in the lumen of the gut but do not degrade it, delivering it intact to the underlying lymphoid cells. The germinal centers of the follicles of the PP are rich in B lymphocytes committed to producing IgA (Jones and Cebra 1974); they do not, however, mature into IgA-producing plasma cells in the Peyer's patches, but serve importantly as a pool of cells that are capable of migrating to distant mucosal sites.

This ability of B cells from the Peyer's patches to home to, and repopulate, distant mucosal sites in irradiated animals was first noted in the early 1960s (Jacobsen et al. 1961) and the studies were subsequently extended in a number of laboratories (e.g., Craig and Cebra 1971). In a mouse study, labeled, adoptively-transferred mesenteric lymph node (MLN) cells homed to MLN, gut, cervix, vagina, uterus, and mammary glands and were predominantly IgA in their phenotype, while peripheral lymph node (PLN) cells preferentially homed back to PLN and produced IgG (McDermott and Bienenstock 1979). Studies in various animal species have also demonstrated the appearance of specific antibodies in sites remote from oral immunization (Challacombe and Lehner 1979; Forrest et al. 1992; Goldblum et al. 1975; Montgomery et al. 1976). In humans, this work has included the classic studies by Ogra and colleagues using Sabin polio vaccine (Ogra and Karzon 1969; Ogra and Ogra 1973) and by Mestecky and coworkers with bacterial antigen (Mestecky et al. 1978). The term "mucosa-associated lymphoid tissues" (MALT) was introduced by Bienenstock and Befus (1980) to describe the immune cell traffic between mucosal tissues.

In brief, immature surface membrane IgM-positive B cells in the Peyer's patch "switch" to become surface membrane IgA-positive under the influence of cognate antigen, special "switch" T cells, dendritic cells, and T-cell-derived cytokines (McGhee et al. 1993). These committed cells exit the Peyer's patches and travel to the mesenteric lymph nodes; here they mature further prior to entering the bloodstream via the lymph and thoracic duct, thence homing to, and repopulating, distant mucosal sites. An elegant study by Czerkinsky and colleagues provides support for the notion of a common mucosal system in man: *Streptococcus mutans*-specific, IgA-producing cells were isolated from blood seven days after oral immunization and seven days prior to the appearance of antigen-specific IgA in saliva and tears (Czerkinsky et al. 1987). It should also be noted that, in the mouse, an alternative source of precursor IgA plasmacytes is the peritoneal cavity (Husband and Gowans 1978); these peritoneal cavity-derived B cells have recently been shown to be Ly-1 CD5 positive (Kroese et al. 1988).

Cellular Mucosal Immunity

The mucosal organs also provide a substantial reservoir of T cells, which are located in three major areas: the organized lymphoid tissue (GALT, BALT), the lamina propria, and the epithelium. The T cells of the Peyer's patches are predominantly of the CD4 phenotype and one of the major roles for these T cells is thought to be regulation of IgA responses (McGhee et al. 1993). *In vitro* experiments in which Peyer's patch B cells were activated with lipopolysaccharide resulted in a four- to six-fold increase in IgA production in the presence of activated T cells from PP; if the T cells were splenic in origin, however, IgG and IgM production were increased (Elson et al. 1979).

Studies at the University of Alabama are currently dissecting the dynamics of the B and T cell interactions in the Peyer's patch (see Mestecky and McGhee 1993 for review). Cytokines that seem to have a key role in this environment are interleukin 5 (IL-5) and interleukin 6 (IL-6). In the murine model, IL-5 selectively enhanced IgA production (Beagley et al. 1989; Bond et al. 1987; Murray et al. 1987) and IL-6-induced terminal differentiation of activated B cells and increased IgA synthesis in *in vitro* systems (Beagley et al. 1989). These cytokines are synthesized by T lymphocytes of the Th2 subset (Mosmann and Coffman 1989; Romagnani 1992), a subset shown through ELISPOT assay to be overrepresented in PP T cells and lamina propria compared to blood (McGhee et al. 1993). However, TH1-type cytokines (γ-interferon, TNF β) are also produced by T lymphocytes at mucosal surfaces, especially at sites of infection.

The T cells in the lamina propria are also predominantly CD4-positive memory (CD45RO+) cells (Brandtzaeg et al. 1989); in contrast, approximately 85 percent of the intraepithelial cells (IELs) are of the CD8 phenotype (Janossy et al. 1980; Jarry et al. 1990). In humans, the majority of intestinal T cells express the $\alpha\beta$ T cell receptor (TCR) (Brandtzaeg et al. 1989; Halstensen et al. 1989); in mice, a substantial proportion of the IELs are TCR positive (Itohara et al. 1990). Mouse studies strongly suggest that the $\alpha\beta$TCR cells in the lamina propria and epithelium of the mucosa are derived from T cells in organized lymphoid tissue, indicating that there is committed trafficking of T cells from inductive sites to the various mucosa. Adoptive transfer experiments with labeled T cells from Peyer's patch and mesenteric lymph node have shown a preferential homing back to gut mucosa (Guy-Grand et al. 1978); infection of Peyer's patch with reovirus results in the appearance of reovirus-specific CD8+ cytotoxic IEL (London et al. 1989); and T cells isolated from breast milk respond better to enteric antigens than do peripheral blood T cells from the same donor (Ada 1993).

Recent studies have identified receptors on lymphocytes that are involved in homing to, and possibly maintaining localization within, mucosal-associated organs. The integrin $\alpha4\beta7$ (LPAM-1), expressed on most naive murine (CD45RA+) T cells and a subset of memory (CD45RO+) T cells, mediates binding to Peyer's patch high endothelial venules (HEV), but not peripheral lymph node HEV (Holzmann et al. 1989). The ligand for LPAM-1 is the immunoglobulin superfamily adhesion molecule MADCAM-1 that is expressed on mucosal venules, and the interaction between the two is thought to play an important role in lymphocyte homing to mucosal sites (Berlin et al. 1993). In both man and mouse, an integrin has been identified that is almost exclusively expressed by T cells residing in the mucosa. This is also a $\beta7$ integrin, but it is co-expressed with a unique α chain. In the mouse it is known as the αM290$\beta7$ integrin (Kilshaw and Murant 1991) and in humans as the HML-1 antigen, αe$\beta7$ integrin, or CD103 (Cerf-Benussan et al. 1992; Parker et al. 1992). Murine studies suggest that this molecule is induced after mucosal localization, since αM290$\beta7$-positive cells are abundant in the various mucosae but rare in spleen or lymph node (Kilshaw and Murant 1990; Quayle et al. 1994). The *in vitro* addition of transforming growth factor beta (TGF-β) to stimulated lymph node cells increases expression of the $\beta7$ subunit and changes the associated $\alpha4$ subunit to αM290; this has been hypothesized as the possible mechanism of induction in the mucosa (Kilshaw and Murant

1991). Another hypothesis is that αM290v7 plays a role in adhesion, modulating or focusing effector cell activity (Kilshaw and Murant 1991).

MUCOSAL IMMUNOLOGY OF THE
HUMAN GENITAL TRACT IN FEMALES

Plasma cells are present in the greatest concentration in the subepithelial layers of the human endocervix, but substantial numbers are also seen in the ectocervix, vagina, and fallopian tubes (Kutteh et al. 1993; Kutteh and Mestecky 1994). Approximately 70 percent of the plasmacytes are IgA positive and, of these, 50–75 percent of cells co-label for J chain, indicating that the majority of local IgA synthesis is polymeric. Of the IgA positive cells, 40 percent are of the IgA2 subclass, indicating an A1/A2 ratio similar to that of the lower intestine. Plasmacytes are rarely detected in the ovary, endometrium, or myometrium (Kutteh et al. 1993; Kutteh and Mestecky 1994), but secretory component is expressed on the epithelial cells of the villi of the fallopian tubes and the cervical glandular epithelium, suggesting that all the elements for local production and transport of sIgA are present at those sites (Kutteh et al. 1993; Kutteh and Mestecky 1994).

Infection with *Neisseria gonorrhoeae, Trichomonas vaginalis,* or *Candida albicans* also results in an increase in plasma cell numbers on the endocervical region, predominantly of the IgA class (Chipperfield and Evans 1972). Similarly, acute and chronic salpingitis is associated with elevated plasmacyte numbers in the fallopian tubes that are also predominantly IgA-positive (Kutteh et al. 1990); interestingly, plasma cell numbers in tissues with evidence of healed salpingitis were similar to those of normal healthy tissue.

Although there have been a number of studies of immunoglobulin concentrations and isotypes in female genital tract secretions, the data remain conflicted. This may be due to differences among species and other confounding variables such as the secretion collected, technique of collection, hormonal influences, reproductive status, and concomitant infections present in the tract. In addition, cervicovaginal secretions presumably contain "spillover" from uterine secretions. Quantitative analysis of cervical mucus from over 100 healthy women revealed the presence of IgG, IgM, and IgA in this secretion, with IgG the major immunoglobulin; the highly significant correlation between albumin and IgG suggested that this was a serum transudate (Tjokronegoro and Sirisinha 1975). Furthermore, while the mean level of IgA was approximately half that of IgG, the majority of this was associated with secretory component and therefore indicative of local production.

Locally produced antigen-specific IgA has also been found in the cervical secretions of women with gonococccal cervicitis, but only IgG was detected in the serum (O'Reilly et al. 1976). In a series of classic mucosal experiments with polio vaccine performed by Ogra and colleagues, women were immunized vaginally, intrauterinally, or intramuscularly with killed (Salk) poliovirus, or orally with live attenuated (Sabin) polio vaccine; the poliovirus-specific antibody response was then measured (Ogra and Ogra 1973). Vaginal immunization resulted in the appearance of IgA and IgG in vaginal secretions, an occasional low IgG response in uterus, and no detectable specific IgA or IgG in serum. In contrast, intrauterine immunization resulted in the appearance of IgG in uterine washings, an occasional low positive in vaginal secretions, undetectable IgA local secretions, and no antibody response in serum. In the women immunized orally or intramuscularly, specific serum IgG and IgA were detected, but the only locally detectable antibody was low-level IgG; the appearance of this was correlated with increasing serum IgG. This correlates well with a primate study in which animals were vaginally or systemically immunized with lipopolysaccharide (LPS) of *Salmonella typhosa*. Vaginal immunization resulted in immunoglobulin responses that were greater in cervical secretions than in serum in the majority of animals; in the systemically immunized animals, however, only 10 percent of the serum response was seen locally (Yang and Schumacher 1979).

In summary, studies indicate that, in humans and primates, there is an efficient local production of IgA in the cervix/vagina in response to antigenic challenge; however, the uterine response is predominantly IgG. Whether the IgG is locally produced or is a serum transudate still remains to be established. Since women who are hysterectomized have IgA levels that are 10 percent of normal, but IgG levels are only decreased by 50 percent, it does appear that there may be a substantial serum contribution. This is supported by a study of hysterectomized mice (Parr and Parr 1989a).

Animal studies have also clearly shown that the mucosal immune system in the female urogenital tract is regulated by sex hormones; in an extensive series of experiments by Wira and associates, local immunoglobulin levels in the reproductive tract were shown to be under the control of estradiol and progesterone (Sullivan and Wira 1984; Wira and Sullivan 1985). Immunoglobulin levels have been reported to decrease at mid-cycle (Yang and Schumacher 1979) and an estrogen-dependent increase of IgA has also been documented (Jalanti and Isliker 1977). Nonetheless, the literature on the effects of the menstrual cycle on local immunoglobulin secretion in both primates and humans is conflicted and needs further study.

The T-cell population of the human and primate female reproductive tract varies considerably from tissue to tissue. In the human endometrium, T cells are rarely seen in the proliferative phase of the menstrual cycle but increase in number in the secretory phase, often forming small aggregates (Bulmer et al. 1988). The majority of these endometrial T cells express the CD8 antigen, particularly those found in the lymphoid aggregates and within the epithelium (Bulmer et al. 1988; Kamat and Isaacson 1986). A unique population of phenotypically unusual CD16[-], CD56[+] natural killer cell-like large granula leukocytes, and CD8-positive intra-epithelial T lymphocytes are found in the ectocervix, the vagina, and the transformation zone (Edwards and Morris 1985; Miller et al. 1992). Substantial infiltrates of CD8- and CD4-positive cells are seen in the stroma of the transformation zone, often in lymphoid aggregates, but T cells are relatively sparse in the stroma of the ectocervix and vagina (Edwards and Morris 1985). The particularly high numbers of T lymphocytes in the transformation zone of the cervix has led some researchers to believe that this is an area of particularly high immunologic activity (Edwards and Morris 1985).

In the endometrium, the predominant antigen presenting cells are macrophages (Bulmer et al. 1988). The vagina and ectocervix are also characterized by the presence of Langerhans cells, bone marrow-derived antigen-presenting cells with dendritic processes that can extend to the epithelial surface. These cells are found only in the epidermis and non-keratinized epithelia (Bjercke et al. 1983; Edwards and Morris 1985; Miller et al. 1992). After activation, Langerhans cells migrate from the epithelium to draining lymph nodes, where they present antigens to T lymphocytes, thereby initiating a specific immune response. Langerhans cells in the epithelium express a phenotype that is characteristically CD1a, MHC class II, Fcγ, CD3 and, to a lesser extent, CD4-positive; following activation, these cells also express a variety of adhesion molecules including ICAM-1 (CD54) and LFA-3 (CD58) (deGraaf et al. 1995). Langerhans cells show marked variation in their distribution, with the highest numbers found in the vulva and ectocervix and lower numbers in the vagina (Edwards and Morris 1985). There is also considerable individual variation in the concentration of Langerhans cells in the human vaginal and ectocervical epithelium, although the variation does not appear to be related to the menstrual cycle.

MUCOSAL IMMUNOLOGY OF THE
HUMAN GENITAL TRACT IN MALES

Until recently, little had been documented on the immunobiology of either the human or primate male reproductive tract. While immunocytochemical evidence for local synthesis of IgA or secretory component has not been seen in normal epididymis, prostate, or seminal vesicles (Brandtzaeg et al. 1993), in autopsy tissues from HIV-positive men with genital-tract inflammation, all three sites stained strongly for secretory component, suggesting that infection/inflammation may up-regulate its expression (Anderson and Pudney 1992).

Further studies are clearly needed to identify the exact origins of immunoglobulin synthesis, as IgA, IgG and IgM can also be detected in semen and sterile prostatic fluid from healthy men (Fowler et al. 1982). Absorption with anti-secretory component results in a 64–100 percent decrease in IgA concentration, indicating that this antibody is in the secretory form and thus is locally derived (Fowler et al. 1982). Levels of all three immunoglobulin types are approximately 10 times higher in prostatic fluid than semen, suggesting that a large proportion of immunoglobulin may be derived from the prostate (Fowler et al. 1982; Fowler and Mariano 1983). However, recent studies suggest that the penile urethra may be the primary source of sIgA in semen from normal men: In penile urethral tissue taken at autopsy from a series of 15 immunologically normal men, epithelial cells were observed to stain strongly for secretory component and numerous IgA positive plasma cells were seen in the submucosa, indicating that the urethra contains all the elements for production of sIgA (Pudney and Anderson 1995). In addition, studies of semen from HIV-positive and normal seronegative men detected high concentrations of sIgA in pre-ejaculatory fluid, suggesting that there is local urethral production and transport of IgA (Haimovici and Anderson 1992). Pathogen-specific secretory IgA has been detected in the semen of men infected with *Chlamydia trachomatis* (Kojima et al. 1988), *Escherichia coli* (Fowler and Mariano 1982), and *Neisseria gonorrhoeae* (McMillan et al. 1979).

On the basis of these findings, it is possible to hypothesize that, while all the components for secretory immunity are present in various areas of the male reproductive tract, only in the presence of overt infection are they brought into play. Such a hypothesis receives indirect support from studies in the mouse: While IgA-positive plasma cells cannot be detected in the urethra of germ-free mice and rats, scattered cells can be seen in the deep urethral glands (Parr and Parr 1989b; Parr et al. 1992). Secretory component staining is also only seen in the urethral glands, suggesting that a low-level constituent production of sIgA may exist. Yet, after oral immunization followed by a local antigen challenge, IgA-secreting plasma cells were readily detectable in the urethra, suggesting that, in fact, local uptake of antigen and/or inflammation can up-regulate production when required (Husband and Clifton 1989). Very importantly, in the same study, chronic drainage of the thoracic lymphatic duct during the postchallenge period abrogated plasma cell appearance in the urethra after local challenge; reinfusion of these cells resulted in the appearance of urinary tract IgA plasmacytes, documenting for the first time that the male genital tract mucosa is part of the common mucosal system.

T lymphocytes are not usually detected in the healthy human testis (El-Demiry et al. 1985 and 1987), but are seen in the rete testis, with CD8+ cells observable within the epithelium and CD4+ cells primarily in the stroma (El-Demiry and James 1988). T cells are also seen in the human urethra, with a predominance of CD8+ cells in the intraepithelial population and a mixture of CD8 and CD4+ cells in the stroma; T cells in the urethra are positive for the integrin $\alpha,^E\beta 7$, an antigen exclusively found on mucosa-associated lymphocytes (Pudney and Anderson 1995). A recent study in mice reported similar findings, with scattered T cells in the urethra positive for the murine mucosa-associated integrin $\alpha M290\beta 7$ (Quayle et al. 1994).

Macrophages are abundant in the human and primate male urogenital tract: in the testicular interstitium, epididymis, the epithelium and connective tissue of the excurrent ducts and accessory glands, and in the penile urethra (El-Demiry et al. 1987; Fowler et al. 1982; Miller et al. 1994; Wang and Holstein 1983). Unlike the female lower urogenital tract, Langerhans cells are rarely detected in the penile urethra, but are abundant in the epithelium of the foreskin (Miller et al. 1994).

Leukocytes are commonly found in the semen of healthy, fertile men (Wolff and Anderson 1988a). Although these cells cross the reproductive tract epithelium, neither the mechanism of migration nor where it takes place along the tract is known. The median number of leukocytes in normal semen is 170,000 but the range is wide—from 9,000 to over 100 million (Wolff and Anderson 1988a). Numbers are elevated in samples from men with evidence of genital-tract inflammation, and a leukocyte count of greater than one million is considered pathologic according to criteria established by the World Health Organization and is associated with decreased sperm parameters and subfertility (Wolff and Anderson 1988b). Various cytokines (TNF-α, IL-6, IL-8) have been detected in seminal fluid from infertile men, indicating that mediators of cellular immunity can also enter male genital tract secretions (Anderson and Hill 1995).

EVIDENCE FOR A COMPARTMENTALIZATION OF THE MUCOSAL IMMUNE SYSTEM

A distinguishing and highly relevant feature of the pathways of immune cell traffic that constitute the common mucosal system is the localization of immune cells at mucosal sites that are distant from the site of mucosal immunization. Studies as early as the 1970s demonstrated the appearance of specific humoral and cellular immunity in respiratory and genital tracts after oral immunization (Ogra and Karzon 1969; Ogra and Ogra 1973). However, many studies have also indicated that optimal mucosal immune responses appear to be obtained by immunization at that mucosal site or an adjacent mucosal locale. The reason for this is unknown, but there are at least two appealing hypotheses. The first is that there are tissue-specific homing receptors additional to those that are specific for generic mucosa. The second is that a depot of antigen is retained locally by macrophages or dendritic cells, resulting in the production of soluble factors that can up-regulate the expression of vascular addressins on the endothelial cells and thence increase the number of lymphocytes homing to this area. If this hypothesis is correct, the administration of antigen in a long-lasting adjuvant would be particularly effective when applied locally.

Examples of compartmentalization are numerous in the genital tract. For example, adoptive transfer of T cells isolated from genital-tract-draining (but not other) lymph nodes (including mesenteric) from mice vaginally immunized with heat-killed herpes simplex virus protected naive mice from vaginal challenge with live virus, verifying that there is also a local homing of T cells (McDermott et al. 1989). Rectal immunization has proved more efficient at stimulating secretory immunity in the genital tract than other mucosal routes, including in one study a vaginal route (Haneberg et al. 1994; Lehner et al. 1992, 1993).

ORAL IMMUNIZATION

A desirable achievement for an immunogen based upon reproductive or STD pathogen antigens would be the induction of both a local and a systemic immune response, the latter appearing to supplement mucosal immunity at least in some tissues. Systemic immunization alone would not fulfill both criteria, except in specific cases such as when an individual has previously been immunized with the antigen "naturally" via the mucosa. Thus, milk samples from lactating Swedish women who were parenterally immunized with cholera vaccine had undetectable anticholera sIgA, but Pakistani women who had naturally been exposed to the bacterium had strong anticholera secretory IgA responses in their milk (Svennerholm et al. 1980). Similar results have also been seen in mice orally immunized with cholera and boosted parenterally (Bloom and Rowley 1979), although a study in rats recorded a parenteral immunization with an oral boosting, using cholera toxoid as the antigen, as the most successful regime in rats (Pierce and Gowans 1975). Thus, depending on the antigen, if natural exposure has recently occurred, or continually occurs, a subcutaneous or intramuscular immunization regime may be suitable. However, in the majority of situations, mucosal immunization with parenteral or mucosal boosting appears to be a most suitable regime.

A possible prediction is that any orally administered vaccine would have fewer adverse side effects than one that is administered systemically. It would also be easier to administer *en masse,* relatively inexpensive since costly injection equipment and highly trained personnel would be unnecessary, and therefore eminently suitable for use in many developing countries. There are, however, a number of difficulties inherent in stimulating mucosal immunity.

First, the mucosal immune system has evolved primarily to avoid sensitization of the individual to antigens in food that escape degradation. As a consequence, the majority of antigenic material is not absorbed so that oral immunization requires substantial amounts of antigen to achieve an immune response. Furthermore, administration of some antigens by the oral route may result in the immunologic unresponsiveness of the systemic immune system on parenteral rechallenge with the same antigen, a phenomenon termed "oral tolerance" and demonstrated in rodent models with a variety of antigens (Challacombe and Tomasi 1980; Mowat 1987). Antigens that are "tolerogenic" tend to be soluble proteins, unlike particulate antigens, particularly viable organisms, that are able to effectively elicit systemic immunity when administered mucosally (de Aizpurua and Russell-Jones 1988). Developing tolerance in T cells is far easier than developing tolerance in B cells (Husby et al. 1994; Titus and Chiller 1981); recent studies in the mouse (Burstein et al. 1992) and in humans (Husby et al. 1994) also showed Th1 type T cells to be more easily "tolerized" than the Th2 subset.

Adjuvants for Mucosal Immunization

There are three keys to any successful oral immunogen: (1) The formulation must achieve survival in the mucosal environment; (2) There must be adequate delivery of antigen to inductive sites; and (3) There must be stimulation of an appropriate protective immune response.

Development of new technology may soon offer a number of possible delivery systems for immunogens, and research into vaccines for enteric, respiratory and, particularly, sexually transmitted diseases will inevitably offer insights into options for mucosal immunization for different purposes.

Mucosally active adjuvants (*adjuvare* = to help) that are administered with antigen increase the immune response to that antigen. This means that development of mucosal vaccines based upon recombinant microbial proteins or synthetically synthesized peptides that otherwise would be only weakly immunogenic becomes a real possibility. Use of an adjuvant decreases the quantity of antigen needed and, therefore, the cost of the vaccine. Finally, different adjuvant formulations can produce qualitatively different immunologic responses. For example, a study in mice showed that while an antigen administered parenterally in Freund's complete antigen stimulated a Th1-type response, in alum the same antigen elicited a Th2 response, indicating both a potential for flexibility among options and the importance of choosing the correct adjuvant for an appropriate immune response (Grun and Maurer 1989).

Live Microorganisms

Live attenuated or genetically engineered organisms that are capable of colonizing mucosal surfaces yet do not cause pathology can provide a continual effective stimulation to the mucosal immune system. For example, live attenuated polio virus (Sabin vaccine) was first reported to effectively induce sIgA in the gastrointestinal tract (Ogra and Karzon 1969) and has been used in successful immunization programs worldwide. Organisms that can be genetically manipulated to express specific antigens from pathogenic species include bacillus Calmette-Guérin (BCG), avirulent *Escherichia coli*, Salmonella and Shigella strains, and Adenovirus. A number of studies have demonstrated induction of local immunity after administration of these organisms (Mestecky 1987).

Of particular interest for induction of genital tract immunity is a genetically modified *Lactobacillus*—the dominant comensal bacteria in the human vagina, with no pathogenic potential whatever—expressing *Chlamydia trachomatis* antigens. Researchers at Queensland University of Technology and the University of Siena have used the guinea pig as an animal model to assess the possibility of exploiting lactobacilli for a human vaccine against pathogens of the female reproductive tract. Preliminary results showed that the recombinant strain had excellent segregational stability in the absence of antibiotic selection and that it also persisted, though only for five days, when administered to the guinea pig vaginal tract (Hafner et al. 1992). The main significance of the work so far is in demonstrating that naturally occurring vaginal lactobacilli can be genetically manipulated.

Though eminently suitable for mucosal vaccination, the use of a live organism is not without problems. The attraction of a live organism as a mucosal vaccine is its ability to colonize and replicate at a mucosal surface, thus providing a constant source of antigen for immune stimulation with consequent long-term effects. However, in the case of immunocontraception, reversibility may be highly desirable and a long-term effect might well be disadvantageous; that would not be the case for protection from sexually transmitted infection. A second, potentially catastrophic disadvantage in connection with an immunocontraceptive would be induction of herd immunity owing to transmission of the organism in secretions; in this instance, inactivated organisms, while less efficient as inducers of mucosal immunity, would be the clear preference.

Cholera Toxin

This toxin, produced by *Vibrio cholera* and the cause of the copious secretion of fluid and electrolytes in cholera disease, consists of five binding (B) subunits in a ring with a single toxin-active (A) subunit. The B subunit binds with high affinity to the ganglioside GM1 expressed on M cells and the A subunit enters the cell where it ADP ribosylates the G_s subunit of adenylate cyclase and increases cAMP formation. Whole cholera toxin is a powerful mucosal adjuvant in mice, promoting isotype switching to IgA and enhancement of IgA production. Unfortunately, in humans, doses as low as 5 μg can promote severe diarrhea. However, recent studies have indicated that, unlike the mouse system, the B subunit can be administered alone, covalently linked to an antigen of choice, and still retain its stimulatory properties (Holmgren et al. 1993). This is probably due to the ability of the B subunit to bind to M cells, thus enhancing uptake of antigen.

Immune Stimulating Complexes (ISCOMs)

Immune-stimulating complexes (ISCOMs) are stable, 30- to 40-nm-diameter particulate complexes of protein antigens incorporated into dodecahedral-shaped structures composed of the adjuvant Quil A (saponin) and lipid. Parenterally administered ISCOMs are highly immunogenic (Mowat et al. 1991; Takahashi et al. 1990) and have been used successfully in animal models to protect against lethal challenge with a number of viruses and parasites (Araujo and Morein 1991; Cook et al. 1990; de Vries et al. 1988). ISCOMs have been shown to elicit antibody, delayed-type hypersensitivity, T-cell proliferative responses, and cytotoxic T lymphocytes (CTLs). The induction of CD8-positive CTLs implies that, unlike other exogenously administered antigen, ISCOMs are able to enter the endogenous pathway of antigen processing and therefore be presented in the context of MHC class I (Mowat et al. 1991). Furthermore, ISCOMs have been found capable of fusing with endosomes within the cytoplasm (Claasen and Osterhaus 1993). Recent studies also show that ISCOMs administered by the oral (Mowat et al. 1991), respiratory (Jones et al. 1988), and vaginal (Thapar et al. 1991) routes can induce both systemic and local immunity.

An alternative strategy for delivery of antigen to the mucosa is to incorporate antigen into an appropriate "carrier" or delivery system. Two of the most suitable carriers are biodegradable microspheres and liposomes. It is worth noting that there are not always definitive boundaries between adjuvants and delivery systems as categories; many compounds can also probably modulate immune response in addition to providing a depot of antigen.

Biodegradable Microspheres

Biodegradable microspheres are being evaluated clinically as possible vehicles in a mucosal delivery system. These particles may be constructed of poly(DL-lactide-coglycolide), a copolymer made of the same class of material as resorbable sutures. Antigen is dispersed homogeneously within the copolymeric matrix and the resulting product is a stable powder that is easily reconstitutable.

Microspheres can also be made in different sizes for different effects. In an elegant study by Eldridge and colleagues, mice were orally immunized with different diameter particles incorporating staphylococcal enterotoxin B (SEB). The results were that particles less than 5 μm in diameter very quickly entered the systemic circulation, those between 5 and 10 μm in diameter were retained by the macrophages in the Peyer's patch dome region for a substantial time period, and a combination of sphere sizes (1–10 μm plus 20–50 μm) produced a substantially greater plasma IgG anti-toxin titre at 60 days than when either of the two size ranges was administered individually (Eldridge et al. 1991). This ability to effectively prime and boost immune response in a single administration can also be achieved by changing the ratio of lactide to glycolide in the polymer.

Mucosal immunization with biodegradable microspheres has achieved specific systemic and secretory immune responses, as well as the generation of cytotoxic T lymphocytes (CTLs) (Eldridge et al. 1991; O'Hagan et al. 1992, 1993). The microspheres abrogate the need for use of a live organism and, because they lack surface antigen, potential problems with preexisting sIgA are circumvented.

Liposomes

Liposomes are synthesized globules composed of concentric phospholipid bilayers encapsulating the substance to be delivered. They can be made from biodegradable components common to all mammalian membranes (Edelman 1980), were originally developed for the delivery of biologically active substances, and have been used to deliver a variety of antigens by several parenteral routes (Buiting et al. 1992). Liposomes are avidly phagocytosed by macrophages and *in vitro* studies have shown that antigen is effectively delivered to CD4+ T cells (Alving and Richards 1990). A small number of studies have indicated that liposomes are effective when administered via the mucosal route; for example, antigens of *Streptococcus mutans* delivered in liposomes have been found to enhance specific salivary IgA (Michalek et al. 1985; Wachsmann et al. 1983).

Hybrid Mucosal Immunogens

Combinations of mucosal delivery systems and adjuvants may prove to be the most effective way of inducing strong mucosal immunity. An example of this is a vaccine consisting of recombinant simian immunodeficient virus (SIV) gag p27 antigen expressed as hybrid Ty-virus-like particles (Ty-VLP) that are chemically coupled to cholera toxin B subunit. The vaccine has been used successfully for oral/vaginal and oral/rectal immunization regimes in macaques, inducing serum and local antibody and T cell proliferative responses in draining lymph nodes after oral and rectal immunization regimes (Lehner et al. 1992, 1993). Presumably the B subunit allows specific binding to the M cell, while the particle formulation of the vaccine allows a continual depot of antigen. Cytokines such as IL-1, IL-2, and IL-6 have also been incorporated into various formulations as "co-adjuvants" for boosting immune responses (Abraham and Shah 1992; Duits et al. 1993).

Optimal Immunization Strategies for the Female Reproductive Tract

Two murine studies of intrauterine plus systemic immunization regimes with sperm or sperm antigens have reported reduced fertility parameters (Haimovici and Anderson 1992; Shelton and Goldberg 1986). Numerous reports have indicated that vaginal immunization in both humans and animals results in the production of sIgA (Ogra and Ogra 1973; O'Hagan et al. 1992; McAnulty and Morton 1978; Thapar et al. 1990; Yang and Schumacher 1979). A number of studies have reported that titres of antibody were rather low after vaginal immunization and, in the murine model, it has been found that injection of antigen into the pelvic presacral space resulted in a much higher local antibody titre (Parr and Parr 1989a; Thapar et al. 1990). In another study in which epididymal sperm were injected via the intraperitoneal route, fertility was shown to be decreased, although local antibodies were not measured (Tung et al. 1979).

The success of these regimes may be due to activation of the resident peritoneal Ly-1 positive cells, which then populate the genital tract as they do in the gut (Kroese et al. 1988). Alternatively, antigen may be gaining access to the draining lymph nodes of the genital tract. If this is so and an alternative induction site were to be immunized, this would circumvent the need for antigen to cross the vaginal epithelium, which appears to be a significant barrier to uptake (Parr and Parr 1989a). Although lymphoid nodules do seem to be present in the human vagina, lymphoid tissue there is, in total, much sparser than it is in gut, so that induction of immune response through that route would be predicted to be much less efficient. In fact, in mice, rectal immunization with cholera was far more successful at inducing specific IgA in the vagina than was vaginal immunization (Haneberg et al. 1994). A study in rhesus monkeys with an SIV p27 vaccine expressed as Ty-VLP and conjugated to cholera toxin utilized an oral plus vaginal boosting regime and successfully induced vaginal sIgA and IgG, serum IgG, and IgA and T cells located in genital-tract-draining lymph nodes that proliferated to p27 (Lehner et al. 1992). The effectiveness of this approach was probably due to the fact that oral immunization introduced antigen to, and mobilized, the very substantial gut lymphocyte population, while the local application induced a "local" homing. Rectal immunization alone can also induce good sIgA titres in vaginal secretions, for two possible reasons: First, the rectal mucosa is endowed with numerous lymphoid follicles that allow very effective induction of the immune response; second, as discussed earlier, the genital tract and rectum are adjacent mucosae and share draining lymph nodes.

Optimal Immunization of the Male Reproductive Tract

A limited number of studies have demonstrated that infection or inflammation in the male reproductive tract leads to the appearance of specific IgA. Furthermore, numerous T cells are seen in the urethral mucosa and semen, particularly during times of inflammation. It would appear impractical at this time to target the urethra as a route of mucosal vaccination. However, a study of nine male rhesus monkeys, sequentially immunized ororectally with SIV p27 expressed as Ty-VLP and conjugated to cholera toxin, successfully induced serum IgA and IgG, rectal sIgA p27 antibodies, and T cells isolated from draining lymph nodes, blood, and spleen that proliferated specifically to the antigen (Lehner et al. 1993). This was contrasted with intramuscular immunization, which could only induce serum antibodies and antigen-specific proliferation in blood and spleen T cells. Urethral washings were not examined, but data from rectal immunization in the female does suggest that rectal or sequential oral-rectal immunization should induce genital tract immunity. Furthermore, in the mouse, the male lower genital tract and the rectum have also been shown to share draining lymph nodes (Quayle et al. 1994).

Cellular versus Antibody-mediated Immunity and Infertility

IgA, as well as IgG-type antisperm and antiovarian antibodies, have been detected in infertility patients and are implicated as a cause of reproductive failure (see Best and Hill 1995 for review). However, it has become apparent recently that antisperm cellular immunity, mediated by cytokines, may also play a major role in immunologic fertility. Cellular immune responses to sperm have been detected in male and female infertility patients (Anderson and Hill 1995; McShane et al. 1985; Metter and Schirwani 1975) and are known to cause infertility in animal models (Haimovici et al. 1992; Naz and Metha 1989; Shelton and Goldberg 1986). Furthermore, TH1-type cytokines associated with cellular immunity (i.e., γ-interferon, tumor necrosis factors α and β) are toxic to preimplantation embryos, trophoblast cells, and sperm when present in high concentrations and some of these cytokines also inhibit hormone synthesis by granulosa and Leydig cells (see Anderson and Hill 1995 for review). Finally, there has long been a clinical association between genital tract infections and infertility, an effect that may be due to: 1) adjuvant effects of microbial antigens; and/or 2) local production of TH1-type cytokines, which damage "innocent bystander" reproductive cells (Anderson and Hill 1995).

CONCLUSIONS

The conclusions that follow relate to both Parts 1 and 2 of this set of paired papers on the subject of barriers to conception and infection and the mucosal immune system as a key entity in the "construction" of such barriers. It is clear that more research is required to determine whether or not a mucosal immunization strategy will produce the effects that are desired, whether contraceptive, anti-infective, or both. However, the following points can be made that suggest avenues for the next wave of research:

1. The uterus does not have a significant secretory IgA defense system, but is permeable to systemic immunoglobulins. Therefore, reproductive function occurring at this site may be better blocked by systemically-administered vaccines. However, other regions of the tract (cervix, vagina, fallopian tube) appear to have a strong local secretory immune component, so that an immunization regime targeting events that occur at these sites (especially sperm migration and fertilization) should have a mucosally targeted component to take advantage of this local defense mechanism.

2. The penile urethra appears to be the principal site of mucosal immunity in the male genital tract. Since it is not yet clear where or how local immuity can be induced at this mucosal site, more studies of the male genital tract will be essential.

3. In both males and females, a primary oral immunization followed by repeated local boosting (rectal, vaginal, or urethral) would appear to have the best chance of being successful. Local boosters could possibly be provided by self-

administered suppositories and a boosting effect might also be produced by reproductive processes themselves.

4. Relatively little is known about cell-mediated immune (CMI) responses within the male or female genital tracts and their potential effects on fertility. Although chronic CMI responses may be associated with undesirable side effects such as delayed-type hypersensitivity and irreversibility, CMI responses to infrequent or low antigen exposures could provide a powerful adjunct mechanism for mucosally targeted immunization.

5. More needs to be known about how secreted antibodies function in mucus to protect the human mucosal surfaces. Despite evidence that antibodies can be highly effective at blocking mucosal transmission of both infectious agents and sperm, both sperm and STD pathogens have evolved mechanisms for successful exchange between sexual partners—mechanisms that evade immune defenses in mucosal secretions—of which one of the most challenging is the common evasion mechanism of antigenic variability, which enables pathogens to stay a step ahead of host immune responses. A potential, though surely challenging, research direction would be to seek combinations of pathogen-specific monoclonal antibodies and pan-semen or other anti-human surface antigenic monoclonal antibodies that could defeat these evasive actions and ultimately provide effective broad-spectrum protection against STDs and pregnancy (Cone and Whaley 1994).

REFERENCES

Abraham E, S Shah. Intranasal immunization with liposomes containing IL-2 enhances polysaccharide antigen-specific pulmonary secretory antibody response. Journal of Immunology 149:3719–3726, 1992.

Ada GL. The induction of immunity at mucosal surfaces. IN Local Immunity in Reproductive Tract Tissues. PD Griffin, PM Johnson, eds. Oxford, UK: Oxford University Press. 1993.

Alving CR, RL Richards. Liposomes containing lipid A: A potent nontoxic adjuvant for a human malaria sporozoite vaccine. Immunology Letters 25:275–279, 1990.

Anderson DJ. Mechanisms of HIV-1 transmission via semen. Journal of NIH Research 4:104–108, 1992.

Anderson DJ. Cell mediated immunity and inflammatory processes in male infertility. Archives of Immunology and Therapeutic Experiments 38:79–86, 1990.

Anderson DJ, JA Hill. Cytokines in the reproductive tract that affect fertility. Mucosal Immunology Update 2:6–15, 1995.

Anderson DJ, J Pudney. Mucosal immune defense against HIV-1 in the male urogenital tract. Vaccine Research 1:143, 1992.

Anderson DJ, EJ Yunis. "Trojan Horse" leukocytes in AIDS. New England Journal of Medicine 309:984–985, 1983.

Araujo FG, B Morein. Immunization with *Trypanosoma cruzi* epimastigote antigens incorporated into ISCOMS protects against lethal challenge in mice. Infectious Immunology 59:2909–2914, 1991.

Beagley KW, JH Eldridge, F Lee, et al. Interleukins and IgA synthesis: Human and mouse IL-6 induce high rate of IgA secretion in IgA committed B cells. Journal of Experimental Medicine 169:2133–2148, 1989.

Berkley S. The public health significance of sexually transmitted diseases in HIV infection in Africa. IN AIDS and Women's Health: Science for Policy and Action. L Chen, et al., eds. New York: Plenum Press. 1991.

Berlin C, EL Berg, MJ Briskin, et al. α4β7 integrin mediates lymphocyte binding to the mucosal vascular addressin MAdCAM-1. Cell 74:185–195, 1993.

Besredka A. De la vaccination contre les états typhoides par la voie buccale. Annales de l'Institut Pasteur 33:882–903, 1919.

Besredka A. Local Immunization. Baltimore: Williams and Wilkins. 1927.

Best CL, JA Hill. Natural infertility due to immunological factors. IN Birth Control Vaccines. R Raghupathy, GP Talwar, eds. Austin, TX: RG Landes. 1995.

Bienenstock J, AD Befus. Mucosal immunology. Immunology 41:249–270, 1980.

Bjercke S, H Scott, LR Braathen, et al. HLA-DR expressing Langerhans-like cells in vaginal and cervical epithelium. Acta Obstetrica Gynecologica Scandinavica 585–589, 1983.

Bloom LD, D Rowley. Local immune response in mice to *Vibrio cholerae*. Australian Journal of Experimental Biology and Medical Science 57:313–323, 1979.

Bockman DE, MD Cooper. Pinocytosis by epithelium associated with lymphoid follicles in the bursa of Fabricus, appendix, and Peyer's patches: An electron microscopic study. American Journal of Anatomy 136: 455–478, 1973.

Bond MW, B Strader, TR Mosmann, et al. A mouse T cell product that preferentially enhances IgA production. 2. Physicochemical characterization. Journal of Immunology 139:3691–3696, 1987.

Bourinbaiar AS, S Lee-Huang. Comparative *in vitro* study of contraceptive agents with anti-HIV activity: Gramicidin, nonoxynol-9 and gossypol. Contraception 49:131–137, 1994a.

Bourinbaiar AS, S Lee-Huang. Acrosin inhibitor, 4'-acetamidophenyl 4-guanidinobenzoate, an experimental vaginal contraceptive with anti-HIV activity. Contraception 51:319–322, 1994b.

Bourinbaiar AS, R Nagorny. Effect of serine proteinase inhibitor, N-a-tosyl-L-lysyl-chloro-methylketone (TLCK) on cell-mediated and cell-free HIV-1 spread. Cellular Immunology 155:230–236, 1994.

Brandtzaeg P. Human secretory immunoglobulin M: An immunochemical and immunohistochemical study. Immunology 29: 559–570, 1975.

Brandtzaeg P. Two types of IgA immunocytes in man. Nature/New Biology 243:142–143, 1973.

Brandtzaeg P, V Bosnes, TS Halstensen, et al. T lymphocytes in human gut epithelium express preferentially the alpha/beta antigen receptor and are CD45/UCHL-1 positive. Scandinavian Journal of Immunology 30:23–128, 1989.

Brandtzaeg P, E Christiansen, F Muller, et al. Humoral immune response patterns of human mucosae, including the reproductive tracts: The induction of immunity at mucosal surfaces. IN Local Immunity in Reproductive Tract Tissues. PD Griffin, PM Johnson, eds. Oxford, UK: Oxford University Press. 1993.

Brandtzaeg P, I Fjellanger, ST Gjeruldsen. Human secretory immunoglobulins. I. Salivary secretions from individuals with normal or low levels of serum immunoglobulins. Scandinavian Journal of Haematology, Supplement 12: 1–83, 1970.

Brandtzaeg P, I Fjellanger, ST Gjeruldsen. Immunoglobulin M: Local synthesis and selective secretion in patients with Immunoglobulin A deficiency. Science 160:789–791, 1968.

Buiting AMJ, N van Rooijen, E Claasen. Liposomes as antigen carriers and adjuvants *in vivo*. Research in Immunology 143:541–548, 1992.

Bulmer JN, DP Lunny, SV Hagin. Immunohistochemical characterization of stromal leukocytes in nonpregnant human endometrium. American Journal of Reproductive Immunology 17: 83–90, 1988.

Burstein HJ, CM Shea, AK Abbas. Aqueous antigens induce *in vivo* tolerance selectively in IL-2 and IFN-gamma-producing (Th1) cells. Journal of Immunology 148:3687, 1992.

Cerf-Benussan N, B Begue, J Gagnon, et al. The human intraepithelial lymphocyte marker HML-1 is an integrin consisting of a β7 subunit associated with a distinctive α chain. European Journal of Immunology 22:73–277, 1992.

Challacombe SJ, T Lehner. Salivary antibody responses in rhesus monkeys immunized with *Streptococcus mutans* by the oral, submucosal or subcutaneous routes. Archives of Oral Biology 24:917–925, 1979.

Challacombe SJ, TB Tomasi. Systemic tolerance and secretory immunity after oral immunization. Journal of Experimental Medicine 152:1459–1472, 1980.

Chantler E, R Sharma, D Sharman. Changes in cervical mucus that prevent penetration by spermatozoa. Society for Experimental Biology 43:325–336, 1989.

Chipperfield EJ, BA Evans. The influence of local infection on immunoglobulin formation in the human endocervix. Clinical Experiments in Immunology 11:219–223, 1972.

Claasen I, A Osterhaus. The ISCOM structure as an immune-enhancing moiety: Experience with viral systems. Research in Immunology 143:531–541, 1993.

Claypool LE. The challenges ahead: Implications of STDs/AIDS for contraceptive research. IN Contraceptive Research and Development, 1984 to 1994: The Road from Mexico City to Cairo and Beyond. PFA Van Look, G Pérez-Palacios, eds. Delhi: Oxford University Press. 1994.

Cohen MS, RD Weber, PA Mardh. Genitourinary mucosal defenses. IN Sexually Transmitted Diseases (2nd ed.). KK Holmes, P-A Mardh, PF Sparling et al. eds. New York: McGraw-Hill. 1990.

Cone RA, KJ Whaley. Monoclonal antibodies for reproductive health: Part I, Preventing sexual transmission of disease and pregnancy with topically applied antibodies. American Journal of Reproductive Immunology 32:114–131, 1994.

Cook RF, T O'Neill, E Strachan, et al. Protection against lethal equine herpes virus type 1 (subtype 1) infection in hamsters by immune stimulating complexes (ISCOM) containing the major viral glycoproteins. Vaccine 8:491–496, 1990.

Corner A-M, MM Dolan, SL Yankell, et al. C31G, a new agent for oral use with potent antimicrobial and antiadherence properties. Antimicrobiological Agents and Chemotherapy 32:350–353, 1988.

Cornes JS. Number, size and distribution of Peyer's patches in human small intestine. Gut 6:225–233, 1965.

Crabbe PA, AO Carbonara, JF Heremans. The normal human intestinal mucosa a major source of plasma cells containing A-immunoglobulin. Laboratory Investigation 14:235–248, 1965.

Craig SW, JJ Cebra. Peyer's patches: An enriched source of precursors for IgA producing immunocytes in the rabbit. Journal of Experimental Medicine 134:188–200, 1971.

Czerkinsky C, SJ Prince, SM Michalek, et al. IgA antibody-producing cells in peripheral blood after antigen ingestion: Evidence for a common mucosal system. Proceedings of the National Academy of Sciences, USA 84: 2449–2453, 1987.

D'Cruz OJ, HA Pereira, GG Haas. Sperm immobilizing activity of a synthetic bioactive peptide 20–44 of 37-kDa cationic antimicrobial protein (CAP37) of human neutrophils. Journal of Andrology 16:432–440, 1995.

de Aizpurua HJ, GJ Russell-Jones. Oral vaccination: Identification of classes of proteins that provoke an immune response upon oral feeding. Journal of Experimental Medicine 167:440–451, 1988.

DeClercq E. Antiviral agents: Characteristic activity spectrum depending on the molecular target with which they interact. Advances in Virus Research 42:1–55, 1993.

deGraaf JH, RYJ Tamminga, WA Kamps, et al. Expression of cellular adhesion molecules in Langerhans cell histiocytosis and normal Langerhans cells. American Journal of Pathology 147:1161–1171, 1995.

de Vries P, RS van Binnendijk, et al. Measles virus fusion protein presented in an immune-stimulating complex (ISCOM) induces haemolysis-inhibiting and fusion-inhibiting antibodies, virus-specific T cells and protection in mice. Journal of General Virology 69:549–559, 1988.

de Waal A, AV Goes, A Mensink, et al. Magainins affect respiratory control, membrane potential and motility of hamster spermatozoa. Federation of European Biological Societies Letters 293:219–223, 1991.

Devlin MC, BN Barwin. Barrier contraception. Advances in Contraception 5:197–204, 1989.

Duits AJ, A van Puijenbroek, H Vermuelen, et al. Immunoadjuvant activity of a liposomal IL-6 formulation. Vaccine 11:777–781, 1993.

Dunbar BS, MG O'Rand, eds. A Comparative Overview of Mammalian Fertilization. New York: Plenum Press. 1991.

Edelman R. Vaccine adjuvants. Review of Infectious Disease 2:370, 1980.

Edelstein MC, JE Gretz, TJ Bauer, et al. Studies on the *in vitro* spermicidal activity of synthetic magainins. Fertility and Sterility 55:647–649, 1991.

Edwards JNT, HB Morris. Langerhans cells and lymphocyte subsets in the female genital tract. British Journal of Obstetrics and Gynaecology 92:974–982, 1985.

El-Demiry MIM, TB Hargreave, A Busuttil, et al. Immunocompetent cells in human testis in health and disease. Fertility and Sterility 48:470–479, 1987.

El-Demiry MIM, TB Hargreave, A Busuttil, et al. Lymphocyte sub-populations in the male genital tract. British Journal of Urology 57:769–774, 1985.

El-Demiry MIM, K James. Lymphocyte subsets and macrophages in the male genital tract in health and disease. European Journal of Urology 14:226–235, 1988.

Eldridge JH, JK Staas, JA Meulbroek, et al. Biodegradable microspheres as a vaccine delivery system. Molecular Immunology 3:287–294, 1991.

Elias CJ, L Heise. The Development of Microbicides: A New Method of HIV Prevention for Women (Working Papers No. 6). New York: The Population Council. 1993.

Elson CO, JA Heck, W Strober. T-cell regulation of murine IgA synthesis. Journal of Experimental Medicine 149:632–643, 1979.

Foldesy RG, RE Homm, SL Levinson, et al. Multiple actions of a novel vaginal contraceptive compound, OR 13904. Fertility and Sterility 45:550–555, 1986.

Forrest BD, DJA Shearman, JT LaBrooy. Specific immune reponses in humans following rectal delivery of live typhoid vaccines. Vaccine 8:209–212, 1992.

Fowler JE, DL Kaiser, M Mariano. Immunologic response of the prostate to bacteriuria and bacterial prostatitis: Part 1. Immunoglobulin concentrations in prostatic fluid. Journal of Urology 128:158–164, 1982.

Fowler JE, M Mariano. Immunoglobulin in seminal fluid of fertile, infertile, vasectomy and vasectomy reversal patients. Journal of Urology 129:869–872, 1983.

Fowler JE, M Mariano. Immunologic response of the prostate to bacteruria and bacterial prostatitis. II. Antigen specific immunoglobulin in prostatic fluid. Journal of Urology 128:165–170, 1982.

Franek J, J Libich, V. Kubin. Mechanisms of antibacterial immunity of mucous membranes. Folia Microbiologia 29:375–384. 1984.

Ganz T, RI Lehrer. Defensins. Current Opportunities in Immunology 6:584–589, 1994.

Gay FP. Local resistance and local immunity to bacteria. Physiology Reviews 4:191–214, 1924.

Goldblum RM, S Ahlstedt, B Carlsson, et al. Antibody forming cells in human colostrum after oral administration. Nature 257:797–799, 1975.

Greenwood S, AJ Margolis. "Outercourse." Advances in Planning and Parenting 15:126–128, 1981.

Grun JL, PH Maurer. Different T helper cell subsets elicited in mice utilizing two different adjuvant vehicles: The role of endogenous interleukin 1 in proliferative responses. Cell Immunology 121:134–145, 1989.

Guy-Grand D, C Griscelli, P Vassalli. The mouse gut T lymphocyte, a novel type of T cell: Nature, origin and traffic in mice in normal and graft-versus-host conditions. Journal of Experimental Medicine 169:1277–1294, 1978.

Hafner L, C Rush, P Timms. Lactobacilli: Vehicles for antigen delivery to the female urogenital tract. IN Abstract book of the 7th International Congress of Mucosal Immunology, Prague, Czechoslovakia, August 1992.

Haimovici F, DJ Anderson. Antifertility effects of antisperm cell-mediated immunity in mice. Journal of Reproductive Immunology 22:281–298, 1992.

Hallenberger S, V Bosch, HJ Angliker, et al. Inhibition of cleavage activation of HIV-1 glycoprotein gp160. Nature 360:358–361, 1992.

Halpern MS, ME Koshland. Novel subunit in secretory IgA. Nature 228:1276–1278, 1970.

Halstensen TS, H Scott, P Brandtzaeg. Intraepithelial T cells of the TCR gamma/delta+ CD8- and V delta1/J delta 1+ phenotypes are increased in coeliac disease. Scandinavian Journal of Gastro-enterology 30:665–672, 1989.

Haneberg B, D Kendall, HM Amerongen, et al. Induction of specific IgA in small intestine, colon-rectum, and vagina measured with a new method for collection of secretions from local mucosal surfaces. Infectious Immunology 62(1):15–23, 1994.

Hanson LA. Comparative immunological studies of the immune globulins of human milk and of blood serum. International Archives of Allergy and Applied Immunology 18:241–267, 1961.

Haslett S. Barrier methods of contraception. Nursing Standard 4:24–27, 1990.

Hatcher RA, DL Warner. New condoms for men and women, diaphragms, cervical caps, and spermicides: Overcoming barriers to barriers and spermicides. Current Opinions in Obstetrics and Gynecology 4:513–521, 1992.

Hattori T, A Koito, KJ Takatsuki, et al. Involvement of tryptase-related cellular protease(s) in human immunodeficiency virus type 1 infection. Federation of European Biochemical Societies Letters 248:48–52, 1989.

Holmgren J, N Lycke, C Czerkinsky. Cholera toxin and cholera toxin B subunit as oral-mucosal adjuvant and antigen vector systems. Vaccine 11:1179–1184, 1993.

Holzmann B, BW McIntyre, ILWeissman. Identification of a murine Peyer's patch-specific lymphocyte homing receptor as an integrin molecule with an α chain homologous to human VLA-4a. Cell 56:37–46, 1989.

Homm RE, GE Doscher, EG Hummel, et al. Relative antifertility activity of three vaginal contraceptive products in the rabbit: Relationship to *in vitro* data. Contraception 13:479–488, 1976.

Homm RE, RG Foldesy, DW Hahn. ORF 13904, a new long-acting vaginal contraceptive. Contraception 32:267–274, 1985.

Hornick CL, F. Karush. Antibody affinity-III: The role of multivalency. Immunochemistry 9:325–340, 1972.

Husband AJ, VL Clifton. Role of intestinal immunization in urinary tract defence. Immunology and Cell Biology 67:371, 1989.

Husband AJ, JL Gowans. The origin and antigen-dependent distribution of IgA containing cells in the small intestine. Journal of Experimental Medicine 148:1146, 1978.

Husby S, J Mestecky, Z Moldoveanu, et al. Oral tolerance in humans: T cell but not B cell tolerance after antigen feeding. Journal of Immunology 152:4663–4670, 1994.

Isaacs CE, S Kashyap, WC Heird, et al. Antiviral and antibacterial lipids in human milk and infant formula feeds. Archives of Diseases in Children 65:861–864, 1990.

Itohara S, AG Farr, JJ Lafaille, et al. Homing of a γδ thymocyte subset with homogeneous T-cell receptors to mucosal epithelia. Nature 343:754–757, 1990.

Jacobsen LO, EK Marks, EL Simmons, et al. Immune response in irradiated mice with Peyer's patch shielding. Proceedings of the National Academy of Sciences, USA 108:487–493, 1961.

Jalanti R, H Isliker. Immunoglobulins in human cervico-vaginal secretions. International Archives of Allergy and Applied Immunology 53:402–409, 1977.

Janossy G, N Tidman, ES Selby, et al. Human T lymphocytes of the inducer and suppressor type occupy different microenvironments. Nature 288:81–84, 1980.

Jarry A, N Cerf-Benussan, N Brousse, et al. Subsets of CD3+ (T cell receptor alpha/beta or gamma/delta) and CD3-lymphocytes isolated from normal human gut epithelium display phenotypical features different from their counterparts in peripheral blood. European Journal of Immunology 20:1097–1103, 1990.

Jefferson WL. Non-ionic surfactant spermicidal agents. British Journal of Family Planning 11:131–135, 1986.

Jones PD, JJ Cebra. Restriction of gene expression in B lymphocytes and their progeny: 111. Endogenous IgA and IgM on the membranes of different plasma cell precursors. Journal of Experimental Medicine 140:966–976, 1974.

Jones PP, R Tha Hla, B Morein, et al. Cellular immune responses in the murine lung to local immunisation with influenza A virus glycoproteins in micelles and immunostimulatory complexes (ISCOMs). Scandinavian Journal of Immunology 27:645–652, 1988.

Kamat BR, PG Isaacson. The immunocytochemical distribution of leukocytic subpopulations in human endometrium. American Journal of Pathology 127:66–73, 1986.

Kaminski JM, NA Nuzzo, L Bauer, et al. Vaginal contraceptive activity of aryl 4-guanidinobenzoates (acrosin inhibitors) in rabbits. Contraception 32:183–189, 1985.

Katz DH, JF Marceletti, MH Khalil, et al. Antiviral activity of 1-docosanol, an inhibitor of lipid-enveloped viruses including herpes simplex. Proceedings of the National Academy of Sciences, USA 88:10825–10829, 1991.

Katz DH, JF Marceletti, LE Pope, et al. n-Docosanol: Broad spectrum antiviral activity against lipid-enveloped viruses. Annals of the New York Academy of Sciences 724:472–488, 1994.

Kilshaw PJ, SJ Murant. Expression and regulation of β7(β) integrins on mouse lymphocytes: Relevance to the mucosal immune system. European Journal of Immunology 21:2591–2597, 1991.

Kilshaw PJ, SJ Murant. A new surface antigen on intraepithelial lymphocytes in the intestine. European Journal of Immunology 20:2201–2207, 1990.

Klebanoff SJ. Effects of the spermicidal agent nonoxynol-9 on vaginal microbial flora. Journal of Infectious Diseases 165:19–25, 1992.

Klebanoff SJ, RW Coombs. Viricidal effects of *Lactobacillus acidophilus* on human immunodeficiency virus type 1: Possible role in heterosexual transmission. Journal of Experimental Medicine 174: 289–292, 1991.

Koito A, T Hattori, T Murakami, et al. A neutralizing epitope of human immunodeficiency virus type 1 has homologous amino acid sequences with the active site of inter-a-trypsin inhibitor. International Immunology 1:613–618, 1989.

Kojima H, S-P Wang, C-C Kuo, et al. Local antibody in semen for rapid diagnosis of *Chlamydia trachomatis* epididymitis. Journal of Immunology 140:528–531, 1988.

Kreiss J, E Ngugi, K Holmes, et al. Efficacy of nonoxynol-9 contraceptive sponge use in preventing heterosexual acquisition of HIV in Nairobi prostitutes. Journal of the American Medical Association 268:477–482, 1992.

Krieger JN, MF Rein. Canine prostatic secretions kill *Trichomonas vaginalis*. Infectious Immunology 37:77–81, 1982.

Kroese FGM, EC Butcher, AM Stall, et al. Many of the IgA producing plasma cells in the murine gut are derived from self-replenishing precursors in the peritoneal cavity. International Immunology 1:75–84, 1988.

Kutteh WH, RP Edwards, AC Menge, et al. IgA immunity in female reproductive tract secretions. IN Local Immunity in Reproductive Tract Tissues. PD Griffin, PM Johnson, eds. Oxford, UK: Oxford University Press, 1993.

Kutteh WH, C Kutteh, RE Blackwell, et al. Secretory immune system of the female reproductive tract. II. Local immune system in normal and infected fallopian tube. Fertility and Sterility 54:51–55, 1990.

Kutteh WH, J Mestecky. Secretory immunity in the female reproductive tract. American Journal of Reproductive Immunology 31:40–46, 1994.

Lehner T, LA Bergmeier, C Panagiotidi, et al. Induction of mucosal and systemic immunity to a recombinant simian immunodeficiency viral protein. Science 258:1365–1369, 1992.

Lehner T, R Brookes, C Panagiotidi, et al. T- and B-cell functions and epitope expression in nonhuman primates immunized with simian immunodeficiency virus antigen by the rectal route. Proceedings of the National Academy of Sciences, USA 90:8638–8642, 1993.

Lehrer RI. Defensins: Antimicrobial and cytotoxic peptides of mammalian cells. Annual Review of Immunology 11:105–128, 1993.

Lenaerts V, R Gurny. Bioadhesive Drug Delivery Systems. Boca Raton, FL: CRC Press. 1990.

London SD, JJ Cebra, DH Rubin. Intraepithelial lymphocytes contain virus-specific MHC-restricted precursors after gut mucosal immunization with reovirus serotype 1/Lang. Regional Immunology 2:99–105, 1989.

Ma JK-C, A Hiatt, M Hein, et al. Generation and assembly of secretory antibodies in plants. Science 268:716–719, 1995.

Mann J, DJM Tarantola, TW Netter, eds. A Global Report: AIDS in the World. Cambridge, MA: Harvard University Press. 1992.

Mardh P-A, S Colleen, J Sylwan. Inhibitory effect on the formation of chlamydial inclusions in McCoy cells by seminal fluid and some of its components. Investigations in Urology 17:510–513, 1980.

Masters WH, VE Johnson. Human Sexual Response. New York: Bantam Books. 1980.

Mauck CK, M Cordeo, HL Gabelnick, et al., eds. Barrier Contraceptives: Current Status and Future Prospects. New York: Wiley-Liss. 1994.

Mayer KH, DJ Anderson. Issue of the day: Heterosexual HIV transmission. Infectious Agents and Disease 4:273–284, 1995.

Mazanec MB, JG Nedrug, et al. A three-tiered view of the role of IgA in mucosal defense. Immunology Today 14:430–435, 1993.

McAnulty PA, DB Morton. The immune response of the genital tract of the female rabbit following local and systemic immunization. Clinical Laboratory Immunology 1:255–260, 1978.

McCune JM, LB Rabin, MB Feinberg, et al. Endoproteolytic cleavage of gp160 is required for the activation of human immunodeficiency virus. Cell 53:5–57, 1988.

McDermott MR, J Bienenstock. Evidence for a common mucosal system. 1. Migration of B immunoblasts into intestinal, respiratory and genital tissues. Journal of Immunology 122:1892–1898, 1979.

McDermott MR, CH Goldsmith, KL Rosenthal, L Brais. T lymphocytes in genital lymph nodes protect mice from intravaginal infection with Herpes Simplex type 2. Journal of Infectious Diseases 159:460–466, 1989.

McGhee JR, KW Beagley, K Fujihashi, et al. Regulatory mechanisms in mucosal immunity: Roles for T helper cell subsets and derived cytokines in the induction of IgA responses. IN Local Immunity in Reproductive Tract Tissues. PD Griffin, PM Johnson, eds. Oxford, UK: Oxford University Press. 1993.

McGhee JR, J Mestecky, MT Dertzbaugh, et al. The mucosal immune system: From fundamental concepts to vaccine development. Vaccine 10:75–88, 1992.

McMillan A, G McNeillage, H Young. Antibodies to *Neisseria gonorrhoeae:* A study of the urethral exudates of 232 men. Journal of Infectious Diseases 140:89–95, 1979.

McShane PM, I Schiff, DE Trentham. Cellular immunity to sperm in infertile women. Journal of the American Medical Association 253:3555–3558, 1985.

Mestecky J. The common mucosal immune system and current strategies for induction of immune responses in external secretions. Journal of Clinical Immunology 7:265–276, 1987.

Mestecky J, JR McGhee. The secretory IgA system. IN Local Immunity in Reproductive Tract Tissues. PF Griffin, PM Johnson, eds. Oxford, UK: Oxford University Press. 1993.

Mestecky J, JR McGhee. Oral immunization: Past and present. IN Current Topics in Microbiology and Immunology: New Strategies of Oral Immunization. J Mestecky, JR McGhee, eds. Berlin: Springer Verlag. 1989.

Mestecky J, JR McGhee, RR Arnold et al. Selective induction of immune responses in external secretions. Journal of Clinical Investigation 61:731–737, 1978.

Mestecky J, J Zikan, W Butler. Immunoglobulin M and secretory immunoglobulin A: Evidence for a common polypeptide chain different from light chains. Science 171:1163–1165, 1971.

Metter L, D Schirwani. Macrophage migration inhibitory factor in female sterility. American Journal of Obstetrics and Gynecology 121:117–120, 1975.

Michaels EB, EC Hahn, AJ Kenyon. Effect of C31G, an antimicrobial surfactant, on healing of incised guinea pig wounds. American Journal of Veterinary Research 44:1378–1381. 1983.

Michalek SM, I Morisaki, IL Gregory, et al. Oral adjuvants enhance salivary IgA responses to purified *Streptococcus mutans* antigens. Protides Biology of Fluids 32:47–52, 1985.

Miller CJ, JR McGhee, MB Gardner. Biology of disease: Mucosal immunity, HIV transmission and AIDS. Laboratory Investigation 68:129–145, 1992.

Miller CJ, P Vogel, NJ Alexander, et al. Pathology and localization of SIV in the reproductive tract of chronically infected male rhesus macaques. Laboratory Investigation 70:255–262, 1994.

Mims CA. The Pathogenesis of Infectious Disease. London: Academic Press. 1988.

Montgomery PC, J Cohn, ET Lally. The induction and characterization of secretory IgA molecules. Advances in Experimental Medicine and Biology 45:453–462, 1976.

Moore KS, S Wehrli, H Roder, et al. Squalamine: An aminosterol antibiotic from the shark. Proceedings of the National Academy of Sciences, USA 90:1354–1358, 1993.

Mosmann TR, RL Coffman. Th1 and Th2 cells: Different patterns of lymphokine secretion lead to different functional properties. Annual Review of Immunology 145–173, 1989.

Mowat AM. The regulation of immune responses to dietary protein antigens. Immunology Today 8:93–98, 1987.

Mowat AM, AM Donachie, G Reid, et al. Immune-stimulating complexes containing Quil A and protein antigen prime class 1 MHC-restricted T lymphocytes *in vivo* are immunogenic by the oral route. Immunology 72:317–322, 1991.

Murray PD, DT McKenzie, SL Swain, et al. Interleukin 5 and interleukin 4 produced by Peyer's patch T cells selectively enhance immunoglobulin A expression. Journal of Immunology 139:2669–2674, 1987.

National Research Council. Neem: A Tree for Solving Global Problems. Washington, DC: National Academy Press. 1992.

Naz RK, K Metha. Cell-mediated immune responses to sperm antigens: Effect on mouse sperm and embryos. Biology of Reproduction 41:533–542, 1989.

Neurath AR, S Jiang, N Strick, et al. Bovine beta-lactoglobulin modified by 3-hydroxyphatalic anhydride blocks the CD4 cell receptor for HIV. Nature Medicine 2:230–234, 1996.

Niruthisard S, RE Roddy, S Chutivongse. Use of nonoxynol-9 and reduction in rate of gonococcal and chlamydial cervical infections. Lancet 339:1371–1375, 1992.

Niruthisard S, RE Roddy, S Chutivongse. The effects of frequent nonoxynol-9 use on the vaginal and cervical mucosa. Sexually Transmitted Diseases 18:176–179, 1991.

Norman LR, J Cornett. Discussing nonpenetrative sexual activities as safer sex alternatives for HIV prevention with HIV-infected clients. Presentation at workshop sponsored by the Centers for Disease Control, Washington, DC, 1995.

Norsigian J. Feminist perspective on barrier use. IN Barrier Contraceptives: Current Status and Future Prospects. CK Mauck, M Cordero, HL Gabelnick, et al., eds. New York: Wiley-Liss. 1994.

O'Hagan DT, JP McGhee, J Holmgren, et al. Biodegradable microparticles for oral immunization. Vaccine 11:149–154, 1992.

O'Hagan DT, D Rafferty, S Wharton. Intravaginal immunization in sheep using a bioadhesive microsphere antigen delivery system. Vaccine 11:660–664, 1993.

O'Reilly RJ, L Lee, BG Welch. Secretory IgA antibody responses to *Neisseria gonorrhoeae* in the genital tract secretions of infected females. Journal of Infectious Diseases 133:113–125, 1976.

Ogra PL, DT Karzon. Distribution of poliovirus antibody in serum, nasopharynx and alimentary tract following segmental immunization of lower alimentary tract with poliovirus. Journal of Immunology 102:1423–1427, 1969.

Ogra PL, SS Ogra. Local antibody response to polio vaccine in the human genital tract. Journal of Immunology 110:1307–1311, 1973.

Owen RL, AL Jones. Epithelial cell specialization within Peyer's patches: An ultrastructural study of intestinal lymphoid follicles. Gastroenterology 66:189–203, 1974.

Parker CM, KL Cepek, GJ Russell, et al. A family of β7 integrins on human mucosal lymphocytes. Proceedings of the National Academy of Sciences, USA 89:1924–1928, 1992.

Parr MB, EL Parr. A comparison of antibody titres in mouse uterine fluid after immunization by several routes, and the effect of the uterus on antibody titres in vaginal fluid. Journal of Reproduction and Fertility 89:619–625, 1989a.

Parr MB, EL Parr. Immunohistochemical localization of secretory component and immunoglobulin A in the urogenital tract of the male rodent. Journal of Reproduction and Fertility 85:115–124, 1989b.

Parr MB, HP Ren, LD Russell, et al. Urethral glands of the male mouse contain secretory component and immunoglobulin A plasma cells and are targets of testosterone. Biology of Reproduction 47:1031–1039, 1992.

Patton DL, SK Wang, CC Kuo. *In vitro* activity of nonoxynol-9 on HeLa 229 cells and primary monkey cervical epithelial cells infected with *Chlamydia trachomatis*. Antimicrobial Agents and Chemotherapy 36:1478–1482, 1992.

Pierce NF, JL Gowans. Cellular kinetics of the intestinal immune response to cholera toxoid in rats. Journal of Experimental Medicine 142:1550, 1975.

Potts M. The urgent need for a vaginal microbicide in the prevention of HIV transmission. American Journal of Public Health 84:890–891, 1994.

Pudney J, DJ Anderson. Immunology of the human male urethra. American Journal of Pathology 147:155–165, 1995.

Quayle AJ, J Pudney, D Muñoz, et al. Characterization of T lymphocytes and antigen presenting cells in the murine male urethra. Biology of Reproduction 51:809–820, 1994.

Quigg JM. Development and evaluation of pH sensitive bioerodible polymers for the controlled release of vaginal contraceptive agents. PhD dissertation, University of Illinois at Chicago, 1991.

Quigg JM, IF Miller, SR Mack, et al. Development of polyurethane sponge as a delivery system for aryl 4-guanidinobenzoates. Contraception 38:487–497, 1988.

Raff HV, C Bradley, W Donaldson, et al. Comparison of functional activities between IgG1 and IgM class-switched human monoclonal antibodies reactive with group b *streptococci* or *Escherichia coli* K1. Journal of Infectious Diseases 163:346–354, 1991.

Romagnani S. Induction of Th1 and Th2 responses: A key role for the "natural" immune response? Immunology Today 13:379–381, 1992.

Rosenberg MJ, AJ Davison, JH Chen et al. Barrier contraceptives and sexually transmitted diseases in women: A comparison of female-dependent methods and condoms. American Journal of Public Health 82:669–674, 1992.

Rosenberg MJ, W Rojanapithayakorn, PJ Feldblum, et al. Effect of the contraceptive sponge on chlamydial infection, gonorrhea, and candidiasis: A comparative clinical trial. Journal of the American Medical Association 257:2308–2312, 1987.

Rush CM, LM Hafner, P Timms. Lactobacilli: Vehicles for antigen delivery to the female urogenital tract. Advances in Experimental Medicine and Biology 371B:1547–1552, 1995.

Sadownik A, G Deng, V Janout, et al. Rapid construction of a squalamine mimic. Journal of the American Chemical Society 117:6138–6139, 1995.

Schonwetter BS, ED Stolzenberg, MA Zasloff. Epithelial antibiotics induced at sites of inflammation. Science 267:1645–1648, 1995.

Sharman D, E Chantler, M Dukes, et al. Comparison of the action of nonoxynol-9 and chlorhexidine on sperm. Fertility and Sterility 45:259–264, 1986.

Shedlovsky L, D Belcher, I Levenstein. Titrations of human seminal fluid with acids and alkalis and their effects on the survival of sperm motility. American Journal of Physiology 136:535–541, 1942.

Shelton JA, E Goldberg. Local reproductive tract immunity to sperm-specific lactate dehydrogenase-C4. Biology of Reproduction 35:873–876, 1986.

Sherwood JK, L Zeitlin, KJ Whaley, et al. Controlled release of antibodies for long-term topical passive immuno-protection of female mice against genital herpes. Nature Biotechnology 14:468–471, 1996.

Sobrero AG. Use and effectiveness of condoms, diaphragms, cervical cap, vaginal sponge, and spermicides. IN Gynecology and Obstetrics, Vol. 6. GI Zatuchni, JJ Laferla, JJ Sciarra, eds. Philadelphia: J.B. Lippincott. 1989.

Stein Z. HIV prevention: An update on the status of methods women can use. American Journal of Public Health 83(10):1379–1382, 1993.

Stein Z. HIV prevention: The need for methods women can use. American Journal of Public Health 80:460–462, 1990.

Stone KM. HIV, other STDs, and barriers. IN Barrier Contraceptives: Current Status and Future Prospects. CK Mauck, M Cordero, HL Gabelnick, et al., eds. New York: Wiley-Liss. 1994.

Stratton P, NJ Alexander. Prevention of sexually transmitted infections. Infectious Disease Clinics of North America 7(4):841–859, 1993.

Sullivan DA, CR Wira. Hormonal regulation of immunoglobulins in the uterus: Uterine response to multiple estradiol treatments. Endocrinology 114:650–658, 1984.

Svennerholm A-M, LA Hanson, J Holmgren, et al. Different secretory immunoglobulin A antibody responses to cholera vaccination in Swedish and Pakistani women. Infectious Immunology 30:427–430, 1980.

Takahashi H, T Takeshita, B Morein, et al. Induction of CD8+ cytotoxic T cells by immunization with purified HIV-1 envelope protein in ISCOMS. Nature 344:873–875, 1990.

Talwar GP, S Garg, R Singh, et al. Praneem polyherbal cream and suppositories. IN Barrier Contraceptives: Current Status and Future Prospects. CK Mauck, M Cordero, HL Gabelnick, et al. New York: Wiley-Liss. 1994.

Thapar MA, EL Parr, JJ Bozzola, et al. Secretory immune responses in the mouse vagina after parenteral or intravaginal immunization with an immunostimulating complex (ISCOM). Vaccine 9:129–133, 1991.

Thapar MA, EL Parr EL, MB Parr. Secretory immune response in mouse vaginal fluid after pelvic, parenteral or vaginal immunization. Immunology 70:121–125, 1990.

Thormar H, CE Isaacs, HR Brown, et al. Inactivation of enveloped viruses and killing of cells by fatty acids and monoglycerides. Antimicrobial Agents in Chemotherapy 31:27–31, 1987.

Titus RG, JM Chiller. Orally induced tolerance. International Archives of Allergy and Applied Immunology 65:323–338, 1981.

Tjokronegoro A, S Sirisinha. Quantitative analysis of immunoglobulins and albumin in secretion of female reproductive tract. Fertility and Sterility 26:413–417, 1975.

Tomasi TB, EM Tan, A Soloman, et al. Characteristics of an immune system common to external secretions. Journal of Experimental Medicine 121:101, 1965.

Tomasi TB, S Ziegelbaum. The selective occurence of gamma 1A globulins in certain body fluids. Journal of Clinical Investigation 42:1552–1560, 1963.

Trussell J. Contraceptive efficacy of barrier contraceptives. IN Barrier Contraceptives: Current Status and Future Prospects. CK Mauck, M Cordero, HL Gabelnick, et al., eds. New York: Wiley-Liss. 1994.

Tsai C-C, KE Follis, A Sabo et al. Prevention of SIV infection in macaques by (R)-9-(2 phosphonylmethoxypropyl) adenine. Science 270:1197–1199, 1995.

Tung KSK, EH Goldberg, E Goldberg. Immunobiological consequence of immunization of female mice with homologous spermatozoa: Induction of infertility. Journal of Reproductive Immunology 1:145–158, 1979.

Voeller B, DJ Anderson. Heterosexual transmission of HIV. Journal of the American Medical Association 31:27–31, 1992a.

Voeller B, DJ Anderson. pH and related factors in the urogenital tract and rectum that affect HIV-1 transmission. Mariposa Occasional Paper No. 16, Topanga, CA, 1992b.

Wachsmann D, JP Klein, M Scholler, et al. Local and systemic immune response to orally administered liposome-associated soluble *S. mutans* cell wall antigens. Immunology 54:189–193, 1983.

Walter BA, GA Digenis et al. High-performance liquid chromatographic (HPLC) analysis of oligomeric components of the spermicide nonoxynol-9. Pharmacology Research 8:409–411, 1991a.

Walter BA, AA Hawi et al. Solubilization and *in vitro* spermicidal assessment of nonoxynol-9 and selected fraction using rabbit spermatozoa. Pharmacology Research 8:403–408, 1991b.

Wang YE, A-F Holstein. Intraepithelial lymphocytes in the human epididymis. Cell and Tissue Research 233:517–521, 1983.

Wasserheit JN. Epidemiological synergy: Interrelationships between human immunodeficiency virus infection and other sexually transmitted diseases. Sexually Transmitted Diseases 19:61–77, 1992.

Wiley JA, SJ Herschkorn, N Padian. Heterogeneity in the probability of HIV transmission per sexual contact: The case of male-to-female transmission in penile-vaginal intercourse. Statistics in Medicine 8:93–102, 1988.

Wira CR, CP Sandoe. Effect of uterine immunization and estradiol on specific IgA and IgG antibodies in uterine, vaginal and salivary secretions. Immunology 68:24–36, 1989.

Wira CR, DA Sullivan. Estradiol and progesterone regulation of IgA, IgG and secretory component in cervico-vaginal secretions of the rat. Biology of Reproduction 32:90–95, 1985.

Wolff H, DJ Anderson. Immunologic characterization and quantitation of leukocyte subpopulations in human semen. Fertility and Sterility 49:497–504, 1988a.

Wolff H, DJ Anderson. Male genital tract inflammation associated with increased numbers of potential human immunodeficiency virus host cells in semen. Andrologia 20:404–410, 1988b.

Yang SL, GFB Schumacher. Immune response after vaginal application of antigens in the rhesus monkey. Fertility and Sterility 32:588–598, 1979.

Zaneveld LJD. Vaginal contraception since 1984: Chemical agents and barrier devices. IN Contraceptive Research and Development, 1984 to 1994: The Road from Mexico City to Cairo and Beyond. PFA Van Look, G Pérez-Palacios, eds. Delhi: Oxford University Press. 1994a.

Zaneveld LJD. Vaginal contraceptive efficacy: Animal models. IN Barrier Contraceptives: Current Status and Future Prospects. CK Mauck, M Cordero, HL Gabelnick, et al., eds. New York: Wiley-Liss. 1994b.

Zaneveld LJD, AK Bhattacharyya, DS Kim, et al. Primate model for the evaluation of vaginal contraceptives. American Journal of Obstetrics and Gynecology 129:368–372, 1977.

Zaneveld LJD, RT Robertson, WL Williams. Synthetic enzyme inhibitors as antifertility agents. Federation of European Biochemical Societies Letters 11:345–347, 1970.

Zheng H-Y, TM Alcorn, MS Cohen. Effects of H_2O_2-producing lactobacilli on *Neisseria gonorrhoeae* growth and catalase activity. Journal of Infectious Diseases 170:1209–1215, 1994.

E

Agendas and Participants in Committee Workshops

Workshop on Contraceptive Research and Development and the Frontiers of Contemporary Science

December 8–9, 1994

Room 130, Cecil and Ida Green Building
2001 Wisconsin Avenue, NW
Washington, DC 20015

Thursday, December 8, 1994

8:45 a.m. **WELCOME**
Allan Rosenfield, chair
Polly Harrison

9:00 a.m. **OPENING REMARKS**
Kenneth Shine
Mahmoud Fathalla

9:30 a.m. **MALE CONTRACEPTION**
William Bremner, overview
Frank French
David Hamilton
Geoffrey Waites

10:15 a.m. **MENSES INDUCERS**
Paul Van Look, overview
Horacio Croxatto

11:00 a.m. **BARRIERS AGAINST STD/HIV AND HIV ATTACHMENT-PREVENTION**
Nancy Alexander, overview
Lourens Zaneveld

11:45 a.m. **VACCINES**
Paul Primakoff, overview
John Herr

12:30 p.m. **LUNCH**

1:30 p.m. **New Thoughts About Old Ideas**
Henry Gabelnick

2:00 p.m. **AREA 1—BASIC GENETICS**
Genetic screening and mapping, gene expression, and
transcription factors
Moderator:
Bert O'Malley
Principals:
Walter Gilbert
Donald McDonnell
David Page
Allen Spradling

3:30 p.m. **AREA 2—CONTROL/ACTION**
Signal transduction, releasing factors, RAFT proteins, ion channels,
peptide receptors, and steroid hormone synthesis
Moderator:
Jerome Strauss
Principals:
Bertil Hille
Andrés Negro-Vilar
Neena Schwartz
Roy Smith
Robert Stein

5:00 p.m. **ADJOURN**

6:00 p.m. **Reception/Buffet**

Friday, December 9, 1994

9:00 a.m. **AREA 3—PRE-FERTILIZATION TO FERTILIZATION**
Apoptosis, ovulation and the ovaries, meiotic and mitotic cell cycles, mammalian fertilization, molecular basis of gamete interaction, and signalling pathways
Moderator:
David Garbers
Principals:
Aaron Hsueh
William Lennarz
JoAnne Richards
Patricia Saling
Debra Wolgemuth

10:30 a.m. **AREA 4—POST-FERTILIZATION TO IMPLANTATION**
Angiogenesis, apoptosis, and implantation (cytokine function, integrin biology, and trophoblast invasion)
Moderator:
Susan Fisher
Principals:
Mina Bissell
Michael Harper
Judah Folkman
Bruce Lessey

12:00 p.m. **LUNCH**

1:00 p.m. **AREA 5—METHODOLOGIES**
Combinatorial chemistry, appropriate modelling
Walter Moos
Jeffrey Harris

1:30 p.m. **AREA 6—INFECTIOUS DISEASES AND IMMUNOLOGY**
Deborah Anderson
Jiri Mestecky

3:00 p.m. **REVIEW PANEL**
Horacio Croxatto
Egon Diczfalusy
Bert O'Malley

4:00 p.m. **ADJOURN**

Saturday, December 9, 1994

8:30 a.m.   **Executive Session of the Committee**

12:00 p.m. **ADJOURN**

WORKSHOP PARTICIPANTS

Nancy J. Alexander
Chief, Contraceptive Development
    Branch
Center for Population Research
National Institute for Child Health
    and Human Development
National Institutes of Health

Deborah J. Anderson
Associate Professor
Harvard Medical School
Fearing Research Laboratory

Felice M. Apter
Center for Population, Health, and
    Nutrition
Bureau for Global Programs
U.S. Agency for International
    Development

Hedia Belhadj El Ghouayel
Technical and Evaluation Division
United Nations Population Fund

Balbir Bhogal
Director of Immunology
Zonagen, Inc.

Gabriel Bialy
Acting Deputy Director
Center for Population Research
National Institute for Child Health
    and Human Development
National Institutes of Health

Mina J. Bissell
Director
Life Sciences Division
Lawrence Berkeley Laboratory

William J. Bremner
Professor and Vice Chairman
Department of Medicine
University of Washington

Donald D. Brown
Director
Department of Embryology
Carnegie Institute of Washington

Nancy L. Buc
Partner
Buc and Beardsley
Washington, DC

Peter F. Carpenter
Founder/Director
Mission and Values Institute
Stanford University

Willard Cates, Jr.
Director, Division of Training
Centers for Disease Control and
    Prevention

Rebecca J. Cook
Associate Professor
Faculty of Law
University of Toronto

Horacio B. Croxatto
Professor
Instituto Chileno de Medicina

Egon Diczfalusy
Professor Emeritus
Karolinska Hospital

Laneta Dorflinger
Director
Clinical Trials Division
Family Health International

Richard H. Douglas
Vice President for Corporate
   Development
Genzyme Corporation

Mahmoud F. Fathalla
Senior Advisor for Biomedical and
   Reproductive Health Research
The Rockefeller Foundation,
   and
Professor of Obstetrics and
   Gynaecology
Assiut University

Susan J. Fisher
Professor and Chair
Division of Oral Biology
University of California at San
   Francisco

Jonathan J. Fleming
General Partner
Matrushka Venture Capital (MVC)

Judah M. Folkman
Professor of Pediatrics
Harvard Medical School

Frank S. French
Director
Laboratories for Reproductive Biology
Department of Pediatrics
School of Medicine
University of North Carolina at
   Chapel Hill

Henry L. Gabelnick
Director and Principal Investigator
Contraceptive Research and
   Development (CONRAD) Program
Professor, Department of Obstetrics
   and Gynecology
Eastern Virginia Medical School

David L. Garbers
Professor of Pharmacology
Howard Hughes Medical Institute
University of Texas Southwestern
   Medical Center

Walter Gilbert
Professor
Harvard University
The Biological Laboratories

Allan Goldhammer
Director for Research Activities
Biotechnology Industry Organization
   (BIO)

David W. Hamilton
Professor and Head
Department of Cell Biology and
   Neuroanatomy
University of Minnesota

Michael J.K. Harper
Professor
Department of Obstetrics and
   Gynecology
Baylor College of Medicine

Jeffrey D. Harris
Director of Molecular Biology
Zonagen, Inc.

Polly F. Harrison
Study Director
Division of Health Sciences Policy
Institute of Medicine

John M. Herr, Jr.
Professor of Cell Biology
Director, Center for Recombinant
   Gamete Vaccinology
University of Virginia Medical
   School

Bertil Hille
Professor
Department of Physiology
University of Washington

Gregory F. Hollis
Director
Cellular and Molecular Biology
Merck Research Laboratories

Aaron J.W. Hsueh
Professor
Department of Obstetrics and
   Gynecology
Stanford University Medical Center

Timothy Kanaley
Research Assistant
Division of Health Sciences Policy
Institute of Medicine

William J. Lennarz
Department of Biochemistry and Cell
   Biology
State University of New York

Bruce A. Lessey
Department of Obstetrics and
   Gynecology
University of North Carolina

Dennis W. Lincoln
Director
Reproductive Unit, Edinburgh
Medical Research Council

Carolyn Makinson
Program Officer
Population Program
Andrew W. Mellon Foundation

Donald P. McDonnell
Associate Professor of Pharmacology
Duke University Medical Center

Jiri Mestecky
Professor
Department of Microbiology
University of Alabama

Walter H. Moos
Chemical Therapeutics Research
Chiron Corporation

David C. Mowery
Associate Professor of Business and
   Public Policy
University of California at Berkeley

Andrés F. Negro-Vilar
Director
Women's Health Research Institute,
   and
Vice President
Wyeth-Ayerst Research

Allan C. Spradling
Staff Member
Howard Hughes Medical Institute
Carnegie Institute of Washington

Jacqueline Sherris
Editor, *Outlook*
Program for Appropriate Technology
in Health (PATH)

Robert Stein
Senior Vice President, and
Chief Scientific Officer
Ligand Pharmaceuticals

Jerome F. Strauss, III
Professor and Director
Center for Research on Women's
Health
University of Pennsylvania

Laura Tangley
Science Writer for the Institute of
Medicine

Paul Van Look
Associate Director
Special Programme of Research,
Development, and Research
Training in Human Reproduction
World Health Organization

Geoffrey M.H. Waites
President, International Society for
Andrology

Kevin J. Whaley
Research Scientist
Department of Biophysics
Johns Hopkins University

Debra J. Wolgemuth
Professor of Human Genetics and
Development
College of Physicians and Surgeons
Columbia University

Lourens J. D. Zaneveld
Research Director
Women's Health Research Center
Professor
Department of Obstetrics and
Gynecology, and Department of
Biochemistry
Rush University, St. Luke's Medical
Center

Bai-ge Zhao
Director
Shanghai Institute of Planned
Parenthood Research

Agenda

Workshop on Private-Sector Participation in Contraceptive Research and Development: Opportunities, Challenges, Strategies

May 11–12, 1995

Room 130, Cecil and Ida Green Building
2001 Wisconsin Avenue, NW
Washington, DC 20015

Thursday, May 11, 1995

8:45 a.m.   **Welcome**
Introduction of Participants
Adoption of Agenda and Timetable
Allan Rosenfield, *Chair*

(All presentations on the rest of Day 1 will be of a length that will permit ample time for discussion.)

SESSION 1: WHAT WE HAVE DONE SO FAR

9:15 a.m.   **Thoughts and Conclusions from Bellagio Conference,
April 10–14, 1995, on Public- and Private-Sector Collaboration
in Contraceptive Research and Development**
Mahmoud Fathalla

10:00 a.m. **Findings from IOM Workshop on Contraceptive Research and
Development and the Frontiers of Science, December 8–9, 1994**

The Farther Frontier
David Garbers

The Middle Ground
Andrés Negro-Vilar

11:00 a.m. **Break**

SESSION 2: CHALLENGES AND QUESTIONS

11:15 a.m. **Defining the Market:**

What Are the Needs?
Jacqueline Forrest

What Is the Market?—Measures and Calculations
William Sheldon

12:15 p.m. **Lunch**

1:30 p.m. **The Legal and Regulatory Scene:**

Changes and Perspectives at the FDA
Philip Corfman

Tort Reform Update
Ellen Flannery

2:30 p.m. **Industry Perspectives: A Panel Discussion**
Robert Essner
Michael Kafrissen
Hans Vemer
Guenter Stock

3:45 p.m. **Break**

4:00 p.m. **Instructions to Working Groups: Objectives and Framework for Discussions**
Allan Rosenfield/Polly Harrison

(The composition of each Working Group will be balanced among the expertises and backgrounds of the participant group as a whole. A set of draft questions for the Groups is attached to this agenda.)

4:30 p.m. **What Are the Most Important Political Perspectives in the United States and How Might These Be Taken into Account?**
The Honorable Nita M. Lowey
The Honorable Constance A. Morella

5:30 p.m.   **ADJOURN**

BUFFET RECEPTION

7:30 p.m.   **Brief Meeting of Each Working Group to Organize Itself and Marshal Initial Thoughts**

Friday, May 12, 1995

8:45 a.m.   **Reconvene Briefly in Room 130 for trouble-shooting, questions, clarifications, et cetera.**

9:00 a.m.   **Working Groups (continued) and Preparation of Working Group Reports**

12:00 p.m. **Lunch**

1:00 p.m.   **Working Group Presentations by Rapporteurs**
Response Panel and Discussion
Conclusions, Recommendations, Followup

[A panel of individuals with expertise in the areas addressed on Day 1 will react to the conclusions and recommendations reported by each group, and moderate comments from the workshop audience as a whole.]

4:00 p.m.   **ADJOURNMENT**

4:15 p.m.   **Meeting of Committee and Sponsors**

5:15 p.m.   **FULL ADJOURNMENT**

WORKSHOP PARTICIPANTS

Nancy J. Alexander**
Chief, Contraceptive Development
Center for Population Research
National Institute for Child Health and
   Human Development
National Institutes of Health

Hedia Belhadj-El Ghouayel*
Technical and Evaluation Division
United Nations Population Fund

Willem Bergink
Program Manager for Reproductive
   Medicine
Organon International B.V.

Seth Berkley**
Acting Director for Health Sciences
The Rockefeller Foundation

Enriqueta C. Bond
President
The Burroughs Wellcome Fund

Lance Bronnenkant
President and Chief Executive Officer
Finishing Enterprises, USA

Donald D. Brown*
Director
Department of Embryology
Carnegie Institute of Washington

Barbara Brummer
Advanced Care Products

Nancy L. Buc*
Partner
Buc, Levitt, and Beardsley

Stephanie Burns
Manager, FDA and Women's Health
Dow Corning Corporation

Peter F. Carpenter*
Founder/Director, Mission and Values
   Institute
Visiting Scholar, Center for
   Biomedical Ethics
Stanford University

Willard Cates, Jr.*
Director
Division of Training
Epidemiology Program Office
Centers for Disease Control and
   Prevention

James Cavanaugh
President
HealthCare Investment Corporation

Scott Chappel
Senior Scientific Advisor
Ares-Serono

Michael Cohen
Scientific Director
Applied Medical Research, Ltd.

Philip A. Corfman
Supervisory Medical Officer for
   Fertility and Maternal Health
U.S. Food and Drug Administration

Rebecca J. Cook*
Associate Professor, Faculty of Law
University of Toronto

---

*Committee Member
**Sponsor Representative

Horacio B. Croxatto*
Professor
Instituto Chileno de Medicina
  Reproductiva

Bernard M. Dickens
Professor, Faculty of Law, Faculty of
  Medicine
Centre of Criminology and Centre for
  Bioethics
University of Toronto

Laneta Dorflinger
Family Health International

Richard H. Douglas*
Vice President, Corporate
  Development
Genzyme Corporation

Robert Essner
President
Wyeth-Ayerst Laboratories

Mahmoud F. Fathalla**
Senior Advisor for Biomedical and
  Reproductive Health Research
The Rockefeller Foundation, and
Professor of Obstetrics and
  Gynaecology
Assiut University

Diane Feldman
Vice President for Over-the-Counter
  Business
Syntex Corporation

Alan Ferguson
Atlas Venture

Mary Flack
Parke-Davis Pharmaceutical Research
Warner-Lambert Co.

Ellen Flannery
Partner
Covington and Burling

Jonathan Fleming
Matrushka Venture Capital (MVC)

Jacqueline D. Forrest
Director of Research
The Alan Guttmacher Institute

Adrian Fugh-Berman**
Contraceptive Development Branch
National Institute for Child Health
  and Human Development
National Institutes of Health

Henry L. Gabelnick**
Director
Contraceptive Research and
  Development (CONRAD) Program
Professor, Department of Obstetrics
  and Gynecology
Eastern Virginia Medical School

David L. Garbers
Patrick E. Haggerty Distinguished
  Chair in Basic Biomedical Science
Howard Hughes Medical Institute
University of Texas Southwestern
  Medical Center at Dallas

Philip Gevas
President and Chief Executive Officer
Aphton Pharmaceuticals

Michael J.K. Harper*
Professor, Department of Obstetrics
  and Gynecology
Baylor College of Medicine

Polly F. Harrison
Study Director
Division of Health Sciences Policy
Institute of Medicine

Robert Howells
Director, Population Initiative
The Wellcome Trust

Leonard Jacob
Executive Vice President and Chief
  Operating Officer
Magainin Pharmaceuticals

Michael Kafrissen
Vice President for Clinical Affairs
Ortho-McNeil

Timothy Kanaley
Research Assistant
Division of Health Sciences Policy
Institute of Medicine

David H. Katz
Chief Executive Officer and President
Lidak Pharmaceuticals

Walter Klemann
Head, Strategic Business Unit,
  Fertility Control and Hormone
  Therapy
Schering AG

Susan Lambert
Vice-President
J&J Development Corporation
Ortho-McNeil Pharmaceutical

Samuel Lin
Assistant Surgeon General (Ret.), US
  Public Health Service, and
Executive Director, Federal Medical
  Affairs
The Upjohn Company

Ernest Loumaye
Corporate Ob/Gyn Director
Medical Affairs Department
Serono Corporation

Carolyn Makinson**
Program Officer
Population Program
Andrew W. Mellon Foundation

Donald Patrick McDonnell*
Associate Professor of Pharmacology
Department of Pharmacology
Duke University Medical Center

Jonathan Miles Brown
Director of Technical Marketing
Martek Biosciences

Jonathan Missner
Vice President, Operations
Applied Medical Research, Ltd.

David C. Mowery*
Professor of Business and Public
  Policy
Walter A. Haas School of Business
University of California at Berkeley

Andrés Negro-Vilar
Director, Women's Health Research
  Institute, and
Vice President
Wyeth-Ayerst Research

Felicia Stewart
Deputy Assistant Secretary for
  Population Affairs
Department of Health and Human
  Services, Public Health Service

Pamela Stratton**
Special Assistant in Gynecology and
  Clinical Research
Contraceptive Development Branch
National Institute of Child Health and
  Human Development
National Institutes of Health

Laura Tangley
Science Writer for the Institute of
  Medicine

Wylie Vale*
Professor
The Clayton Foundation Laboratories
  for Peptide Biology
The Salk Institute

Hans M. Vemer
Director of Research and Medical
  Director
Organon International B.V.

David Woo
President and Chief Scientific Officer
Immunotherapy Corporation

Craig Wright
Vice President of Research and
  Development
Novovax

Lourens J. D. Zaneveld
Research Director
Women's Health Research Center
Professor, Department of Obstetrics
  and Gynecology, and Department
  of Biochemistry
Rush University, Rush-St. Luke's
  Medical Center

Bai-ge Zhao*
Director
Shanghai Institute of Planned
  Parenthood Research

F

Committee Biographies

Hedia Belhadj-El Ghouayel, MD, is Technical Officer in the Reproductive Health Branch in the Technical and Evaluation Division, United Nations Population Fund (UNFPA). She obtained her MD from the Faculty of Medicine of Tunis and a specialist degree in endocrinology and metabolic diseases from the Universities of Tunis and Paris. Dr. Belhadj was UNFPA country director for Yemen, Oman, and Djibouti (1991–1993) and program officer for the Arab States and Europe (1989–1991). From 1985 to 1988, Dr. Belhadj was a Tietze Fellow at the Population Council's Center for Biomedical Research, working on clinical studies for development of contraceptive technologies and basic research in reproductive physiology.

Donald D. Brown, MD, is Director of the Department of Embryology, the Carnegie Institute of Washington. He earned his MD from the University of Chicago. Dr. Brown is a Fellow of the American Academy of Arts and Sciences, the American Society of Cell Biology, and the National Academy of Sciences of the United States. He has earned numerous awards, including the Honorary Doctor of Science, University of Cincinnati (1992); the Feodor Lynen award from the University of Miami Winter Symposium (1987); and the Louisa Gross Horwitz Award from Columbia University and the Rosenstiel Award in Basic Biomedical Science from Brandeis University in 1985.

Nancy L. Buc is Partner in the law firm of Buc and Beardsley in Washington, DC, and earned her LLB from the University of Virginia. In 1980–1981 she was Chief Counsel for the United States Food and Drug Administration, prior to which she was Partner in the law firm of Weil, Gotshal, and Manges. Her awards include the LLD *honoris causa* from Brown University (1994), Distinguished Service Award from the Federal Trade Commission (1972), and the Secretary's Special Citation and Award of Merit from the USFDA (1981). Ms. Buc is on the boards of directors of the Alan Guttmacher Institute and Women's Legal Defense Fund and on the editorial boards of the *Food Drug and Cosmetic Law Journal* and *Journal of Products Liability.*

Peter F. Carpenter, MBA, is a public policy/public service fellow at the Mission and Values Institute; Adjunct Professor, Department of Epidemiology and Biostatistics, McGill University; and Visiting Scholar, Center for Biomedical Ethics, Stanford University. He is a graduate of Harvard University and received his MBA from the University of Chicago in 1965. From 1976 to 1992, Mr. Carpenter worked for the ALZA Corporation, where he served as president for eight years. He has served on the IOM Committee to Study Decision-Making on Biomedical Innovations, Committee on the Social and Ethical Impact of Advances in Biomedicine, and Committee to Study Medications Development and Research at the National Institute on Drug Abuse.

Willard Cates, Jr., MD, MPH, is Corporate Director of Medical Affairs at Family Health International, prior to which he served as Director, Division of Training, Epidemiology Program Office, Centers for Disease Control; from 1982 to 1991 he served as director of CDC's Division of Sexually Transmitted Diseases and HIV. He earned his MPH and MD at the Yale University School of Medicine. Dr. Cates is a member of the NAS Committee on Population study of Reproductive Health in Developing Countries and has served several Institute of Medicine study committees beginning in 1975. He is a member of the Board of Overseers for the *American Journal of Epidemiology,* Associate Editor of *Sexually Transmitted Diseases,* and is on the editorial advisory board for the *Journal of Reproductive Health Medicine* and *Venereology.*

Rebecca J. Cook, JD, JSD, is Professor, Faculty of Law, University of Toronto, and Adjunct Associate Professor in the Division of Population and Family Health at the Columbia University School of Public Health. She received her JSD at the Columbia University School of Law and her JD at Georgetown University Law Center. She serves on the editorial advisory boards of *Drug Regulation and Reproductive Health, Family Planning Perspectives, Journal of Third World Legal Studies,* and *Reproductive Health Matters.* She is a member of the Scientific and Ethical Review Group of the Human Reproduction Programme of the World Health Organization, International Women's Rights Action Watch, and Profamilia Servicios Legales para Mujeres in Bogotá, Colombia.

Horacio B. Croxatto, MD, is President of the Chilean Institute of Reproductive

Medicine and Professor of Reproductive Physiology at the Catholic University of Chile. He received his MD at the School of Medicine of the Catholic University of Chile. Dr. Croxatto is a member of several Chilean medical and research societies, the American Society of Reproductive Medicine, and the Society for the Study of Reproduction. He has authored numerous articles in scientific journals and invited book chapters on oviductal physiology and on contraceptive development.

Richard H. Douglas, PhD, is Vice-president for Corporate Development, the Genzyme Corporation, and has served the corporation as Vice-president for Scientific Development and Director for New Product Development. Prior to holding these positions, Dr. Douglas was Manager of Protein Chemistry Research at Genzyme Integrated Genetics, whose Protein Engineering group combined protein chemistry, molecular biology, and molecular modeling for rational drug design to produce novel proprietary therapeutic molecules. Dr. Douglas earned his PhD in biochemistry from the University of California at Berkeley, after which he held a Postdoctoral Research Fellowship at the California Institute of Technology under Dr. Leroy Hood, focusing on immunology, immunochemistry, molecular biology, and protein microsequencing.

Michael J. K. Harper, PhD, ScD, is presently Professor of Obstetrics and Gynecology at Eastern Virginia Medical School. He also served as Professor at the Baylor College of Medicine Center for Reproductive Medicine and Department of Obstetrics and Gynecology, where his research centered on maternal recognition of pregnancy; chemical mediators such as platelet-activating factor (PAF) and leukemia inhibitory factor (LIF). His previous experience as Technical Officer at ICI (now Zeneca) Pharmaceutical involved research on antihormonal agents for contraception and cancer therapy and the discovery of tamoxifen, a widely used antiestrogen. Dr. Harper has consulted for the World Health Organization, U.S. Agency for International Development, National Institute of Child Health and Development, National Science Foundation, and Andrew W. Mellon Foundation. His many publications include *Birth Control Technologies: Prospects by the Year 2000*.

Donald P. McDonnell, PhD, is Associate Professor of Pharmacology at Duke University Medical Center. He earned his PhD in cell biology from Baylor College of Medicine in 1987. Between 1991 and 1994 he served as Associate Director, then Director and Head of Molecular Biology at Ligand Pharmaceuticals. Dr. McDonnell has received numerous investigator awards, is on the editorial board of *Molecular Endocrinology*, and referees articles for *Endocrinology, Science, Nature, Proceedings of the National Academy of Sciences USA*, and several other scientific journals. He holds patents on several screening assays for steroid hormone receptor agonists and antagonists and has published numerous articles in scientific journals, most recently on the topic of nuclear hormone receptors as targets for new drug discovery.

David Mowery, PhD, is Professor of Business and Public Policy at the Walter A. Haas School of Business at the University of California, Berkeley. His research deals with the economics of technological innovation and effects of public policies on innovation. He earned his PhD in economics from Stanford University and was a postdoctoral research fellow at the Harvard Business School. In 1987–1988, Dr. Mowery served as study director for the National Academy of Sciences Panel on Technology and Employment and, in 1988, as a Council on Foreign Relations Internal Affairs Fellow in the Office of the United States Trade Representative. Among Dr. Mowery's publications are *Technology and the Pursuit of Economic Growth; Alliance Politics and Economics; Technology and Employment: Innovation and Growth in the U.S. Economy;* and *International Collaborative Ventures in U.S. Manufacturing.*

Judy Norsigian is Codirector of the Boston Women's Health Book Collective and a consultant to the Massachusetts Department of Public Health, the Contraceptive Research and Development program (CONRAD), World Health Organization, and National Institutes of Health. She was on the board of the National Women's Health Network and now serves on the editorial board for the journal *Women and Health.* In addition to her work at the Health Collective, she has served on numerous advisory boards and committees for the International Childbirth Education Association, the American Public Health Association, the New England Research Institute, the Planned Parenthood League of Massachusetts, and Family Health International. Ms. Norsigian also served on the National Research Council/Institute of Medicine Committee on Contraceptive Development (1987–1990).

Sandra Panem, PhD, is President, Vector Fund Management, prior to which she was Vice-president and Portfolio Manager at Oppenheimer Management Corporation (1992–1994) and Vice-president at Salomon Brothers (1986–1992). She earned her PhD in microbiology at the University of Chicago. Dr. Panem served as Program Officer for the Alfred P. Sloan Foundation (1966–1968), Guest Scholar at The Brookings Institute (1985–1986), Science Advisor at the US Environmental Protection Agency (1983–1985), and Research Associate and Assistant Professor at the University of Chicago (1971–1982). She is a member of the Board of Directors of the National Center for Human Genome Resources and the Board of Governors of the New York Academy of Sciences.

Allan Rosenfield, MD, FACOG (Committee Chair) is Dean of the Columbia University School of Public Health, Joseph R. DeLamar Professor of Public Health, and Professor of Obstetrics and Gynecology. He received his MD from

Columbia University. Dr. Rosenfield was the Population Council representative and advisor to the Ministry of Public Health in Bangkok, Thailand, and Assistant Director of the Technical Assistance Division at Population Council headquarters in New York City between 1967 and 1975. He has contributed over 100 articles to professional journals and is a Fellow of the American College of Obstetrics and Gynecology, American Public Health Association, and American Fertility Society.

Bennett M. Shapiro, MD, is Executive Vice-president for Worldwide Basic Research, Merck Research Laboratories. He earned his MD at Jefferson Medical College. Before joining Merck, Dr. Shapiro was on the faculty of biochemistry at the University of Washington (1971–1990) and Chairman of the Biochemistry Department (1985–1990). Between 1968 and 1970 he was a visiting scientist at the Institut Pasteur, Paris, and US Public Health Service surgeon and, from 1965 to 1968, research associate at the National Institutes of Health. He is a member of the American Society of Biologists and Chemists, American Society of Cell Biology, and American Society of Development Biology.

Wylie W. Vale, PhD, is Head of the Clayton Foundation Laboratories for Peptide Biology at the Salk Institute and has been Professor at the Institute since 1980 and serves on its Board of Trustees and as Chairman of Faculty. Of his many named lectures and awards, the most recent is the Vincent du Vigneaud Award of the American Peptide Society (1992). Dr. Vale has been President of the Endocrine Society (1992–1993), the NIDDK Council of Scientific Advisors, and Board of Directors of the Laurentian Hormone Conference, and now serves as Vice-president of the International Society for Neuroendocrinology. Dr. Vale was elected to the US National Academy of Sciences in 1992. The most recent of his numerous scientific publications are concerned with corticotropin-releasing factor and activin receptors.

Bai-ge Zhao, PhD, is Director of the Shanghai Institute of Planned Parenthood Research. She earned her PhD at the University of Cambridge, UK. Prior to that she was Director of the WHO Collaborating Center for Research in Human Reproduction and the National Laboratory for Contraceptives and Devices Research (1990–1994) and Deputy Director of the Medical Section of Shanghai Science and Technology Commission (1984–1985). Dr. Zhao was named Outstanding Woman and Scientist in Shanghai and Outstanding Postgraduate in China. Her basic research in mechanisms of hormone action, signal transduction, and gene expression in aspects of reproductive process, as well as her work with RU 486 and implant technologies, earned her the National Prize for Progress in Science and Technology. She is a member of the New York Academy of Sciences.

Glossary

Abortion   The expulsion or extraction of the products of conception from the uterus before the embryo or fetus is capable of independent life. Abortions may be spontaneous or induced. Spontaneous abortions are commonly called miscarriages. Induced abortions are voluntary interruptions of pregnancy or therapeutic abortions. Incomplete abortion occurs when some products of conception, usually the placenta, remain inside the uterus. Missed abortion is when the fetus has died in utero and some or all of the nonliving products of conception remain in the uterus.

Abortion, unsafe   A procedure for terminating an unwanted pregnancy either by persons lacking the necessary skills or in an environment lacking the minimal medical standards or both.

Abstinence   Refraining from sexual intercourse.

Adhesion   Abnormal sticking together of body tissues, usually by bands of scar tissue which form between two tissues following inflammation.

Amenorrhea   The absence or suppression of menstruation. This state is normal before puberty, after menopause, and during pregnancy and lactation.

Amenorrheic women   Women who are already pregnant, or who have just had a child and their menses have not yet returned.

Androgen   Generic term for an agent, usually a hormone (e.g., testosterone), that stimulates activity of the accessory male sex organs, encouraging development of male sex charcteristics, or prevents changes in the latter that follow castration. Androgens are produced chiefly by the testes but also by the adrenal cortex and the ovary.

495

Anemia   A reduction in the quantity of red blood cells per unit volume of blood to below normal levels.

Antibody   A protein produced by B lymphocytes in response to contact with an antigen from a foreign microorganism and triggered by T lymphocytes. Antibodies attach themselves to the foreign antigen, and to nothing else. This signals other elements of the immune system, including monocytes and macrophages, to destroy the invading organism.

Antigen   1. Any substance capable of reacting with the products of an immune response, that is, specific antibodies, or sensitized T-lymphocytes or both. 2. An extruding molecule on the surface of a cell, microorganism, toxin or other foreign body which is capable, under appropriate conditions, of inducing a specific immune response when coming into contact with a lymphocyte or antibody.

Azoospermia   Absence of living sperm in semen.

Barrier method   A contraceptive method that establishes a physical or chemical barrier between the sperm and ovum, e.g., condom, diaphragm, foam, sponge, cervical cap. Some of the barrier contraceptives are used in conjunction with a spermicidal agent.

Biotechnology   The collection of industrial processes that involve the use of biological systems. For some of these industries, the processes involve the use of genetically engineered organisms.

Capacitation   The process by which sperm become capable of penetrating an egg, which occurs in the female reproductive tract.

Cervical cap   Small latex or plastic cap that covers the cervix. Users of this barrier method of birth control must spread spermicidal cream or jelly inside the cap.

Chancroid   A sexually transmitted disease caused by the *Hemophilus ducreyi* bacterium and characterized by a soft sore on the genitals which becomes painful and discharges pus.

Chlamydia trachomatis   A microorganism that can cause vaginitis, urethritis, cervitis, pelvic inflammatory disease, and lymphogranuloma venereum (LGV). Women with positive chlamydia cultures are more likely to have the following: cervical discharge (yellow or green), erythema, ectopy, friability, and white blood cells on microscopic evaluation of cervical secretions. Also called chlamydia, mucopurulent cervicitis, and nongonococcal urethritis (in men).

Coitus   Entry or penetration of the penis into the vagina. Also called intercourse or copulation.

Complication   A difficult factor or issue often appearing suddenly or unexpectedly.

Conception   Generally the beginning of pregnancy. Conception is usually equated with the fertilization of the ovum by the sperm, but is sometimes equated with the implantation of the fertilized ovum in the uterine lining.

Condom   A cylindrical sheath of latex, polyurethane, or sheep intestine worn over the penis during intercourse as a barrier method of contraception and as a prophylactic against sexually transmitted disease. Some condoms contain a spermicide to kill sperm to decrease the risk of pregnancy should a condom break or should semen leak over the outer rim of the condom. Also called a rubber.

Contraception   As a means of logical progression, contraception is necessarily anything that acts against conception, and therefore, anything that prevents the success of fertilization or implantation.

Contraceptive immunogen   All molecular constructs or organoids meant to directly elicit an immune reaction for birth control.

Contraceptive prevalence rate   The percentage of women currently using a contraceptive method.

Contraindications   Describe patients who should not receive a drug because, for one reason or another, the risks of taking it are likely to outweigh the benefits.

Corpus luteum   The structure which develops from the ovarian follicle once a ripened ovum has been expelled. It produces progesterone to prepare the endometrium for implantation. During the second half of the cycle, if conception does not occur, the corpus luteum degenerates, leaving visible scars called the corpora albicans. If pregnancy does occur, the corpus luteum persists and functions through the first half of the pregnancy. During pregnancy it is stimulated by human chorionic gonadotropin (HCG).

Cyst   A walled sac containing gas, liquid, or semi-solid material.

Depo-Provera   Injectable form of medroxyprogesterone acetate.

Desired total fertility rate (DTFR)   Hypothesized estimate of what the Total Fertility Rate (TFR) would be in different populations if women were to realize their wishes and bear exactly the number of children they preferred.

Diaphragm   The soft, rubber, dome-shaped device worn over the cervix and used with spermicidal jelly or cream for contraception. Diaphragms are circular, shallow, rubber domes with a firm but flexible outer rim that fit between the posterior vaginal wall (posterior fornix) and the recess behind the pubic arch. Sizes vary from 50 to 105 mm in diameter.

Douche   Cleansing the vaginal canal with a liquid; not an effective means of birth control or STD prevention.

Dysmenorrhea   Painful menstruation. Usually cramping midline lower abdominal pain. May be associated with low back pain, nausea, diarrhea, or upper thigh pain.

Ectopic   Out of place; an ectopic pregnancy occurs when the embryo implants outside the uterus, usually in the fallopian tube. Much less commonly, implantation may occur in the endocervical canal, on the ovary, or within the abdominal cavity.

Egg   An ovum; a female gamete; an oocyte; a female reproductive cell at any stage before fertilization.

Ejaculation   Expulsion of semen from the penis.

Endocrine glands   Ductless glands which secrete hormones into the bloodstream.

Endometrium   The mucous inner lining of the uterus.

Epididymis   A coiled tubular structure where sperm cells mature and are nourished, and which connects the testes to the vas deferens.

Estrogen   The primary female hormones; any natural or artificial substance that induces estrogenic activity, more specifically, the hormones estradiol and estrone produced by the ovary. Estrogens are produced chiefly by the ovary but also by the adrenal cortex, the testis, and the placenta.

Failure rate   The number of pregnancies occurring per 100 users per year.

Fecund   Potentially fertile.

Fecundity   1. Possessing the power or quality conducive to producing offspring. 2. Exposed to the risk of conception.

Fertility norm   Desired or ideal number of children.

Fetus   The developing conceptus after 7 to 8 weeks postfertilization (the end of the embryonic period) until birth.

Fibrocystic breast disease   Benign breast tumor(s) involving multiple cysts in the terminal ducts and acini of the breast. Believed to be estrogen dependent. Breast cancer is twice as common in women with some types of fibrocystic breast disease. Also known as cystic mastitis, chorionic cystic breast disease, cystic hyperplasia, and cystic adenosis.

Follicle   A small secretory sac or cavity. One type of follicle is an ovarian follicle which is a very small sac in the ovary in which an ovum matures and from which the egg is released.

Follicle stimulating hormone (FSH)   Anterior pituitary hormone which stimulates the ovary to ripen egg follicles. FSH stimulates sperm production in the males testes.

Gonadotropin   A substance having an affinity for, or stimulating effect on, the gonads. There are three varieties: anterior pituitary, chorionic (from pregnant women's urine), and equine (from the serum of pregnant horses).

Gonads   An organ that produces sex cells (e.g., the testis and ovary).

Gossypol   A derivative of the cottonseed plant that induces infertility in males; being used experimentally as a male contraceptive in China. Also known to have spermicidal properties when employed as a vaginal contraceptive.

Homologue Likeness short of identity in structure or function between parts of different organisms due to evolutionary differentiation from the same or a corresponding part of a remote ancestor.

Hormone A "messenger" molecule of the body that helps coordinate the actions of various tissues. Hormones produce a specific effect on the activity of cells remote from their point of origin.

Human chorionic gonadotropin (HCG) A glycoproteinaceous hormone produced by the placenta which maintains the corpus luteum and causes it to secrete estrogen and progesterone. Measured in urine and blood to detect pregnancy.

Human immunodeficiency virus (HIV) A virus that causes AIDS. It causes a defect in the body's immune system by invading and then multiplying within white blood cells.

Hypothalamus Part of the brain just above the pituitary which helps to regulate basic functions such as sleep, appetite, body temperature, fertility. The hypothalamus is influenced by higher cortical levels of the brain and controls hormone production by the pituitary.

Immune system The body's system of protection against infection or penetration by microorganisms, toxins or small particles. Elements of the immune system include white blood cells and the cells, immunoglobin proteins and hormones they produce, such as macrophages, antibodies and lymphokines.

Immunocontraceptive methods All contraceptive methods based on interference of some step of the reproductive process by products of an immune reaction, be it antibodies or cells.

Immunogen Any substance that is capable of eliciting an immune response.

Implantation The process whereby an ovum 6 or 7 days after fertilization burrows into the lining of the uterus and attaches itself firmly. Successful implantation is essential to the development of the embryo.

Infertility Failure, voluntary or involuntary, to produce offspring. Primary infertility: The woman has never conceived despite cohabitation, exposure to the possibility of pregnancy, and the wish to become pregnancy for at least 12 months (World Health Organization definition). Secondary infertility: The woman has previously conceived but is subsequently unable to conceive despite cohabitation, exposure to the possibility of pregnancy, and the wish to become pregnant for at least 12 months (WHO).

Injectable contraceptives Hormonal contraceptives given by injection. Two examples of injectable progestins are Depo-Provera (DMPA or depot medroxyprogesterone acetate), and norethindrone enanthate.

Intended pregnancy One that was wanted at the time, or sooner, irrespective of whether or not contraception was being used.

Interval insertion All other instances of insertion of the IUD excluding post-placental insertion.

Intrauterine device (IUD)   A flexible, usually plastic device inserted into the uterus to prevent pregnancy. May contain metal (generally copper) or hormones for added effectiveness. It produces a local sterile inflammatory response caused by the presence of a foreign body in the uterus which causes lysis of the blastocyst and sperm, and/or the prevention of implantation. IUDs may also prevent fertilization due to deleterious effects on spermatozoa as they pass through the uterus.

KAP   Knowledge, attitude and practices
Knockout   Inactivation of a gene.

Luteinizing hormone (LH)   Anterior pituitary hormone which causes a follicle to release a ripened ovum and become a corpus luteum. In the male it stimulates testosterone production and the production of sperm cells.

Menopause   Cessation of menstruation; i.e., the last episode of physiologic uterine bleeding. After menopause, a woman is naturally infertile. Surgical menopause refers to the removal of a woman's ovaries before natural menopause occurs.
Menses   Menstrual flow.
Microbicide   An agent that inactivates or kills microbes.
Minipill   Oral contraceptive containing no estrogen and generally less than 1 mg of a progestational agent per pill.
Miscarriage   The interruption of the implantation of the embryo in the woman's womb. The fertilized ova that are never implanted and simply lost with the next menstrual cycle are not considered miscarriages or abortions because it is free floating and not being "carried" by the female body.
Mistimed conception   One that was wanted by a woman at some time, but which occurred sooner than wanted.
Myometrium   The muscle layer of the uterus.

Oogenesis   Formation and maturation of the egg.
Oral contraceptives (OC)   Various progestin/estrogen or progestin compounds in tablet form taken by mouth; the pill. Estrogenic and progestational agents have contraceptive effects by influencing normal patterns of ovulation, sperm or ovum transport, cervical mucus, implantation, or placental attachment.
Osteoporosis   An abnormal softening, porousness, or reduction in the quantity of bone, resulting in structural fragility. Causes appear to include estrogen deficiency, prolonged immobilization, and adrenal hyperfunction, which result in more bone resorption than formation.
Ovaries   The female gonads; glands where ova are formed; also the primary source of female hormones, estrogen and progesterone.

Ovulation   The release of an ovum from the ovarian follicle in the ovary during the female cycle.

Ovum   The egg cell.

Oxytocin   A hormone produced by the pituitary gland. As the baby suckles, impulses are sent to the posterior pituitary. The hormone oxytocin is released causing the milk let-down reflex. Oxytocin also causes the uterine muscles to contract.

Pathogen   A microbe capable of causing disease.

Pelvic inflammatory disease (PID)   Inflammation of the pelvic structures, especially the uterus and tubes, whose precipitating or contributing cause quite often is a sexually transmitted disease, e.g., gonorrhea, chlamydia, or both. Also called pelvic infection, polymicrobial pelvic infection, tubal infection, and salpingitis.

Perfect use   When the directions for use of a contraceptive method are followed and the method is used correctly for every act of intercourse.

Perimenopause   Traditionally defined as the few (three to five) years surrounding a woman's last menstrual period; more recently it is being defined as beginning more than a decade before frank menopause, in the mid-thirties and early forties, coincident with the initiation of ovarian decline.

Periodic abstinence methods   Contraceptive methods that rely on timing of intercourse to avoid the ovulatory phase of a woman's menstrual cycle; also called fertility awareness or natural family planning. 1. The basal body temperature (BBT) method uses daily temperature readings to identify the time of ovulation. 2. In the ovulation or Billings methods, women identify the relationships of changes in cervical mucus to fertile and infertile days. 3. The sympto-thermal method charts changes in temperature, cervical mucus, and other symptoms of ovulation (e.g., intermenstrual pain).

Pituitary gland   A small gland located at the base of the brain beneath the hypothalamus; serves as one of the chief regulators of body functions, including fertility. Most endocrine glands in the body are controlled by the pituitary. Also known as the hypophysis.

Post-placental insertion   1. Manual post-placental IUD insertion which occurs immediately following delivery of the placenta. 2. immediate postpartum insertion occurs during the first week after delivery.

Postpartum   After childbirth.

Potential reproductive years   Years between menarche and menopause.

Pregnancy   The interval from the completion of implantation of the blastocyst in the uterus until parturition.

Progesterone   A steroid hormone produced by the corpus luteum, adrenals, or placenta. It is responsible for changes in the uterine endometrium in the second half of the menstrual cycle which are preparatory for implantation of the fertilized ovum, development of maternal placenta after implantation, and development of mammary glands.

Progestins   A large group of synthetic drugs that have a progesterone-like effect on the uterus.

Prostaglandin   Refers to a group of naturally occurring, chemically related long-chain fatty acids that have certain physiological effects (stimulate contraction of uterine and other smooth muscles, lower blood pressure, affect action of certain hormones). When prostaglandins are produced as the endometrial lining degenerates, they may cause mild to severe menstrual cramps, diarrhea, nausea, and vomiting. Oral contraceptives diminish the prostaglandins released by the endometrial lining, decreasing menstrual cramps in users.

Prostate   A pale, firm, partly muscular, partly glandular body that surrounds the base of the male urethra in man and other mammals and discharges its viscid opalescent secretion through ducts opening into the floor of the urethra.

Puberty   The age when sex organs become functionally operative and secondary sex characteristics develop. Puberty is defined as the state or quality of being first capable of bearing offspring or the period at which sexual maturity is reached. The dictionary says the age of puberty is commonly designated legally as 14 years for boys and 12 years for girls. For a girl, puberty means producing an ovum, and for a boy it is manufacturing spermatozoa. Secondary sexual characteristics in girls include breasts development, enlargement of the hips, and the development of axillary and pubic hair. In boys they include appearance of pubic, facial, and axillary hair; growth of the penis, testicles and scrotum; and deepening of the voice.

Reproductive intentions   Intentions to postpone or terminate childbearing.

Saturation mutagenesis   Selectively mutating all genes within a species by mutating one gene per individual of the species until all the genes are mutated. Then the function of the genes can be determined.

Semen   The thick, whitish fluid which normally contains sperm and seminal secretions and is ejected during ejaculation.

Seminal vesicles   Two glandular structures located behind the prostrate gland which secrete a component of semen.

Sexually transmitted diseases (STD)   Any disease that is communicated primarily or exclusively through intimate sexual contact. Sexually transmitted diseases have been estimated to cause from 20% to 40% of infertility in the U.S. STDs can adversely affect fertility by three primary mechanisms; pregnancy wastage, prenatal deaths, and damage to male or female reproductive capacity. Also called venereal disease or VD, sexually transmitted infections or STIs, or sexually transmitted reproductive tract infections or RTIs.

Side effect   An effect of a drug other than the one it was administered to evoke.

Spacing intentions Preferred length of the next birth interval.

Sperm Male reproductive cell.

Sperm antigens Substances on or in the sperm that in certain circumstances elicit the production of antibodies.

Spermatogenesis The formation of spermatozoa.

Spermicide A chemical substance that kills sperm, marketed in the form of foam, cream, jellies, and suppositories used for contraception. The spermicides used in almost all currently marketed spermicides are surfactants, surface-active compounds that destroy sperm cell membranes.

Sponge The light fibrous skeleton of certain aquatic animals used as an absorbent. Natural sea sponges have been used for centuries as contraceptives. In 1983 the U.S. Food and Drug Administration approved a vaginal contraceptive sponge, the Today sponge, a polyurethane sponge that contains 1 gram of the spermicide nonoxynol-9, which is available without a prescription.

Sterilization (Tubal ligation, Vasectomy) A surgical procedure which leaves the male or female incapable of reproduction. Sterilization is the most commonly employed method of birth control in the world.

Steroidogenesis The natural production of steroids. The usual progression of hormones is from progesterone and other progestins to androgens to estrogens.

Testosterone Male sex hormone produced in the testes.

Transgenesis Introduction of a gene.

Unintended pregnancy One that was not wanted at the time conception occurred, irrespective of whether contraception was being used.

Unwanted conception One that occurred when the woman did not want to have any more pregnancies at all.

Uterus The hollow, pear-shaped, muscular, elastic reproductive organ where the fetus develops during pregnancy.

Vagina The 3- to 5-inch long muscular tube leading from the external genitals of the female to the uterus. The external opening, called the introitus, may be diminished by a membrane called hymen. Sometimes called the birth canal, the vagina is the passageway through which babies are born and menstrual fluid flows. The vagina widens and lengthens during sexual arousal.

Validity A principle of epidemiology used in connection with screening tests, which consists of sensitivity (ability to identify correctly those who have a given disease) and specificity (ability to identify correctly those who do not have a given disease).

Vas deferens The tube through which sperm pass from the epidydimis to the ejaculatory duct and then into the urethra. It is this tube which is interrupted in the male sterilization procedure called vasectomy. Also called ductus deferens.

Vasectomy   A surgical procedure in which segments of the vas deferens are removed and the ends tied to prevent passage of sperm. Vasectomy should be regarded as permanent, although reversal is possible in some cases.

Withdrawal (coitus interruptus)   Removing the penis from the vagina just prior to ejaculation.

Women in fertile age (WIF)   Females of childbearing age, typically defined as between ages 15 and 44 or between ages 15 and 49.

Zygote   The fertilized egg before it starts to divide.

Index

Index